Implant Restorations: A Step-by-Step Guide

2nd Edition

Implant Restorations: A Step-by-Step Guide

2nd Edition

Carl Drago, DDS, MS
Gundersen Lutheran Medical Center
LaCrosse, Wisconsin

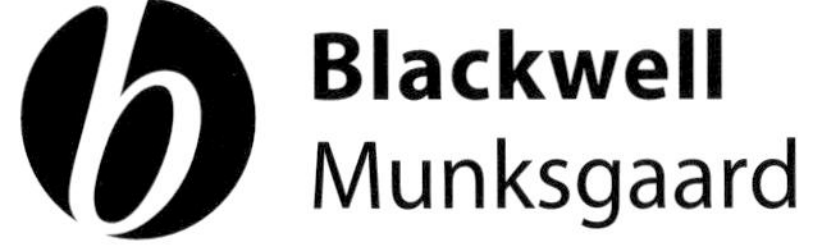

Carl Drago is Clinical Science Editor of the Journal of Prosthodontics, the journal of the American College of Prosthodontists. He has had a practice limited to fixed, removable, and implant prosthodontics since 1981, and practices as a prosthodontist at the Gundersen Lutheran Medical Center in LaCrosse, Wisconsin. He has also held positions as Assistant Clinical Professor at the University of Texas Dental School at San Antonio. He is a Diplomate of the American Board of Prosthodontics (ABP).

Editorial Offices:
Blackwell Publishing Professional,
2121 State Avenue, Ames, Iowa 50014-8300, USA
Tel: +1 515 292 0140
9600 Garsington Road, Oxford OX4 2DQ
Tel: 01865 776868

Blackwell Publishing Asia Pty Ltd,
550 Swanston Street, Carlton South,
Victoria 3053, Australia
Tel: +61 (0)3 9347 0300

Blackwell Wissenschafts Verlag, Kurfürstendamm 57, 10707
Berlin, Germany
Tel: +49 (0)30 32 79 060

First published 2007 by Blackwell Munksgaard, a Blackwell Publishing Company

Library of Congress
Cataloging-in-Publication Data
Drago, Carl J.
Implant restorations : a step by step guide / Carl J. Drago. — 2nd ed.
p. ; cm.
Includes bibliographical references and index.
ISBN-13: 978-0-8138-2883-1 (alk. paper)
1. Dental implants. I. Title.
[DNLM: 1. Dental Implantation, Endosseous—methods.
2. Dental
Abutments. 3. Jaw, Edentulous—surgery. WU 640 D759i 2006]
RK667.I45D73 2006
617.6′92—dc22

2006009527

ISBN-13: 978-0-8138-2883-1

Printed and bound in Singapore by Markono Print Media Pte Ltd

For further information on
Blackwell Publishing, visit our website:
www.blackwellpublishing.com

The last digit is the print number: 9 8 7 6 5 4

With great respect,
I humbly dedicate this book to
Richard J. Lazzara, DMD, MScD, and
Keith D. Beaty, BS (Civil Engineering)

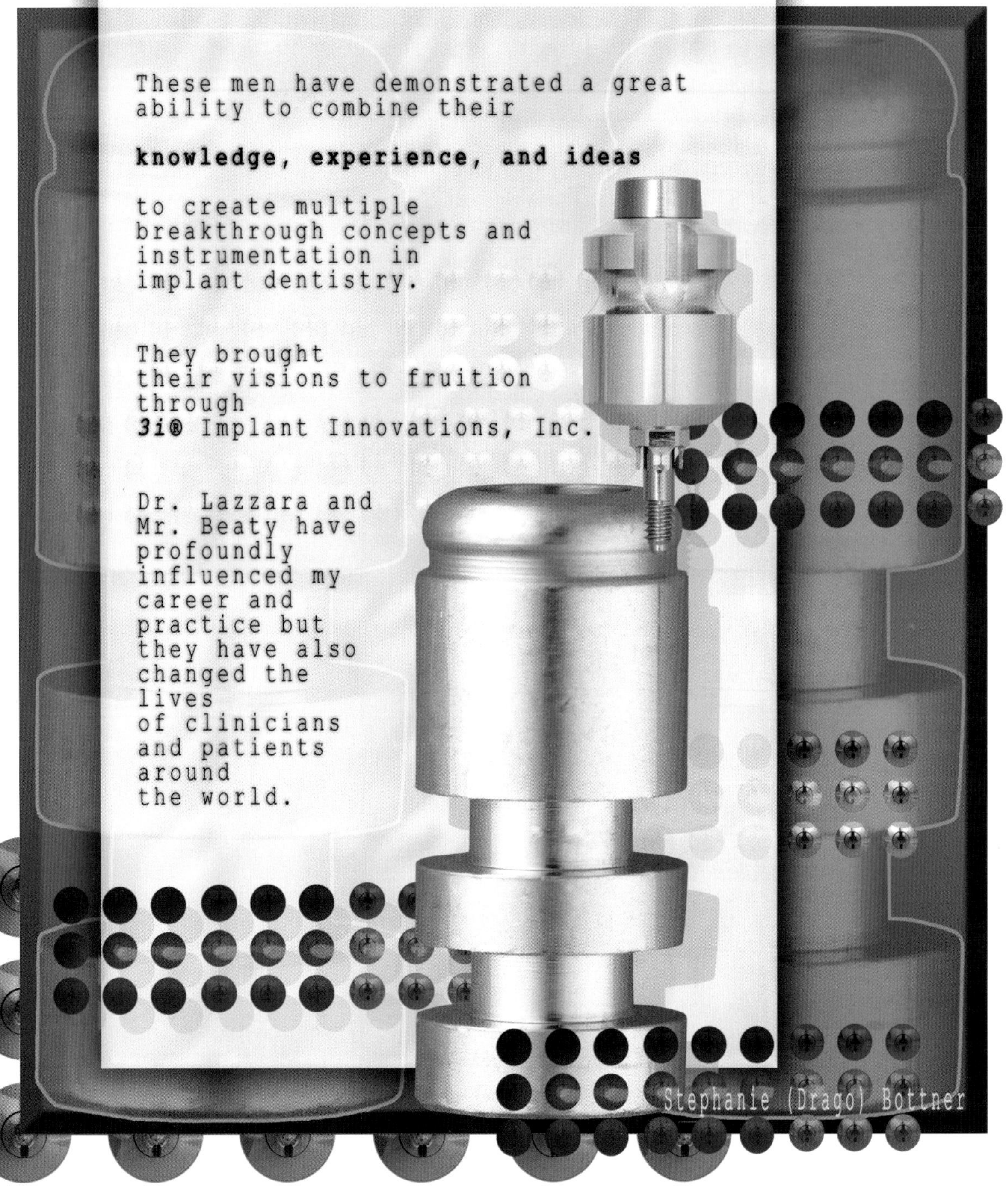

These men have demonstrated a great ability to combine their

knowledge, experience, and ideas

to create multiple breakthrough concepts and instrumentation in implant dentistry.

They brought their visions to fruition through ***3i*®** Implant Innovations, Inc.

Dr. Lazzara and Mr. Beaty have profoundly influenced my career and practice but they have also changed the lives of clinicians and patients around the world.

Stephanie (Drago) Bottner

Table of Contents

Contributors

C. Garry O'Connor, DDS, MS
Gundersen Lutheran Medical Center
1900 South Avenue
LaCrosse, WI 54601

Phone: 608 775 2696
Fax: 608 775 4430
cgoconno@gundluth.org

Paul J. Kelly, DMD, MS
Arizona Maxillofacial Surgeons PC
6755 East Superstition Springs Blvd
Suite 103
Mesa, AZ 85206

Phone: 480-830-5866
Fax: 480-807-0606
Email: pkelly@azoralsurgery.com

Formerly, Chief Resident, Oral and Maxillofacial Surgery
Gundersen Lutheran Medical Foundation

Foreword

Dr. Carl Drago is an educator and practitioner with a vision to share his experiences with dental colleagues. His first book, *Implant Restorations: A Step-by-Step Guide for Dentists,* illustrated his approach for multiple, basic implant case reconstructions. Carl now supports your move to the next level with this book. Each clearly written chapter continues your growth in implant placement and reconstruction with insightful treatment plans, explanations, and solutions for patients requesting implant restorations. Dr. Drago describes our multidisciplinary team approach for the total care of implant patients.

Carl explains the communication between clinicians and laboratory technicians on an appointment-by-appointment basis. He discusses the restorative options, his billing program, loading protocols, implant component selection, work orders, and clinical procedures for each case type. The patient's aesthetics and functional goals are identified and their accomplishments in each case are his measure of success. This book will expand your practice and enjoyment of implant dentistry. Include it with your favorite texts that define the way you practice.

C. Garry O'Connor, D.D.S., M.S.
Chairman, Department of Dental Specialists
Gundersen Lutheran Medical Center
2006

Acknowledgments

The author would like to acknowledge the assistance of the following people in development of this textbook:

Gundersen Lutheran Department of Prosthodontics
LaCrosse, Wisconsin

Nan Dreves, RDH, BS
Stephanie Gerlach
Andrew Gingrasso
Carole Jose
Nicole Stakston
Jamie Tranberg
Mary Rumble, RDH

Gundersen Lutheran Department of Periodontics
LaCrosse, Wisconsin

Linda Sing
Michelle Wruck
Mary Johnson Benchina
Amy Bergey
Mary Ellen Freisinger
Cheryl Olson
Linda Pampuch
Claudia Devens, RDH
Amy Moriarty, RDH

Gundersen Lutheran Department of Oral Surgery
LaCrosse, Wisconsin

P. Michael Banasik, DDS
Ajit Pillai, DMD
Paul J. Kelly, DMD, MS

Implant Innovations, Inc. (All "product shot" photographs courtesy of Implant Innovations, Inc.)
Palm Beach Gardens, Florida

Lisa Adams, Associate Manager of Marketing Communications
Hannah Johnson, Director of Corporate Communications
Stephanie Schoenrock, Territory Manager, Wisconsin
Russ Bonafede, Vice President of Global Marketing
Steve Schiess, President

Family and Friends
Matthew Brisgal Drago
Betty Drago
Stephanie Drago Bottner
Eleanor Drago Severson
Jill Jensen
Kara Kelly
Candace O'Connor, DDS
Connie O'Connor

3i® Registered Trademarks (5/10/05)
ASYST®
Certain®
EP®
GingiHue® Post
Implant Innovations, Inc.®
Immediate Occlusal Loading®
IOL®
OSSEOTITE®
OSSEOTITE® Certain®
OSSEOTITE NT®
OSSEOTITE XP®

3i® Trademarks™ (5/10/05)
ARCHITECH PSR™
CAM StructSURE™ Precision Milled Bars
DIEM™
Encode™
Gold Standard ZR™
Gold-Tite™
Patient Specific Restorations™
Prep-Tite™
Prevail™
Provide™
QuickSeat™ Connection
Twist Lock™
ZiReal™ Post

The preceding registered trademarks and trademarks are registered to Implant Innovations, Inc.®, Palm Beach Gardens, Florida. For clarity, the author did not identify each specific product with its specific trademark symbol each time the product was mentioned. This list serves notice that the above are registered to Implant Innovations, Inc.®.LOCATOR® is a registered trademark of Zest Anchors, Inc.

Implant Restorations: A Step-by-Step Guide

2nd Edition

Chapter 1: Introduction to Implant Dentistry

INTRODUCTION

The successful, long-term clinical use of dental endosseous implants requires some type of biologic attachment of implants to bone. In 1969 Brånemark and others defined this process as osseointegration (Brånemark and others 1977). This process has been subsequently studied by numerous authors and has come to identify the functional stability of the endosseous implant/bone connection (Davies 1998). The histology and biomechanics of osseointegration is beyond the scope of this text; the reader is referred to other sources for further information and increased understanding relative to osseointegration.

Treatment of edentulous or partially edentulous patients with endosseous implants requires a multidisciplinary team approach. This team generally consists of an implant surgeon, restorative dentist and dental laboratory technician. Each team member needs to be aware that implant dentistry is a restorative-driven service and the ultimate success of implant treatment will be measured, at least in part, by the aesthetic and functional results as perceived by patients. The design of the prosthesis, whether it be a single implant retained crown or a full-arch prosthesis, will have a major impact on the number, size, and position of the implant(s) that will be used in a particular treatment plan. Treatment planning for implant dentistry must therefore begin with the restorative phase prior to considering the surgical phases of treatment.

Brånemark and co-workers introduced a two-stage surgical protocol into North America in 1982 (Zarb 1993). Numerous, long-term clinical studies have proven the efficacy of titanium, endosseous implants (Adell 1981; Sullivan and Sherwood 2002; Friberg and Jemt 1991; Testori and Del Fabbro 2002). Many clinicians now consider osseointegration of dental implants to be predictable and highly effective in solving clinical problems associated with missing teeth (Davarpanah and Martinez 2002).

PURPOSE OF TEXTBOOK

The purpose of this textbook is to provide clinicians and dental laboratory technicians with a step-by-step approach to the treatment of certain types of edentulous and partially edentulous patients with dental implants. Six types of patient treatments are featured. The treatments are illustrated with emphasis on diagnosis and treatment planning, restorative dentist/implant surgeon communication and restorative treatments, on an appointment-by-appointment basis. Implant components are identified for each specific appointment. Laboratory procedures and work orders are also included. Implant loading protocols are discussed for each particular case presentation.

The biologic and theoretical aspects of osseointegration are not reviewed. Osseointegration is defined as clinically immobile implants; absence of peri-implant radiolucencies as assessed by an undistorted radiograph; mean vertical bone loss less than 0.2 mm annually after the first year of occlusal function; absence of pain, discomfort and infection (Smith and Zarb 1989). Clinical verification of osseointegration can be difficult at best. Some implants that have been considered successful at the second surgical or impression appointments have subsequently failed prior to or after completion of the prosthetic portion of treatment. Zarb and Schmitt (1990) have found that "late failures" occurred 3.3% of the time in patients with mostly edentulous mandibles. Naert and Quirynen (1992) published a report that contained data from partially edentulous patients, maxillae and mandibles. They reported late failures of 2.5%. Late failures are important to clinicians and patients because of the additional expense and treatment that patients may elect to undergo in replacing prostheses on failed implants.

This text concentrates on how clinicians may successfully incorporate implant restorative dentistry into their practices. A team approach is emphasized among members of the implant team: restorative dentists, implant surgeons, dental laboratory technicians, dental assistants and office staff. Appointment sequencing, laboratory work orders and fee determination for restorative dentists are also discussed, including identification of fixed overhead, implant components, laboratory costs and profit margins.

Clinicians have multiple implant systems to choose from. There are similarities and differences among systems, including but not limited to macroscopic surface morphology, implant/abutment connections, diameters, thread pitch, and screw hex/morphology. This textbook illustrates the surgical and restorative components manufactured by ***3i®***, Implant Innovations, Inc., Palm Beach Gardens, FL. The author is not a representative of Implant Innovations, Inc., and purchased all the components that were used. The principles described in this textbook should be applicable to other implant manufacturers.

ECONOMICS OF IMPLANT DENTISTRY

One of the major reasons cited by general dentists relative to including or excluding implant dentistry in their practices is the cost involved in dental implant treatment. Levin has reported that more than 35% of patients referred

TABLE 1.1. Costs/Fees/Profits Associated with a 3-Unit Porcelain Fused-to-Metal Fixed Partial Denture (FPD)

Chair Time	Fixed Overhead	Laboratory Expenses	Fees
Preparations		Casts	$ 50
Impression		Dies	$ 25
Provisional Restoration		Articulation	$ 25
1.75 hours	$350/hr = $613	FPD	$775
			$875
FPD Insertion			
.75 hours	$350/hr = $263		
TOTALS	**$876**		**$ 875**
Professional Fee			$2700
Costs (fixed overhead and laboratory expenses)			$1751
Profit (fees less costs)			$ 949
Profit per hour ($949/2.5 hrs)			$ 380

from general dentists to oral surgeons or periodontists for implant dentistry never actually make the appointment (Levin 2004). He has recommended that financing be offered to every implant patient because it is not known which patients will require financing for treatment and which ones will not. Levin considered that financing was no longer an option; it should be considered a necessity. He reported that clients of The Levin Group significantly increased their levels of case acceptance by making financing options available to patients.

Levin (2005) described a comprehensive approach to dentistry that included four significant parts:

1. The comprehensive exam
2. Tooth-by-tooth exam
3. Cosmetic exam
4. Implant exam

Levin identified implant dentistry for his general practitioner clients as an enormous growth opportunity and also stated that more than half of general dentists do not restore a single implant in any given year. Implant dentistry not only improves the lives of patients but also can be a significant profit center for dental practices. Because implant dentistry generally is not covered by dental insurance, Levin stated that implants should be viewed as an opportunity to increase the elective portions of dental practices.

Implant treatment may be divided into treatment of partially edentulous and edentulous patients. Partially edentulous patients may warrant treatment involving the replacement of one tooth or they may require replacement of multiple teeth (Table 1.1). Patients will frequently call for "comparison shopping." A common question is, "How much will an implant cost?" Patients may also request the costs of a single crown for comparison purposes. It is the responsibility of the dental staff to make sure patients know that in order to make fair comparisons, patients must compare the costs associated with a 3-unit fixed partial denture (FPD) or similar prosthesis to the costs of an implant retained restoration replacing one tooth (Tables 1.2 and 1.3).

Implant dentistry should also be profitable for restorative dentists. Initially, as with other new technologies that require the acquisition of learned, skilled behaviors, implant restorative dentistry may not be as profitable as other aspects of restorative dentistry. Restorative dentists should expect a learning curve relative to diagnosing; treatment planning and treatment in implant restorative dentistry. With practice and reasonable efforts on behalf of the dentist and staff, implant dentistry may become one of the most profitable aspects of general practice.

Predictability of Fixed Prosthodontics

The goal of prosthodontic treatment is to provide aesthetic and functional replacements for missing teeth on a long-term basis. Clinicians would like to attain these goals with restorations that have a predictable prognosis, minimal biologic trauma and at reasonable cost. For the majority of restorative dentists, there are multiple advantages to conventional fixed prosthodontic therapy: familiarity with protocols, techniques, and materials. There are also multiple limitations associated with conventional fixed prosthodontics: tooth preparation and soft tissue retraction, potential pulpal involvement, recurrent caries, and periodontal disease. Missing teeth may be predictably replaced with fixed partial dentures, but there are increased stresses and demands placed on the abutment teeth.

In 1990, more than four million fixed partial dentures were placed in the United States (ADA Survey, 1994). It may be surprising to note that there is little long-term research on the longevity of these restorations, and comparisons

TABLE 1.2. Costs/Fees/Profits Associated with an Implant-Retained Crown (Premachined Abutment/PFM Crown)

Chair Time	Fixed Overhead	Laboratory Expenses		Fees
		Casts	$ 45	
Impression		Articulation	$ 15	
		PFM crown	$275	
		Mill abutment	$ 75	
.5 hours	$350/hr = $175	Sub Total	$410	
		Implant Components		
		Healing abutment	$ 36	
		Impression Coping	$ 45	
		Analog	$ 21	
		Pre-machined abutment	$ 90	
		Lab screw	$ 14	
		Abutment Screw	$ 54	
		Sub Total	$260	
Crown Insertion				
.5 hours	$350/hr = $175			
TOTALS	$350			$ 670
Professional Fee				$1400
Costs (fixed overhead and laboratory expenses)				$1020
Profit (fees less costs)				$ 380
Profit per hour	($380/1 hr)			$ 380

Note: Because the profit per hour is equivalent to the 3-unit FPD but the clinical time required is significantly less, restorative dentists can be more profitable with implant dentistry by seeing more patients.

Healing abutments, impression copings, and lab screws may be used multiple times; therefore, costs will be decreased for each succeeding case and profits will be increased. Analogs should not be re-used.

TABLE 1.3. Comparison of Costs, Fees, and Profits Per Hour for 3-Unit FPD versus Single-Unit Implant-Retained Crown

	Fixed Overhead	Laboratory And Implant Components Costs	Fees	Profit/HR
3-Unit FPD	$876	$875	$2700	$380
Implant Restoration	$350	$275	$1400	$380

Note: Implant-retained crown needs to be compared to the costs for a 3-unit FPD in order to accurately compare the costs associated with replacing a single missing tooth.

between studies cannot be easily accomplished due to the lack of established parameters (Mazurat 1992). Authors have reported on the failure rates of FPDs over time, but the definitions of failures are inconsistent: recurrent caries, fractured porcelain, broken rigid connectors, loss of periodontal attachment (Schwartz and Whitsett 1970; Reuter and Brose 1984; Walton, Gardner, and Agar 1986; Foster 1990; Randow and Glantz 1993).

Fixed partial dentures have documented long-term success. Scurria (1998) performed a meta-analysis of multiple published studies and documented success rates as high as 92% at 10 years and 75% at 15 years. Other authors have recorded failure rates of 30% or more for FPDs at 15–20 years (Lindquist and Karlsson 1998). A key point that should be recognized from these reports is that it is important for clinicians to realize that for younger patients, fixed partial dentures may need to be replaced 2–3 times during their lifetimes.

In a concise literature review, Priest (1996) reviewed multiple papers to compare the efficacy of implant-retained crowns and conventional fixed partial dentures over time. He found that although FPDs were assumed to demonstrate predictable longevity, failure rates have been reported from 20% over a three-year time, to 3% failures over 23 years. Implant longevity, on the other hand, appears to be more promising and generally displays more narrow ranges of failures: 9% over three years to 0% over 6.6 years. Priest cautioned that failure rates for FPDs and implant-retained crowns cannot be easily compared among studies because parameters had not been established and that replacing missing teeth is a complex issue. There is sufficient data for single-tooth implant retained restorations to be used as a functional and biologic method for satisfactory tooth replacement.

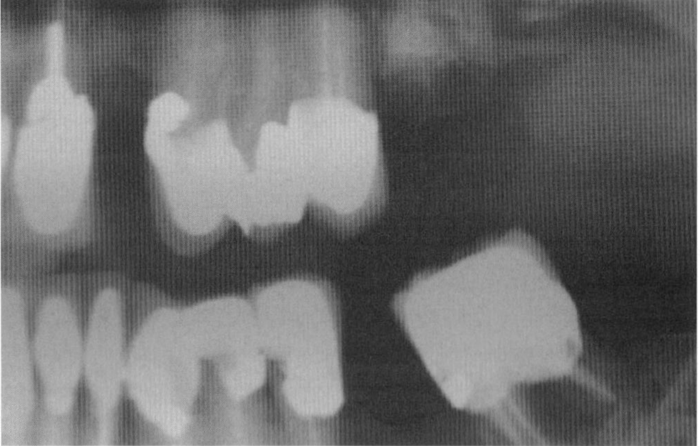

Figure 1.1. Radiograph of mandibular molar that may be considered for use as the distal abutment for a 3-unit FPD. It has been treated endodontically and restored with a crown. There are recurrent caries beneath the mesial margin.

DEVELOPMENT OF PROGNOSIS FOR TEETH: EXTRACT OR MAINTAIN

A question often asked by clinicians and patients relates to the viability and prognosis of maintaining compromised teeth. Even with the advances in implant dentistry since the 1970s, the predictability of implants is still not 100%. Therefore, it may still be difficult to recommend the extraction of a tooth with a compromised prognosis and replace it with a dental implant. The American Academy of Periodontology's position paper on dental implants stated that all patients should be informed as to the risks and benefits of implant and alternative treatment prior to implant placement and restoration (AAP Position Paper 2000).

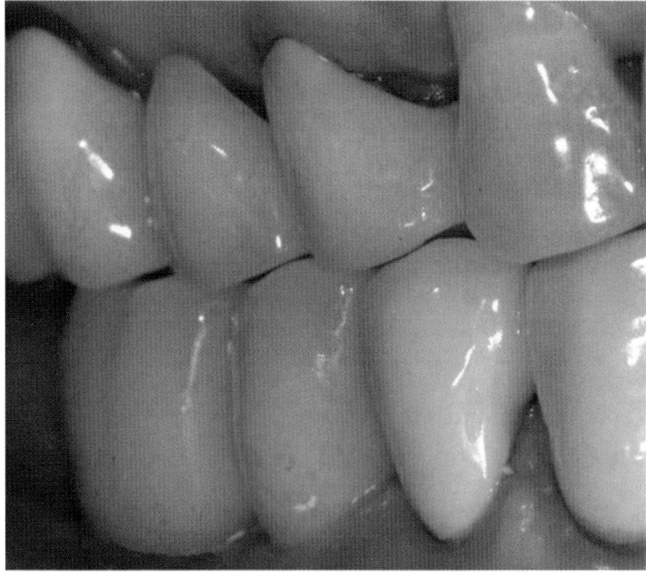

Figure 1.2. Clinical view of implant-retained crowns replacing the mandibular right second premolar and first molar.

O'Neal and Butler discussed the clinical and economic factors that clinicians should consider in making decisions relative to extraction and implant placement versus retention of compromised teeth (O'Neal and Buler 2002). They divided the clinical issues into four basic categories:

1. The heavily restored tooth
2. The furcation-involved tooth
3. The periodontal-prosthesis patient
4. Difficult aesthetic cases

The Heavily Restored Tooth

This type of tooth may have been damaged as a result of blunt trauma, dental caries, or multiple dental restorations (Figure 1.1). In Figure 1.1, this mandibular molar has been treated endodontically and had moderate bone loss and dental caries. The long-term prognosis for this tooth would be poor if used as the distal abutment for a 3-unit fixed partial denture. The treatment choices for this patient could include a mesial root amputation, osseous surgery and a

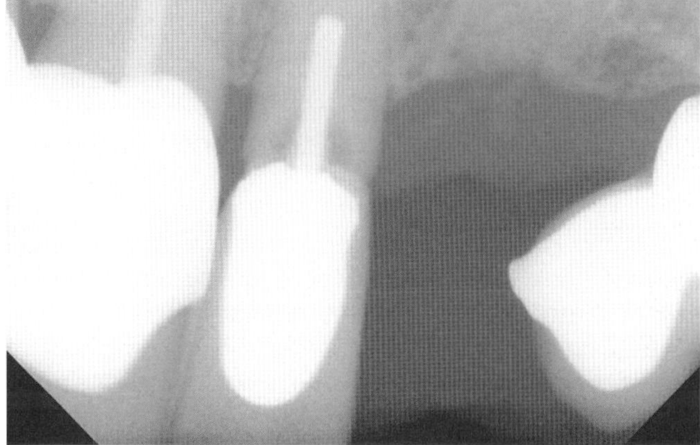

Figure 1.3. Radiograph of a maxillary lateral incisor with previous endodontic therapy. The post retained the crown.

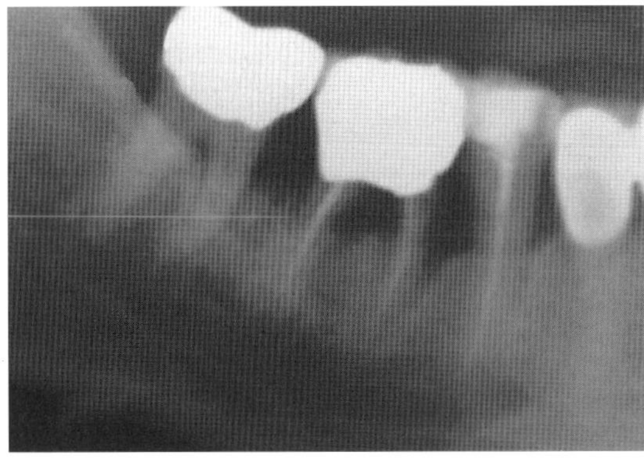

Figure 1.4. Radiograph of mandibular right posterior segment that demonstrates advanced bone loss around the first molar. This tooth was a poor candidate for root resection and an abutment for a 3-unit FPD.

new 3-unit FPD. Or, the tooth could be extracted, the socket grafted with bone or a bone substitute, and the extraction site allowed to heal prior to placing an implant and implant restoration (Figure 1.2). The prognosis for the latter choice is much better and may be more conservative than the first treatment option.

The clinical condition exemplified by Figure 1.3 is also frequently encountered in clinical practice: an incompletely fractured tooth with previous endodontic therapy where the crown was held in place by a post. Numerous authors have suggested that the axial walls of tooth preparations for endodontically treated teeth should include at least 1 mm of dentin in order to provide the requisite ferrule effect needed for predictable retention for the crown, even in the presence of a post (Fan, Nicholls and Kois 1995; Libman and Nicholls 1995; Sorenson and Engelman 1990). Crown lengthening procedures can be accomplished in order to obtain greater access to dentin for increased retention of the crown, but the surgery is associated with moderate to significant surgical morbidity and is accomplished at the expense of the supporting bone.

The Furcation Involved Tooth

Posterior teeth with advanced bone loss are the most commonly lost teeth. Hirschfeld studied natural teeth over a 22-year period and found that 31.4% of molars and 4.9% of single rooted teeth were lost (Hirschfeld and Wasserman 1978). Therefore, decisions to retain or extract posterior teeth generally involve molars. Both maxillary and mandibular molar teeth exhibit concavities associated with multiple roots. The anatomy may also be compromised with recurrent caries and lateral canals. In Figure 1.4, the mandibular right first molar has had previous endodontic therapy, advanced bone loss around both roots and in the furcation, mobility, and was uncomfortable for the patient. The patient's chief complaint was related to the discomfort that she was feeling anytime she attempted to chew on the right side. Yet she did not feel that she wanted to have this tooth extracted. Even with a root resection, this tooth had a poor prognosis as an abutment for an FPD. A more appropriate choice would be extraction, grafting, and placement of one implant to replace the missing molar.

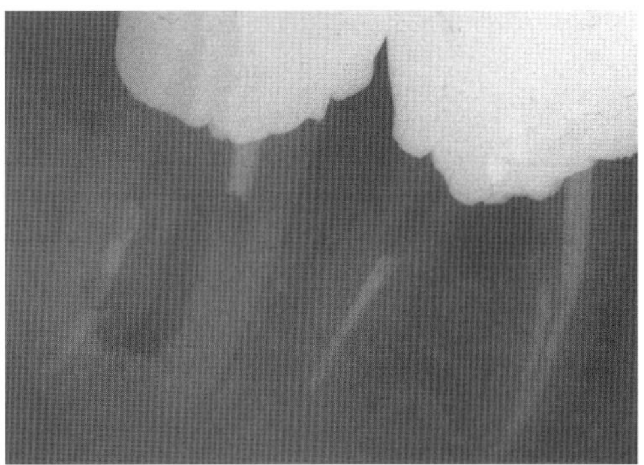

Figure 1.5. Radiograph after endodontic therapy for the mandibular right first and second molars prior to resection of the second molar's mesial root.

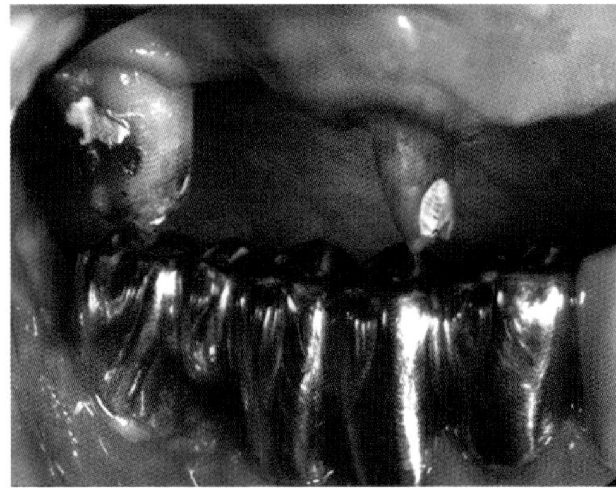

Figure 1.6. Mandibular FPD cemented in place.

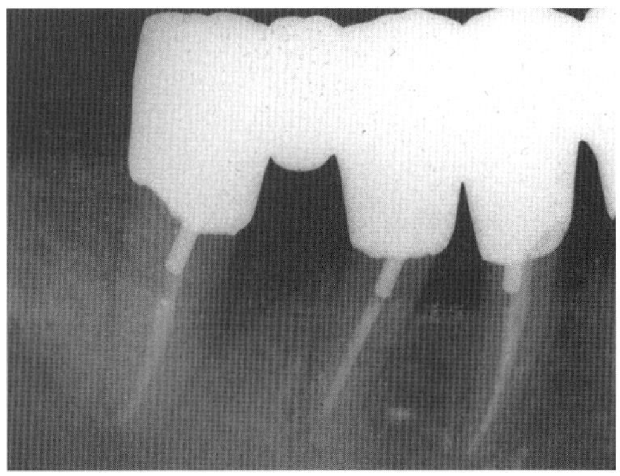

Figure 1.7. Radiograph at FPD try-in appointment, post extraction of the mesial root of the mandibular second molar.

The most common causes of failure in posterior, furcation-involved teeth have been reported to be recurrent caries and endodontic failure (Buhler 1994). When clinical success is likely, root resection procedures can be clinically and financially sound. In Figures 1.5–1.7, compromised

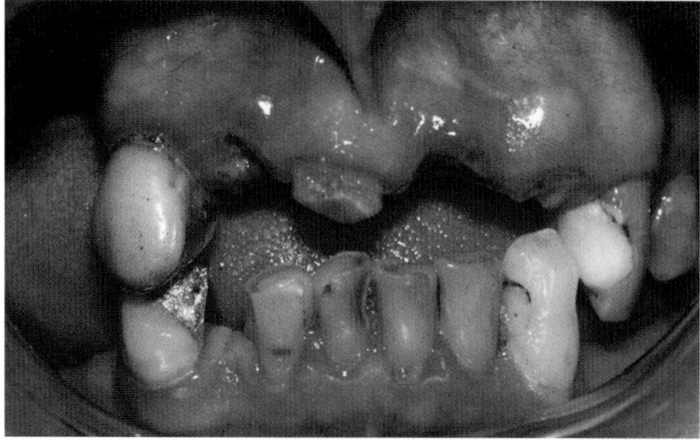

Figure 1.8. Pre-operative anterior view of centric occlusion.

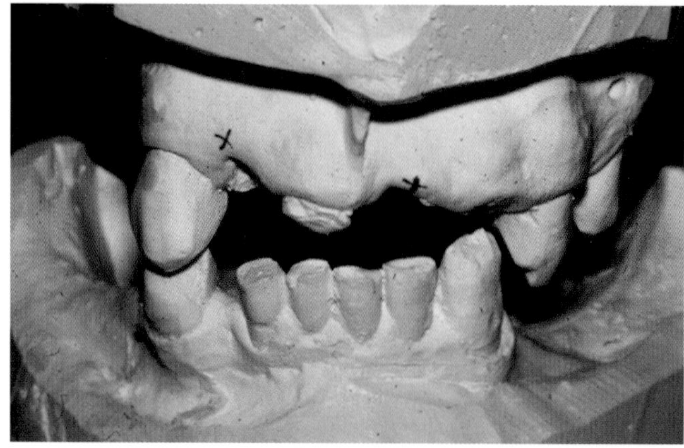

Figure 1.10. Pre-operative diagnostic articulator mounting. Vertical dimension of occlusion has not been changed.

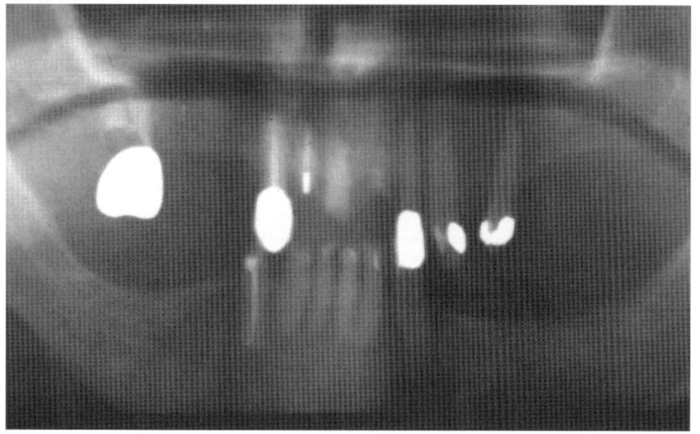

Figure 1.9. Pre-operative panoramic radiograph.

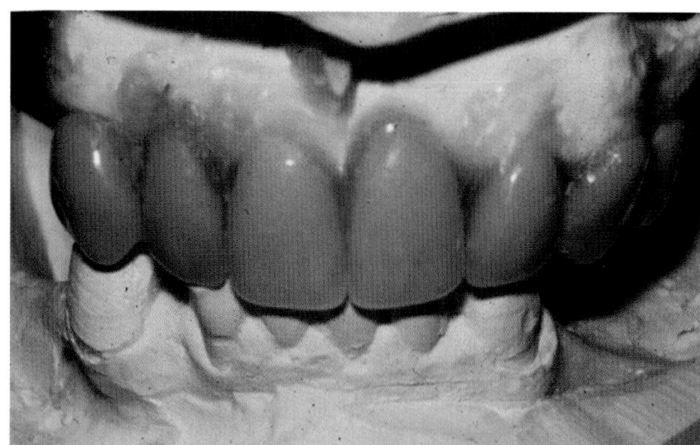

Figure 1.11. Diagnostic wax patterns; incisal plane of mandibular teeth has been modified.

mandibular molars were treated with endodontic therapy, posts, root resections and a fixed periodontal splint. The postoperative radiograph was taken 15 years after the prosthesis was inserted. This treatment can be considered an unqualified success.

The Periodontal Prosthesis Patient

Dentistry has witnessed tremendous advances in treatment alternatives for the severely compromised dentition. In the 1960s and 1970s these advances resulted in the salvaging of many teeth that were formerly extracted (Yalisove and Dietz 1977). Conventional fixed and removable prosthodontic treatments were not applicable to treat severely compromised dentitions, especially in cases in which there were multiple missing teeth and moderate to advanced bone loss. Amsterdam defined the sophisticated dental therapy to treat such patients as periodontal prosthesis (Amsterdam 1974). Periodontal prosthesis is the treatment required to stabilize and retain dentitions that have been weakened by the loss of alveolar bone and multiple teeth. In the past, periodontal prostheses were the primary means to treat these debilitated dentitions. Today the use of dental implants has decreased the frequency for these complex patients to be treated with periodontal prosthesis (Nevins 1993).

This patient presented to the author in 1988 with multiple missing teeth, an end-to-end dental occlusion, moderate to advanced bone loss, and a severe gag reflex (Figure

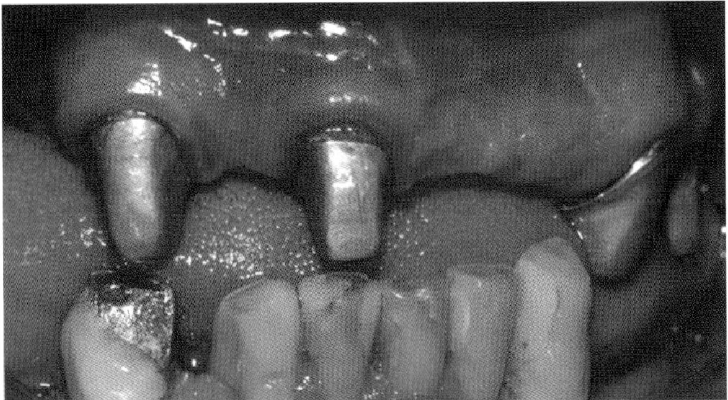

Figure 1.12. Clinical anterior view with maxillary copings in place.

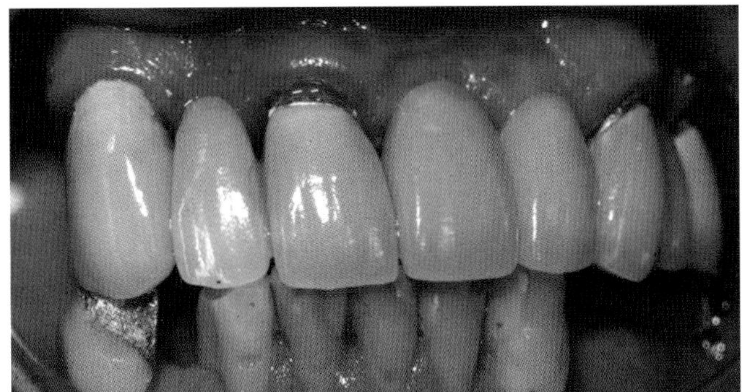

Figure 1.13. Periodontal prosthesis in place at insertion.

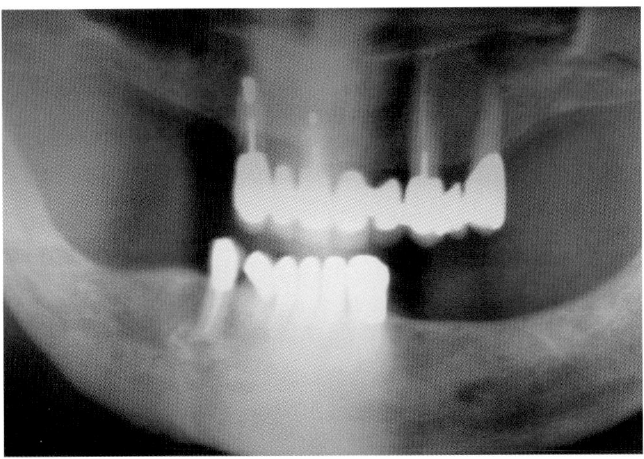

Figure 1.14. Post-operative panoramic radiograph.

1.8). Treatment consisted of thorough radiographic and physical examinations (Figure 1.9). The treatment plan called for diagnostic articulator mountings (Figure 1.10), diagnostic wax patterns (Figure 1.11), extraction of several hopeless teeth, periodontal osseous and soft tissue surgery, and a maxillary periodontal prosthesis (Figures 1.12, 1.13, 1.14). The mandibular incisal plane was recontoured

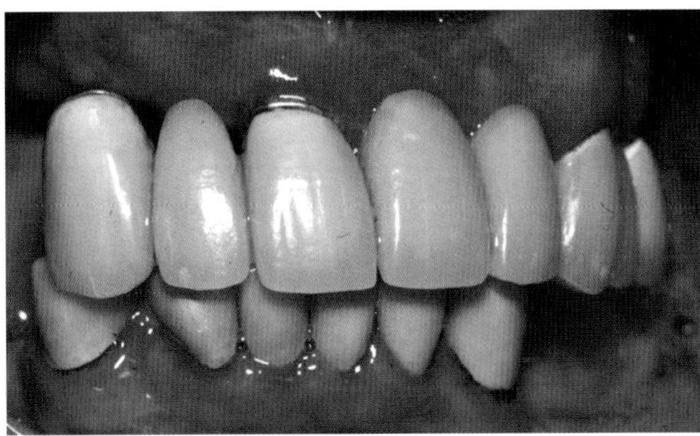

Figure 1.15. Clinical anterior view eight years post insertion. Maxillary right cuspid needed to be extracted secondary to a combined periodontal/endodontic lesion.

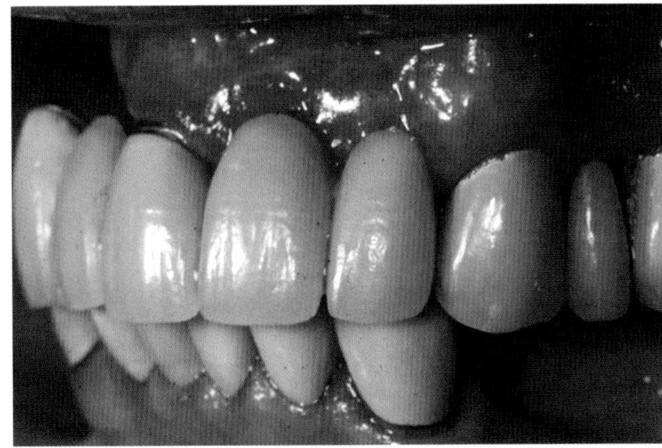

Figure 1.16. Clinical left lateral view two years post extraction of maxillary right cuspid (10 years post insertion of original prosthesis). Note the amount of alveolar ridge resorption gingival to the cuspid pontic.

in conjunction with the maxillary reconstruction and the mandibular teeth were restored with individual crown restorations.

The patient functioned comfortably for several years and then presented with a problem with the maxillary right canine eight years post insertion. (Figure 1.15) This tooth was diagnosed as having a combined periodontal/endodontic lesion. The periodontal prosthesis was tapped off and the cuspid was extracted. The periodontal prosthesis was re-cemented and remained in place for an additional eight years (the last recall appointment). Note the amount of residual ridge resorption gingival to the cuspid pontic (Figure 1.16).

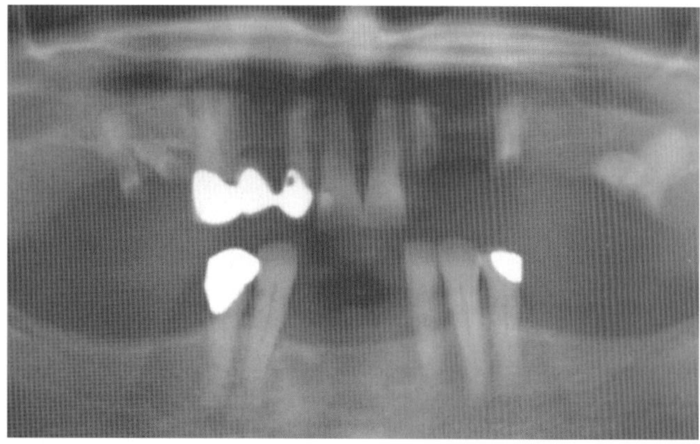

Figure 1.17. Pre-operative panoramic radiograph demonstrating severe dental caries, moderate bone loss, and multiple missing teeth.

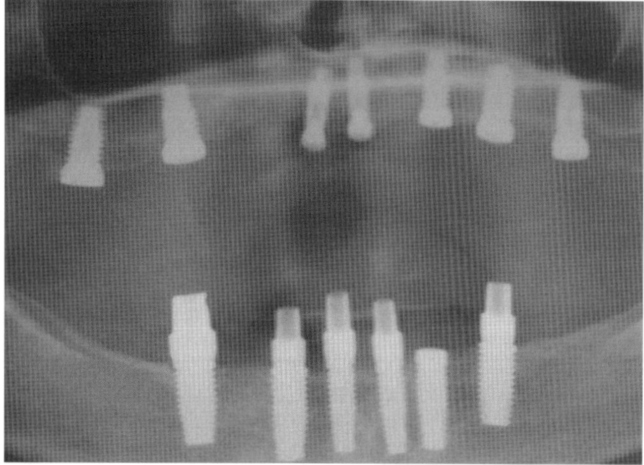

Figure 1.18. Intra-operative panoramic radiograph post maxillary and mandibular implant placement.

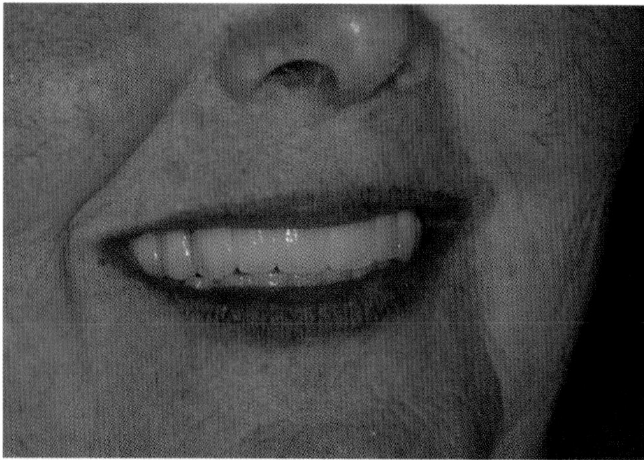

Figure 1.19. Clinical view of patient from Figures 1.17 and 1.18, smiling with fixed maxillary and mandibular implant restorations.

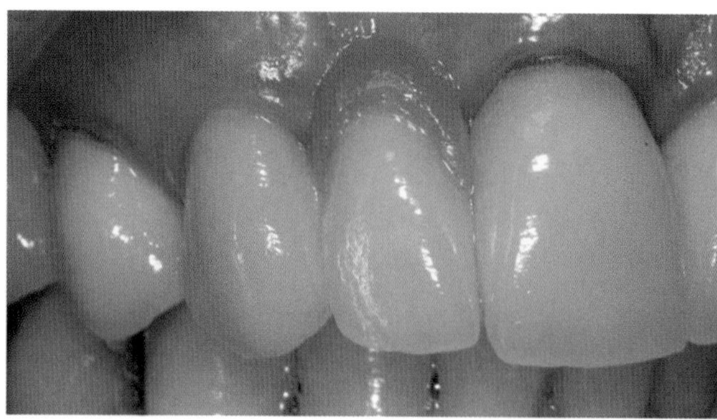

Figure 1.20. Clinical view of a patient missing a maxillary right lateral incisor who had inadequate bone volume for implant placement and did not want to have bone grafting accomplished in order to have an implant-retained crown. The missing lateral incisor was replaced with a 3-unit FPD.

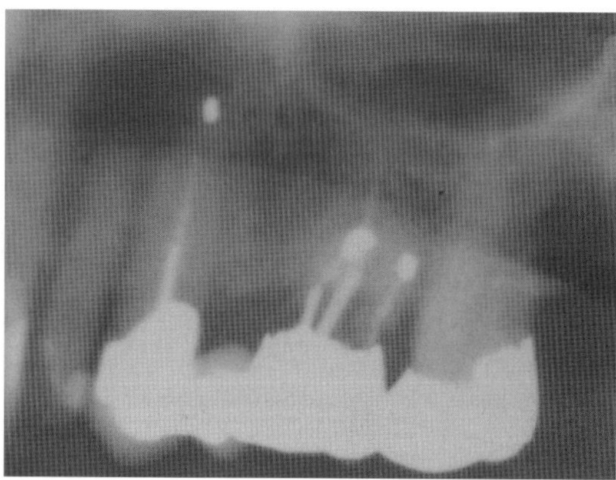

Figure 1.21. Radiograph of a patient with a nonrestorable maxillary left first molar, pneumatized maxillary sinus, and inadequate bone volume for implant placement.

If this patient presented to a dentist today, the preceding treatment certainly could be offered as a treatment alternative. The morbidity associated with the periodontal surgery, endodontic surgery and all the complexities of the fixed prosthodontic treatment probably would outweigh the morbidities involved in extraction of the teeth, grafting as needed, placement of implants, and implant prosthetic treatment with either fixed or removable prosthodontics. The net, long-term results with fixed implant-retained restorations would probably be more predictable on a long-term basis than the results that could be obtained with periodontal prosthesis (Figures 1.17, 1.18, 1.19).

Difficult Aesthetic Cases

Replacement of anterior teeth with dental implants is probably one of the greatest challenges that the dental implant team will face. There are numerous factors to consider in order to fabricate aesthetic, long-term, functional restorations: bone quality and bone quantity, gingival symmetry,

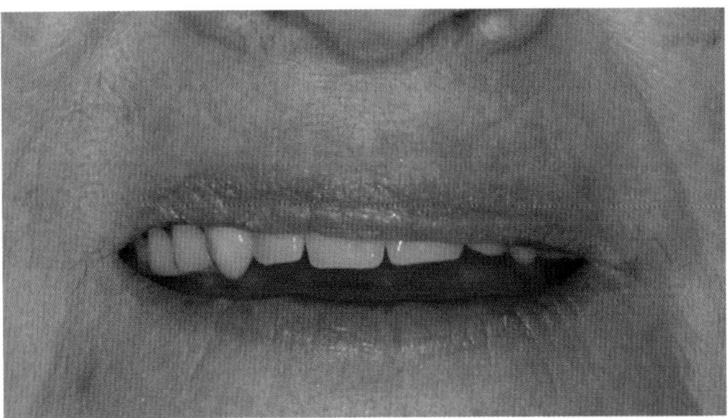

Figure 1.22. This patient had lost her maxillary anterior teeth 10 years previous to this photograph. The anterior and posterior occlusal planes were at different levels. There was inadequate lip support.

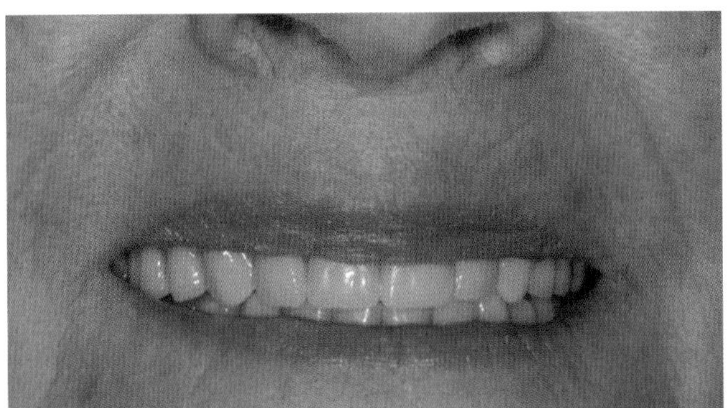

Figure 1.23. This is the same patient as in Figure 1.22. The posterior teeth were restored with crowns and maxillary anterior teeth were replaced with a new removable partial denture that provided more lip support and incisal display of the teeth with smiling.

three-dimensional orientation of the edentulous space and adjacent teeth, presence or absence of inter dental papillae, and location of the lip during speaking, smiling, and at rest. Dentists and patients have come to expect excellent aesthetic and functional results in the anterior regions of the mouth (Chang and Odman 1999).

However, implant-retained restorations may not always be the most appropriate treatment option. Fixed and removable partial dentures may still be viable options for patients who need to replace anterior teeth (Figure 1.20). In the case of multiple missing teeth, anatomical limitations, and inadequate bone volume, a fixed partial denture may be more appropriate if bone grafting is needed (Figure 1.21). In the case of multiple missing teeth and significant alveolar ridge resorption, a removable partial denture with a labial acrylic resin flange may be the treatment of choice in order to provide patients with the requisite lip support (Figures 1.22, 1.23).

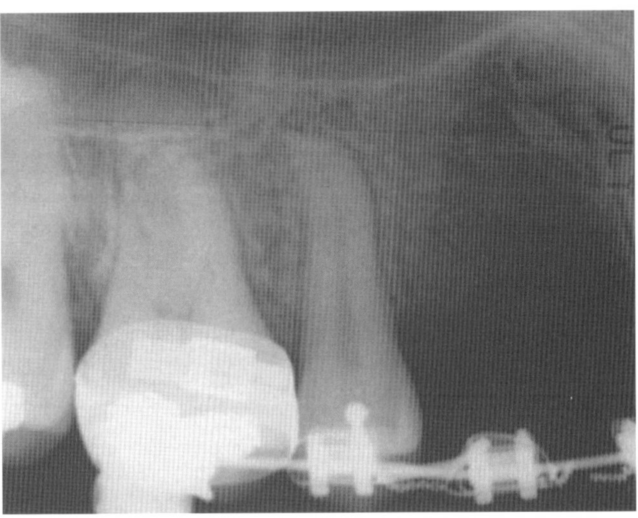

Figure 1.24. Pre-operative periapical radiograph of the maxillary right quadrant that demonstrates adequate bone volume for implant placement to replace the missing teeth (maxillary right first premolar and cuspid).

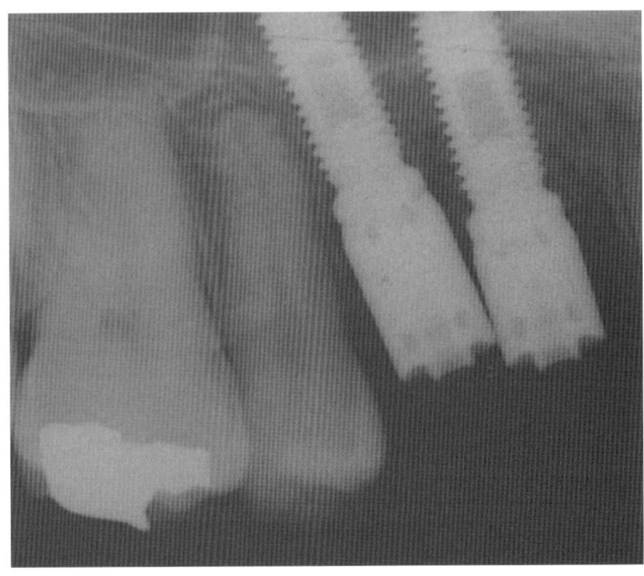

Figure 1.25. Postoperative radiograph of two implants that were placed too close together and too high into the alveolus.

For aesthetic restorations, implants must be placed in optimal positions, not where there is available bone (Garber 1995). Implant placement must also be viewed in three dimensions: mesio/distal; facial/lingual; and occlusal/cervical. Deficient sites need to be augmented with bone and soft tissue as needed in order to insure proper implant placement. In this instance, there appeared to be adequate bone volume for implant placement on the periapical radiograph (Figure 1.24). However, the bone was deficient vertically, but the implants were placed anyway (Figure 1.25). In spite of multiple problems associated with implant

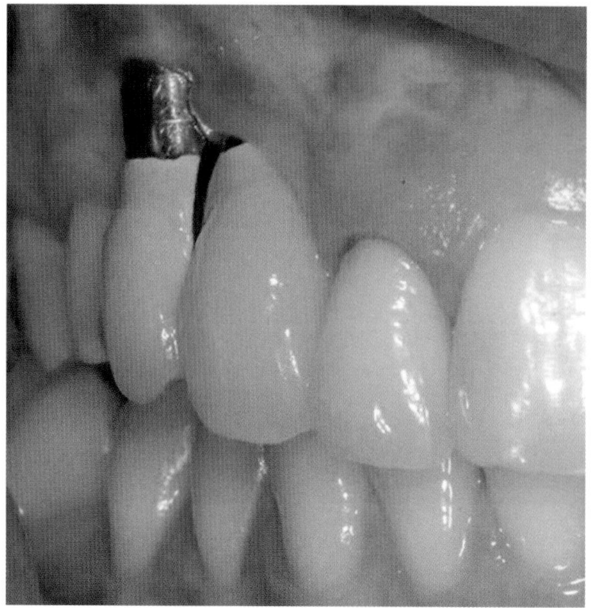

Figure 1.26. Clinical view of the patient in Figure 1.25. Note the contours of the implant-retained crowns secondary to less-than-optimal implant placement.

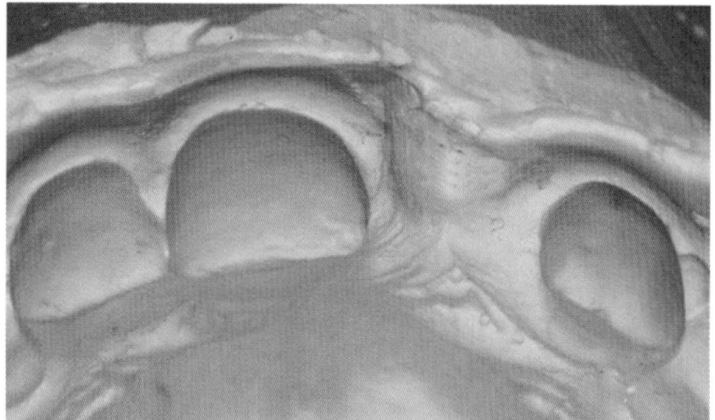

Figure 1.27. Pre-operative occlusal view of a maxillary diagnostic cast demonstrating a Class I horizontal ridge defect.

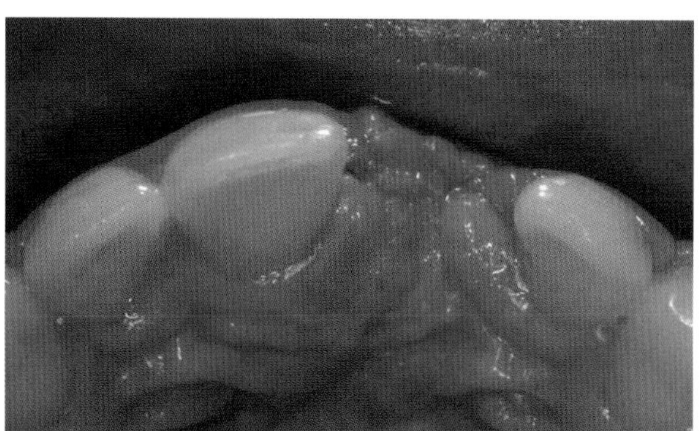

Figure 1.28. Ten-week postoperative clinical view of patient in Figure 1.27 demonstrating increase in buccal/lingual width of the edentulous ridge.

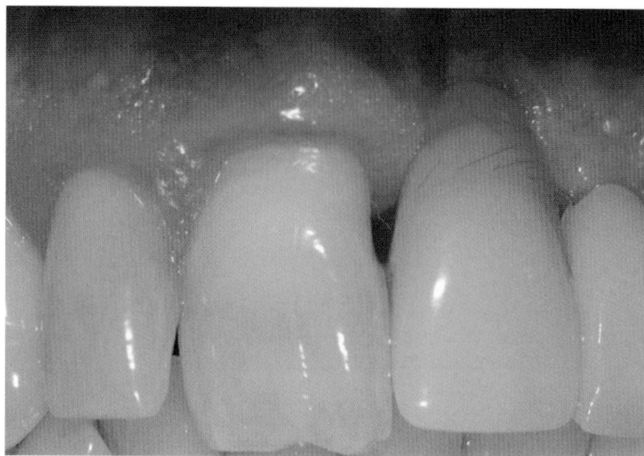

Figure 1.29. Clinical view of transitional partial denture that did not replace the missing hard and soft tissues associated with the missing maxillary left central incisor.

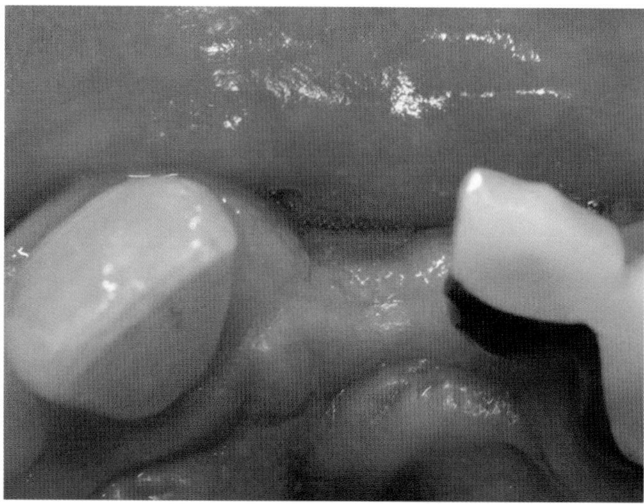

Figure 1.30. Clinical occlusal view demonstrating the horizontal component of the defect that will have to be addressed prior to or during implant placement.

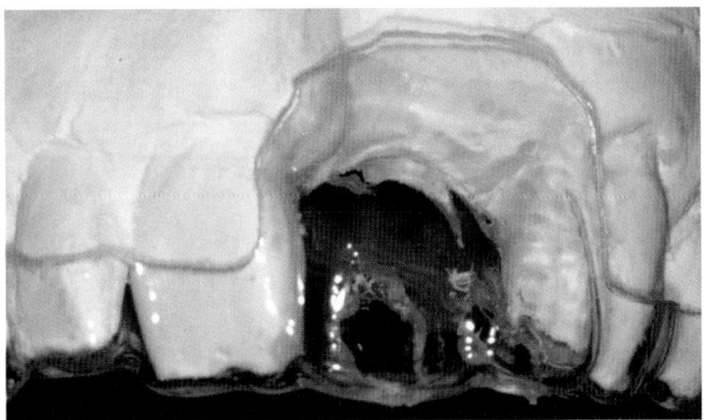

Figure 1.31. Surgical guide on the diagnostic cast may be appropriate for the surgeon to use during the augmentation portion of the surgical treatment.

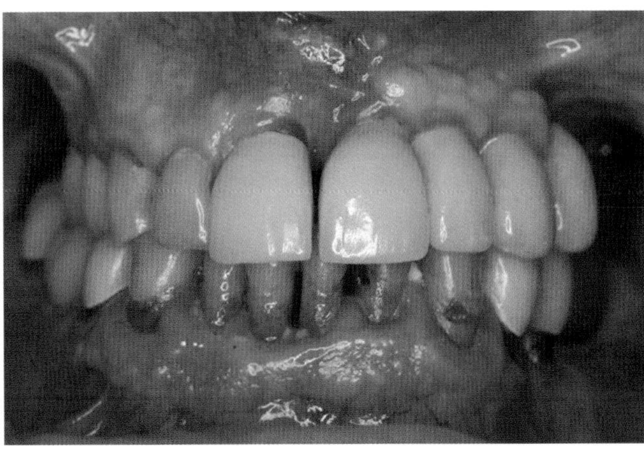

Figure 1.32. Pre-operative clinical view of a patient with advanced periodontitis and a significant dental malocclusion who did not wish to maintain his dentition.

placement, location and lack of keratinized tissues around the premolar implant, this patient has adapted to the restorations and maintained them 10 years post implant insertion (Figure 1.26).

Restoration of edentulous spaces in aesthetic zones with dental implants should probably not be undertaken by surgeons and restorative dentists with limited implant experience (Weisgold and Arnoux 1997). Thorough pre-operative diagnostic work ups are especially warranted prior to embarking on treatment in the anterior maxillae (Hess and Buser 1998). Ridge deformities have been classified into three types: Class I—loss of buccal/lingual width; Class II—loss of vertical height; Class III—combination of Class I and II (Seibert 1983). Bone regeneration is now well accepted by dentistry. The horizontal Class I defect is predictable to treat (Figures 1.27, 1.28). Augmentation procedures do add time and expense to overall treatment.

This removable partial denture does not restore the restorative volume required for an aesthetic replacement of the missing maxillary central incisor. The defect is significant in both the vertical and horizontal planes (Figure 1.29). In this case, the ill-fitting partial denture can be diagnostic for the surgeon by giving him/her an idea as to the volume of material required to eliminate the defect (Figure 1.30). A surgical guide would be beneficial even if an implant cannot be placed at the time of bone grafting (Figure 1.31).

DEVELOPMENT OF PROGNOSIS FOR THE DENTITION

Diagnosis and treatment planning for patients with compromised dentitions can be one of the more daunting challenges facing dental practitioners. A process should be developed that assists practitioners in formulating treatment plans that are evidenced based, predictable, and as practical as possible. Accurate diagnoses are critical for success and need to be identified relative to periodontal disease, occlusion (skeletal and dental), and other anatomical considerations (maxillary sinus, inferior alveolar canal, and so on).

Patients who present with moderate to advanced periodontitis will probably have several potential treatment options: periodontal surgery with grafting, membranes, antimicrobial therapy, and so on; selective extraction and replacement with removable or fixed prostheses supported by natural teeth; selective extraction and replacement with removable or fixed prostheses supported by dental implants; or full arch extractions and prosthetic replacement (Figure 1.32).

Certainly an argument could be made for the patient in Figure 1.32 that with selective extraction, periodontal therapy, and fixed/removable prosthodontic treatment, the dentition could be salvaged and maintained for a given number of years. However, what would the morbidity and expense be for the required treatments and how long should the patient reasonably expect the reconstruction to last? Wang and Burgett (1994) studied the influence of furcation involvement on tooth loss over a period of eight years. They reported that with and without furcation involvement, 23% and 13% respectively were lost after eight years. Other authors have reported similar findings (Hirschfeld and Wasserman 1978; McFall 1982; Goldman and Ross 1986). Findings such as these may make it difficult for clinicians to recommend intensive periodontal and fixed prosthodontic therapy to patients for whom the support for the reconstruction is dependent on compromised molars.

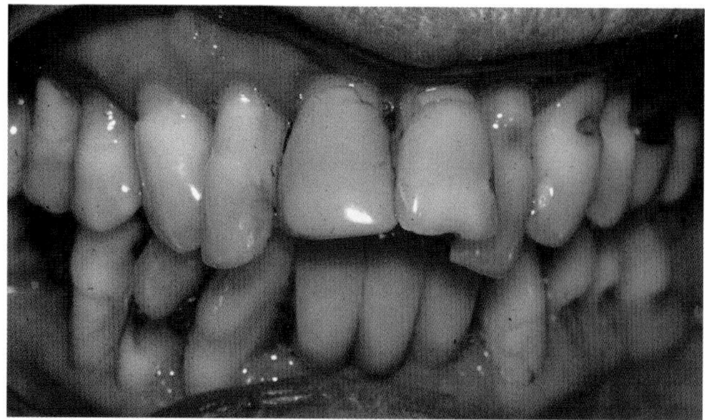

Figure 1.33. Pre-operative clinical view of a patient three years post-periodontal surgery.

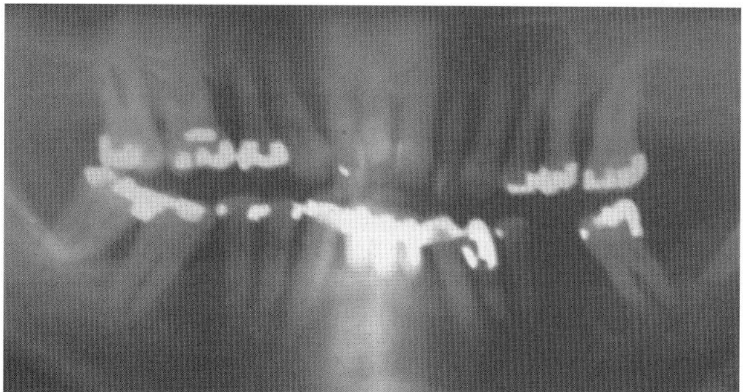

Figure 1.34. Panoramic radiograph corresponding to Figure 1.33.

In another case of a debilitated dentition, a patient presented three years post periodontal surgery (Figure 1.33, 1.34). She spent approximately 20 minutes per day brushing, flossing, and rubber tipping in and around all her teeth. The teeth were still sensitive, prone to food impaction, and unattractive. Selective extractions could have been performed and the missing teeth could have been replaced with fixed or removable prostheses. The patient did not wish to spend any more time or money on maintaining her teeth and she opted to have the teeth extracted and replaced with complete dentures. She healed uneventfully from the extractions and then proceeded with implant placement and reconstruction with a maxillary complete denture and mandibular fixed hybrid prosthesis (Figure 1.35).

Morrow and Brewer (1980) presented a treatment planning concept for the debilitated dentition prior to the advent of implant dentistry as we know it today. They considered the use of overdentures if four or fewer retainable teeth remained in a dental arch. They considered fixed or removable partial dentures, or a combination, if more than four teeth remained. They stressed that the number four was not immutable and that treatment planning required flexibility as to the number and position of the abutments for overdentures. Morrow and Brewer recognized that overden-

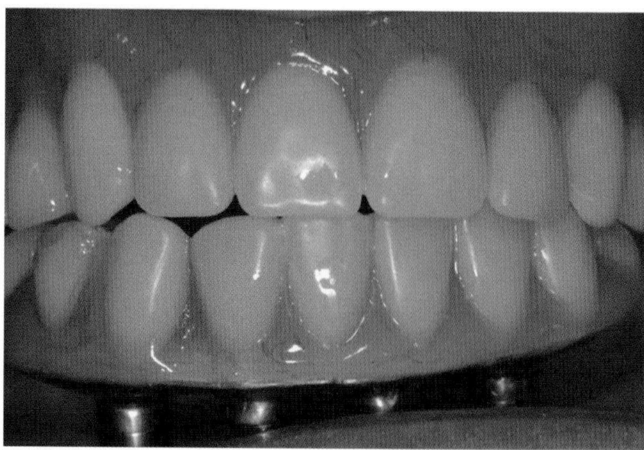

Figure 1.35. Postoperative clinical view of patient in 1.33 with definitive maxillary complete denture and mandibular fixed hybrid implant prosthesis.

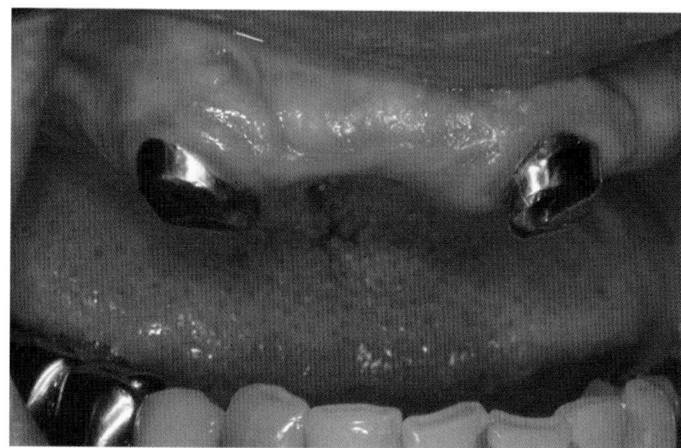

Figure 1.36. Clinical view of a patient eight years post insertion of a maxillary overdenture supported by two overdenture abutment teeth. This patient has lost a minimal amount of bone in the anterior maxillae secondary to the retention of these two abutment teeth.

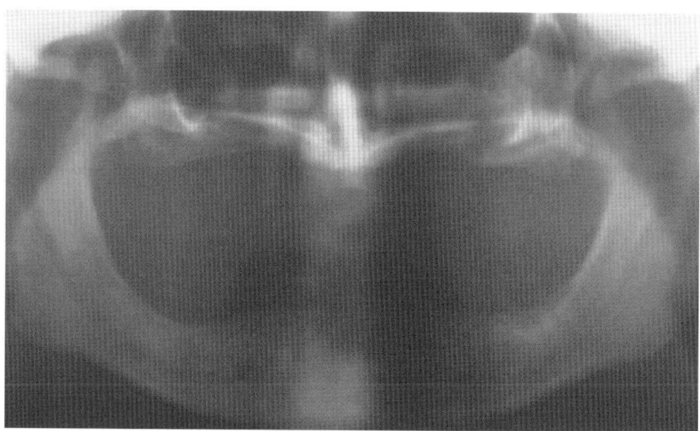

Figure 1.37. Panoramic radiograph of a patient who lost his maxillary teeth 25 years prior to this radiograph. The mandibular teeth were lost two years prior to this radiograph. Note the significant bone resorption that has occurred in the maxillae compared to how little bone has resorbed in the mandible.

tures were not appropriate for every patient, but they also stated that there were few situations in which complete dentures were preferable to overdentures, because they routinely saw the results of long-term edentulism and the difficulties associated with adaptation to complete dentures (Figures 1.36 and 1.37).

SUMMARY

Clinicians must constantly update their knowledge and clinical skills in order to provide state of the art care to patients. Clinicians are responsible for gathering the data required for an accurate diagnosis of patients' conditions. They are also required to provide treatment options to patients that are evidenced based, predictable, and as harmless as possible. Financial considerations also need to be taken into account by patients and clinicians. The treatment planning process will become less problematic for clinicians who keep their knowledge and skills current, perform comprehensive examinations, and provide evidenced-based treatment options. Patients will also benefit by having the treatments performed that are best for them at the time the decision was made.

BIBLIOGRAPHY

Adell, R, Lekholm, U, Rockler, B, Brånemark, PI. 1981. A 15-year study of osseointegrated implants in the treatment of the edentulous jaw. *Int J Oral Surg* 10:387–416.

American Academy of Periodontology. 2000. Position paper-Dental implants in periodontal therapy. *J Periodontol* 71:1934–1942.

American Dental Association Survey Center, 1994. Changes in dental services rendered, 1959–1990. In: *1990 Survey of Dental Services Rendered*. Chicago: American Dental Association: 24–38.

Amsterdam, M, 1974. Periodontal prosthesis; twenty-five years in retrospect. *Alpha Omegan*, December 1974.

Brånemark, P-I, Hansson B, Adell, R, Breine U, Lindstrom, J, Hallen, O, Ohman A, 1977. Osseointegrated implants in the treatment of edentulous jaws. Experience from a 10-year period. *Scand J Plast Reconstr Surg* 16:1–132.

Buhler, H, 1994. Survival rates of hemisected teeth: an attempt to compare them with survival rates of alloplastic implants. *Int J Periodontics Restorative Dent* 14:536–543.

Chang, M, Odman, P, Wennstrom J, Andersson, B. 1999. Esthetic outcomes of implant-supported single-tooth replacements assessed by the patient and by prosthodontists. *Int J Prosthodont* 12:335–341.

Davarpanah M, Martinez H, Etienne D, Zabalegui I, Mattout P, Chiche F, Michel J, 2002. A prospective multicenter evaluation of 1583 ***3i***® implants: 1- to 5-year data. *Int J Oral Maxillofac Implants* 17(6):820–828.

Davies, J, 1998. Mechanisms of endosseous integration. *Int J Prosthodont* 11:391–401.

Fan, P, Nicholls, J, Kois, J, 1995. Load fatigue of five restoration modalities in structurally compromised premolars. *Int J Prosthodont* 8:213–220.

Foster, L, 1990. Failed conventional bridge work from general dental practice: clinical aspects and treatment needs of 142 cases. *Br Dent J* 168:199–201.

Friberg, B, Jemt, T, Lekholm, U, 1991. Early failures in 4641 consecutively placed Brånemark dental implants: a study from stage I surgery to the connection of completed prostheses. *Int J Oral Maxillofac Implants* 6:142–146.

Garber, D, 1995. The esthetic implant letting the restoration be the guide. *J Am Dent Assoc* 12:319–325.

Goldman, M, Ross, I, Goteiner, D, 1986. Effect of periodontal therapy on patients maintained for 15 years or longer. A retrospective study. *J Periodontol* 57:347–353.

Hess, D, Buser, D, Dietschi, D, Grossen, G, Schonenberger, A, Belzer, U, 1998. Esthetic single-tooth replacement with implants: a team approach. *Quintessence Int* 29:77–86.

Hirschfeld, L, Wasserman, B, 1978. A long-term survey of tooth loss in 600 treated periodontal patients. *J Periodontol* 49:225–237.

Levin, R, 2004. Implant dentistry and patient financing. *Implant Dent* 13(1):10.

Levin, R, 2005. A comprehensive approach to dentistry. *Compendium* 26:764–765.

Limban, W, Nicholls, J, 1995. Load fatigue of teeth restored with cast post and cores and complete crowns. *Int J Prosthodont* 8:155–161.

Lindquist, E, Karlsson, S, 1998. Success rate and failures for fixed partial dentures after 20 years of service. Part I. *Int J Prosthodont* 11:133–138.

Mazurat, R, 1992. Longevity of partial, complete and fixed prostheses: a literature review. *J Can Dent Assoc* 58:500–504.

McFall, W, 1982. Tooth loss in 100 treated patients with periodontal disease. *J Periodontol* 53:539–549.

Morrow, R, Brewer, A, 1980. *Overdentures*. St. Louis, C V Mosby Co., 27.

Nevins, M, 1993. Periodontal prosthesis reconsidered. *Int J Prosthodont* 6:209–217.

O'Neal, R, Butler, R, 2002. Restoration or implant placement: a growing treatment planning quandary. *J Periodontol* 30(1):111–122.

Priest, G, 1996. Failure rates of restorations for single-tooth replacement. *Int J Prosthodont* 9:38–45.

Randow, K, Glantz PO, Zoger, B, 1986. Technical failures and some related clinical complications in extensive fixed prosthodontics. *Acta Odontol Scand* 44:241–255.

Reuter, J, Brose, M, 1984. Failures in full crown retained dental bridges. *Br Dent J* 157:61–63.

Schwartz, N, Whitsett, L, Berry, T, Stewart, J, 1970. Unserviceable crowns and fixed partial dentures: life-span and causes for loss of serviceability. *J Amer Dent Assoc* 81:1395–1401.

Scurria, M, Bader, J, Shugars, D, 1998. Meta-analysis of fixed partial denture survival: prostheses and abutments. *J Prosthet Dent* 79:459–464.

Seibert, J, 1983. Reconstruction of deformed, partially edentulous ridges, using full thickness onlay grafts. Part I: technique and wound healing. *Compend Contin Educ Dent* 301:437–453.

Smith, D, Zarb, G, 1989. Criteria for success of osseointegrated endosseous implants. *J Prosthet Dent* 62:67–72.

Sorenson, J, Engelman, M, 1990. Ferrule design and fracture resistance of endodontically treated teeth. *J Prosthet Dent* 63:529–536.

Sullivan DY, Sherwood RL, Porter SS, 2002. Long-term performance of OSSEOTITE® implants: a 6-year follow-up. *Compendium* 22(4):326–333.

Testori T, Del Fabbro M, Feldman S, 2002. A multicenter prospective evaluation of 2-months loaded Osseotite implants placed in the posterior jaws. 3-year follow-up results. *Clin Oral Implants Res* 13:154–161.

Walton, J, Gardner, F, Agar, J, 1986. A survey of crown and fixed partial denture failures: length of service and reasons for replacement. *J Prosthet Dent* 56:416–421.

Weisgold, A, Arnous, J, Lu, J, 1997. Single-tooth anterior implant: a word of caution. *J Esthet Dent* 9:225–233.

Yalisove, I, Dietz, J, 1977. *Telescopic Prosthetic Therapy: Periodontal Prosthesis, Fixed and Removable.* Philadelphia, George F. Stickley Co., p. 7.

Zarb, G, 1993. Proceedings of the Toronto Conferences on Osseointegration in Clinical Dentistry. *J Prosthet Dent* 49:50–55.

Zarb, G, Schmitt, A, 1990. The longitudinal clinical effectiveness of osseointegrated dental implants: The Toronto study. Part 1:Surgical results. *J Prosthet Dent* 63:451–457.

Chapter 2: Implants and Implant Restorative Components

INTRODUCTION

Dental implant treatment requires a different, precise terminology that is unique to implant dentistry. Clinicians must learn the proper terms for implants and implant restorative components to facilitate communication among the members of the implant team: surgeons, restorative dentists, dental laboratory technicians, third-party payers, patients, and implant manufacturers.

All of the implants illustrated in this textbook have been manufactured by Implant Innovations, Inc.®, Palm Beach Gardens, Florida. The internal connection implants are trademarked as OSSEOTITE® Certain® Implants. The external connection implants have been trademarked as OSSEOTITE® Implants.

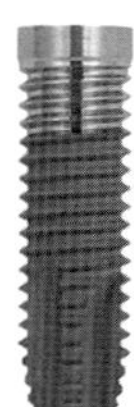

Figure 2.1. Profile view of threaded ***3i®***, 4.0 mm X 11.5 mm OSSEOTITE® Certain® implant (IOSS411).

Figure 2.2. Profile view of threaded ***3i®***, 4.0 X 11.5 mm OSSEOTITE external hex implant (OSS411).

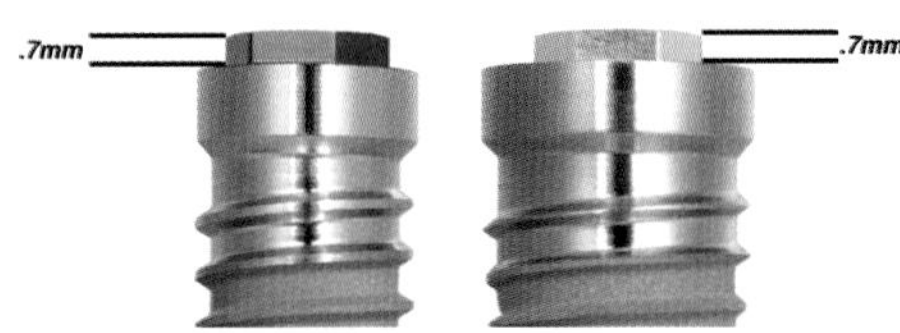

Figure 2.3. Profile view of OSSEOTITE® external hex implant. Vertical measurement of external hex measures 0.7 mm. (4.1 mm restorative platform left; 5.0 mm restorative platform right).

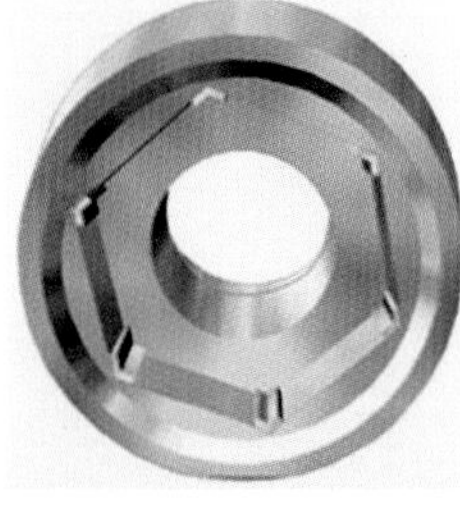

Figure 2.4. Apical view of pre-machined abutment with a 4.1 mm restorative platform. Flat surface to flat surface of the hex measures 2.7 mm. Microstops (Gold Standard ZR®) have been machined into the corners of the hex in UCLA Abutments and GingiHue® Posts.

IMPLANTS

Implants are the components that are placed into patients' bone with the intent of achieving osseointegration. Osseointegration was originally defined by Brånemark as ". . . the direct structural and functional connection between ordered, living bone and the surface of a load carrying implant" (Brånemark 1985). The surgical placement of endosseous implants initiates a complex series of biologic events associated with wound healing: inflammation, proliferation and maturation (Zoldos and Kent 1995).

Healing of bone and soft tissue around endosseous implants is a dynamic process and is the result of numerous factors, among them: surgical, atraumatic technique; design of the osteotomy; host immune system; macroscopic and microscopic design of dental implants; fit of the implant into the osteotomy; wound dehiscence; and loading protocol. For optimal performance, dental implants should have appropriate mechanical strength, biocompatibility, and biostability in humans (Cook and Kay 1987). Further discussion of the biology of osseointegration is beyond the scope of this textbook. The reader is referred to other sources for further discussion.

Clinicians may choose implants from any number of manufacturers. Implants may be made from various materials, but commercially pure titanium or titanium alloy have enjoyed extraordinary clinical results. Dental implants come in various sized diameters and lengths, with various macroscopic thread designs, surface treatments, and implant/abutment connections. This textbook features the implants manufactured by ***3i®***, Implant Innovations, Inc.®, Palm Beach Gardens, Florida. All the catalogue numbers and implant and restorative components refer to products made by ***3i®***.

Dental implants manufactured by ***3i®*** have threaded external surfaces for both the tapered and cylindrical implant designs (Figures 2.1, 2.2) The original external hex implant design consisted of a six-sided hex .7 mm tall; a flat-to-flat surface measurement of 2.7 mm; and a restorative platform that measured 4.1 mm (Figures 2.3, 2.4). Dental

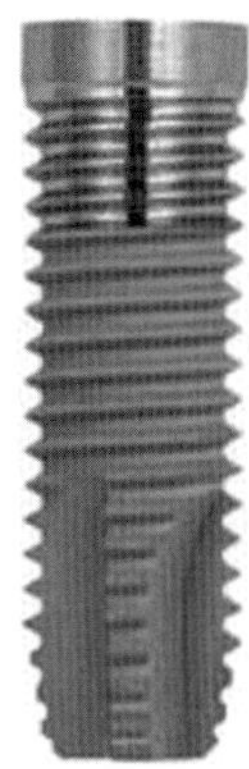

Figure 2.5. Profile view of 3.25 mm diameter internal connection implant. This implant expands to a 3.4 mm restorative platform (IOSM311).

Figure 2.6. Profile view of 4.0 mm diameter internal connection implant. This implant expands to a 4.1 mm restorative platform (IOSS411).

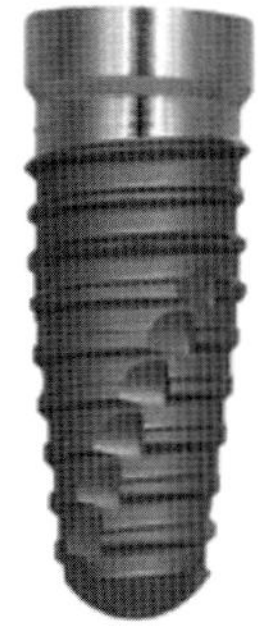

Figure 2.7. Profile view of 5.0 mm diameter internal connection implant (INT511).

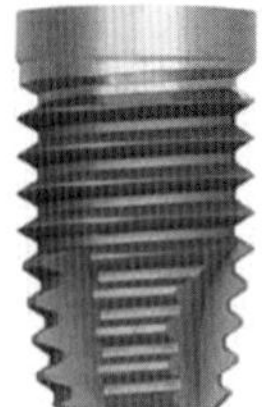

Figure 2.8. Profile view of 6.0 mm diameter internal connection implant (INT611).

TABLE 2.1. Implant Lengths and Catalogue Numbers (4 mm Diameter) for OSSEOTITE® Certain® Implants

Length (mm)	OSSEOTITE® Certain® Implants	OSSEOTITE® Certain® NT Implants
8.5	IOSS485	INT485
10.0	IOSS410	INT410
11.5	IOSS411	INT411
13.0	IOSS413	INT413
15.0	IOSS415	INT415
18.0	IOSS418	N/A
20.0	IOSS420	N/A

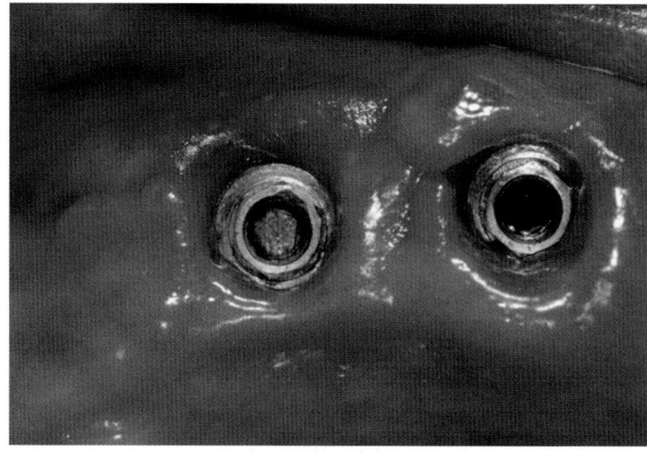

Figure 2.9. Clinical photograph of a broken abutment screw inside an external hexed implant.

implants are available in multiple diameters: 3.4, 4.0, 5.0, and 6.0 mm (Figures 2.5, 2.6, 2.7, 2.8).

Increasing the length of dental implants will also increase the amount of bone in contact with dental implants. Dental implants are generally made in increments of approximately 2 mm (Table 2.1).

IMPLANT/ABUTMENT CONNECTIONS

Osseointegration of dental implants has proven to be predictable in clinical practice (Adell and Lekholm 1981; Davarpanah 2001). The original design for implant restorations per the Brånemark protocol called for screw-retained prostheses. It was not unusual for these restorations to become loose secondary to screw loosening or screw fracture (McGlumphy and Huseyin 1995; Jemt and Lacey 1991). However, there have been more recent reports that have demonstrated a decreased number of screw failures for implant-retained restorations (Zarb and Schmitt 1990; Levine and Clem 1999).

Mollersten and others reported on the effect of implant/abutment joints on the strength and failure modes of implants from several different implant manufacturers (Mollersten and Lockowandt 1997). They found that the strength of the implant/abutment connections varied significantly depending on the length or depth of the connections. Low joint depths or lengths (<2.3 mm) were correlated with failures at lower forces; large/thicker joint depths (>5 mm) were correlated ($r = 0.959$) with failures at higher levels. The lowest failure was measured at 138 N for a connection that was 0.8 mm long. The highest failure was recorded at 693 N for a connection that measured 6.0 mm in length.

EXTERNAL IMPLANT/ABUTMENT CONNECTIONS

The original Brånemark protocol called for the placement of several external hexed implants for restoration of edentulous jaws. The implants were rigidly splinted together with metal castings attached to the implant abutments with retaining screws. The external hex of the original implants was designed to drive implants into their respective osteotomies (Beaty 1994). It was not designed as an antirotation component for single-unit implant restorations. The external hex measured 0.7 mm in height and was not designed to withstand masticatory forces on single, screw-retained crowns (Binon 1995; Jemt 1993).

Implant manufacturers compensated for this design by changing the type of screw used for attaching abutments to implants—geometry, height, and surface area; improved machining between implants and implant restorative components; and application of appropriate torque to the screws (Finger and Castellon 2003). The goals of any modification in the original external hex designs were to improve the stability of the implant/abutment connection on a long-term basis. According to Finger and Castellon, there are at least 20 different implant/abutment connection designs that have been approved by the Food and Drug Administration for sale in the United States (Finger and Castellon 2003).

Clinical success with external hexed implants is dependent on precise machining between implants and implant restorative components and the stability of screw joints. Screw joints are found wherever two implant components are tightened or held in place by screws. The screw joint will fail (the screw will loosen) if outside forces are greater than the ability of the screw to keep the units tight. Forces attempting to disengage the screw joint are called joint separating forces. Those forces attempting to keep the joint together are called clamping forces. There are two primary factors involved in maintaining screw joints: maximum clamping forces and minimal separation forces.

In any external hex implant system, the screw joint includes the abutment, abutment screw, and implant. As the abutment screw is tightened or torqued, a compressive clamping force is generated between the abutment and implant. An equal, but opposite, tensile force is generated between the abutment screw and abutment. This force is referred to as the joint preload, or simply preload (Sakaguchi and Sun 1994). Schulte (1994) measured the external hex dimensions of six implant systems and obtained the ranges and coefficients of variance. Smaller ranges and variances suggested more accurate machining and better quality control. The ranges for the widths of the external hexes for all companies were 0.00030 for ***3i***® to 0.00140 for Nobelpharma. Schulte concluded that there were differences in quality control among the various implant systems as determined by the external hex measurements, but that larger sample sizes and different batches may make a difference in the results.

Torque may be defined as a measurable means of developing tension in a screw joint. Tightening involves the application of torque. Every screw design has a specific preload/torque relationship depending on the material used in the screw and the design of the screw head.

Preload is induced into the abutment screw when the screw is torqued during tightening. Preload keeps the abutment and implant together by producing a clamping force between the screw head and its seat inside the abutment. As torque is applied to the abutment screw, the abutment screw actually elongates, which places the screw shank and screw threads in tension. The elastic recovery of the screw actually creates the clamping force between the abutment and implant. This concept is of great clinical significance because the resistance of the abutment to displacement or screw joint failure is a function of preload or the clamping forces between the abutment and implant (Figure 2.9).

Within the last several years, implant manufacturers have introduced prefabricated or machined abutments that were designed for use with cement-retained crowns (Keith and Miller 1999). Cement-retained crowns have several advantages over screw-retained crowns. The most important is that there is no longer a need to develop a screw access opening in the occlusal or facial surface of the

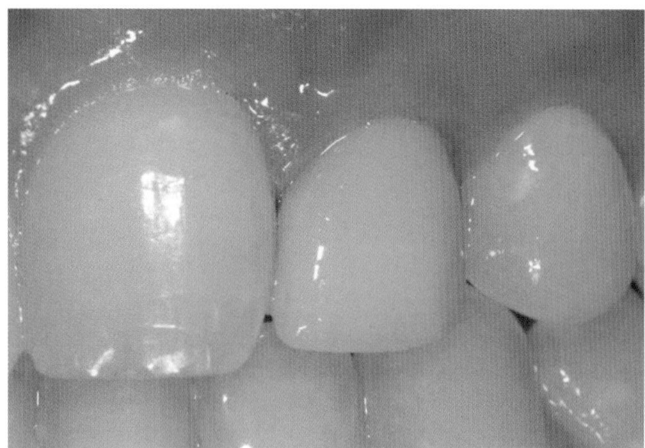

Figure 2.10. Facial view of an implant cement-retained crown replacing the maxillary left lateral incisor.

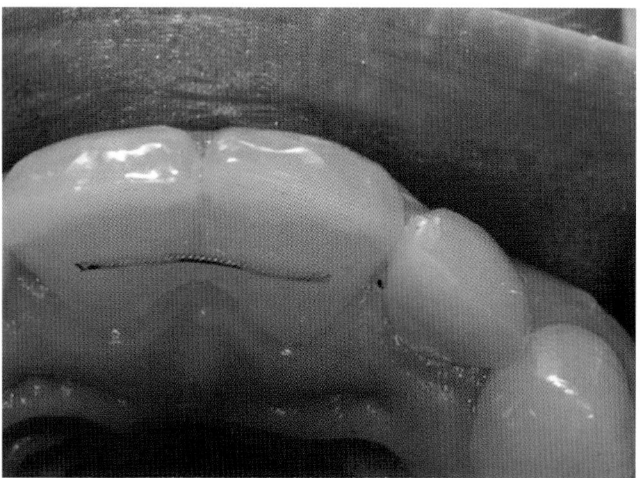

Figure 2.11. Occlusal view of the implant cement-retained crown in Figure 2.10. Note the lack of a screw access opening on the palatal surface.

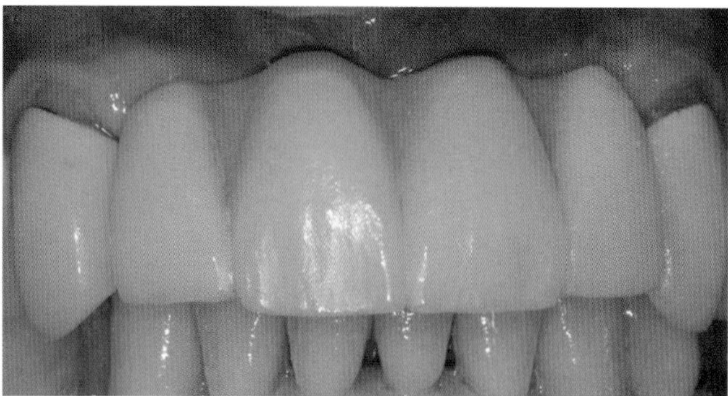

Figure 2.12. Facial view of an implant screw-retained fixed partial denture (inserted 1992) replacing the maxillary incisors.

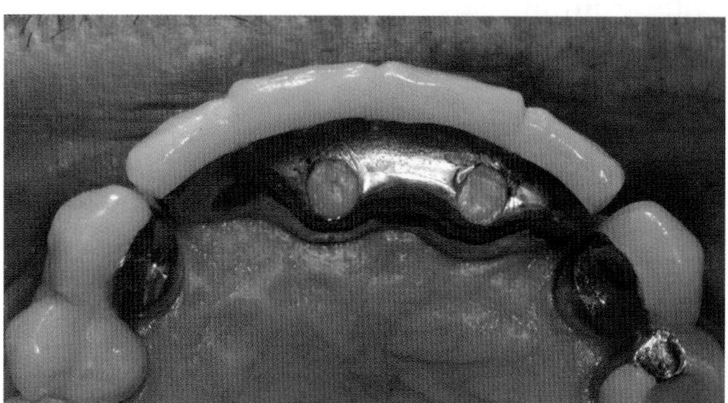

Figure 2.13. Occlusal view of the implant screw-retained fixed partial denture in Figure 2.12. Note that the screw access openings provide access to the abutment screws without interfering with the facial aesthetics of the prosthesis.

implant crown restoration (Figures 2.10, 2.11). However, cement-retained crowns are not as retrievable as screw-retained crowns in the event that the abutment and/or crown have to be repaired (Figures 2.12, 2.13). One survey of commercial dental laboratories suggested that the number of screw-retained restorations was decreasing (Marinbach 1996).

One of the keys to successful long-term implant restorations is the stability of the implant/abutment connection. Rodkey (1977) pointed out that the type of finish on screws could have a significant effect on the tension induced by a given torque. Implant manufacturers have altered the materials in the screws as well as the surface of abutment screws in an attempt to prevent or minimize screw loosening (Robb and Porter 1998; Porter and Robb 1998; Steri-Oss 1968). Martin and Woody (2001) tested the rotational angles in implant/abutment connections with various abutment screws and preloads. They found that the abutment screws with enhanced surfaces reduced the coefficient of friction and produced greater rotational angles and preload values than screws made from conventional gold and titanium alloys.

In review, external implant/abutment connections have proven to be successful in clinical use (Drago 2003; Eckert and Wollan 1998). This connection has a long, successful history in clinical implant dentistry and is still a viable choice for clinicians. This textbook features implant restorations utilizing the external hex implant/abutment connection of the OSSEOTITE® Implant System and the internal implant/abutment connection of the OSSEOTITE® Certain® implant system.

INTERNAL IMPLANT/ABUTMENT CONNECTIONS

One of the first internal implant/abutment connections was designed with a 1.7 mm internal hex below a 0.5 mm wide 45° bevel (Niznick 1983). This system was designed to distribute masticatory forces deeper within the implant, which would protect the abutment screw from excess occlusal

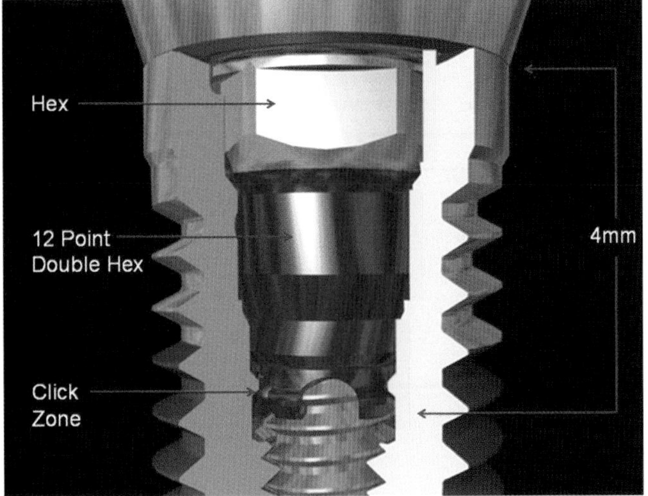

Figure 2.14. Cross section diagram of OSSEOTITE® Certain® implant illustrating 4 mm length of internal connection.

TABLE 2.2. Force Required to Break Implant/Abutment Connections

Implant/Abutment Connection	Force (Ncm) to Break Implant/ Abutment Connection
Internal connection-abutment screw torqued to 35 Ncm	774.7 Ncm
Internal connection-abutment screw torqued to 20 Ncm	767.1 Ncm
External connection-abutment screw torqued to 35 Ncm	648.4 Ncm
Internal connection-no screw	519.9 Ncm

loading. This internal implant/abutment connection provided greater strength to the implant/abutment joint (Niznick 1991) when compared to the strengths of external hex implant/abutment connections.

The OSSEOTITE® Certain® implant internal connection is 4 mm long (Figure 2.14). These connections also feature intimate contact along a significant length of the connection that provides increased lateral stability to the implant/abutment connection (Niznick 1991; Mollersten and Lockowandt 1997).

Laboratory testing has demonstrated that the internal connection implant/abutment connection is stronger than the external hex implant/abutment connection (Implant Innovations 2003). The testing was conducted by placing 30° static loads to abutments connected to their respective implants with abutment screws torqued to a known level of preload. The internal connection implant/abutment connections failed at 767 Ncm of force. The external hex implant/abutment connections failed at 648 Ncm. It is important to note that the abutment screw for the internal connection was a hexed abutment screw tightened to 20 Ncm of preload. The external implant/abutment connection was maintained with square abutment screws torqued to 35 Ncm of preload (Table 2.2).

The OSSEOTITE® Certain® implant system features several design changes that should facilitate predictable restorable treatment. The hexed abutment screw measures 1.95 mm from the occlusal aspect of the screw to the screw seating surface (Figure 2.15). This allows clinicians and laboratory technicians great flexibility in abutment preparation, decreasing the risk of abutment wall fracture or fenestration (Figure 2.16). The long implant/abutment connection

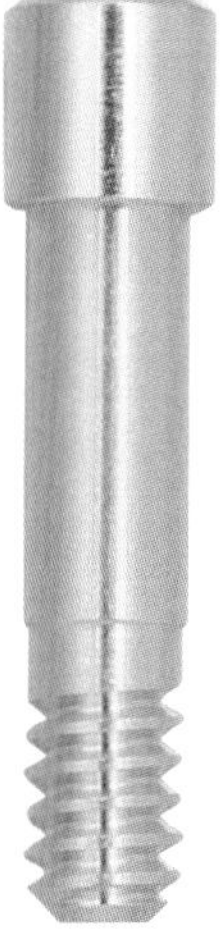

Figure 2.15. Cross-section of an abutment screw (IUNIHG) for the OSSEOTITE® Certain® implant illustrating height of hex abutment screw.

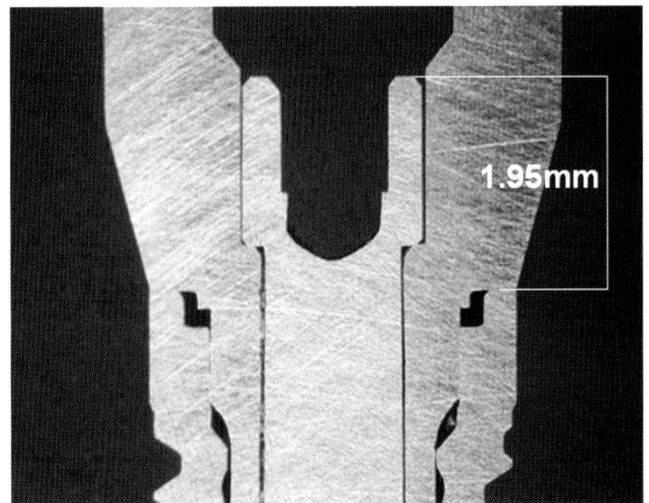

Figure 2.16. Cross-section of GingiHue® Post (OSSEOTITE® Certain® Implant System) demonstrating sufficient axial wall thickness for preparation.

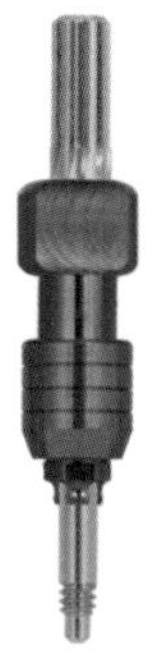

Figure 2.17. Pick-up implant impression coping (OSSEOTITE® Certain® Implant System, IIIC12). This impression coping features a 4 mm connection that allows clinicians to positively seat the coping into the implant with little risk of inaccurate seating.

allows clinicians to positively seat impression copings and abutments into their appropriate positions (Figure 2.17). This internal connection also features audible and tactile feedback (QuickSeat™ Connection) during abutment and impression coping insertion by way of a "click" associated with flexure of fingers at the apical ends of the restorative components (Figure 2.18). The connection also features a 6/12 internal connection that has a hex and 12-point double hex. The hex serves two functions: It engages the driver tip for mountless delivery during implant placement and it provides anti-rotation for all straight abutments. The 12-point double hex provides rotational positioning every 30° for the 15° Pre-angled GingiHue® Post (Figure 2.19).

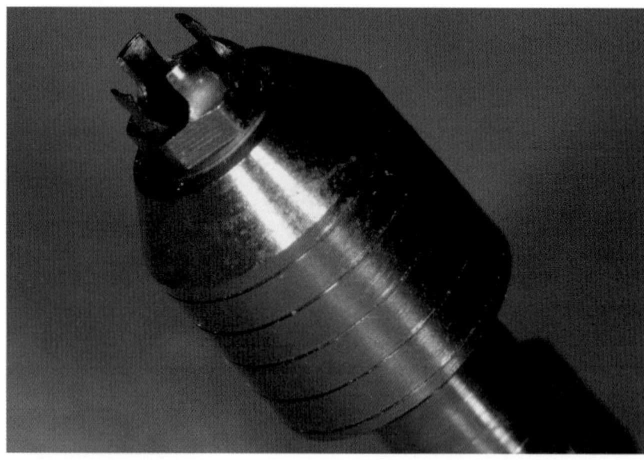

Figure 2.18. Pick-up implant impression coping (OSSEOTITE® Certain® Implant System, IIIC12) with four fingers at the apical end of the coping that provide an audible click when seated into an implant or implant analog.

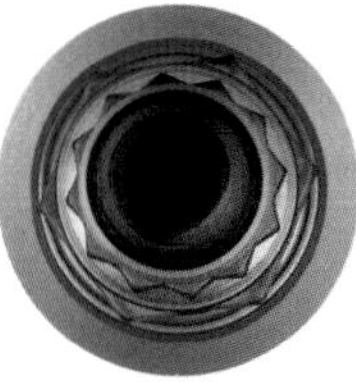

Figure 2.19. Occlusal view of OSSEOTITE® Certain® Implant System internal connection. The 12-point double hex is apical to the hex at the occlusal portion of the implant.

Several impression techniques have been described that provide accurate casts for development of implant frameworks (Sutherland and Hallam 1990; Loos 1986; Taylor 1990). Vigolo and Fonzi (2004) studied the accuracy of implant impression techniques with the OSSEOTITE® Certain® implant system. They found that improved accuracy of the master cast was achieved when the square, pick-up implant impression copings were joined together with autopolymerizing acrylic resin for multiple, splinted implant restorations.

HEALING ABUTMENTS

EP® Healing Abutments

Originally, abutments and gold cylinders were designed for use in edentulous patients. Clinicians were frustrated with the limitations of the components to provide aesthetic, natural-looking implant restorations (Jansen, 1995). Most implant components were 4–5 mm in diameter; many teeth were larger than the components. A maxillary central incisor generally has a CEJ diameter between 6 and 8 mm (Linek 1949). With the original components there were several millimeters difference in size between the implant components and maxillary central incisors. Laboratory technicians were asked to make implant restorations with natural contours and in many cases had to add ridge laps to the restorations to mimic the contours of the adjacent natural teeth.

An implant abutment emergence profile similar to that of a natural tooth is required to support and contour the peri-implant soft tissues (Saadoun 1995). The cylindrical shapes of the implants must be changed to more anatomically correct cross sections by the time the implant restorations reach the gingival margins, reflecting the root structure of the teeth being replaced (Weisgold and Arnoux 1997). Lazzara considered dimensions and contours of implant-retained crown restorations and the stability of the gingival margins surrounding implant restorations to be the two primary concerns in assuring durable aesthetics in implant restorations (Lazzara 1993).

EP® Healing Abutments were designed as part of The Emergence Profile System® to guide soft tissue healing after implant placement in single-stage surgical protocols or after implants had been uncovered in two-stage surgical protocols (Implant Innovations 1993) (Figures 2.20, 2.21, 2.22). They are available for all implant restorative platforms. EP® Healing Abutments were designed with collar heights between 2 and 8 mm and 3.4, 4.1, 5, 6, and 7.5 mm diameters (Figure 2.23) (Table 2.3 through 2.6).

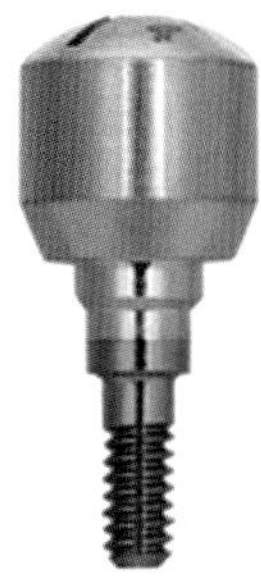

Figure 2.20. Five mm EP® Healing Abutment (ITHA54) for 4.1 mm diameter internal connection implant. The apical portion of the healing abutment has been color coded blue for 4.1 mm diameter implants

TABLE 2.3. Catalogue Numbers for EP® Healing Abutments for 3.4 mm Diameter OSSEOTITE® Certain® Implants

Emergence Profile	Collar Height	Catalogue Numbers
3.8 mm	2.0 mm	IMHA32
3.8 mm	3.0 mm	IMHA33
3.8 mm	4.0 mm	IMHA34
3.8 mm	6.0 mm	IMHA36

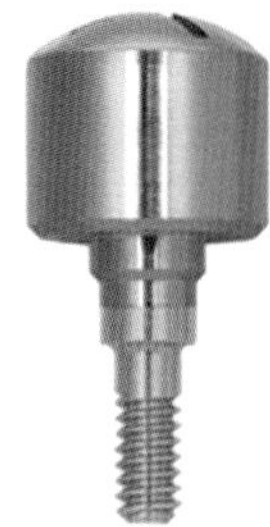

Figure 2.21. Five mm EP® Healing Abutment (IWTH54) for 5.0 mm diameter internal connection implant. The apical portion of the healing abutment has been color coded gold for 5.0 mm diameter implants

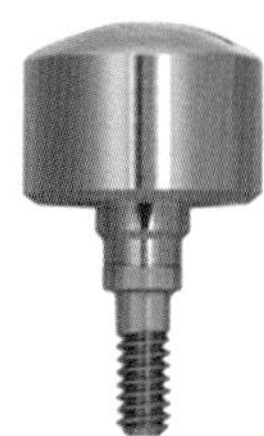

Figure 2.22. Six mm EP® Healing Abutment (IWTH64) for 6.0 mm diameter internal connection implant. The apical portion of the healing abutment has been color coded green for 6.0 mm diameter implants

TABLE 2.4. Catalogue Numbers for EP® Healing Abutments for 4.1 mm Diameter OSSEOTITE® Certain® Implants

Emergence Profile	Collar Height	Catalogue Numbers
4.1 mm	2.0 mm	ITHA42
4.1 mm	3.0 mm	ITHA43
4.1 mm	4.0 mm	ITHA44
4.1 mm	6.0 mm	ITHA46
4.1 mm	8.0 mm	ITHA48
5.0 mm	2.0 mm	ITHA52
5.0 mm	3.0 mm	ITHA53
5.0 mm	4.0 mm	ITHA54
5.0 mm	6.0 mm	ITHA56
5.0 mm	8.0 mm	ITHA58
6.0 mm	3.0 mm	ITHA63
6.0 mm	4.0 mm	ITHA64
6.0 mm	6.0 mm	ITHA66
6.0 mm	8.0 mm	ITHA68
7.5 mm	3.0 mm	ITHA73
7.5 mm	4.0 mm	ITHA74
7.5 mm	6.0 mm	ITHA76
7.5 mm	8.0 mm	ITHA78

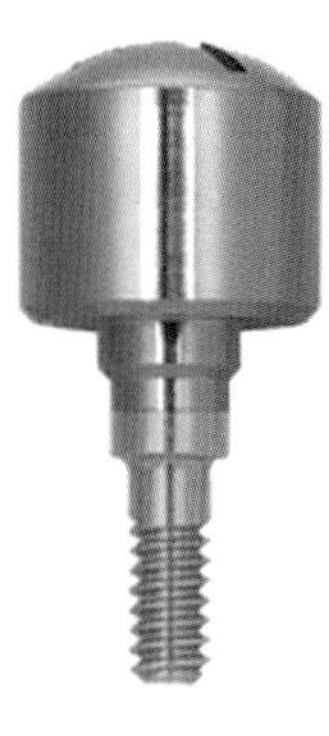

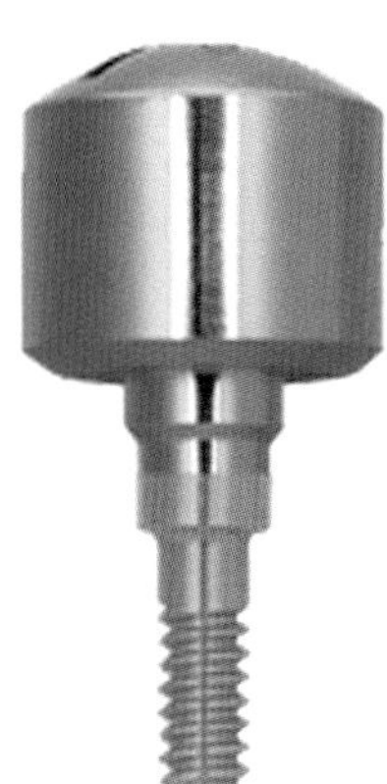

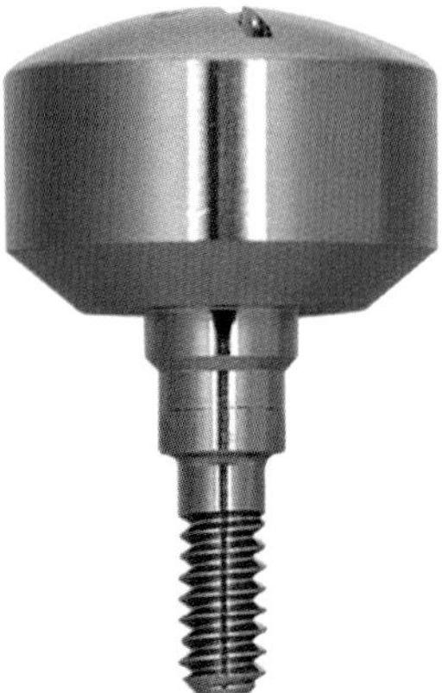

Figure 2.23. Profile view of EP® Healing Abutments for OSSEOTITE® Certain® 5.0 mm implants: 5, 6 and 7.5 mm diameters (left to right). Similar healing abutments are also available for the other implant diameters.

TABLE 2.5. Catalogue Numbers for EP® Healing Abutments for 5.0 mm Diameter OSSEOTITE® Certain® Implants

Emergence Profile	Collar Height	Catalogue Numbers
5.0 mm	2.0 mm	IWTH52
5.0 mm	3.0 mm	IWTH53
5.0 mm	4.0 mm	IWTH54
5.0 mm	6.0 mm	IWTH56
5.0 mm	8.0 mm	IWTH58
6.0 mm	2.0 mm	IWTH562
6.0 mm	3.0 mm	IWTH563
6.0 mm	4.0 mm	IWTH564
6.0 mm	6.0 mm	IWTH566
6.0 mm	8.0 mm	IWTH568
7.5 mm	2.0 mm	IWTH572
7.5 mm	3.0 mm	IWTH573
7.5 mm	4.0 mm	IWTH574
7.5 mm	6.0 mm	IWTH576
7.5 mm	8.0 mm	IWTH578

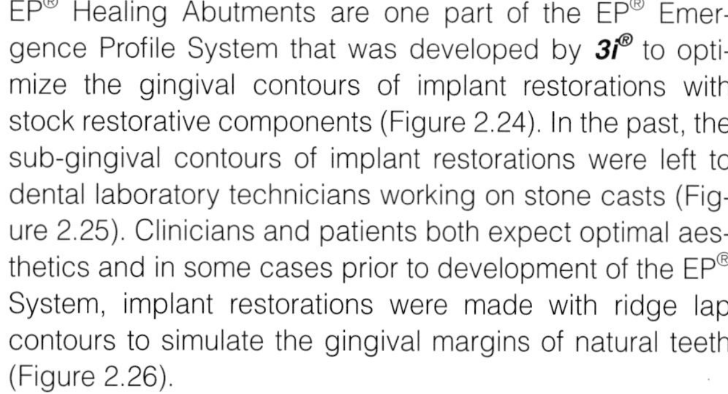

EP® Healing Abutments are one part of the EP® Emergence Profile System that was developed by ***3i®*** to optimize the gingival contours of implant restorations with stock restorative components (Figure 2.24). In the past, the sub-gingival contours of implant restorations were left to dental laboratory technicians working on stone casts (Figure 2.25). Clinicians and patients both expect optimal aesthetics and in some cases prior to development of the EP® System, implant restorations were made with ridge lap contours to simulate the gingival margins of natural teeth (Figure 2.26).

In other instances, implant-retained restorations were made from cylindrical abutments and gold cylinders that had straight emergence profiles (Figure 2.27, 2.28). The subgingival contours for this implant-retained restoration were improved by removing the standard abutment and placing the appropriate healing abutment (THA464, 4.1 mm implant restorative platform, 6 mm EP® diameter, 4 mm height) for soft tissue healing. The definitive crown was cemented to a prefabricated titanium abutment (GingiHue® Post, APP464G) that was prepared in the laboratory (Figures 2.29, 2.30, 2.31).

TABLE 2.6. Catalogue Numbers for EP® Healing Abutments for 6.0 mm Diameter OSSEOTITE® Certain® Implants

Emergence Profile	Collar Height	Catalogue Numbers
6.0 mm	2.0 mm	IWTH62
6.0 mm	3.0 mm	IWTH63
6.0 mm	4.0 mm	IWTH64
6.0 mm	6.0 mm	IWTH66
6.0 mm	8.0 mm	IWTH68
7.5 mm	2.0 mm	IWTH672
7.5 mm	3.0 mm	IWTH673
7.5 mm	4.0 mm	IWTH674
7.5 mm	6.0 mm	IWTH676
7.5 mm	8.0 mm	IWTH678

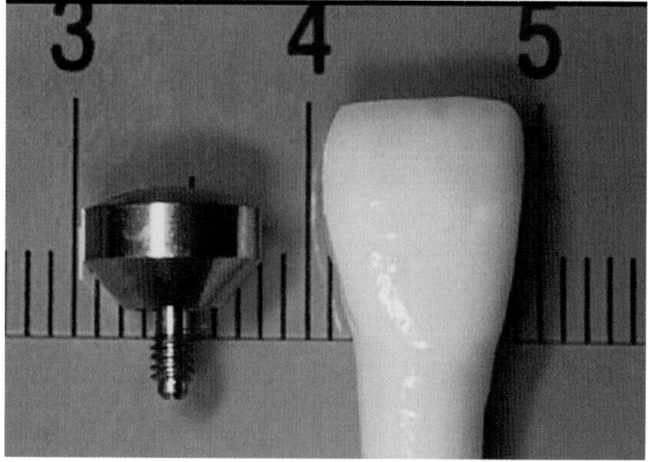

Figure 2.24. 7.5 mm EP® diameter healing abutment (THA74) adjacent to a maxillary central incisor. Note the similarities in the diameters of the abutment and tooth at the CEJ.

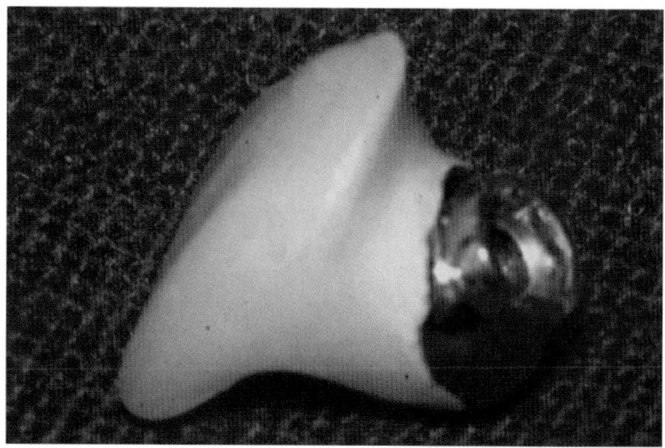

Figure 2.25. Laboratory view of a screw-retained crown that was fabricated to replace a maxillary right cuspid. Note the ridge lap that was developed in the porcelain to simulate the gingival margin of the missing natural tooth.

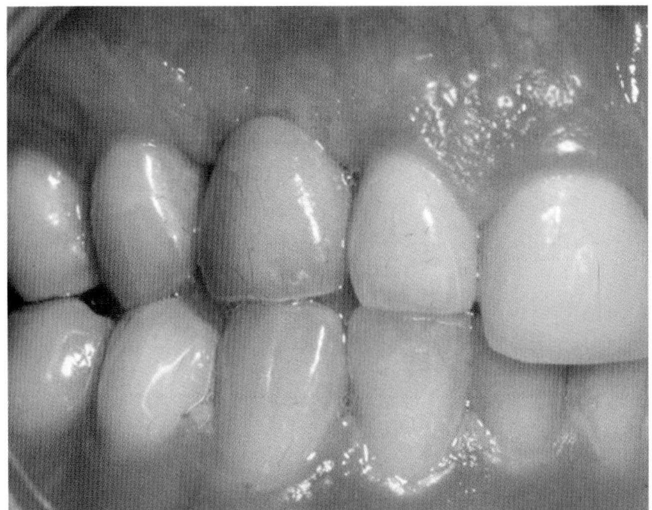

Figure 2.26. Clinical view of the screw-retained crown in place featured in Figure 2.25. Due to the ridge lap design, the gingival contours of the implant restoration mimic the clinical crown heights of the adjacent natural teeth.

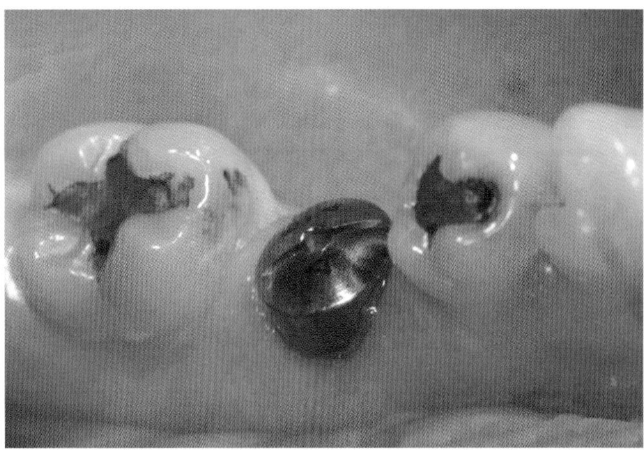

Figure 2.29. Lingual occlusal view with healing abutment (THA46) in place. Optimal sub-gingival contours were established by placing the appropriate size healing abutment consistent with the size of the missing tooth.

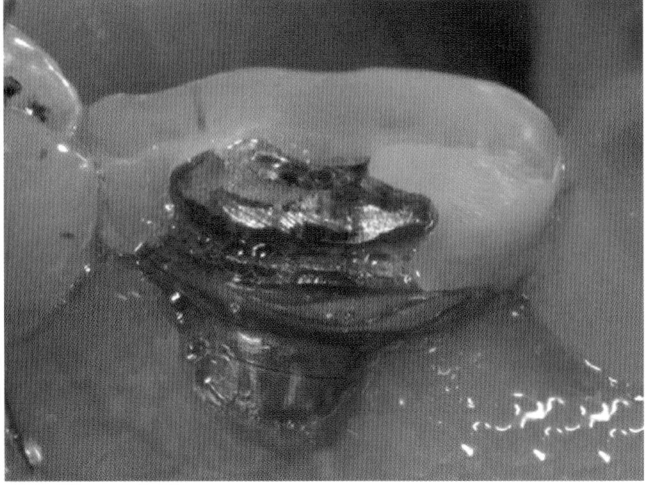

Figure 2.27. Clinical view of a screw-retained crown replacing the mandibular left first molar. The metal coping was cast to a machined gold cylinder that was screwed into a standard abutment.

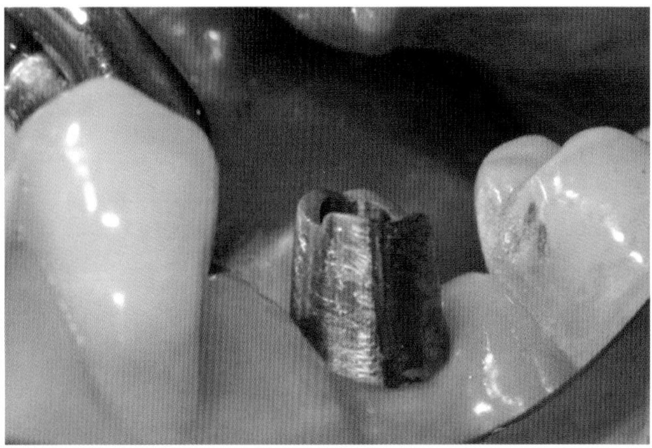

Figure 2.30. Buccal view of pre-machined titanium abutment (APP464G) in place. Emergence profiles were established by the healing abutment.

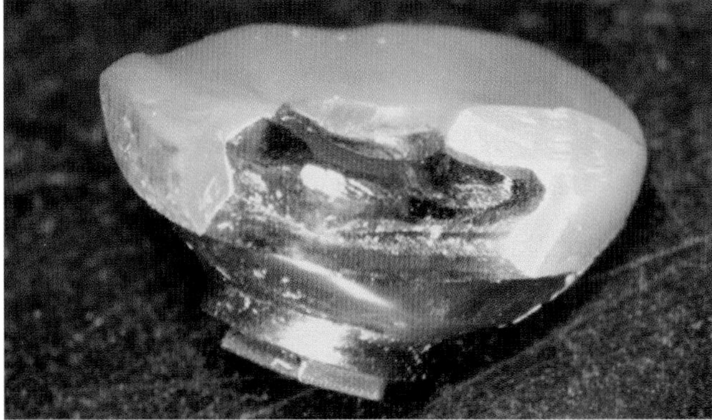

Figure 2.28. Laboratory view of the crown in Figure 2.27. The sub-gingival contours were established by the contours of the standard abutment.

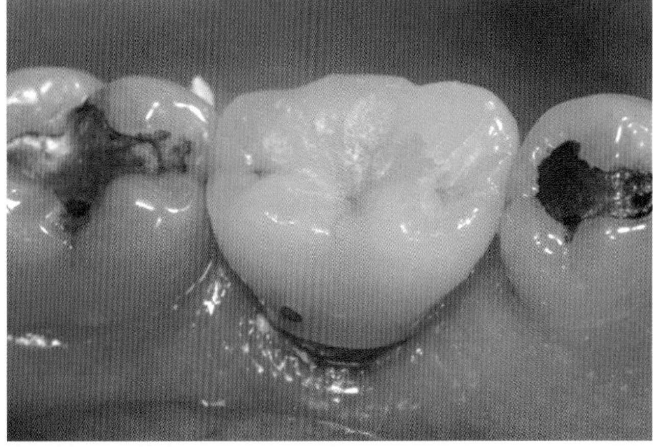

Figure 2.31. Lingual view of definitive crown in place.

Encode™ Healing Abutments

The Encode™ Restorative System has recently been introduced by ***3i®*** (2004). Encode™ Healing Abutments were designed as two-piece components: abutment screws and healing abutments. They are available for both OSSEOTITE® and OSSEOTITE® Certain® implant systems in sizes consistent with the EP® System (Tables 2.7, 2.8, 2.9, 2.10)(Figures 2.32, 2.33). Encode Healing Abutments have codes embedded into the occlusal surfaces that allow development of patient specific abutments through CAD/CAM technology. The codes provide information to a computer relative to the hex position, implant restorative platform, and diameter and collar heights of the Encode Healing Abutments. Encode Healing Abutments will be selected for use by clinicians based on the same criteria already in use with conventional healing abutments (Figures 2.34 and 2.35).

TABLE 2.7. Catalogue Numbers for Encode Healing Abutments for 3.4 mm Diameter Seating Surfaces OSSEOTITE® Certain® and OSSEOTITE® Implant Systems

Emergence Profile (mm)	Collar Height (mm)	OSSEOTITE® Certain® Implants	OSSEOTITE® Implants
3.8	3	IEHA343	EHA343
3.8	4	IEHA344	EHA344
3.8	6	IEHA346	EHA346
3.8	8	IEHA348	EHA348
3.8	3	IEHA353	EHA353
3.8	4	IEHA354	EHA354
3.8	6	IEHA356	EHA356
3.8	8	IEHA358	EHA358

TABLE 2.8. Catalogue Numbers for Encode Healing Abutments for 4.1 mm Diameter Seating Surfaces OSSEOTITE® Certain® and OSSEOTITE® Implant Systems

Emergence Profile (mm)	Collar Height (mm)	OSSEOTITE® Certain® Implants	OSSEOTITE® Implants
4.1	3.0	IEHA443	EHA443
4.1	4.0	IEHA444	EHA444
4.1	6.0	IEHA446	EHA446
4.1	8.0	IEHA448	EHA448
5.0	3.0	IEHA453	EHA453
5.0	4.0	IEHA454	EHA454
5.0	6.0	IEHA456	EHA456
5.0	8.0	IEHA458	EHA458
6.0	3.0	IEHA463	EHA463
6.0	4.0	IEHA464	EHA464
6.0	6.0	IEHA466	EHA466
6.0	8.0	IEHA468	EHA468
7.5	3.0	IEHA473	EHA473
7.5	4.0	IEHA474	EHA474
7.5	6.0	IEHA476	EHA476
7.5	8.0	IEHA478	EHA478

TABLE 2.9. Catalogue Numbers for Encode Healing Abutments for 5.0 mm Diameter Seating Surfaces OSSEOTITE® Certain® and OSSEOTITE® Implant Systems

Emergence Profile (mm)	Collar Height (mm)	OSSEOTITE® Certain® Implants	OSSEOTITE® Implants
5.0	3.0	IEHA553	EHA553
5.0	4.0	IEHA554	EHA554
5.0	6.0	IEHA556	EHA556
5.0	8.0	IEHA558	EHA558
6.0	3.0	IEHA563	EHA563
6.0	4.0	IEHA564	EHA564
6.0	6.0	IEHA566	EHA566
6.0	8.0	IEHA568	EHA568
7.5	3.0	IEHA573	EHA573
7.5	4.0	IEHA574	EHA574
7.5	6.0	IEHA476	EHA576
7.5	8.0	IEHA578	EHA578

TABLE 2.10. Catalogue Numbers for Encode Healing Abutments for 6.0 mm Diameter Seating Surfaces OSSEOTITE® Certain® and OSSEOTITE® Implant Systems

Emergence Profile (mm)	Collar Height (mm)	OSSEOTITE® Certain® Implants	OSSEOTITE® Implants
6.0	3.0	IEHA663	EHA663
6.0	4.0	IEHA664	EHA664
6.0	6.0	IEHA666	EHA666
6.0	8.0	IEHA668	EHA668
7.5	3.0	IEHA673	EHA673
7.5	4.0	IEHA674	EHA674
7.5	6.0	IEHA676	EHA676
7.5	8.0	IEHA678	EHA678

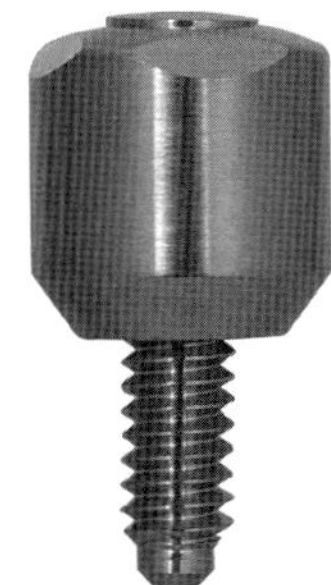
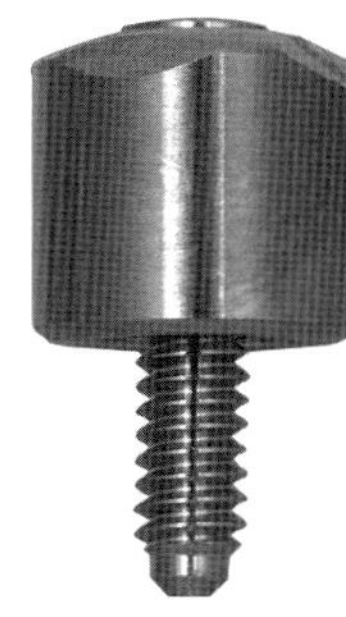
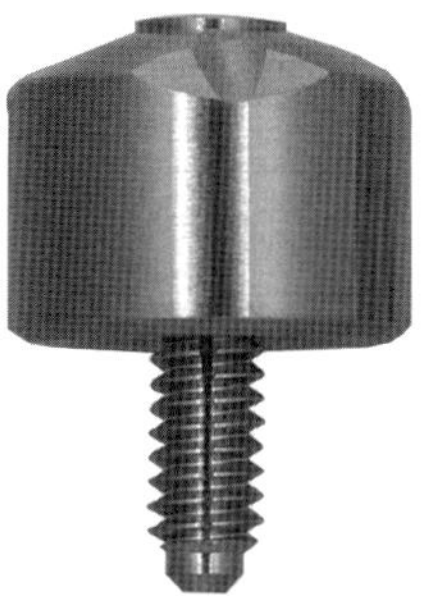

Figure 2.32. Profile views of Encode™ Healing Abutments: 5, 6, and 7.5 mm diameters, 4 mm collar heights for the OSSEOTITE® Implant System (4.1 mm diameter; THA54, THA64, THA74, respectively).

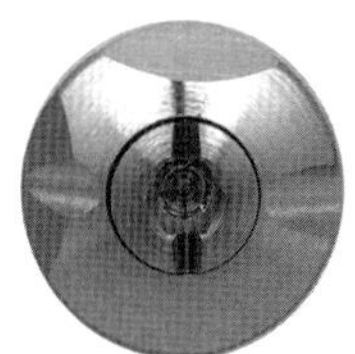
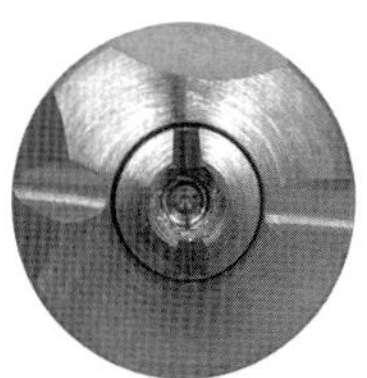
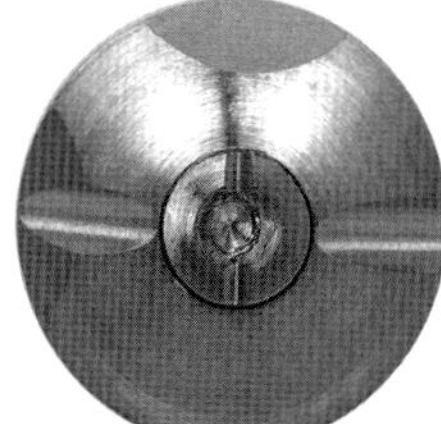

Figure 2.33. Occlusal view of Encode™ Healing Abutments for the OSSEOTITE® Certain® Implant System (4.1 mm diameter): 5, 6, and 7.5 mm diameters (IEHA454, IEHA464, IEHA474, respectively).

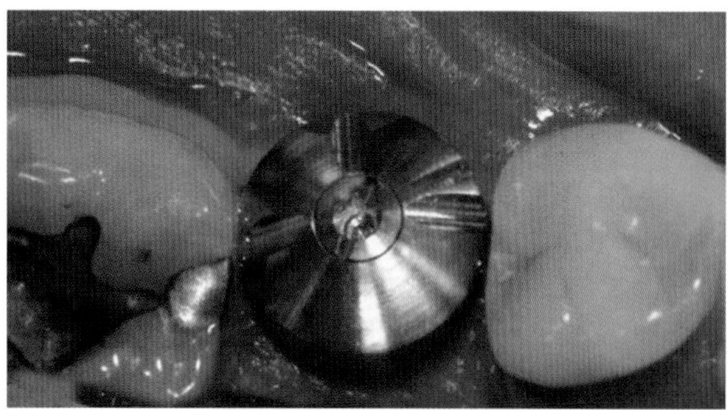

Figure 2.34. Occlusal view of Encode™ Healing Abutment (IEHA464) in place 12 weeks post implant placement for a missing mandibular left second premolar. An optical scanner will read the codes embedded into the occlusal surface of a die of the healing abutment.

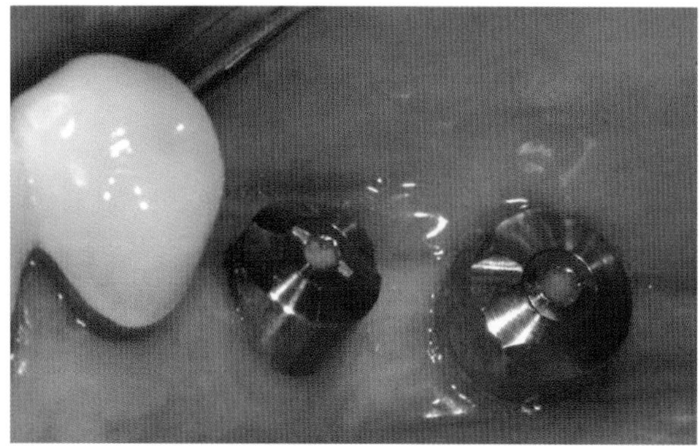

Figure 2.35. Occlusal view of Encode™ Healing Abutments in place 12 weeks post implant placement for missing right mandibular molar and second premolar (IEHA454 anterior, IEHA564 posterior).

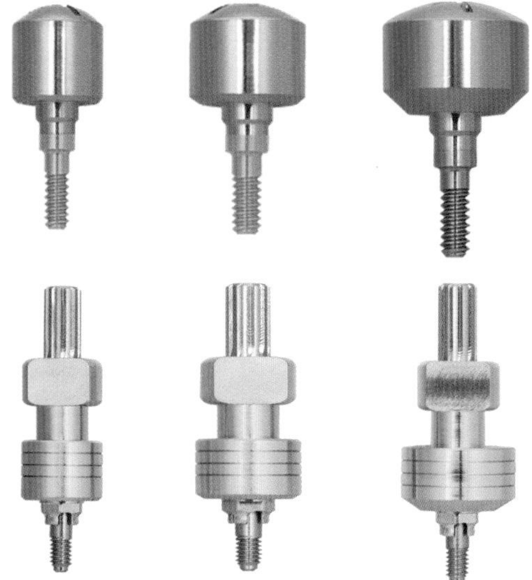

Figure 2.36. Top: Lateral view of EP® Healing Abutments for 5.0 mm diameter OSSEOTITE® Certain® implants (5.6 and 7.5 mm diameters, 4 mm collar heights, IWTH54, IWTH564, IWTH574, left to right, respectively). Bottom: Lateral view of pick-up implant impression copings for 5.0 mm diameter OSSEOTITE® Certain® implants (5, 6, and 7.5 mm diameters; IWIP55, IWIP56, IWIP57, left to right, respectively).

The Encode™ Restorative System has multiple advantages for both clinicians and dental laboratory technicians. Further discussion is featured in Chapters 6 and 9.

IMPRESSION COPINGS

Implant Impression Copings

Definitive implant restorations are best made with indirect techniques using fixed prosthodontic impression materials and techniques. EP® impression copings that correspond to the EP® Healing Abutments described above are available for implants and abutments (Figure 2.36). Impressions can be made that exactly duplicate the clinical soft tissue dimensions in the laboratory and result in crown restorations with optimal emergence profiles made from stock implant restorative components (Figure 2.37, 2.38).

Implant impression copings are placed directly onto the implant restorative platforms; abutment impression copings are placed directly onto standard abutments that have been placed onto implants (Tables 2.11, 2.12). With this system, laboratory technicians do not have to arbitrarily grind or remove material from the master cast to make properly contoured restorations (Figures 2.39, 2.40).

The impression copings that were illustrated in this case were pick-up implant impression copings. Pick-up impression copings require windows or openings in impression trays in order for clinicians to access the screws that retain the copings to the implants (Figures 2.41, 2.42). Twist Lock™ implant impression copings are proprietary for Implant Innovations, Inc.®'s trade name for transfer impression copings. Transfer impression copings remain in the mouth after the impression has set and the impression tray has been removed. Twist Lock™ implant impression copings are available for all implant restorative platforms except for 3.4 mm diameters. They have also been designed per the EP® System (Figure 2.43).

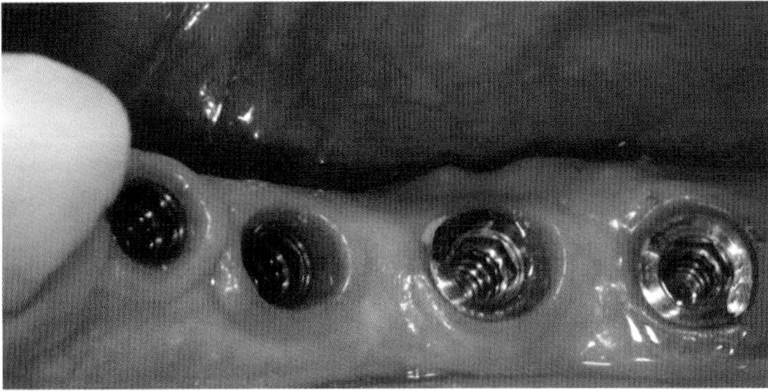

Figure 2.37. Occlusal view of two 4.1 mm and two 5.0 mm OSSEOTITE® Certain® implants in place in the mandibular right posterior quadrant. The emergence profiles were created by the appropriate EP® Healing Abutments.

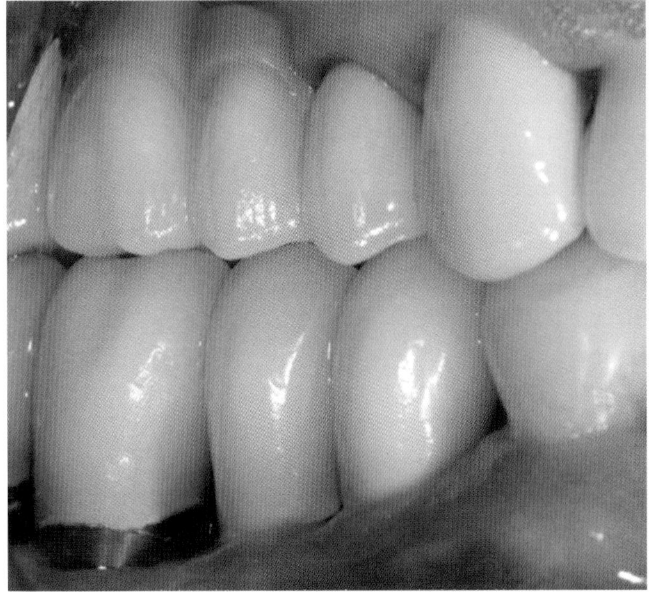

Figure 2.38. Buccal view of crown restorations for the implants in Figure 2.37.

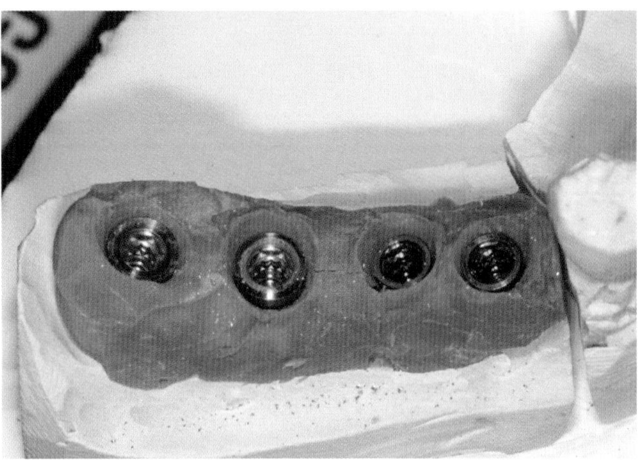

Figure 2.39. Occlusal view of master cast with four implant lab analogs (IILA20, IILAW5) in the mandibular right posterior quadrant. The healing abutments placed at the time of implant placement generated the emergence profiles.

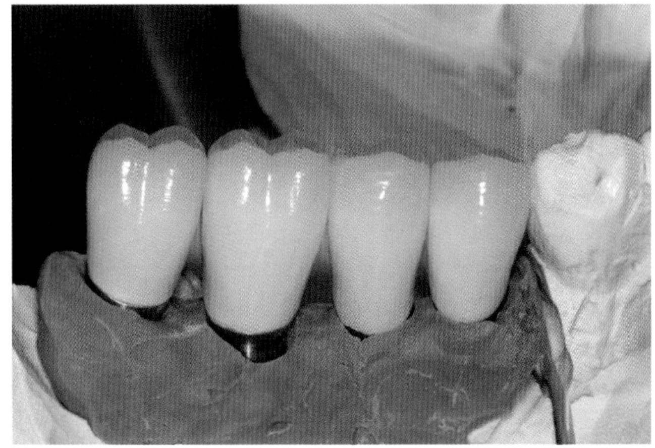

Figure 2.40. Laboratory facial view of four implant-retained crowns from Figure 2.39. Note that the surgeon generated the emergence profiles at the time of implant placement by placing the appropriate healing abutments. The laboratory technician had only to follow those contours to create the crowns.

TABLE 2.11. Implant Impression Copings for 3.4 and 4.1 mm Diameter OSSEOTITE® Certain® Implants

Implant Restorative Platforms (mm)	3.4	4.1	4.1	4.1	4.1
Emergence Profile (mm)	3.8	4.1	5.0	6.0	7.5
Pick Up Impression Copings	IMIC33	IIIC41	IIIC12	IIIC60	IIIC75
Twist Lock™ Impression Coping	N/A	IIIC44	IIIC45	IIIC46	IIIC47

TABLE 2.12. Implant Impression Copings for 5 mm and 6 mm Diameter OSSEOTITE® Certain® Implants

Implant Restorative Platforms (mm)	5.0	5.0	5.0	6.0	6.0
Emergence Profile (mm)	5.0	6.0	7.5	6.0	7.5
Pick Up Impression Copings	IWIP55	IWIP56	IWIP57	IWIP66	IWIP67
Twist Lock™ Impression Coping	IWIT55	IWIT56	IWIT57	IWIT66	IWIT67

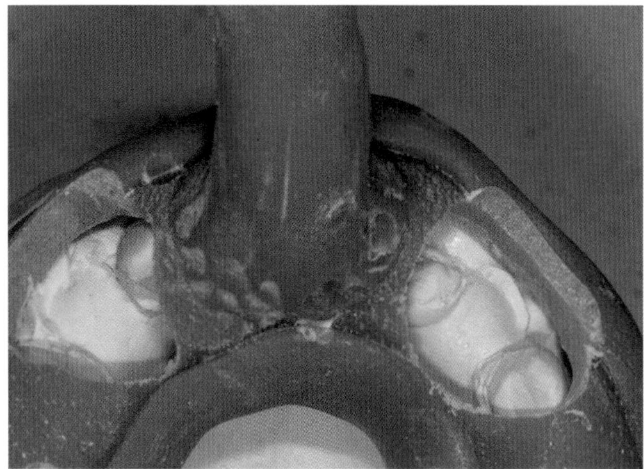

Figure 2.41. Laboratory example of open face tray for implant impression of maxillary right cuspid, maxillary left lateral incisor, and maxillary left cuspid.

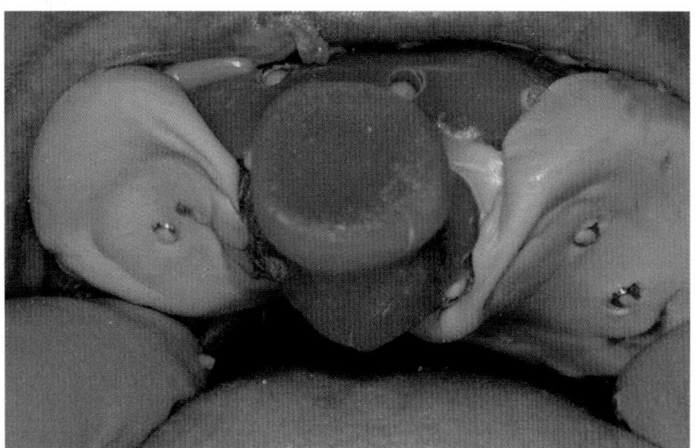

Figure 2.42. Clinical view of impression tray from Figure 2.41 in place. The windows provided the clinician with access to the impression coping screws for loosening prior to removing the impression from the mouth. The implant impression copings remained inside the impression.

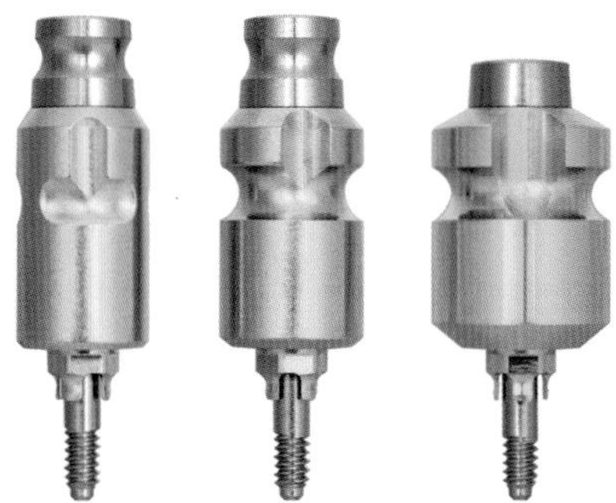

Figure 2.43. Profile view of Twist Lock™ Implant Impression Copings for 5.0 mm diameter OSSEOTITE® Certain® implants: (5, 6, and 7.5 mm emergence profile diameters, IWIT55, IWIT56, IWIT57 left to right).

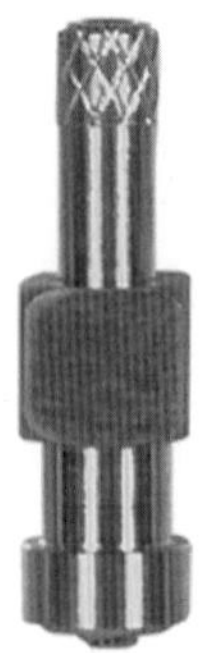

Figure 2.44. Profile view of Pick-Up Standard Abutment Impression Coping for 4.1 and 5.0 implant restorative platforms (SQIC7).

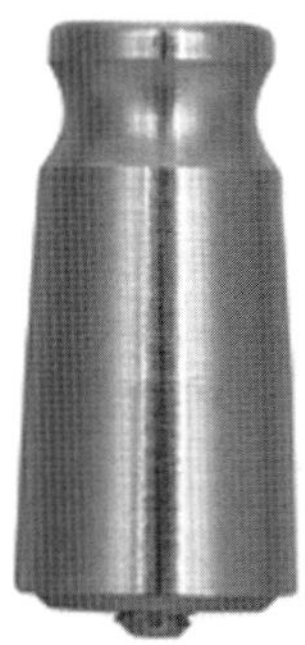

Figure 2.45. Profile view of Twist Lock™ Standard Abutment Impression Coping for 4.1 and 5.0 implant restorative platforms (SIC70).

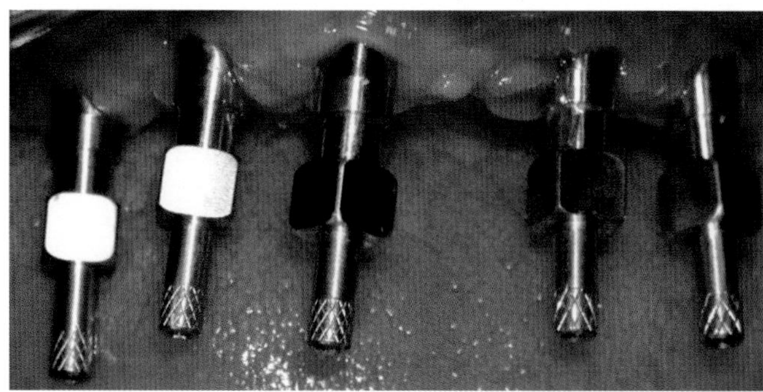

Figure 2.46. Standard Abutment Pick-Up Impression Copings (SQIC7) in place for a maxillary impression.

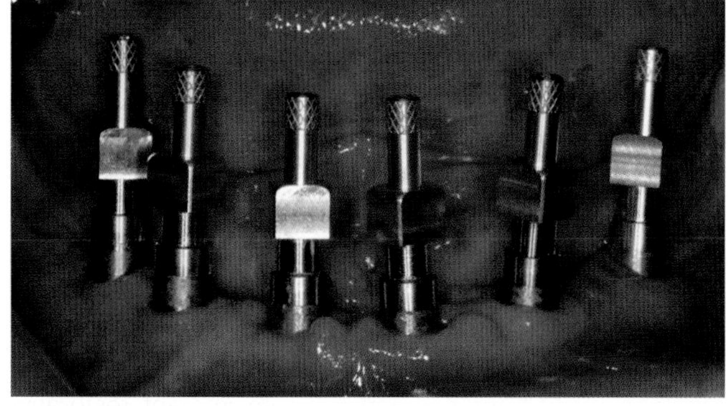

Figure 2.47. IOL® Pick-Up Impression Copings (IOLPIC) in place for a mandibular impression.

TABLE 2.13. Standard Abutment Impression Copings for 4.1 mm and 5 mm Diameter *3i*® Implants

Implant Restorative Platform (mm)	4.1	5.0
Emergence Profile (mm)	4.5	4.5
Pick-Up Impression Coping	SQIC7	SQIC7
Twist Lock™ Impression Coping	SIC70	SIC70

TABLE 2.14. IOL® Abutment Impression Copings for 4.1 mm Diameter *3i*® Implants

Implant Restorative Platform (mm)	4.1
Emergence Profile (mm)	4.5
Pick-Up Impression Coping	IOLPIC
Twist Lock™ Impression Coping	IOLTIC

Abutment Impression Copings

Impression copings are made for standard abutments. Standard Abutments (AB200, AB300, AB400, AB550, AB700) are the implant restorative components that attach directly to implants with abutment screws. Standard Abutments may be used for single- and multi-unit porcelain restorations, implant-retained bars, and within castings for hybrid prostheses. Abutment impression copings (Tables 2.13, 2.14) are available in both pick-up and transfer designs (Figures 2.44, 2.45, 2.46, 2.47).

Abutments

3i® manufactures multiple abutments for use in edentulous and partially edentulous patients. The following abutments are discussed in this textbook:

1. Standard Abutments
2. LOCATOR® Abutments
3. Immediate Occlusal Loading® (IOL®) Abutments
4. GingiHue® Posts
5. ZiReal™ Posts
6. Provide™ Abutments
7. UCLA Abutments
8. Final Encode™ Abutments

Standard Abutments

Standard Abutments are generally used in edentulous patients in which a traditional cast metal framework is used to splint multiple implants together. These abutments require a minimum inter-occlusal clearance of 6.5 mm and a maximum divergence of 30°. Standard abutments have been machined for 4.1 and 5.0 mm implant restorative platforms for OSSEOTITE® Certain® and OSSEOTITE® implant systems (Figure 2.48) (Table 2.15).

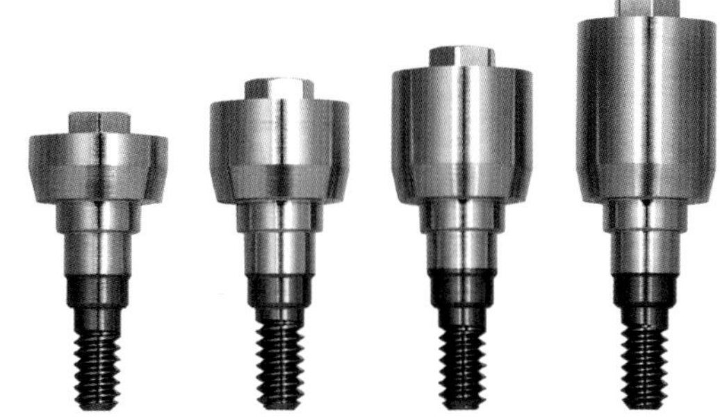

Figure 2.48. Profile view of 4.1 mm diameter OSSEOTITE® Certain® Standard Abutments: IAB200, IAB300, IAB400, IAB550 (2, 3, 4, and 5.5 mm collar heights, left to right).

TABLE 2.15. Standard Abutment Catalogue Numbers for OSSEOTITE® Certain® and OSSEOTITE® Implant Systems

Collar Height (mm)	OSSEOTITE® Certain® Implants	OSSEOTITE® Implants
4.1 mm Implant Restorative Platforms		
2.0	IAB200	AB200
3.0	IAB300	AB300
4.0	IAB400	AB400
5.5	IAB550	AB550
7.0	IAB700	AB700
5.0 mm Implant Restorative Platforms		
2.0	N/A	WAB200
3.0	N/A	WAB300
4.0	N/A	WAB400
5.5	N/A	WAB550

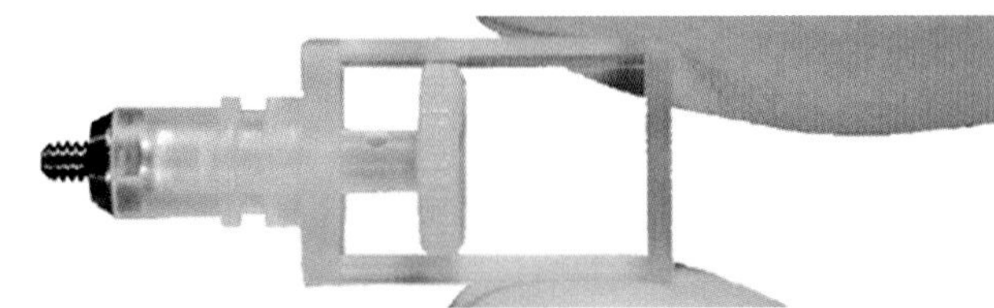

Figure 2.49. Standard Abutments are sold in sterile packages with the ASYST® placement system.

Standard Abutments are manufactured from commercially pure titanium, packaged in sterile containers in a convenient delivery system called ASYST® (Figure 2.49). In clinical use, the abutment screws are generally torqued to 20 Ncm.

LOCATOR® Overdenture Abutments

The LOCATOR® Abutment is ideal for mandibular tissue supported overdentures on two to four implants. These abutments are manufactured from titanium alloy with a gold titanium nitride coating. The housings contained

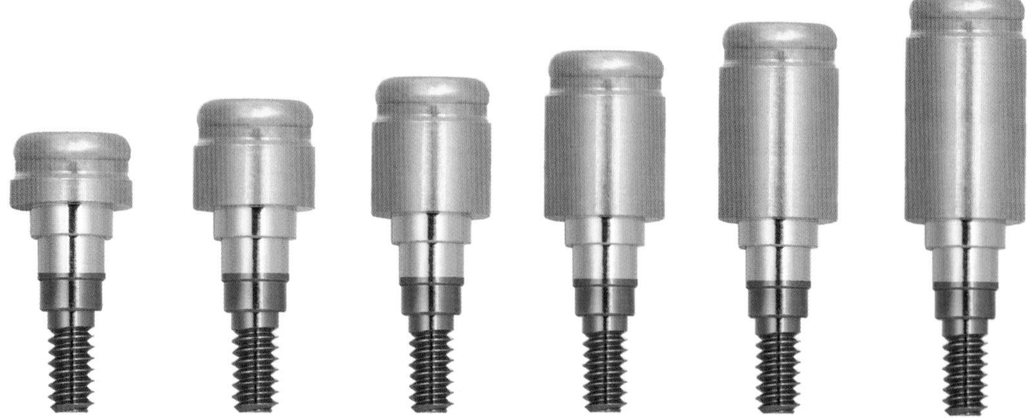

Figure 2.50. Profile view of LOCATOR® Abutments for OSSEOTITE® Certain® implants: ILOA001, ILOA002, ILOA003, ILOA004, ILOA005, ILOA006 (1, 2, 3, 4, 5, and 6 mm collar heights, left to right).

TABLE 2.16. LOCATOR® Abutment Catalogue Numbers for OSSEOTITE® Certain® and OSSEOTITE® Implant Systems

Implant Restorative Platform (mm)	Collar Height (mm)	OSSEOTITE® Certain® Implants	OSSEOTITE® Implants
4.1	1.0	ILOA001	LOA001
4.1	2.0	ILOA002	LOA002
4.1	3.0	ILOA003	LOA003
4.1	4.0	ILOA004	LOA004
4.1	5.0	ILOA005	LOA005
4.1	6.0	ILOA006	LOA006

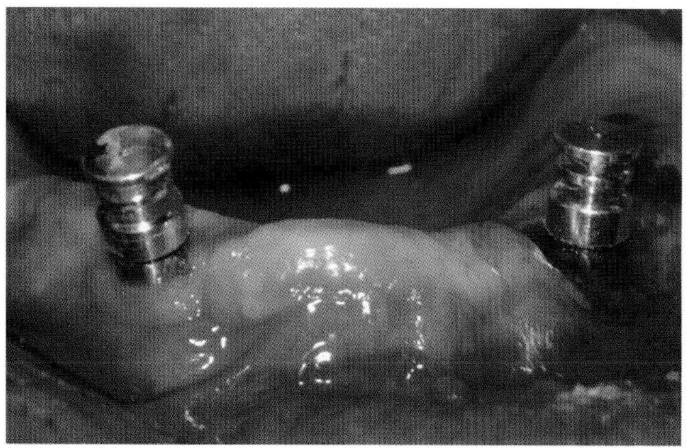

Figure 2.51. Clinical view of two implants with LOCATOR® Abutment Impression Copings (LAIC1) in place. The implants diverge from each other by approximately 25° but were viable for use as overdenture abutments.

within the denture base are made from stainless steel. They are available in multiple collar heights (Figure 2.50), and the smallest LOCATOR® Abutment (ILOA001) is only 3.17 mm in total height (Figure 2.50) (Table 2.16).

It has been the author's experience that patients have demonstrated that they are better able to seat LOCATOR® Abutments than other overdenture abutments even with divergent implant placement. These abutments can be used with nonparallel implant placement of up to 40° (Figure 2.51).

Immediate Occlusal Loading® (IOL®) Abutments

IOL® Abutments are available for 4.1 mm diameter OSSEOTITE® Certain® (one-piece non-hexed) and OSSEOTITE® (two-piece non-hexed) implant systems (Table 2.17). They are manufactured from titanium alloy

TABLE 2.17. Catalogue Numbers for IOL® Abutments for OSSEOTITE® Certain® and OSSEOTITE® Implant Systems

Implant Restorative Platform (mm)	Emergence Profile (mm)	Collar Height (mm)	OSSEOTITE® Certain® Implants	OSSEOTITE® Implants
4.1	4.5	2.0	IIOL20S	IOL20T
4.1	4.5	3.0	IIOL30S	IOL30T
4.1	4.5	4.0	IIOL40S	IOL40T
4.1	4.5	5.5	IIOL55S	IOL55T
4.1	4.5	7.0	IIOL70S	IOL70T

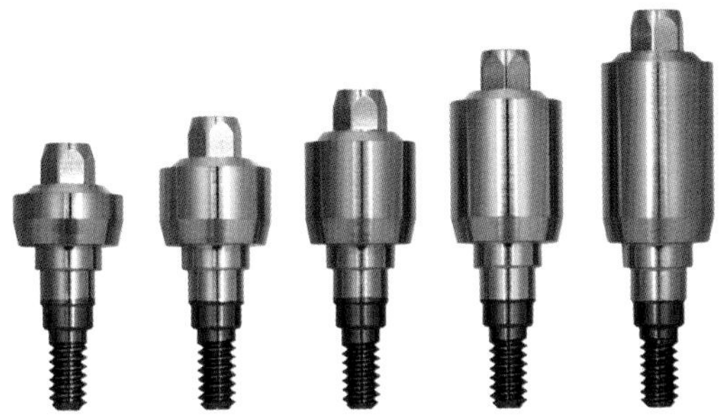

Figure 2.52. IOL® Abutments for OSSEOTITE® Certain® implants: 2, 3, 4, 5.5, and 7 mm collar heights (left to right).

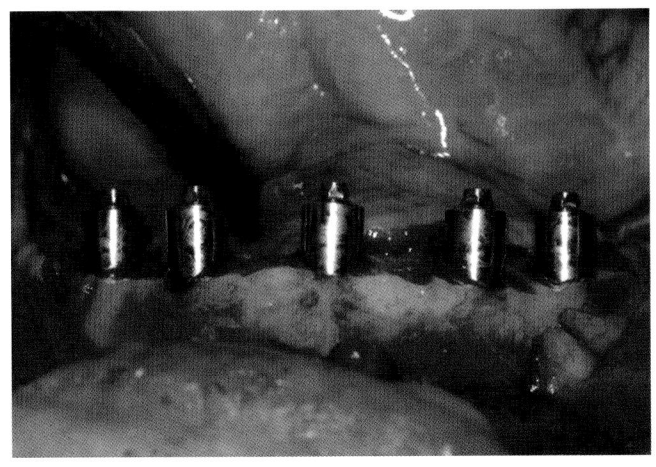

Figure 2.53. Clinical view of 5 IOL® Abutments (IIOL30) in place at the time of implant surgery.

(Figures 2.52, 2.53). Although these components have been specifically designed for use in Immediate Occlusal Loading®, they may also be used as abutments in the traditional, two-stage, unloaded healing protocol.

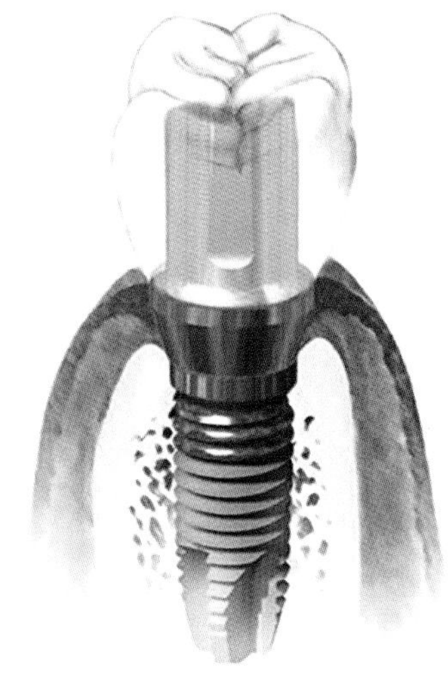

Figure 2.54. Simulation of a GingiHue® Post in place with transparent cement-retained crown for a natural looking, functional restoration.

GingiHue® Posts

3i®'s pre-machined titanium abutments (GingiHue® Posts) have proven to be a versatile, cost-effective addition to the implant restorative dentistry armamentarium. In many cases, they may be used in lieu of custom abutments (Figure 2.54). They have been designed in accordance with the EP® System for natural emergence through the peri-implant soft tissues (5, 6, and 7.5 mm diameters, 2 and 4

TABLE 2.18. Catalogue Numbers for GingiHue® Posts for OSSEOTITE® Certain® and OSSEOTITE® Implant Systems

Seating Surface (mm)	Emergence Profile (mm)	Collar Height (mm)	OSSEOTITE® Certain® Implants-Straight	OSSEOTITE® Certain® Implants-15° Pre-Angled
3.4	3.8	2.0	IMAP32G	IMPAP32G
3.4	3.8	4.0	IMAP34G	IMPAP34G
4.1	5.0	2.0	IAPP452G	IPAP452G
4.1	5.0	4.0	IAPP454G	IPAP454G
4.1	6.0	2.0	IAPP462G	IPAP462G
4.1	6.0	4.0	IAPP464G	IPAP464G
4.1	7.5	2.0	IAPP472G	IPAP472G
4.1	7.5	4.0	IAPP474G	IPAP474G
5.0	5.0	2.0	IWPP552G	IPAP552G
5.0	5.0	4.0	IWPP554G	IPAP554G
5.0	6.0	2.0	IWPP562G	IPAP562G
5.0	6.0	4.0	IWPP564G	IPAP564G
5.0	7.5	2.0	IWPP572G	IPAP572G
5.0	7.5	4.0	IWPP574G	IPAP574G
6.0	6.0	2.0	IWPP662G	IPAP662G
6.0	6.0	4.0	IWPP664G	IPAP664G
6.0	7.5	2.0	IWPP672G	IPAP672G
6.0	7.5	4.0	IWPP674G	IPAP674G
3.4	3.8	2.0	MAP32G	MPAP32G
3.4	3.8	4.0	MAP34G	MPAP34G
4.1	5.0	2.0	APP452G	PAP452G
4.1	5.0	4.0	APP454G	PAP454G
4.1	6.0	2.0	APP462G	PAP462G
4.1	6.0	4.0	APP464G	PAP464G
4.1	7.5	2.0	APP472G	PAP472G
4.1	7.5	4.0	APP474G	PAP474G
5.0	5.0	2.0	WPP552G	PAP552G
5.0	5.0	4.0	WPP554G	PAP554G
5.0	6.0	2.0	WPP562G	PAP562G
5.0	6.0	4.0	WPP564G	PAP564G
5.0	7.5	2.0	WPP572G	PAP572G
5.0	7.5	4.0	WPP574G	PAP574G
6.0	6.0	2.0	WPP662G	PAP662G
6.0	6.0	4.0	WPP664G	PAP664G
6.0	7.5	2.0	WPP672G	PAP672G
6.0	7.5	4.0	WPP674G	PAP674G

mm collar heights) (Table 2.18) (Figure 2.55). They can be prepared intra-orally or in the laboratory on a master cast (Drago 2002) (Figures 2.56, 2.57, 2.58).

ZiReal™ Posts

3i®'s ceramic abutments (ZiReal™ Posts) are indicated in areas where aesthetics is of paramount importance. Metal abutments may cause a gray hue to show through thin, translucent peri-implant soft tissues (Figure 2.59). This coloration may have a negative impact on the overall aesthetic outcome of the implant restoration.

ZiReal™ Posts are manufactured from tetragonal zirconia polycrystals (TZP) that have been extensively used in artificial hip replacements. This material is a combination of zirconia dioxide (ZrO_2) and yttrium-stabilized zirconium oxide (95% and 5%, respectively). These abutments have a flexural strength of more than 900 Mpa. Aluminum oxide (Al_2O_3), used in other commercially available ceramic

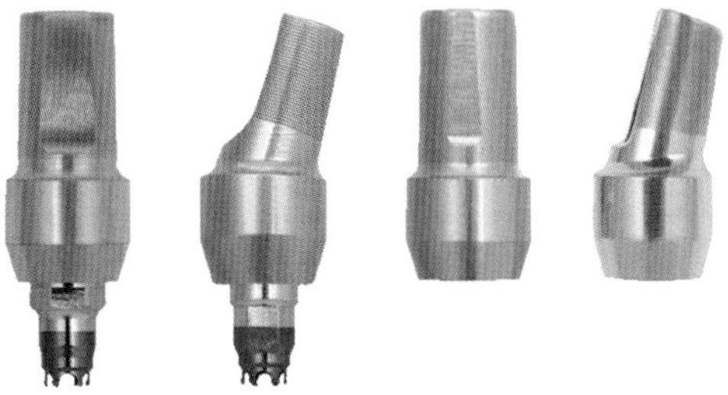

Figure 2.55. GingiHue® Posts (left to right, IAPP454G, IPAP454G, APP454G, PAP454G) for 4.1mm OSSEOTITE® Certain® implants (left) and OSSEOTITE® implants (right).

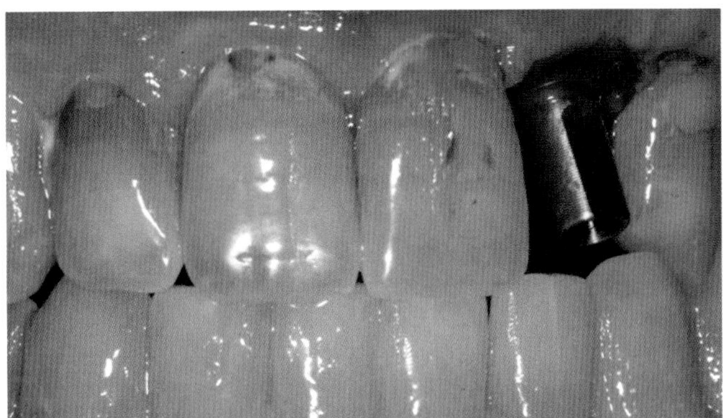

Figure 2.56. Clinical view of GingiHue® Post (IAPP454G) in place at the time an implant was uncovered in the maxillary left lateral incisor location. The flat surface of the abutment was placed on the facial surface.

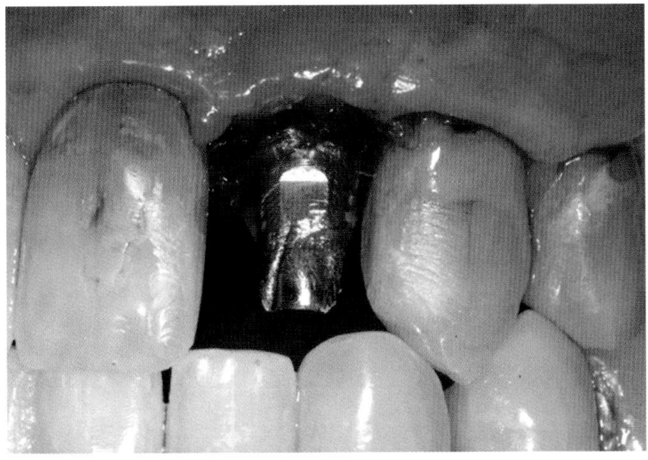

Figure 2.57. Clinical view of GingiHue® Post in Figure 2.56 after it was prepared, prior to fabrication of the provisional crown. It was screwed into the implant with an abutment screw (IUNIHG) torqued to 20 Ncm.

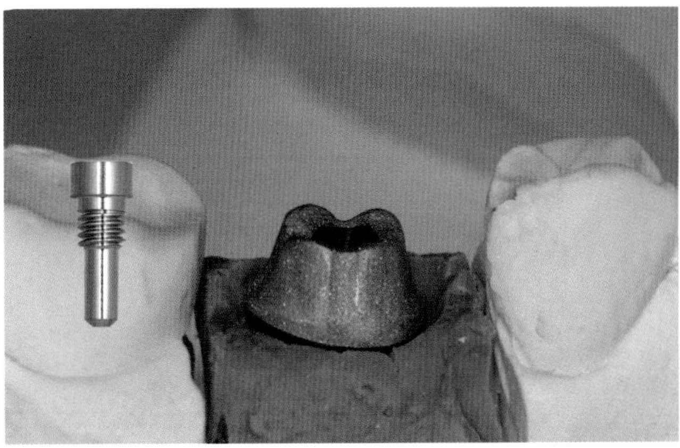

Figure 2.58. Laboratory view of GingiHue® Post (IWPP574G) in place on a master cast in the area of a mandibular right first molar. A dental laboratory technician prepared the abutment on the master cast. The porcelain fused to metal crown was fabricated directly on the abutment. A laboratory try-in screw (IUNIHT) was used during these procedures (inset).

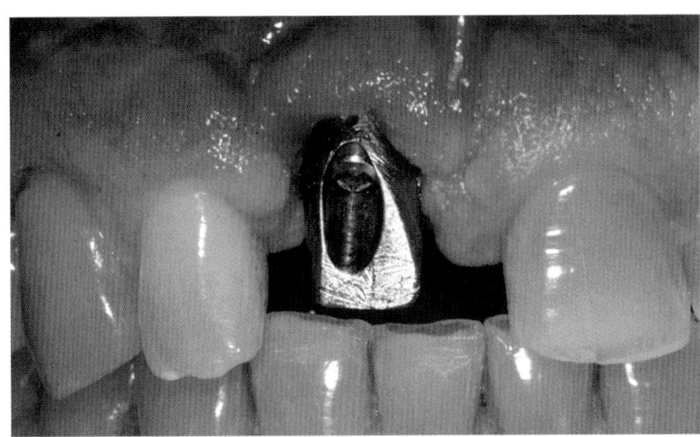

Figure 2.59. Clinical view of titanium abutment in place in maxillary right central incisor site. Note the gray metallic appearance of the distal facial gingival margin.

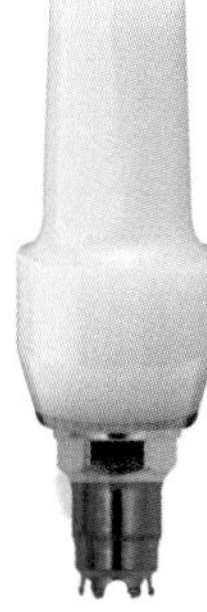

Figure 2.60. ZiReal™ Post demonstrating the titanium cylinder and the zirconia abutment. The height of the cylinder inside the abutment is 1.25 mm. The height of the exposed collar is 0.25 mm.

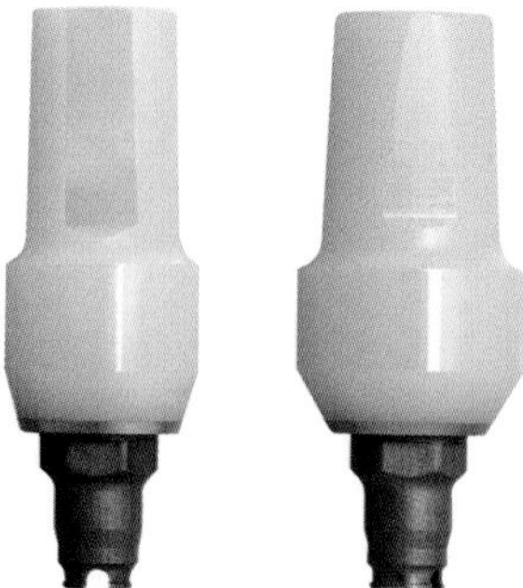

Figure 2.61. ZiReal™ Posts (ICAP454, ICAP464) for 4.1mm OSSEOTITE® Certain® implants (5 and 6 mm EP® diameters).

abutments, has a flexural strength of 500 Mpa (Seghi and Sorenson 1995).

ZiReal™ Posts are unique in that the TZP has been fused with a titanium cylinder (1.25 mm height) that permits a precise metal-to-metal interface between these ceramic abutments and implant restorative platforms. The height of the clinical metal collar is 0.25 mm (Figure 2.60). All-ceramic abutment/implant connections do not have the same high degree of precision that has been reported for metal abutments (Brodbeck 2003).

ZiReal™ Posts have been manufactured for internal and external implant/abutment connections for 4.1 and 5.0 mm implant restorative platforms using the parameters of the EP® System (5, 6, and 7.5 mm EP® diameters) (Figure 2.61) (Table 2.19). They can be used for both single- and multi-unit ceramic restorations with a minimum inter arch space of 6 mm. The maximum angle correction that can be obtained with these abutments is 10°. The axial wall minimum thickness after abutment preparation is 0.3 mm. ZiReal™ Posts may be prepared intra-orally or they may be prepared in the laboratory on a master cast (Bonilla and Sullivan 2003; Drago 2003) (Figures 2.62, 2.63).

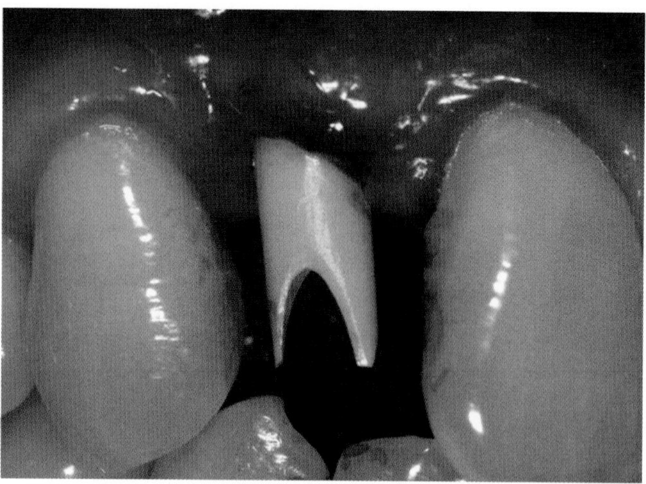

Figure 2.62. Clinical view of ZiReal™ Post (ICAP454) that was prepared intra-orally in the maxillary right lateral incisor site.

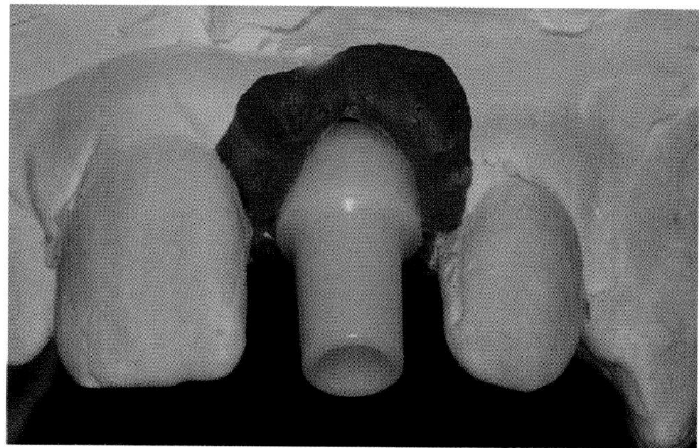

Figure 2.63. Laboratory view of ZiReal™ Post as received from the manufacturer in place for a maxillary left central incisor (IWCAP564). Note the flat side of the abutment (for anti-rotation of the cemented crown) has been placed on the palatal surface and is not visible in this view.

Provide™ Abutments

3i® recently introduced a new abutment: The Provide™ Abutment (Figure 2.64). This abutment provides the implant team with more options and therefore greater flexibility in meeting aesthetic and functional demands of patients with stock, noncustom implant restorative components. Provide™ Abutments give restorative dentists and implant surgeons four different collar heights (1-4 mm) and two different post heights (4.0 and 5.5 mm).

TABLE 2.19. Catalogue Numbers for ZiReal™ Posts for OSSEOTITE® Certain® and OSSEOTITE® Implant Systems

Implant Restorative Platform (mm)	Emergence Profile (mm)	Collar Height (mm)	OSSEOTITE® Certain® Implants	OSSEOTITE® Implants
4.1	5.0	4.0	ICAP454	CAP454
4.1	6.0	4.0	ICAP464	CAP464
5.0	6.0	4.0	IWCAP564	WCAP564
5.0	7.5	4.0	IWCAP574	WCAP574

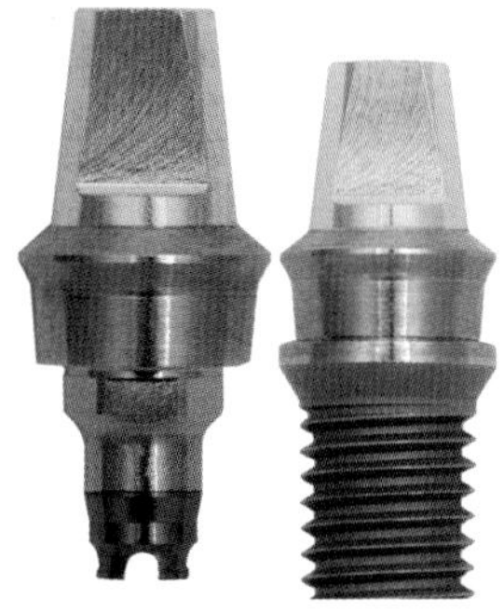

Figure 2.64. Product view of two Provide™ Abutments (IPA4155, IPA4140, left to right).

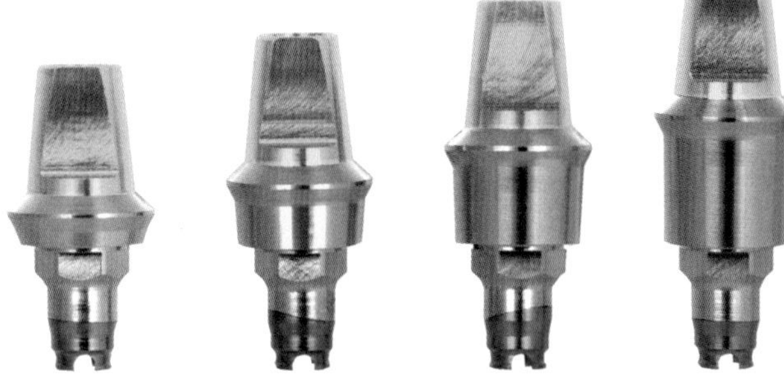

Figure 2.65. Provide™ Abutments 1–4 mm collar height, left to right (IPA4140, IPA4240, IPA4340, IPA4440, left to right).

TABLE 2.20. Catalogue Numbers for the Provide™ Abutment for the OSSEOTITE® Certain® Implant System

Implant Restorative Platform (mm)	Collar Height (mm)	Post Height (mm)	Emergence Profile (mm)	Catalogue Number
4.1	1.0	4.0	4.8	IPA4140
4.1	2.0	4.0	4.8	IPA4240
4.1	3.0	4.0	4.8	IPA4340
4.1	4.0	4.0	4.8	IPA4440
4.1	1.0	5.5	4.8	IPA4155
4.1	2.0	5.5	4.8	IPA4255
4.1	3.0	5.5	4.8	IPA4355
4.1	4.0	5.5	4.8	IPA4455
5.0	1.0	4.0	6.5	IPA5140
5.0	2.0	4.0	6.5	IPA5240
5.0	3.0	4.0	6.5	IPA5340
5.0	4.0	4.0	6.5	IPA5440
5.0	1.0	5.5	6.5	IPA5155
5.0	2.0	5.5	6.5	IPA5255
5.0	3.0	5.5	6.5	IPA5355
5.0	4.0	5.5	6.5	IPA5455
6.0	1.0	4.0	6.5	IPA6140
6.0	2.0	4.0	6.5	IPA6240
6.0	3.0	4.0	6.5	IPA6340
6.0	4.0	4.0	6.5	IPA6440
6.0	1.0	5.5	6.5	IPA6155
6.0	2.0	5.5	6.5	IPA6255
6.0	3.0	5.5	6.5	IPA6355
6.0	4.0	5.5	6.5	IPA6455

Implant surgeons will not need to determine the height of stock abutments at the time of implant placement because this abutment is available in 1, 2, 3, and 4 mm heights (Figure 2.65). OSSEOTITE® Certain® implants can be placed with either single- or two-stage surgical protocols. Abutment selection can be deferred until the tissues have matured, or it can be made at the time of implant placement with the potential of changing the abutment collar height relative to the height of the gingival margins (Table 2.20).

The Provide™ Restorative System provides clinicians with color-coded restorative components within the OSSEOTITE® Certain® Implant System. These abutments are not available in the external hex OSSEOTITE® implant system. These abutments may be used with implant level impressions and prepared in the laboratory. The abutments may also be used with a direct technique and prepared intra-orally. The latter protocol will simplify the restorative procedures by eliminating implant level impressions.

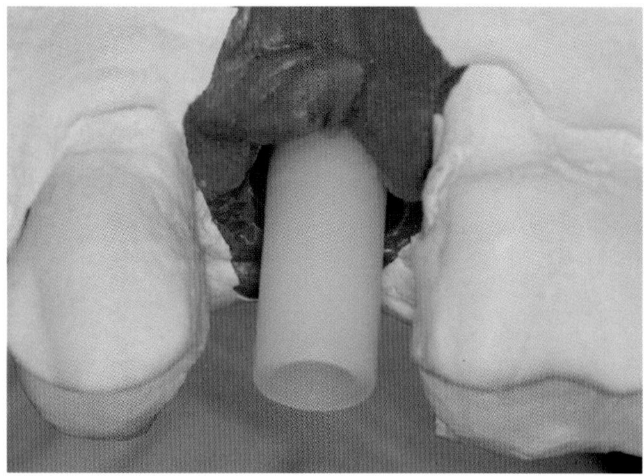

Figure 2.66. Laboratory facial view of UCLA Abutment (IGUCA1C) in place as received from the manufacturer. The titanium cylinder has a precise metal-to-metal fit at the implant/abutment interface.

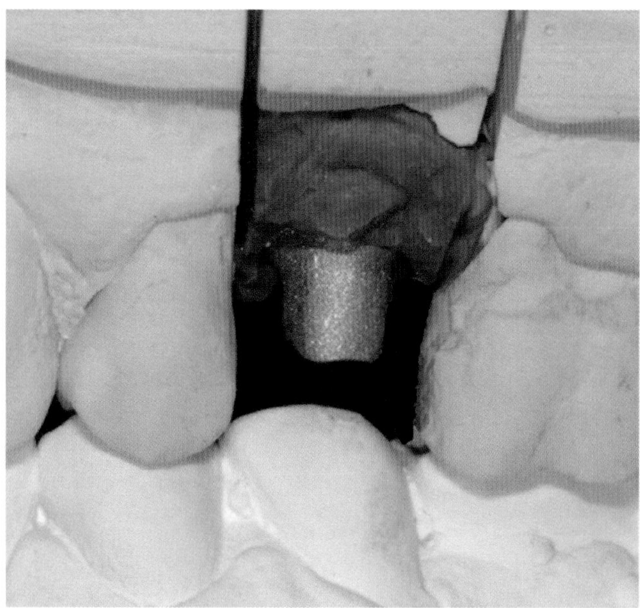

Figure 2.67. This UCLA Abutment was adjusted, waxed, and cast with a noble alloy into the shape of an abutment for a cement-retained crown.

UCLA Abutments

The UCLA Abutment was developed to allow a direct connection between the implant and the implant restoration. These abutments can be used for single- and multiple-unit restorations with a minimum inter-occlusal clearance of 4 mm. They can be used as abutments for cement-retained crowns (Figures 2.66, 2.67, 2.68), as well as one-piece implant restorations screwed directly into implants (Figures 2.69, 2.70, 2.71, 2.72) (Table 2.21).

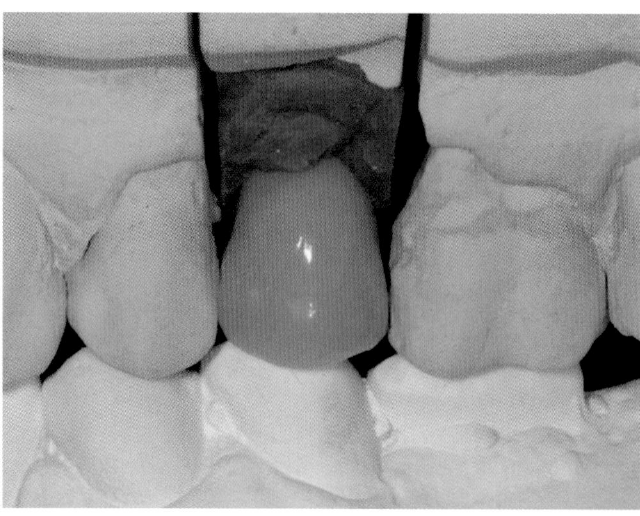

Figure 2.68. Porcelain fused to metal crown and custom UCLA Abutment in place on master cast.

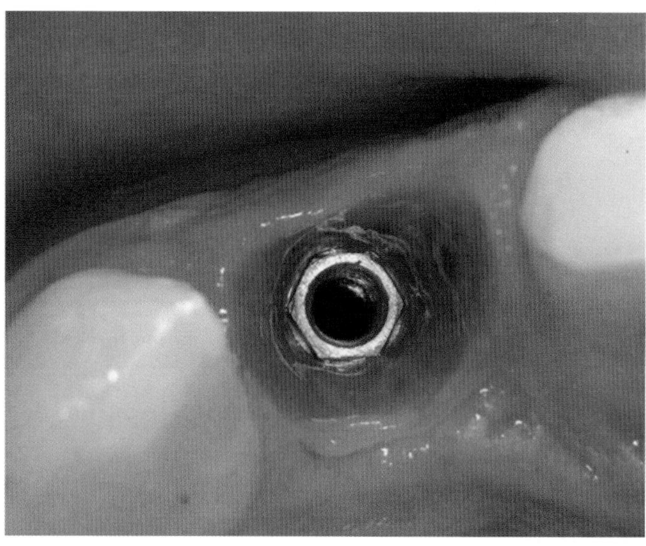

Figure 2.69. Clinical occlusal view of external hex implant 10 years after UCLA Abutment (GUCA1C) was cast as a single-unit, screw-retained implant restoration. The original abutment screw was loose for several months prior to this photograph. Note the redness of the peri-implant sulcular tissues.

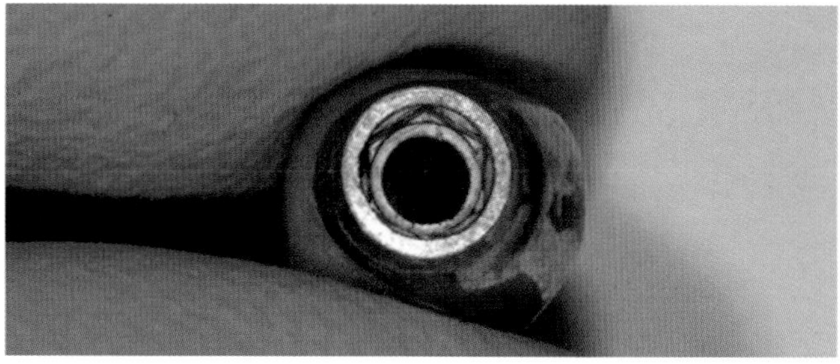

Figure 2.70. Laboratory view of abutment hex from the screw-retained crown in Figure 2.69.

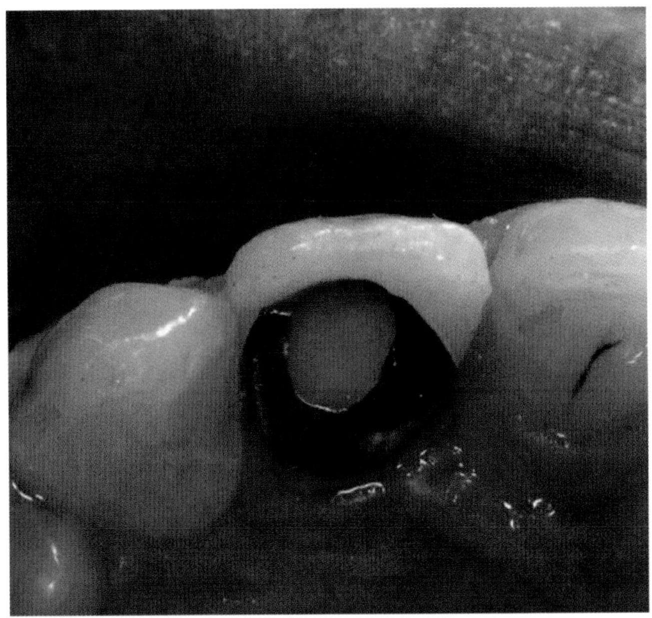

Figure 2.71. Clinical occlusal view of screw access opening on the palatal surface of the implant crown restoration in Figures 2.69 and 2.70. Note the size of the opening that was required to accommodate the head of the abutment screw. The access opening was restored with composite resin.

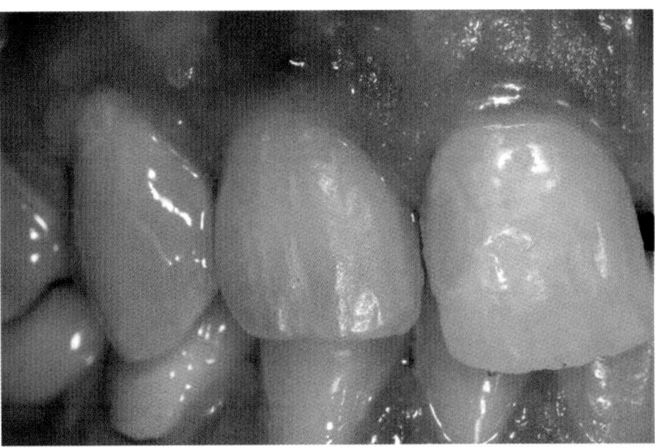

Figure 2.72. Clinical facial view of screw-retained crown replacing the maxillary right lateral incisor. Screw-retained crowns in the aesthetic zone require implant placement that have screw access openings within the palatal surfaces of maxillary restorations.

TABLE 2.21. Catalogue for UCLA Abutments for OSSEOTITE® Certain® and OSSEOTITE® Implant Systems

Implant Restorative Platform (mm)	OSSEOTITE® Certain® Implants	OSSEOTITE® Implants
3.4		
Gold (Hexed)	IMUCG1C	MUCG1C
Gold (Non-Hexed)	NA	NA
4.1		
Gold (Hexed)	IGUCA1C	GUCA1C
Gold (Non-Hexed)	IGUCA2C (includes large diameter Gold-Tite™ Screw)	GUCA2C
Gold (Non-hexed)	IGUCA2T (includes large diameter Ti Screw)	NA
Gold Standard ZR™ (Hexed)	NA	SGUCA1C
5.0		
Gold (Hexed)	IWGA51C	NA
Gold (Non-Hexed)	IWGA52C (includes large diameter Gold-Tite™ Screw)	WGA52C
Gold (Non-Hexed)	IWGA52T (includes large diameter Ti Screw)	NA
Gold Standard ZR™ (Hexed)	NA	SWGA51C
6.0		
Gold (Hexed)	IWGA61C	WGA61C
Gold (Non-Hexed)	IWGA62C (includes large diameter Gold-Tite™ Screw)	WGA62C
Gold (Non-Hexed)	IWGA62T (includes large diameter Ti Screw)	NA
Gold Standard ZR™ (Hexed)	NA	SWGA61C

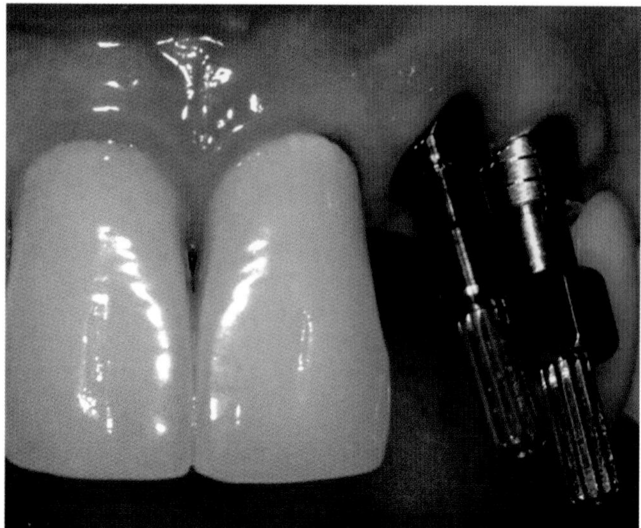

Figure 2.73. Clinical view of implants with impression copings in place replacing the maxillary left lateral incisor and cuspid. Note the facial angulation of the implant impression copings. If the restorations were to be screw-retained, the screw access openings would be in the middle portions of the facial surfaces of the restorations.

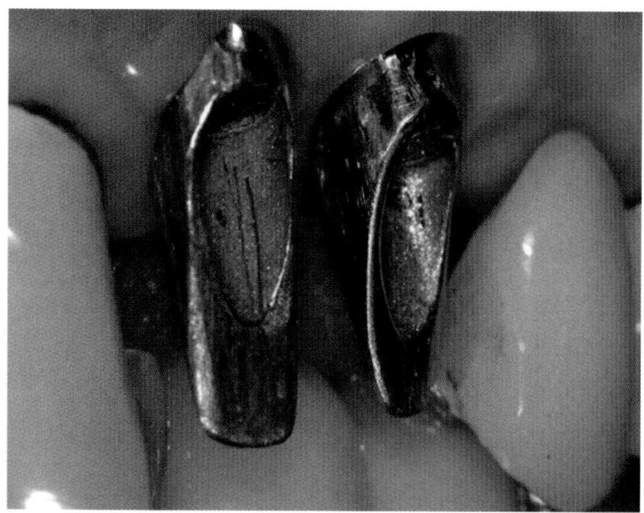

Figure 2.74. Clinical view of custom UCLA Abutments featured in Figure 2.73 in place. Due to amount of inter-occlusal clearance and the 6° axial taper, the nonfacial axial walls provided adequate surface area for satisfactory retention and resistance form for the individual cement-retained restorations.

UCLA Abutments have been manufactured with machined gold palladium cylinders and plastic unitubes. These abutments may be waxed and cast as custom abutments. The heights of the unitubes may be modified depending upon the available inter-occlusal clearance. This allows dental laboratory technicians to correct misaligned implants with up to 30° divergence (Figures 2.73, 2.74). UCLA Abutments are available in hexed and non-hexed configurations (Figure 2.75).

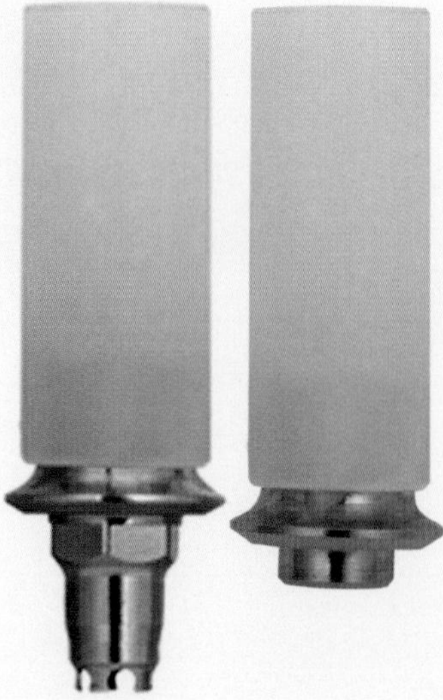

Figure 2.75. Hexed and nonhexed UCLA Abutments (IGUCA1C, IGUCA2C, respectively) for 4.1 mm diameter OSSEOTITE® Certain® Implant System.

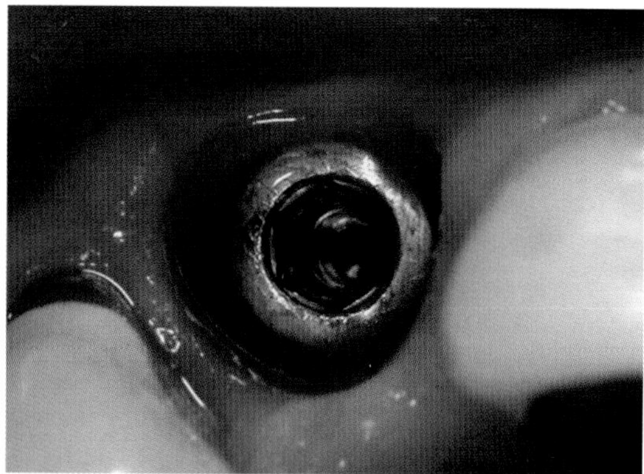

Figure 2.76. Clinical occlusal view of 5.0 mm implant restorative platform in maxillary right cuspid site. The emergence profile of the peri-implant soft tissues was created with a custom provisional implant restoration.

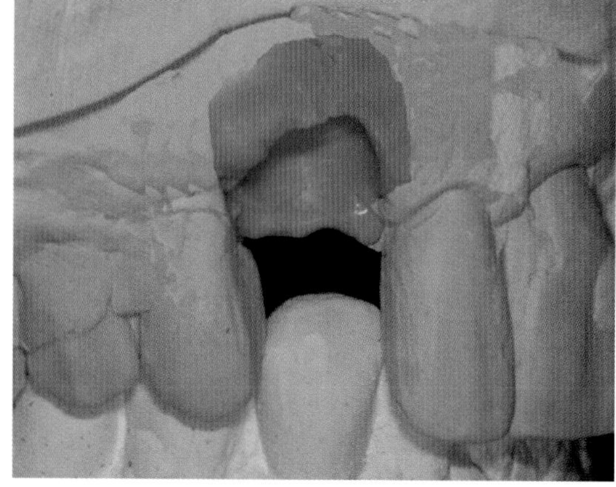

Figure 2.77. Master cast from the impression in Figure 2.76 was mounted against a mandibular cast. The emergence profile was captured in the definitive implant level impression and replicated in poly vinylsiloxane impression material.

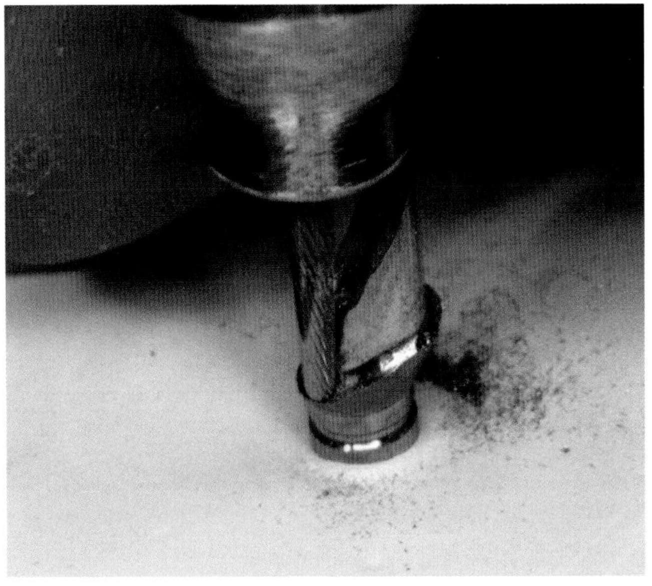

Figure 2.78. A custom UCLA Abutment was developed in wax and cast in a noble alloy. It was milled on a surveyor for minimal axial wall taper. The sub-gingival portions were waxed to fit into the peri-implant space around the implant analog.

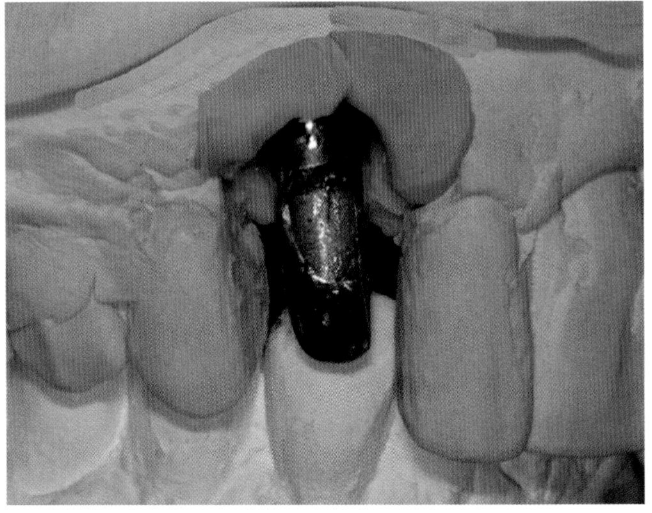

Figure 2.79. Custom cast UCLA abutment in place on master cast. The emergence profiles were originally developed clinically with the provisional restoration. The dental laboratory technician followed these contours to establish optimal anatomic form in the custom abutment.

UCLA Abutments are ideal for use in situations when space is limited and stock, pre-machined abutments will not satisfy aesthetic or functional demands (Lazzara, 1993). These abutments require implant level impressions to develop master casts with implant analogs (Figure 2.76, 2.77). Custom abutments may be fabricated by casting to the UCLA Abutments as received from the manufacturer and milling procedures performed as required by the clinical situations (Figures 2.78, 2.79). Definitive implant crown restorations can be made directly on the custom abutments. The emergence profiles have already been established clinically and this information transferred to the master cast with the implant level impression. The net result is an implant-retained crown with anatomic contours that replicate the contours established by the provisional restoration (Figure 2.80).

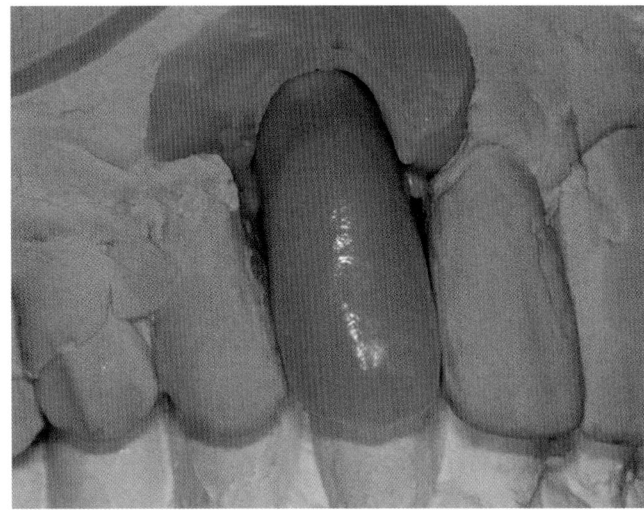

Figure 2.80. A porcelain fused to metal crown was fabricated that replicated the emergence profile of the peri-implant tissues developed with the provisional restoration. The dental laboratory technician was able to follow the contours that were in the master cast to fabricate a crown whose contours had already been determined clinically.

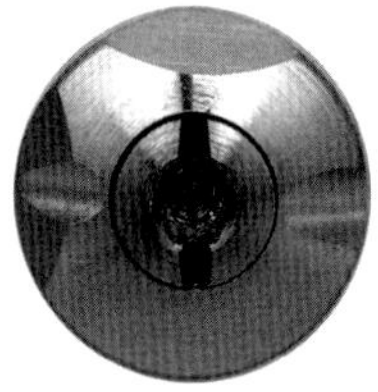

Figure 2.81. Occlusal view of Encode™ Healing abutment (EHA554). Codes have been embedded into the occlusal surfaces that identify the size and location of the implant restorative platform, implant/abutment connection, emergence profile, and height of the healing abutment.

CAD/CAM Abutments (Encode™ Abutments)

Encode™ Healing Abutments have been manufactured with codes embedded into their occlusal surfaces (Figure 2.81). These codes provide the required information for optical scanning and construction of definitive abutments produced with computer-assisted design and computer-assisted milling.

Protocols have been established for fabrication of Encode™ Abutments. In principle, an implant level impression of some type is needed to transfer the position of the implant restorative platform to a cast for fabrication of the

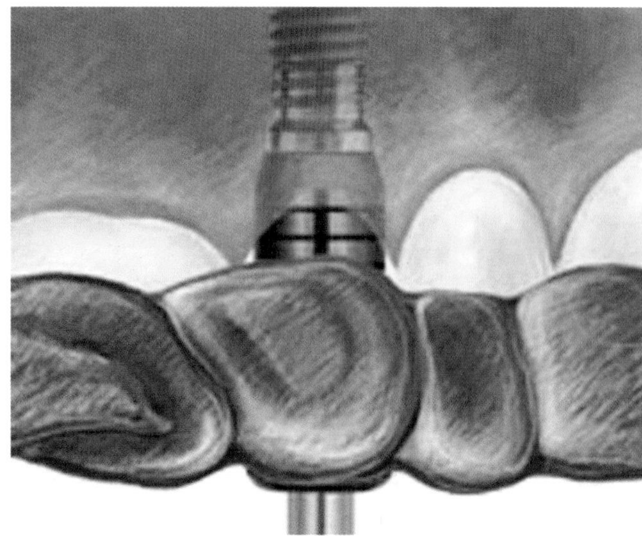

Figure 2.82. Illustration of surgical index: the surgeon, prior to closure of the wound, placed a pick-up implant level impression coping. An index was made that oriented the impression coping to the anatomical contours of the adjacent teeth.

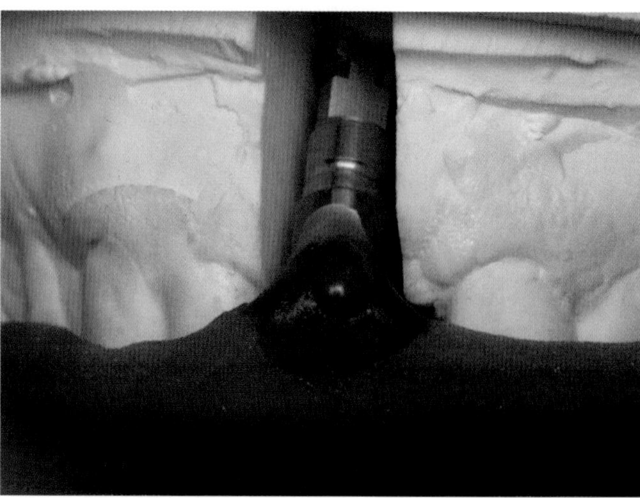

Figure 2.83. Stone was removed from the area corresponding to the implant. An implant analog (ILAW5) was attached to the implant impression coping (WIP55) and the index was refitted to the occlusal surfaces of the adjacent teeth.

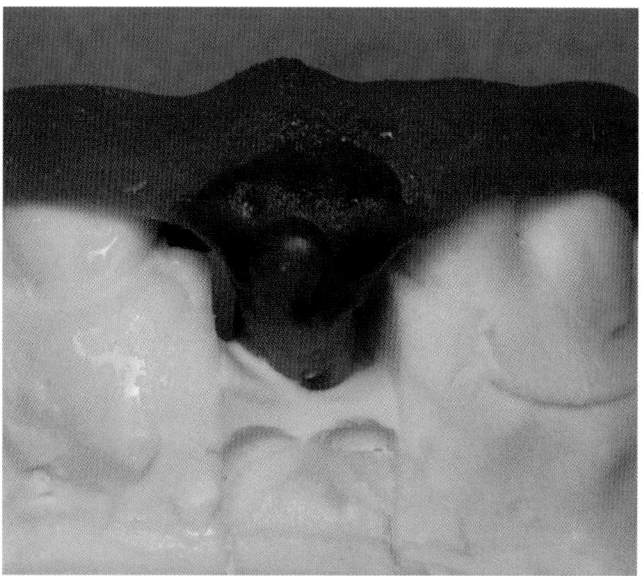

Figure 2.84. The implant analog transferred the precise location of the implant to the diagnostic cast via the surgical index. The gingival margins were not recorded because the wound was not closed at the time the index was made.

crown restoration. This impression may be a surgical index at the time of implant placement (Figure 2.82). Dental stone will then be removed from the cast in the area of the implant; an implant analog will be attached to the impression coping in the index (Figure 2.83) and the analog will be retrofitted to the cast by injecting dental stone into the void around the analog (Figure 2.84).

After osseointegration occurred, a poly vinylsiloxane impression was made of the Encode™ Healing Abutment (Figure 2.85) and the impression was poured in die stone (Fujirock® EP, GC Europe, Leuven, Belgium) (Figure 2.86). This cast was mounted on an articulator with magnetic mounting plates and shipped to ***3i®***. A laser optical scanner was used to scan this cast. A dental laboratory techni-

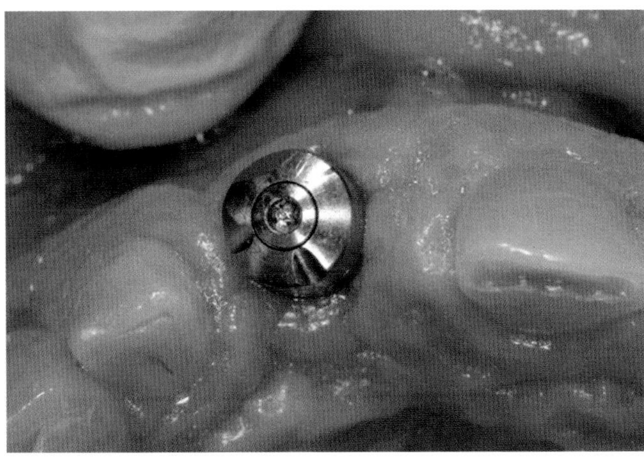

Figure 2.85. Clinical occlusal view of Encode™ Healing Abutment (EHA554) in place.

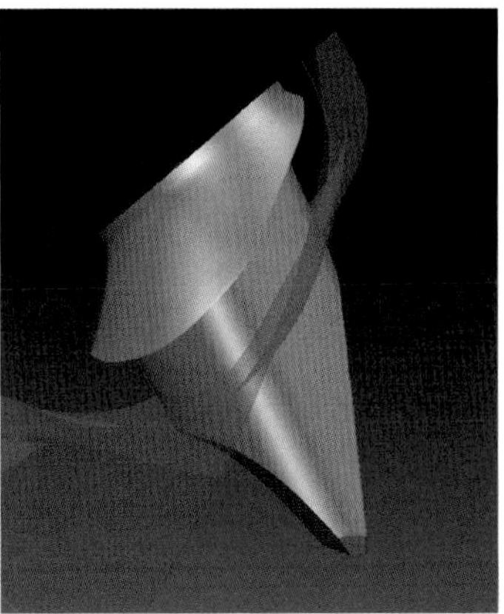

Figure 2.87. Computer-designed, patient-specific abutment in CAD software. The gingival tissues were made translucent to assist in development of the abutment margins.

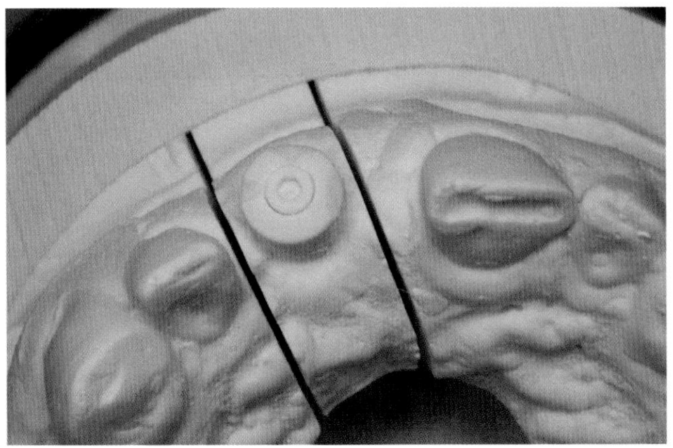

Figure 2.86. Occlusal view of Encode™ Healing Abutment (EHA554) that was replicated in die stone in the master cast.

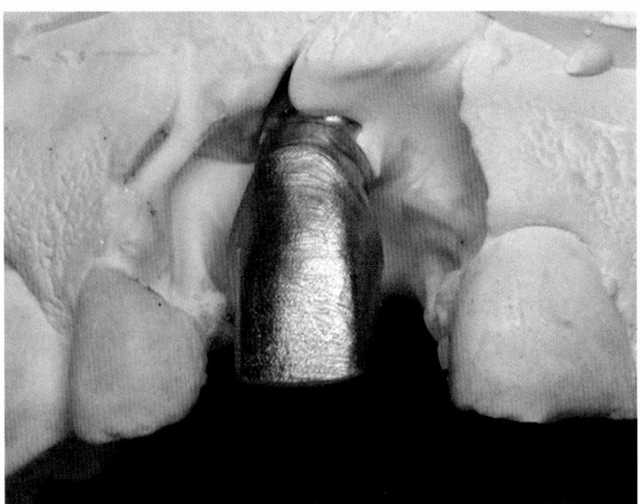

Figure 2.88. Facial laboratory view of cast coping on Final Encode™ Abutment in place on master cast; the soft tissue has been removed from the cast.

cian/computer designer designed the patient specific abutment using a sophisticated software program (Figure 2.87). The Final Encode™ Abutment was milled by a computerized milling machine per the specifications developed in the CAD design (Figure 2.88). The margins were fabricated from the image of the Encode™ Healing Abutment that contained the location of the peri-implant soft tissues. The definitive porcelain fused to metal crown was cemented to the abutment in conventional fashion (Figure 2.89).

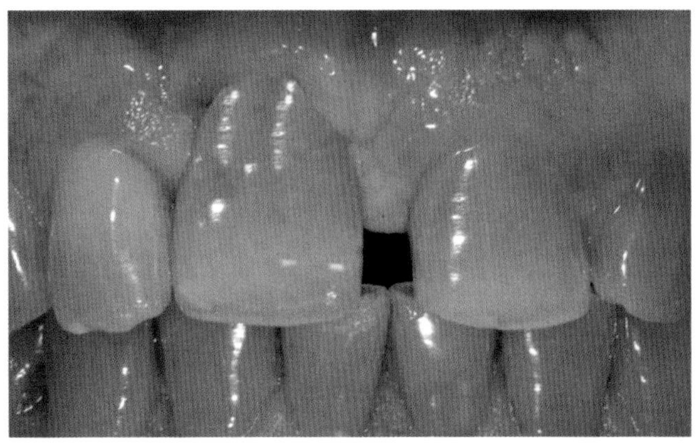

Figure 2.89. Facial clinical view of porcelain fused to metal crown in place on the Final Encode™ Abutment featured in Figure 2.87.

TABLE 2.22. Catalogue Numbers for Abutment Screws for OSSEOTITE® Certain® Implant System

	Gold-Tite™	Titanium	Large Gold-Tite™	Large Titanium
Abutment Screws	IUNIHG	IUNIHT	ILRGHG	ILRGHT
Drivers	PHDO2N, PHDO3N	PHDO2N, PHDO3N	PHDO2N, PHDO3N	PHDO2N, PHDO3N
Driver Tips	RASH3N, RASH8N	RASH3N, RASH8N	RASH3N, RASH8N	RASH3N, RASH8N
Torque	20 Ncm	20 Ncm	20 Ncm	20 Ncm
For Use With	UCLA Abutments, GingiHue® Posts, GingiHue® Posts 15°, Hexed Temporary Cylinders	UCLA Abutments, GingiHue® Posts, GingiHue® Posts 15°, Hexed Temporary Cylinders	Non-Hexed UCLA Abutments, Non-Hexed Temporary Cylinders	Non-Hexed UCLA Abutments, Non-Hexed Temporary Cylinders

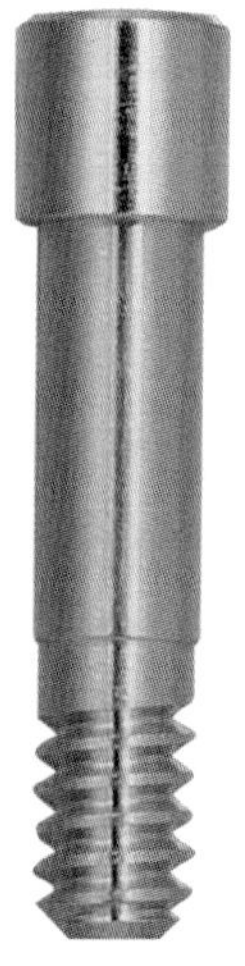

Figure 2.90. Gold-Tite™ Abutment Screw for the OSSEOTITE® Certain® Implant System (IUNIHG).

TABLE 2.23. Catalogue Numbers for Retaining Screws for OSSEOTITE® Certain® Implant System

Screws	GSH20, GSH30
Drivers	PHDO2N, PHDO3N
Driver Tips	RASH3N, RASH8N
Torque	10 Ncm
For Use With	GSH20-Standard Abutment GSH30-Pre-Angled, Standard, conical and TG Hex Abutments

SCREWS (CLINICAL)

Abutment screws have been defined as the screws that connect an abutment to implants (Figure 2.90). Retaining screws have been defined as the screws that retain cylinders to implants (Figure 2.91). In ***3i®***'s implant systems, abutment screws have been designed with slotted, hex, and square heads; retaining screws have been designed with slotted or hex heads. Slotted screws for clinical applications are not illustrated in this text (Tables 2.22, 2.23, 2.24).

3i® has patented a 24-carat-gold, ultra-thin 0.76 μm coating for its abutment and retaining screws called Gold-Tite™. This thin layer of 24-carat gold acts as a dry lubricant that reduces friction and allows approximately 62% more screw-turning during tightening with a given amount of force. This results in increased preloads in the abutment/implant connection and improves the predictability of clinical implant treatment (Figure 2.92).

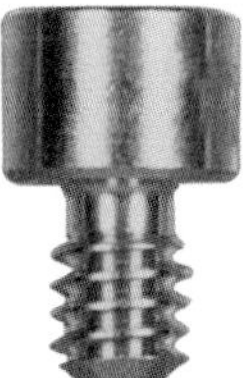

Figure 2.91. Gold-Tite™ retaining screw (GSH30).

TABLE 2.24. Catalogue Numbers for Abutment and Retaining Screws for the OSSEOTITE® Implant System

	Gold-Tite® Square Abutment Screw	**Gold-Tite® Hexed Abutment Screw**	**Titanium Hexed Abutment Screw**	**Gold-Tite® Retaining Screw**
Abutment Screws	UNISG	UNIHG	UNIHT	GSH20, GSH30
Drivers	PSQDON, PSQD1N	PHDO2N, PHDO3N	PHDO2N, PHDO3N	PHDO2N, PHDO3N
Driver Tips	RASQ3N, RASQ8N	RASH3N, RASH8N	RASH3N, RASH8N	RASH3N, RASH8N
Torque	32-35 Ncm	20 Ncm	20 Ncm	10 Ncm
For Use With	UCLA Abutments, GingiHue® Posts, GingiHue® Posts 15°, ZiReal™ Posts, Titanium Cylinders, Pre-Angled Abutments	UCLA Abutments, GingiHue® Posts, GingiHue® Posts 15°, ZiReal™ Posts, Titanium Cylinders, Pre-Angled Abutments	UCLA Abutments, GingiHue® Posts, GingiHue® Posts 15°, ZiReal™ Posts, Titanium Cylinders, Pre-Angled Abutments	GSH20-Standard Abutments, GSH30- Pre-Angled, Standard, Conical and TG Hex Abutments

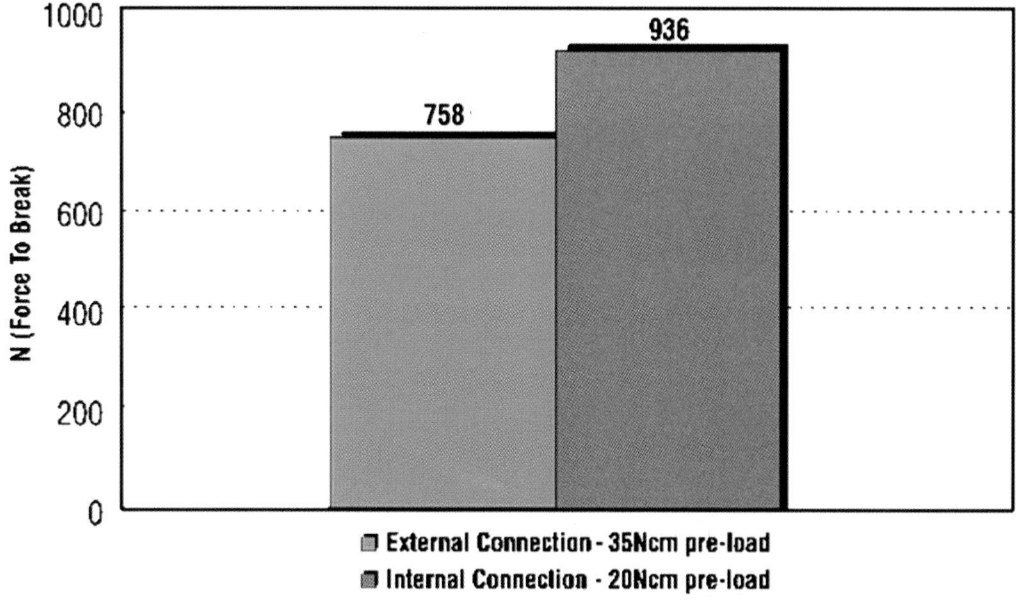

Figure 2.92. Graphic results demonstrating increased preload with applied torque in Gold-Tite™ Abutment Screws.

TABLE 2.25. Catalogue Numbers for *3i*® Gold Cylinders

Implant Restorative Component	Emergence Profile (mm)	4.1 mm Implant Restorative Platform	5.0 mm Implant Restorative Platform
Pick-Up Impression Coping	4.5	SQIC7	SQIC7
Laboratory Analog	4.5	SLA20	SLA20
Gold Cylinder	4.5	SGC30	SGC30
Healing Cap	4.5	TS250	TS250
Retaining Screw	4.5	GSH20, GSH30	GSH20, GSH30

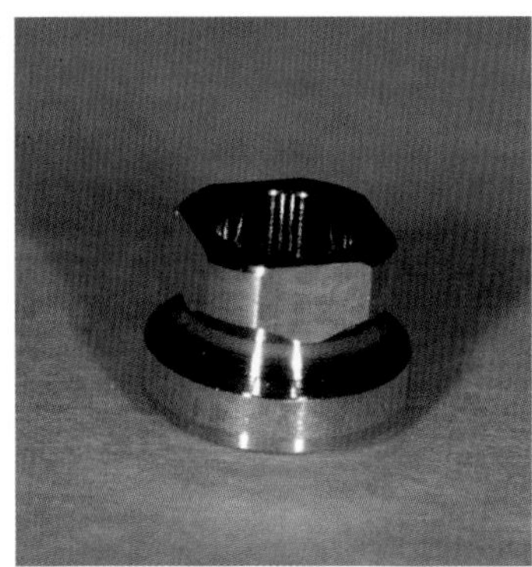

Figure 2.93. Standard Gold Cylinder (SGC30) machined to fit onto standard abutments.

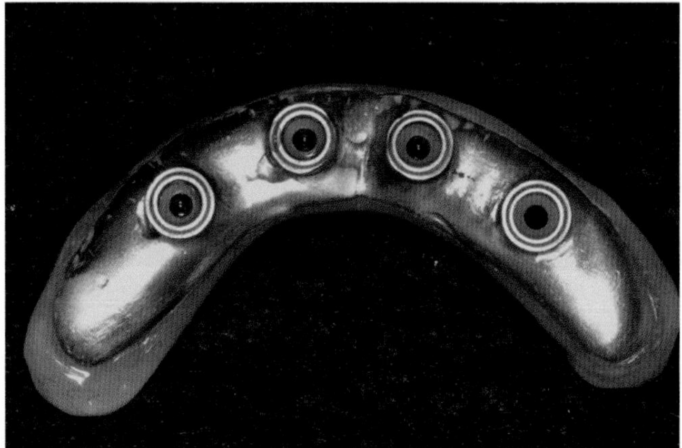

Figure 2.94. The intaglio surface of a cast metal framework for a hybrid prosthesis. The gold cylinders were incorporated into the wax pattern and cast as part of the metal framework. The precise machining was maintained throughout prosthesis fabrication.

TABLE 2.26. Catalogue Numbers for Overdenture and Fixed Hybrid Prostheses

Implant Restorative Platform	4.1 mm	5.0mm
Emergence Profile (mm)	4.5 mm	4.5 mm
Pick-Up Impression Coping	SQIC7	SQIC7
Laboratory Analog	SLA20	SLA20
Polishing Protector	PPSA3	PPSA3
Healing Cap	TS250	TS250
Retaining Screw	GSH20, GSH30	GSH20, GSH30

CYLINDERS

Standard Gold Cylinders

Cylinders (SGC30) are laboratory components that have been machined to fit onto abutments (Figure 2.93)(Table 2.25). They are waxed and cast as part of metal frameworks for implant prostheses (Figure 2.94). Gold cylinders are not generally used for single-unit restorations because optimal emergence profiles cannot be developed with standard abutments. The abutment/cylinder connections are not dependent on the implant/abutment connection type. These components may be used with both internal and external connection implant systems (Table 2.26).

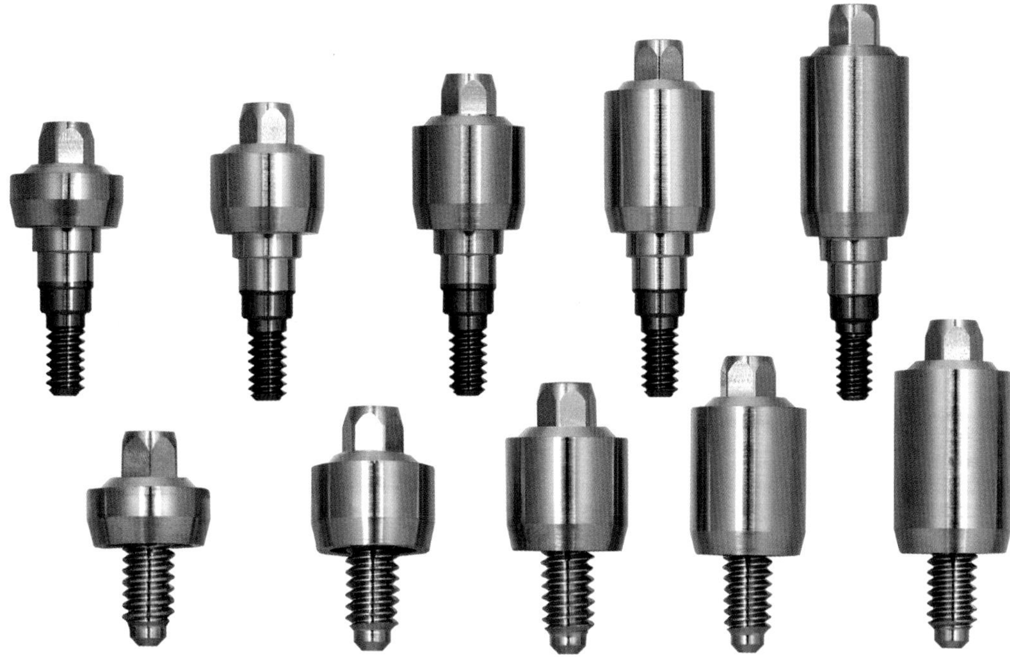

Figure 2.95. IOL® Abutments for the OSSEOTITE® Certain® implant system (top); OSSEOTITE® implant system (bottom): 2, 3, 4, 5.5, and 7 mm collar heights (left to right).

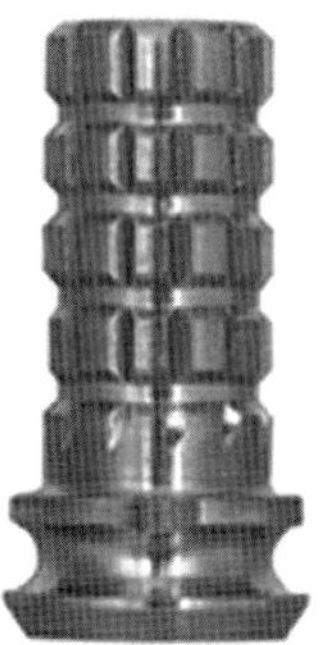
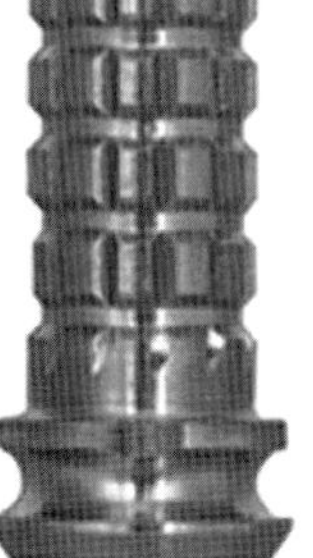

Figure 2.96. IOL® Temporary Cylinder (IOLTC).

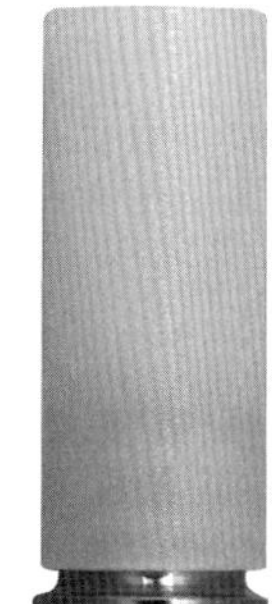

Figure 2.97. IOL® Gold Cylinder (IOLGC).

TABLE 2.27. Catalogue Numbers for Immediate Occlusal Loading® Abutments for 4.1 Implant Restorative Platforms in the OSSEOTITE® Certain® and OSSEOTITE® Implant Systems

Emergence Profile (mm)	Collar Height (mm)	OSSEOTITE® Certain® Implants	OSSEOTITE® Implants
4.5	2.0	IIOL20S	IOL20T
4.5	3.0	IIOL30S	IOL30T
4.5	4.0	IIOL40S	IOL40T
4.5	5.5	IIOL55S	IOL55T
4.5	7.0	IIOL70S	IOL70T

Note: Use PADOO Abutment Driver or RASA3 Driver Tip.

IOL® Abutment Gold Cylinders

IOL® Cylinders were designed specifically for use with Immediate Occlusal Loading® in the edentulous mandible (Figure 2.95). These cylinders are shorter than conical abutments but still provide a positive seating surface for IOL® temporary cylinders and IOL® gold cylinders (Figure 2.96, 2.97). They are manufactured from titanium alloy and are available for both OSSEOTITE® Certain® and OSSEOTITE® Implant Systems (Table 2.27).

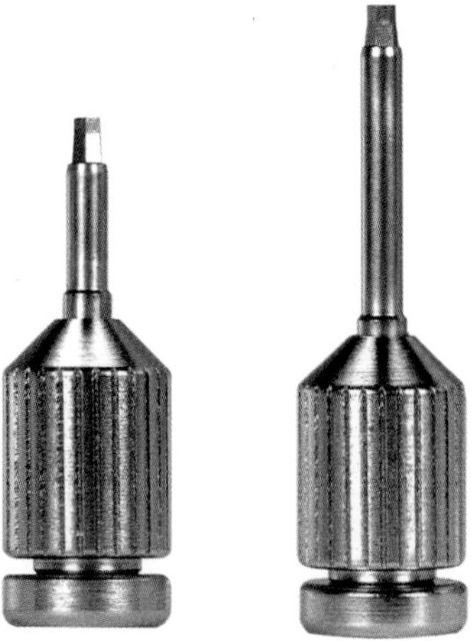

Figure 2.98. Large hex drivers (PHD02N, 17 mm length, left; PHD03N 24 mm length, right).

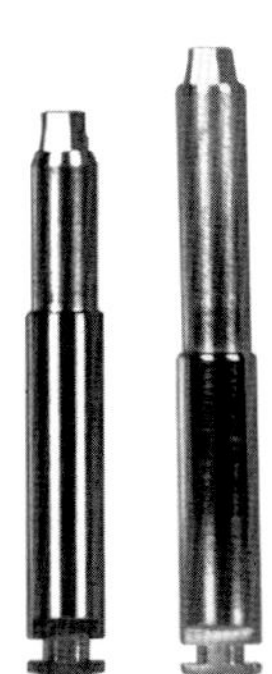

Figure 2.99. Contra-angle driver tips for large hex screws (RASH3N, 24 mm length, left; RASH8N, 30 mm length, right).

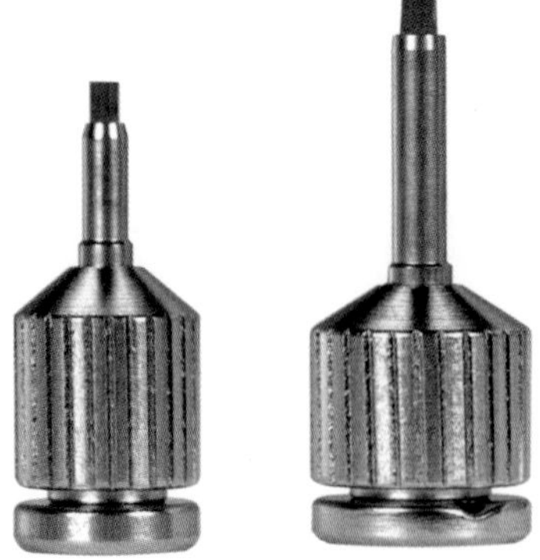

Figure 2.100. Square drivers (PSQD0N, 17 mm, left; PSQD1N, 24 mm, right).

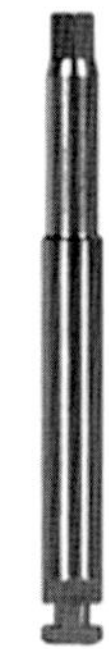

Figure 2.101. Contra-angle driver tip for square screws (RASQ3N, 24 mm length).

DRIVERS AND PLACEMENT INSTRUMENTS

Drivers and placement instruments are the instruments that are used by surgeons, restorative dentists, and dental laboratory technicians in implant dentistry. Some of the drivers may be used with other commercial implant systems. However, this discussion is limited to drivers for ***3i®*** implants.

Large Hex Drivers

Large hex drivers (PHD02N, PHD03N) are used to place healing abutments and tighten hexed abutment and retaining screws (Figure 2.98). These drivers have a patented tip design that allows components to be carried safely via a frictional grip. These drivers have hexagonal tips that measure 1.2 mm (.048 inches) from flat surface to flat surface. The drivers are made from surgical stainless steel.

Large Hex Driver Tips

Driver tips (RASH3N, RASH8N) may be used in contra-angles and torque drivers (Figure 2.99). Driver tips were designed for use with healing abutments and abutment/retaining screws and are also manufactured from surgical stainless steel. These driver tips are used to generate 10 or 20 Ncm of torque to large hex head screws.

Square Drivers

Square drivers (PSQD0N, PSQD1N) were designed for tightening square Gold-Tite™ Abutment screws and Square Try-In screws (Figure 2.100). They are made from surgical stainless steel.

Square Driver Tips

Driver tips (RASQ3N, RASQ8N) may be used in contra-angle and torque drivers (Figure 2.101). These driver tips were designed for use with Gold-Tite™ Square Abutment and Try-In screws and are also manufactured from surgical stainless steel. (Table 2.28). These driver tips are used clinically to generate 32 or 35 Ncm of torque to square head screws.

TABLE 2.28. Catalogue Numbers for Drivers and Driver Tips (Large Hex, Square)

Length	Large Hex Driver	Large Hex Tip	Square Driver	Square Tip
17 mm	PHDO2N	N/A	PSQDON	N/A
24 mm	PHDO3N	RASH3N	PSQD1N	RASQ3N
30 mm	N/A	RASH8N	N/A	RASQ8N
For use with	Healing abutments, Abutment Screws, Retaining Screws	Healing abutments, Abutment Screws,	Square Gold-Tite™ Abutment Screws, Try-In Screws	Square Gold-Tite™ Abutment Screws, Try-In Screws

TABLE 2.29. Catalogue Numbers for Drivers and Driver Tips (Abutments, LOCATOR®)

Length	Abutment Driver	Abutment Tip	LOCATOR® Tip Only
17 mm	PAD00	N/A	N/A
24 mm	PAD24	N/A	LOADT4
30 mm	N/A	N/A	LOADT9
One-size	N/A	RASA3	N/A
For use with	Conical, Standard and IOL® Abutments	Conical, Standard and IOL® Abutments	LOCATOR® Abutments

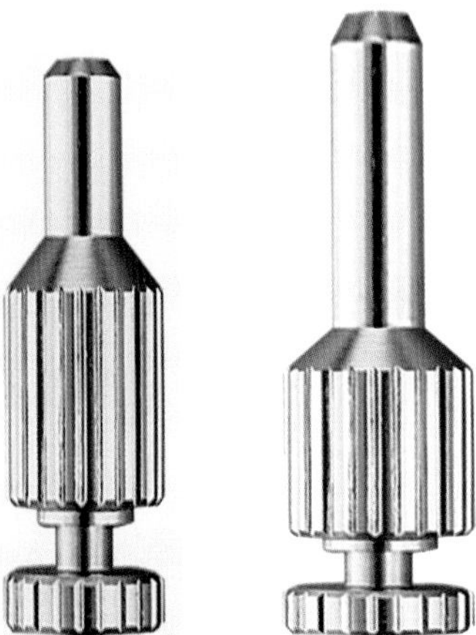

Figure 2.102. Abutment drivers (PAD00, 17 mm length, left; PAD24, 24 mm length, right).

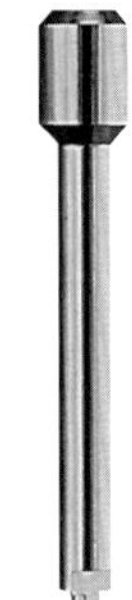

Figure 2.103. Contra-angle driver tip for Conical, Standard and IOL® Abutments (RASA3).

Abutment Drivers

Abutment drivers (PAD00, PAD24) are used to tighten Standard and IOL® Abutments and are also made from surgical stainless steel (Figure 2.102). (Table 2.29).

Abutment Driver Tips

Driver tips (RASA3) may be used in contra-angle and torque drivers (Figure 2.103). These driver tips were designed for use with Standard, Conical, and IOL® Abutment screws and are also manufactured from surgical stainless steel. These driver tips are used to generate up to 20 Ncm of torque to hexed abutment screws. (Table 2.29).

LABORATORY COMPONENTS

Laboratory analogs are replicas of implant restorative platforms and abutments. Analogs need to be manufactured to exact tolerances, because the fit of the final restorations onto the implants is dependent upon, among other factors, the accuracy of the analogs. Binon (1995) measured the machining accuracy of 13 different implant manufacturers' products including implants, abutments, and analogs and found considerable variation in machining accuracy and

TABLE 2.30. Catalogue Numbers For Laboratory Components for the OSSEOTITE® Certain® Implant System

Description	Implant Restorative Platform 3.4 mm	Implant Restorative Platform 4.1 mm	Implant Restorative Platform 5.0 mm	Implant Restorative Platform 6.0 mm
Laboratory Analog	IMMILA	IILA20	IILAW5	IILAW6
Laboratory Holder	ILTAH5	ILTAH7	ILTAH7	ILTAH7
Try In Screws	IUNITS	IUNITS	IUNITS	IUNITS
QuickSeat Activator Tool	IQSA01	IQSA01	IQSA01	IQSA01

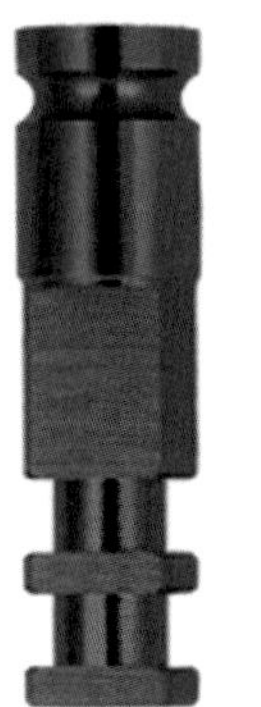
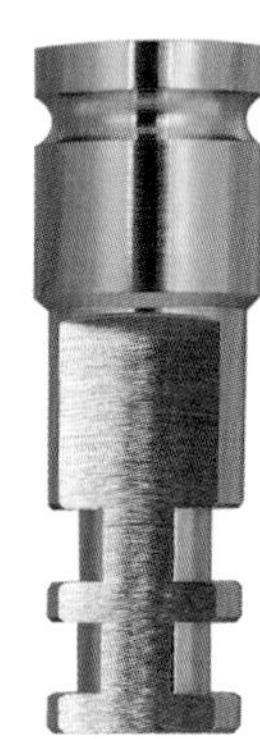

Figure 2.104. 4.1 mm implant analog-left (IILA20); 5.0 mm implant analog-right (IILAW5) for the OSSEOTITE® Certain® Implant System.

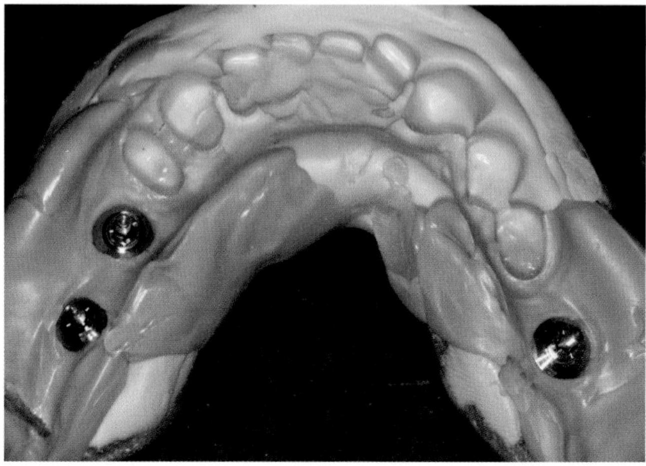

Figure 2.105. Mandibular impression with three internal connection implant impression copings in place. Impression copings and implant analogs are colored coded: blue for 4.1 mm restorative platforms; gold for 5.0 mm restorative platforms.

consistency in the sample implants that he studied. For instance, the mean analog hexagonal extension width (flat surface to flat surface) varied from 2.347 mm to 2.708 mm. Manufacturers had identified this dimension as being 2.7 mm. Binon was convinced that reduction or elimination of these types of discrepancies would decrease rotational movement between implants and abutments and would result in more stable and predictable screw joints. The internal connections of the ScrewVent implant system, although not included in the study with the external connection implant systems, demonstrated the least amount of rotational freedom (1.4° of all of the components and combinations that were tested in Binon's study).

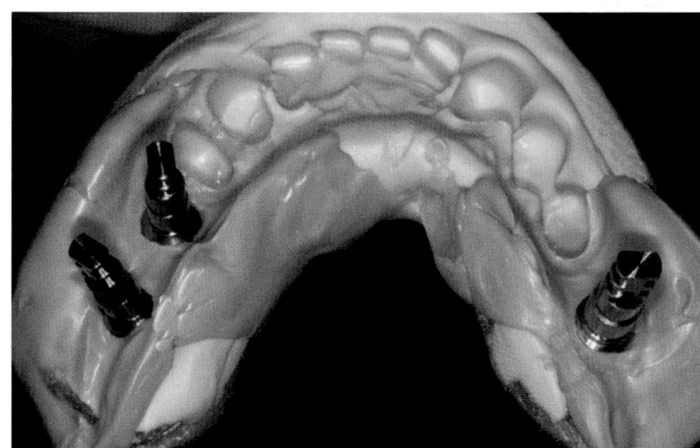

Figure 2.106. Blue (4.1 mm diameter, left) and gold (5.0 mm diameter, right) implant analogs in place on their respective implant impression copings in the mandibular definitive impression.

Implant Analogs

Implant analogs (Figure 2.104, Table 2.30) screw into the apical portions of implant impression copings (IIIC41-blue and IWIP55-gold) via the impression coping screws in the OSSEOTITE® Certain® Implant System (Figures 2.105, 2.106). A resilient impression (polyether) material was injected around the implant impression coping/implant analog junctions and the impression was poured with a Type IV die stone (Figure 2.107). There are machined concavities at the occlusal ends of internal connection implant lab analogs designed to retain the resilient soft tissue material to the implant lab analogs prior to pouring the impression.

Laboratory components are similarly available for the OSSEOTITE® Implant System (Table 2.31).

TABLE 2.31. Catalogue Numbers for Laboratory Components for the OSSEOTITE® Implant System

Description	Implant Restorative Platform 3.4 mm	Implant Restorative Platform 4.1 mm	Implant Restorative Platform 5.0 mm	Implant Restorative Platform 6.0 mm
Laboratory Analog	MMILA	ILA20	ILAW5	ILAW6
Laboratory Holder	LTAH5	LTAH7	LTAH7	LTAH7
Laboratory Try In Screw	UNITS	UNITS	UNITS	UNITS

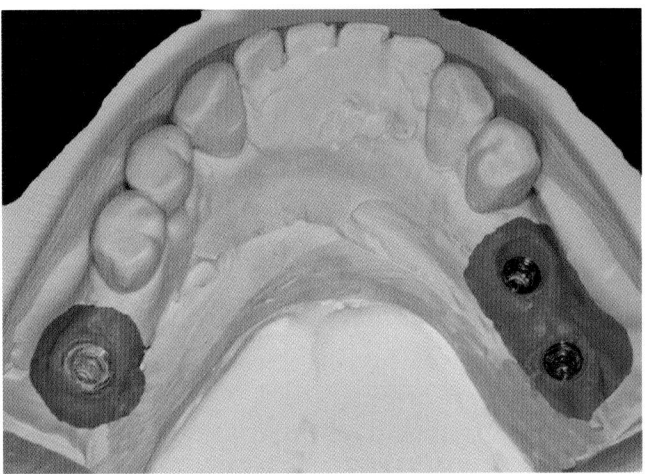

Figure 2.107. Laboratory occlusal view of the master cast from Figures 2.105 and 2.106. The implant analogs have been placed accurately within the master cast in preparation for fabrication of abutments and cement-retained crowns.

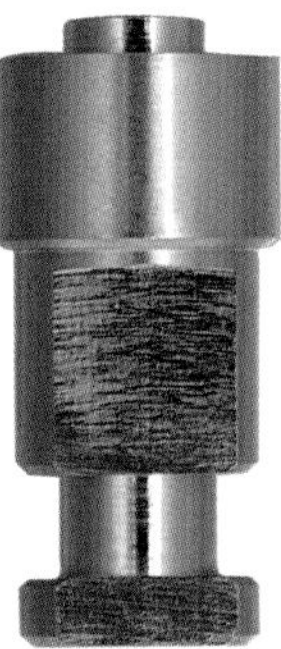

Figure 2.108. Standard Abutment Laboratory Analog (SLA20).

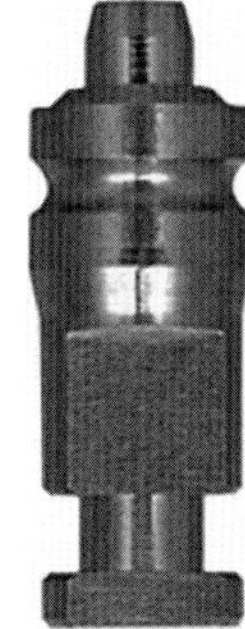

Figure 2.109. IOL® Laboratory Analog (IOLLAS).

Abutment Analogs

Abutment analogs are exact replicas of implant abutments and have to be manufactured to the same high degree of accuracy as implant analogs (Figures 2.108, 2.109, 2.110). Abutment analogs are not specific for internal connection and external hex implant systems in that abutment impression copings identify the location of abutments after they have been placed into the implants. Abutment analogs are generally unique for different implant manufacturers (Table 2.32).

Try-In Screws

Laboratory and clinical try-in screws are available for use by dental laboratory technicians and clinicians for implant

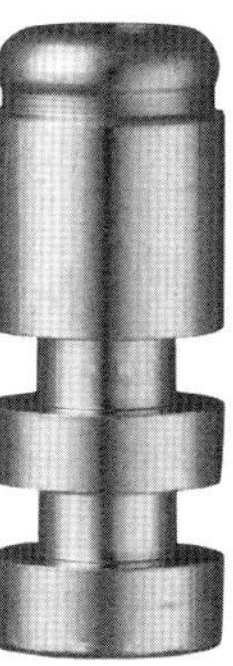

Figure 2.110. LOCATOR® Abutment Analog (LALA1).

TABLE 2.32. Catalogue Numbers for ***3i***® Abutment Laboratory Restorative Components

Abutment Analog	Implant Restorative Platform 4.1 mm	Implant Restorative Platform 5.0 mm	Polishing Protectors
Standard Abutment	SLA20	SLA20	PPSA3
IOL® Abutment	IOLLAS	N/A	IOLPP
LOCATOR® Abutment	LALA1	N/A	N/A

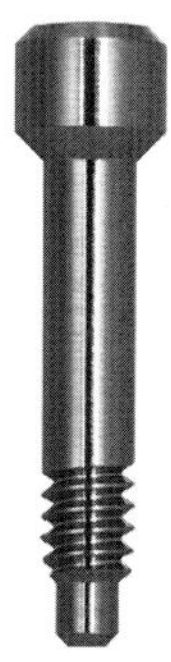

Figure 2.111. Try-In Screw (IUNITS) for OSSEOTITE® Certain® Implant System.

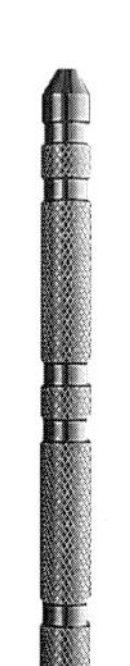

Figure 2.113. Abutment Holder (ILTAH7) for the OSSEOTITE® Certain® Implant System.

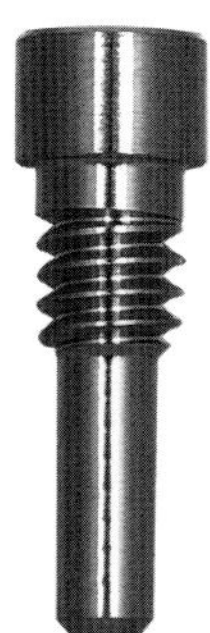

Figure 2.112. Try-In Screw (UNITS) for OSSEOTITE® Implant System.

level laboratory and clinical procedures, respectively (Figures 2.111, 2.112). The tops of the screws are either hexed for the internal connection system or square for use with the external hex implant connection system. This feature allows clinicians to use one type of driver during the clinical appointments because the heads of the try-in screws match the heads of the definitive abutment screws.

Abutment Holders

Laboratory abutment holders are instruments that provide predictable retention of abutments for extra-oral preparation and polishing procedures. They are available for both of ***3i***®'s internal connection and external hex implant systems (Figure 2.113). Dental laboratory technicians and clinicians may securely attach abutments to the holders with try-in screws and be confident that the abutments will remain in place during their procedures (Figures 2.114, 2.115, 2.116). This protocol optimizes clinical chair time because the bulk of the preparation can be accomplished outside the mouth or in the laboratory. This minimizes the need for extensive clinical preparation, is less likely to result in trauma to the peri-implant soft tissue, and is more easily tolerated by patients.

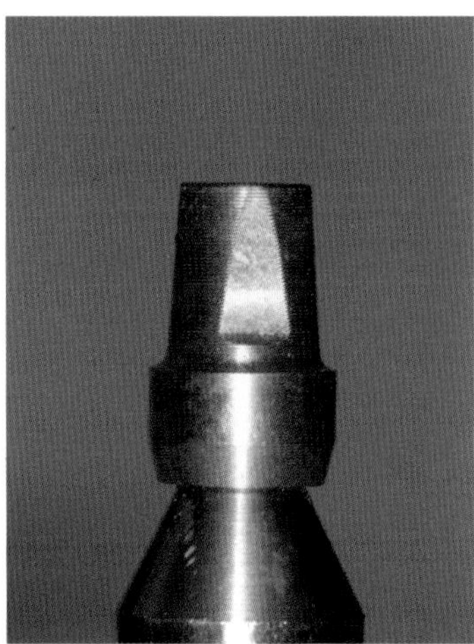

Figure 2.114. GingiHue® Post (WPP564G), as received from the manufacturer, in place on laboratory abutment holder (LTAH7). Note that in spite of the differences between the restorative platforms (the size of the external hex is consistent within the OSSEOTITE® Implant System), a 5 mm diameter abutment fits onto the laboratory abutment holder.

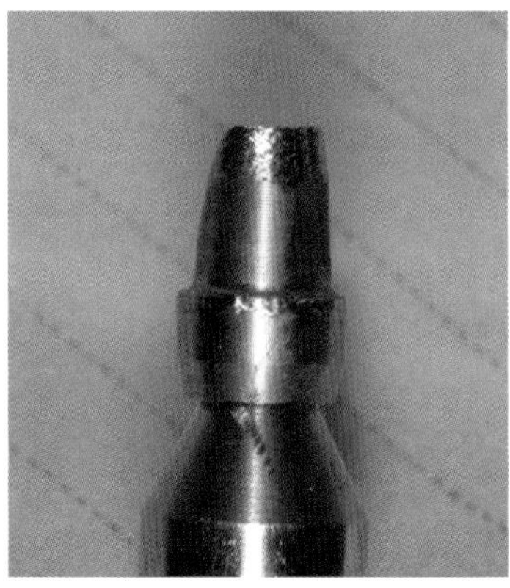

Figure 2.115. The abutment in Figure 2.114 was prepared on the abutment holder and was now ready to be transferred to the implant.

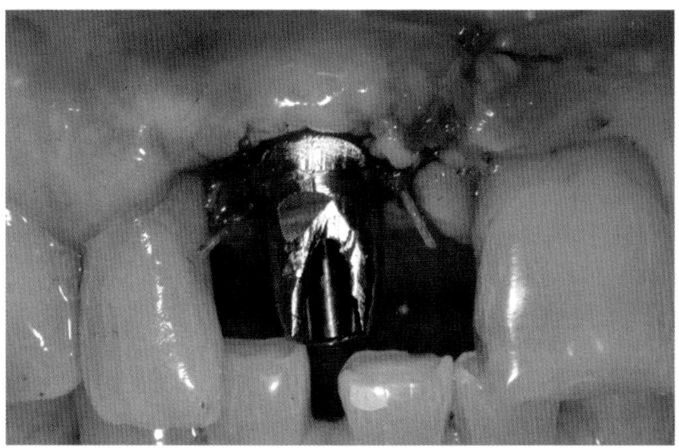

Figure 2.116. GingiHue® Post in place on the implant prior to fabrication of the provisional crown at the time the implant was uncovered.

BIBLIOGRAPHY

Adell, R, Lekholm, U, Rockler, B, Brånemark, P, 1981. A 15-year study of osseointegrated implants in the treatment of the edentulous jaw. *Int J Oral Surg* 2:387–416.

Beaty, K, 1994. The role of screws in implant systems. *Int J Oral Maxillofac Implant* 9 (Special Supplement):52–54.

Binon, P, 1995. Evaluation of machining accuracy and consistency of selected implants, standard abutments and laboratory analogs. *Int J Prosthod* 8(2):162–178.

Bonilla, H, Sullivan, D, 2003. Clinical indications and techniques for the ZiReal post. *Compend Clin Dent Ed* 8:3–7.

Brånemark, P-I, 1985. "Introduction to Osseointegration." In *Tissue Integrated Prostheses. Osseointegration in Clinical Dentistry.* Edited by Brånemark, P, Zarb, G, Albrektsson, T., p. 11. Chicago: Quintessence Publishing Co., Inc.

Brodbeck, U, 2003. The ZiReal Post: a new ceramic implant abutment. *J Esthet Restor Dent* 15:10–24.

Cook, S, Kay, J, Thomas, K, Jarcho, M, 1987. Interface mechanics and histology of titanium and hydroxyapatite-coated titanium for dental implant applications. *Int J Oral Maxillofac Implants* 2:15–23.

Davarpanah, M, 2001. Osseotite implants: a 3-year prospective multi center evaluation. *Clin Implant Dent Rel Res* 3:111–118.

Drago, C, 2001. Prepable ceramic abutments: principles and techniques for the dental laboratory technician. *J Dent Tech* 18:18–22.

Drago, C, 2002. Prepable titanium abutments: principles and techniques for the dental laboratory technician. *J Dent Tech* 19:22–28.

Drago, C, 2003. A clinical study of the efficacy of gold-tite square abutment screws in cement-retained implant restorations. *Int J Oral Maxillofac Implants* 18:273–278.

Eckert, S, Wollan, P, 1998. Retrospective review of 1170 endosseous implants placed in partially edentulous jaws. *J Prosthet Dent* 79:415–421.

Finger, I, Castellon, P, Block, M, Elian, N, 2003. The evolution of external and internal implant/abutment connections. *Pract Proced Aesthet Dent* 15:625–632.

Implant Innovations, Inc. 1993. *The Emergence Profile Brochure.* Palm Beach Gardens, FL.

Implant Innovations, Inc. Department of Biomedical Engineering, 2003. Palm Beach Gardens, FL.

Jansen, C, 1995. Guided soft tissue healing in implant dentistry. *J Calif Dent Assoc* 23:57–60.

Jemt, T, Lacey, W, Harris, D, 1991. Osseointegrated implants for single tooth replacement: a 1-year report from a multicenter prospective study. *Int J Oral Maxillofac Implants* 6:236–245.

Jemt, T, Pettersson, P, 1993. A 3-year follow-up study on single implant treatment. *J Dent* 21:203–208.

Keith, S, Miller, B, Woody, R, Higginbottom, F, 1999. Marginal discrepancy of screw-retained and metal-ceramic crowns on implant abutments. *Int J Oral Maxillofac Implants* 14:369–378.

Lazzara, R, 1993. Managing the soft tissue margin: the key to implant aesthetics. *Pract Perio Aesthet Dent* 5:1–7.

Levine, R, Clem, D, Wilson, T, Higginbottom, F, Solnit, G, 1999. Multicenter retrospective analysis of the ITI implant system used for single-tooth replacement: results of loading for 2 or more years. *Int J Oral Maxillofac Implants* 14:516–520.

Linek, Henry, 1949. *Tooth Carving Manual*, p. 5. New York, NY: Columbia Dentoform Corp.

Loos, L, 1986. A fixed prosthodontic technique for mandibular osseointegrated titanium implants. *J Prosthet Dent* 55:232–242.

Marinbach, M, 1996. The influence of implants on the dental profession through the eyes of a laboratory owner. *Implant Dent* 5:81–83.

Martin, W, Woody, R, Miller, B, Miller, A, 2001. Implant abutment screw rotations and preloads for four different screw materials and surfaces. *J Prosthet Dent* 86:24–32.

McGlumphy, E, Huseyin, A, 1995. Implant screw mechanics. In *Endosseous Implants for Maxillofacial Reconstruction*. Edited by Block, M, Kent, J., p. 151–157. Philadelphia: W. B. Saunders Co.

Mollersten, L, Lockowandt, P, Linden, L, 1997. Comparison of strength and failure modes of seven implant systems: an in vitro test. *J Prosthet Dent* 78:582–591.

Niznick, G, 1983. The Core-Vent™ implant system. The evolution of the osseointegrated implant. *Oral Health* 73:13–17.

Niznick, G, 1991. The implant/abutment connection: the key to prosthetic success. *Compend Cont Dent Educ* 12:932–937.

Porter, S, Robb, T, 1998. Increasing implant-abutment preload by thin-gold coating abutment screws. Implant Innovations, Inc., Engineering, Palm Beach Gardens, FL.

Robb, T, Porter, S, 1998. Increasing abutment rotation by applying thin-gold coating. Implant Innovations, Inc., Engineering, Palm Beach Gardens, FL.

Rodkey, E, 1977. Making fastened joints reliable. . .ways to keep 'em tight. *Assembly Eng* 3:24–27.

Schulte, J, 1994. External hex manufacturing tolerances of six implant systems: a pilot study. *Implant Dent* 3:51–53.

Saadoun, A, 1995. Periimplant tissue considerations for optimal implant results. *Pract Perio Aesthet Dent* 3:53–60.

Sakaguchi, R, Sun, T, Haack, J, 1994. External strain distribution on implant prosthetic components. *J Dent Res* 73:232, Abstract 1045.

Seghi, R, Sorensen, J, 1995. Relative flexural strength of six new ceramic materials. *Int J Prosthod* 8:239–246.

Steri-Oss, 1998. Evaluation of TorqTite surface technology. Number TR01-1148. Steri-Oss Dental Care Co. Yorba Linda, CA.

Sutherland, J, Hallam, R, 1990. Soldering technique for osseointegrated implant prostheses. *J Prosthet Dent* 63:242–244.

Taylor, R, Bergman, G, 1990. Laboratory techniques for the Brånemark system. *Quintessence*:22–30.

Vigolo, P, Fonzi, F, Majzoub, Z, Cordioli, G, 2004. An evaluation of impression techniques for multiple internal connection implant prostheses. *J Prosthet Dent* 92:470–476.

Weisgold, A, Arnoux, I, Lu, J, 1997. Single-tooth anterior implant: a word of caution, Part I. *J Esthet Dent* 6:285–294.

Zarb, G, Schmitt, A, 1990. The longitudinal clinical effectiveness of osseointegrated dental implants: the Toronto study. Part III: problems and complications encountered. *J Prosthet Dent* 64:185–194.

Zoldos, J., Kent, J., 1995. "Healing of Endosseous Implants." In *Endosseous Implants for Maxillofacial Reconstruction*. Edited by Michael S. Block and John N. Kent, p. 65. Philadelphia: W. B. Saunders Co.

Chapter 3: Diagnosis and Treatment Planning in Implant Restorative Dentistry

PATIENT SELECTION

Implant dentistry is similar to conventional dentistry in that the first step of the process consists of data collection. The initial visits in a restorative dental office should include a medical/dental history; complete clinical examination; radiographs and other imaging (CT scan, tomogram, lateral cephalometric radiographs, and so on); and diagnostic casts. The dentist and staff need to develop an appreciation of the patient's goals and expectations of treatment, as well as formulate the diagnosis (or diagnoses) and treatment options.

Age may be a relative contraindication for dental implants, in that patients should have completed their physical growth prior to implant placement (Santos 2002).

Patients will also need to have the requisite amount of bone for the planned treatments, as well as enough space relative to anatomic structures that may interfere with implant placement. Patients who have been edentulous for a significant length of time (Figure 3.1); patients who have had large volumes of the jaws removed and reconstructed associated with cancer surgery (Figures 3.2, 3.3); and patients who have suffered significant localized resorption after the loss of several teeth (Figure 3.4) may present challenges to implant surgeons in order to provide enough bone volume for implant placement.

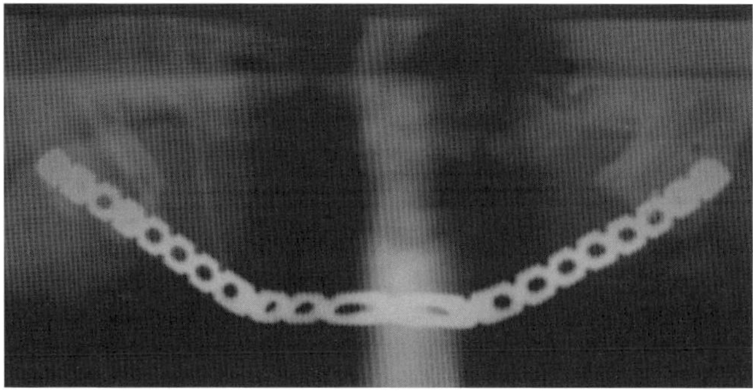

Figure 3.2. Panoramic radiograph of a patient one-week post excision of the anterior two-thirds of his mandible secondary to a diagnosis of a squamous cell carcinoma of the floor of the mouth.

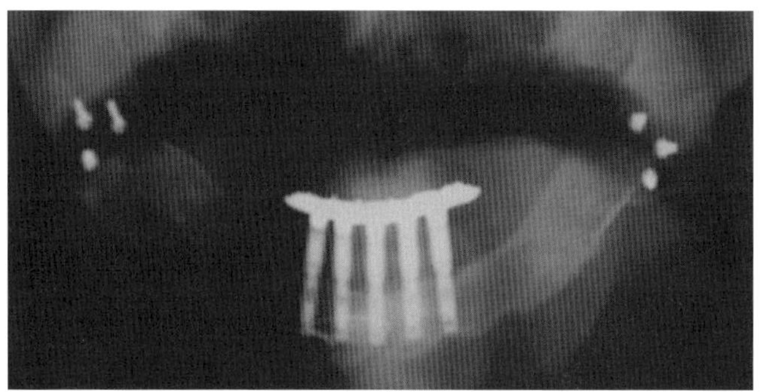

Figure 3.3. Panoramic radiograph of the patient in Figure 3.2. 10 years post insertion of implants and fixed implant-retained prosthesis. This was approximately 14 years post resection and reconstruction of the mandible secondary to removal of the tumor.

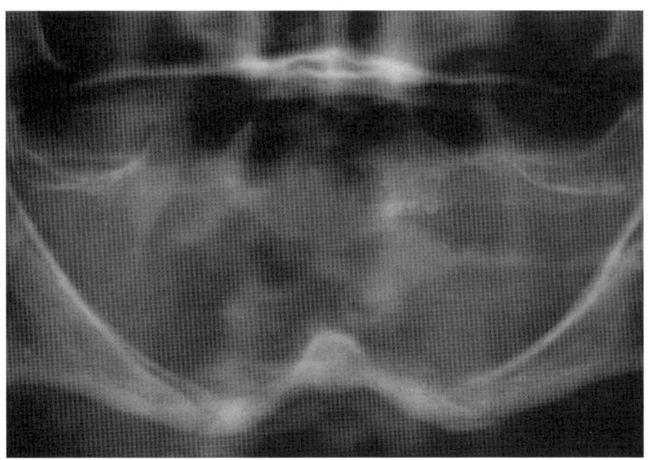

Figure 3.1. Panoramic radiograph of a patient who has been edentulous for 50 years. This radiograph illustrates right and left mandibular fractures.

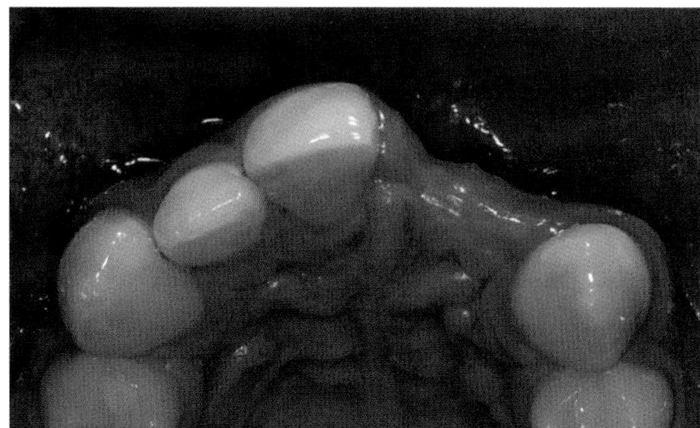

Figure 3.4. Clinical maxillary occlusal view of an anterior maxillary ridge two years after the loss of the maxillary left central and lateral incisors. Note the significant amount of horizontal ridge resorption that has occurred in this period of time.

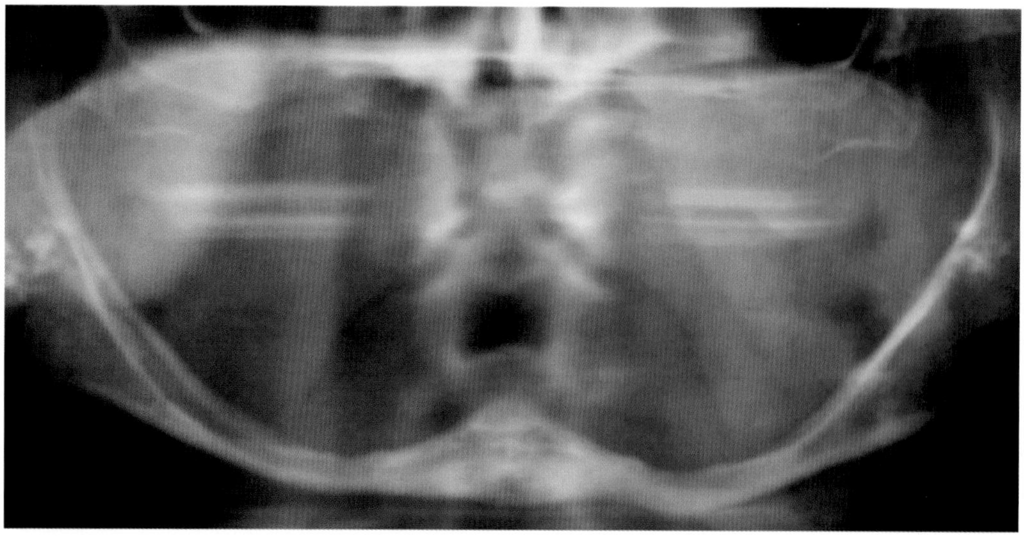

Figure 3.5. Panoramic radiograph of patient who has been edentulous for 40 years. Note the locations of the right and left inferior alveolar canals and their proximity to the crest of the edentulous ridge.

MEDICAL HISTORY

Potential dental implant patients should not be evaluated any differently than other patients in dental practice. A patient's medical status may complicate both the surgical and restorative phases of implant treatment and potentially impact the overall treatment outcomes.

As with any type of surgical procedure, dental implant surgery has risks associated with it: bleeding, infection, and paresthesias. The benefits of the planned treatments must outweigh the risks of the procedures. The American Association of Oral and Maxillofacial Surgeons Parameters of Care (2001) indicated that the standards of care for planned surgical procedures using anesthesia should include:

1. Indications for therapy
2. Therapeutic goals
3. Factors affecting risk
4. Indicated therapeutic standards

Outcome Assessment Indices

Completion of an appropriate medical history questionnaire by the patient and review of it by the surgeon is essential prior to treatment because there may be elements in the history that can influence the surgical portion of the treatment. Medically, most ambulatory patients should be able to tolerate the outpatient surgical procedures associated with dental implants. Active disease that directly or indirectly affects the physiology or anatomy of the head and neck regions would warrant deferral of implant placement until such time as the disease process has been controlled or has resolved.

Absolute contraindications for dental implant treatment on the basis of immediate surgical and anesthetic risks would be limited to patients who are acutely ill, have a terminal illness, have uncontrolled metabolic disease, are pregnant, or have unrealistic expectations (NIH Consensus Statement 1988; Peterson 1998).

The reader is referred to more definitive textbooks on medicine and surgery for more detailed explanations of pathology and medical/surgical management of patients (Peterson 1998).

Diagnostic Procedures

Dental problems that were historically the most difficult to treat can now, many times, be managed with dental implants. The long-term effects of edentulism and alveolar ridge resorption have been well documented (Tallgren 1969, 1972). Partially edentulous patients who have lost multiple molars and been relegated to removable partial dentures can be successfully treated with fixed implant retained restorations if adequate bone exists for implant placement (Guerra and Finger 1995). Patients who have been victimized by trauma and cancer can also be rehabilitated with restorations supported by dental implants (Garlini and Bianchi 2003; Brånemark and Tolman 1998).

Clinical and radiographic evaluations of the implant sites are essential to treatment planning. Implants need to have adequate bone volume for placement, and implant restorations require adequate clinical volume for replacement of the missing teeth (Jansen and Weisgold 1995). Proximity to key anatomic structures may preclude implant placement (Figure 3.5).

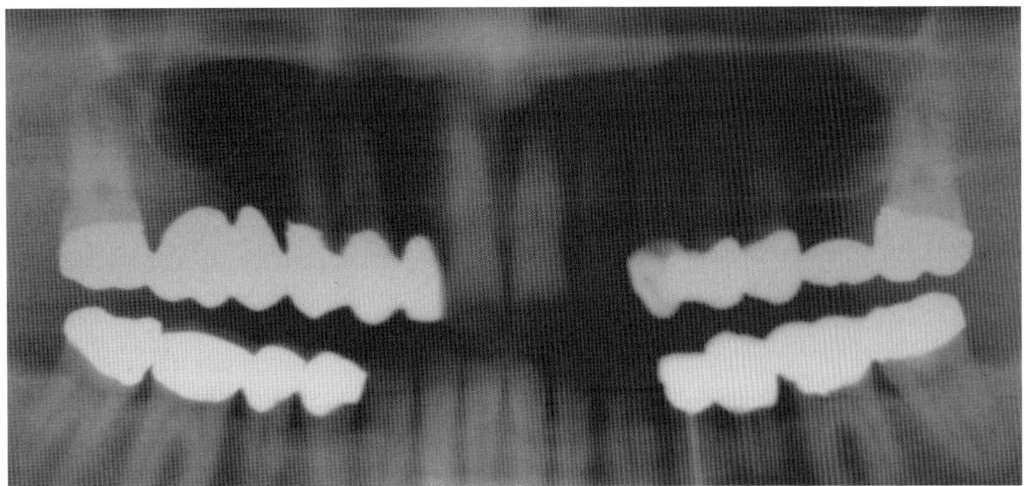

Figure 3.6. Panoramic radiograph of a patient with multiple missing teeth. This radiograph suggested that there was not enough bone volume, without bone grafting, in the right posterior maxilla for implants.

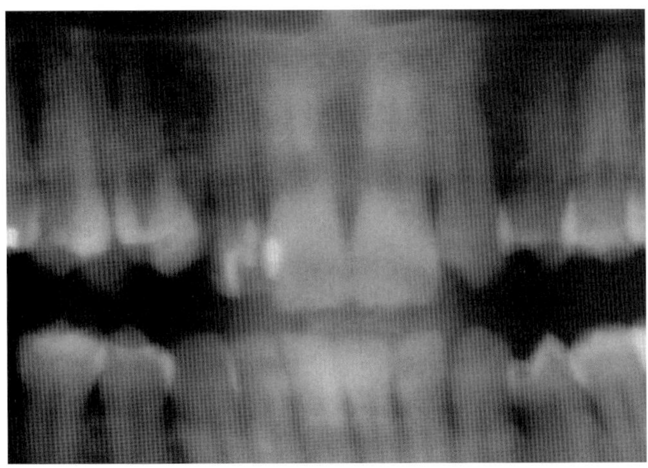

Figure 3.7. Panoramic radiograph of a patient with crowding in the maxillary right posterior quadrant. This radiograph demonstrated compromised restorative volume in the area of the maxillary right first premolar and deciduous cuspid.

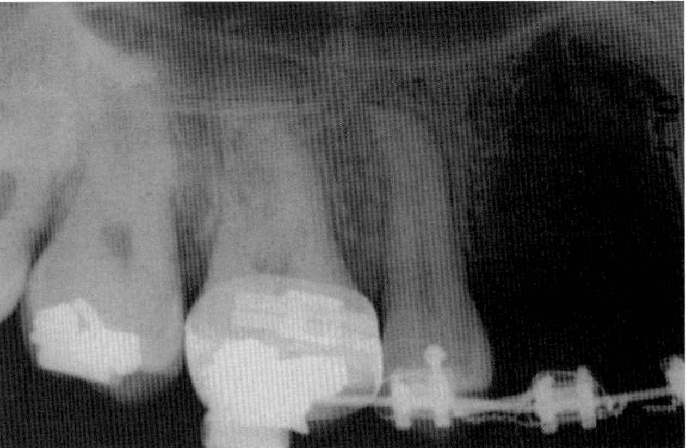

Figure 3.8. Periapical radiograph one month after extraction of the above two teeth (Figure 3.7) that demonstrated adequate mesial/distal dimension for implants to replace the missing teeth.

Radiographs

The best initial radiograph for both edentulous and partially edentulous patients is the panoramic radiograph because it images both jaws in one image (Figure 3.6). However, panoramic radiographs can have significant distortion depending on patient positioning, anatomical contours of the jaws, and other technical considerations (Bellaiche 1997). There are numerous advantages to panoramic radiographs:

1. Both jaws are imaged on one radiograph.
2. They provide an estimate of vertical bone height with a magnification error of approximately 1.3.
3. They are relatively inexpensive.

There are also several limitations associated with panoramic radiographs:

1. Mesial/distal dimensions are not reliable because they can vary as a function of patient positioning and jaw anatomy (Figures 3.7 and 3.8).
2. They do not provide information on the facial/lingual depth of the anatomic structures.
3. They do not provide information on the quality of the cancellous bone.

Periapical radiographs can be useful in identifying the relative parallelism of roots of teeth adjacent to an edentulous space. Accurate, intra-oral radiographs using a paralleling technique allow evaluation of the mesio-distal dimension of

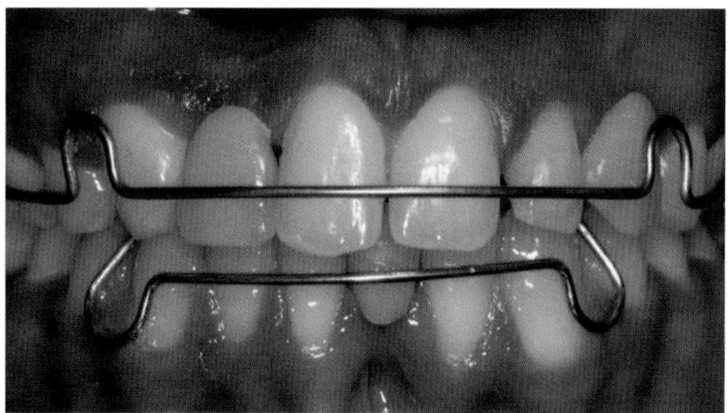

Figure 3.9. Clinical anterior view of a patient immediately after the orthodontic braces had been removed. Note the differences in the mesial/distal widths of the maxillary lateral incisors.

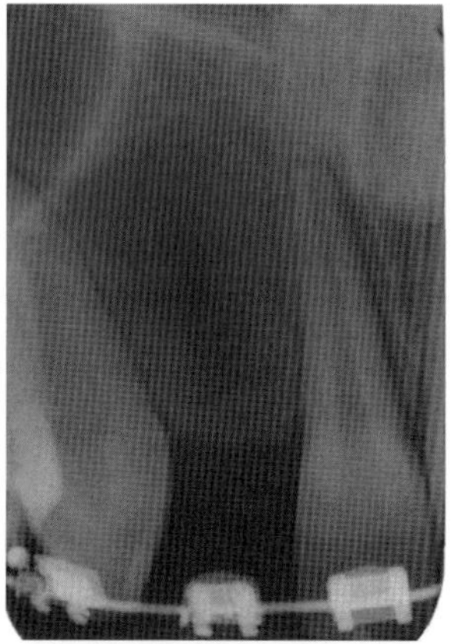

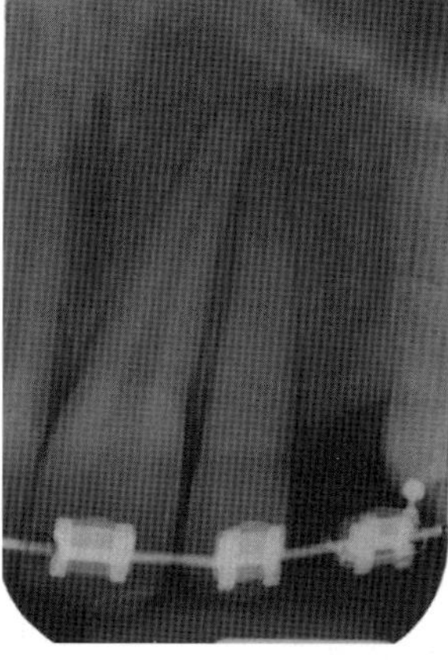

Figure 3.10. Periapical radiographs of the patient in Figure 3.9. Note the limited bone volume available for implant placement in the left cuspid site (bottom). The limited bone volume did not correlate with the size of the clinical pontic on the orthodontic retainer.

the intended implant sites and also provide a preliminary estimate of the vertical bone dimension. The intra-oral paralleling technique provides the best radiographic depiction of the remaining teeth and edentulous sites (Scortecci and Garcias 2001). This can be critical in orthodontic cases in which the clinical crowns of the teeth adjacent to an edentulous site may be aligned correctly but the roots converge and limit the available bone for implant placement (Figures 3.9, 3.10).

CT Scans

Computed tomography (CT) and its computerized dental applications, such as DentaScan® and SIMPLANT®, can be advantageous to restorative dentists and implant surgeons. CT is based on X-radiation of anatomic structures with a highly collimated X-ray beam to obtain "slices" that measure 1 mm in thickness. Following absorption by electronic X-ray sensors, the X-rays are converted to an electronic signal that is digitized and processed by an image reconstruction computer. CT densities can be expressed as Hounsfield units (HU). Cortical bone presents with HU values of 800–2,000; dental enamel and metal presents with HU values of 1,500–3,000 (Rosenfeld and McCall 1996).

CT scans offer clinicians two distinct advantages over conventional radiographs: accurate three-dimensional analysis of bone volume and better visualization of bone architecture (Figures 3.11, 3.12).

There are several limitations of CT scans: motion artifacts caused by patient movement during the scanning process; metal associated artifacts because metal creates concentric bursts or reflections of energy that can be projected into adjacent structures; and limited resolution on reconstructions that involve severely resorbed bone.

CT scans can provide detailed anatomic data that may preclude some surgical procedures and can demonstrate the feasibility of implant placement. CT scans can aid clinicians in more accurate determination on the optimum number, distribution, dimensions and angulation of implants according to the volume and quality of bone (Figures 3.13, 3.14, 3.15, 3.16).

Bellaiche (2001) considered CT scans to be the current gold standard for imaging protocols in implant dentistry. The American Academy of Oral and Maxillofacial Radiology (AAOMR) set forth their own standards in a position paper and stated that some form of cross-sectional imaging should be used for all implant cases (Tyndall and Brooks 2000). According to Friedland (2005), the AAOMR standards did not seem to have much of an impact on the radiographic standard of care for dental implants. The standard of care is frequently determined by clinical practice in academic centers, as well as by what students and residents are taught.

One of the most common types of implant-related lawsuits involves injuries to the inferior alveolar nerve (Givol and Taicher 2002). There are data from other countries that

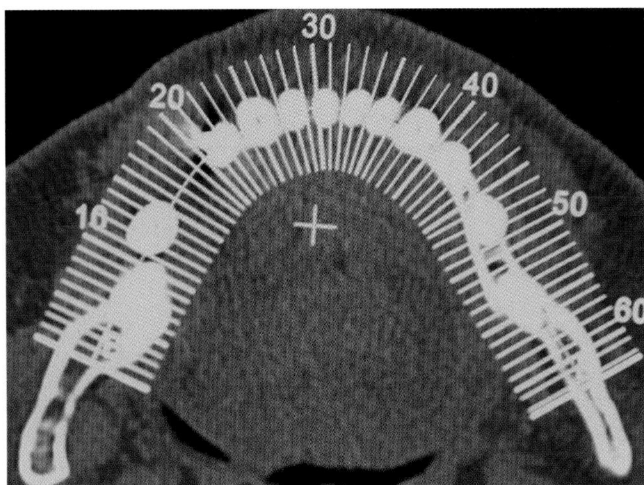

Figure 3.11. Occlusal CT scan that identified by number, 1 mm slices from the left retro molar pad to the right retro molar pad. The numbers that identified the slices are consistent throughout the CT images.

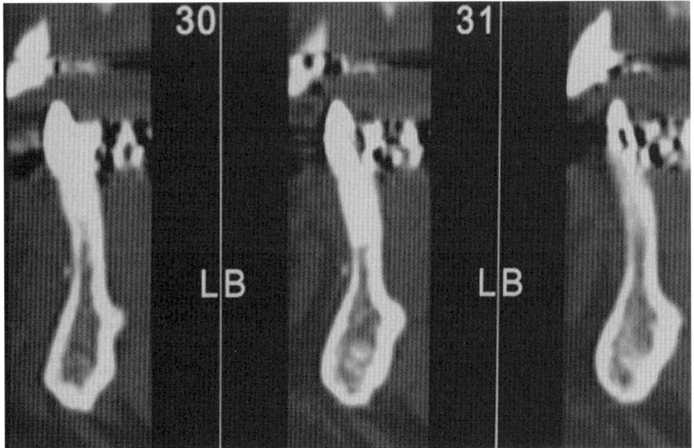

Figure 3.12. Lateral CT oblique slices that were obtained from the anterior mandibular segment of the patient in Figure 3.11. Note the minimum amount of bone covering the facial root surfaces of the incisors and the lack of facial/lingual width within the alveolus.

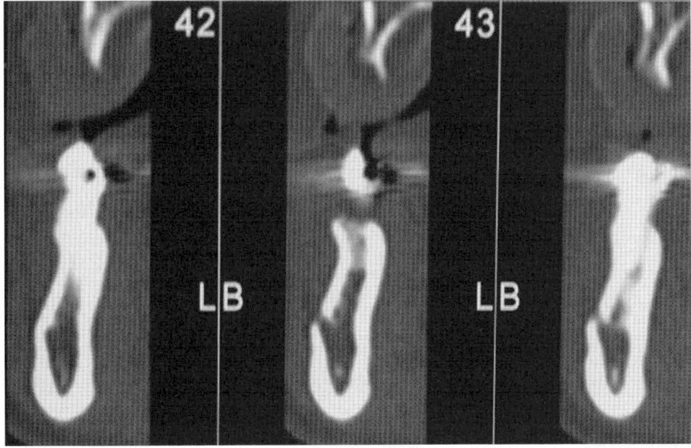

Figure 3.13. Lateral CT oblique slices of a posterior mandibular segment that identified the location of the mental foramen relative to the middle of the edentulous space.

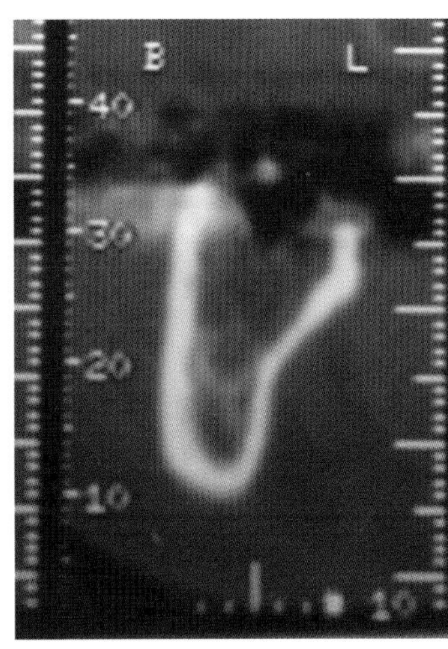

Figure 3.14. Lateral CT oblique slice of a posterior mandibular segment that identified the location of the inferior alveolar canal. The width of the edentulous site superior to the canal was large enough to accommodate a 5 mm diameter implant.

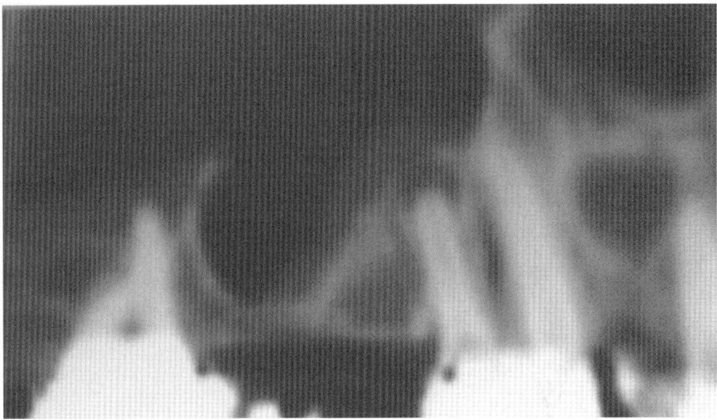

Figure 3.15. Panoramic CT image of a right maxillary sinus with severe pneumatization. This patient would be a candidate for dental implants only if he agreed to undergo a bone graft procedure prior to implant surgery.

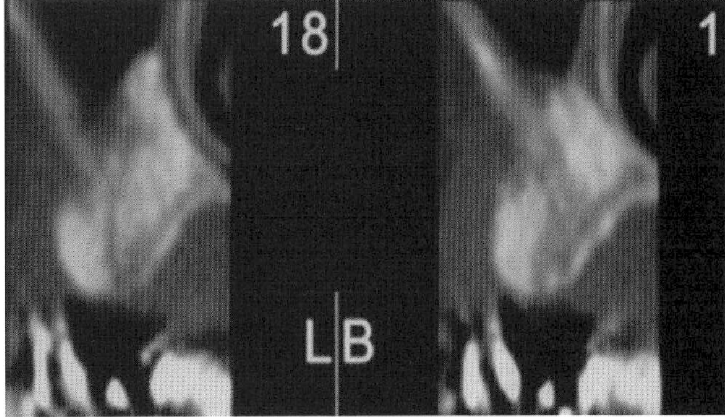

Figure 3.16. Lateral CT oblique slice of the patient in Figure 3.15. Note the increased height and width of the alveolar ridge eight months post bone grafting. There is now adequate bone volume for implant placement.

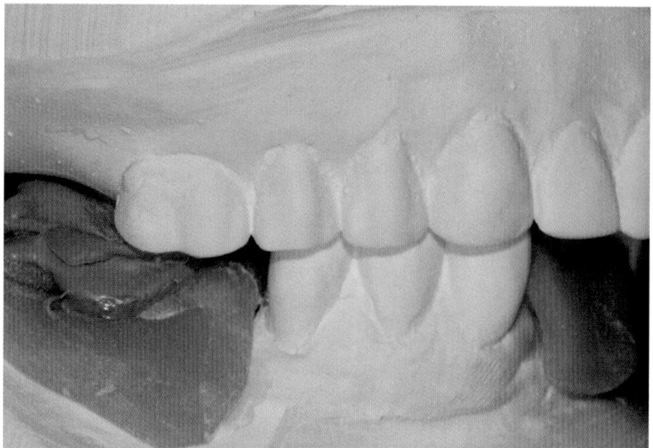

Figure 3.17. These diagnostic casts were mounted at an optimal vertical dimension of occlusion. Due to the minimal number of natural teeth remaining, a mandibular record base was needed for the articulator mounting.

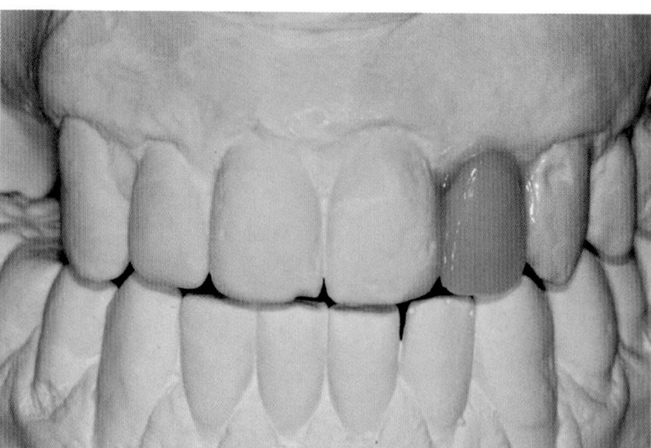

Figure 3.19. For a patient missing a single tooth, diagnostic casts and articulator mountings may still be critical for optimal implant placement and restoration. In this case (end-to-end occlusion) diagnostic casts, wax pattern (denture tooth) and articulator mounting were critical in correctly identifying the position of the implant restoration for the surgeon prior to implant placement.

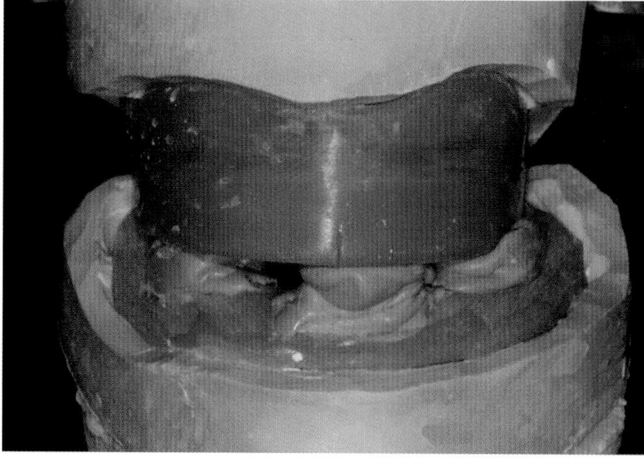

Figure 3.18. For this edentulous patient, the master casts were mounted at the agreed-upon vertical dimension of occlusion and used to evaluate the jaw relationship and the amount of inter-occlusal space available for the implant restorative and denture components.

demonstrate that insurance companies often settle lawsuits associated with these injuries if advanced imaging studies were not performed. For instance, a report from Israel involved 61 implant-related lawsuits. In 53 of those cases, panoramic radiography was the sole imaging modality used, despite the well-known shortcomings of panoramic radiographs (Frederiksen 1995; Kassebaum and Nummikoski 1990). Friedland (2005) was specific in his recommendations that the decision to undergo or forgo cross-sectional imaging studies prior to implant surgery is the patient's decision to make, and the informed consent or denial is critical. The clinician's approach to treatment should be individualized for each patient.

Diagnostic Casts

Diagnostic casts are generally considered to be essential in the treatment planning process. They must be made from accurate impressions of each arch. In partially edentulous and edentulous patients, the casts should be mounted on an articulator at the proposed vertical dimension of occlusion (VDO) (Figures 3.17, 3.18). Diagnostic articulator mountings are no less important for single implant crown restorations (Figure 3.19).

Properly oriented, mounted diagnostic casts will provide clinicians with information relative to the amount of resorption and inter-occlusal space available for implant and prosthetic components, as well as provide the foundation for diagnostic wax patterns that can be used for construction of surgical and CT guides. Diagnostic casts can also be a tremendous teaching aid for patients and their families during consultations.

PHYSICAL EXAMINATION

Definitive treatment begins with a thorough clinical examination. There are several differences in the clinical examinations for dentulous and edentulous patients. The differences relate to the anatomical characteristics associated with resorption of edentulous ridges and the resulting jaw relationships. The goal of the examination process is to

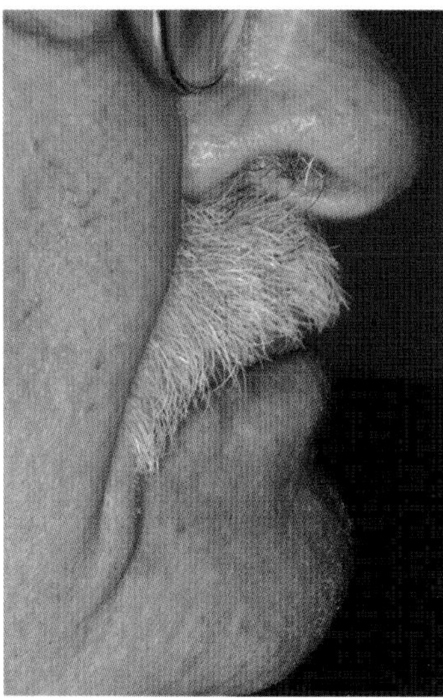

Figure 3.20. Profile view of a patient in centric occlusion with a decreased vertical dimension of occlusion secondary to occlusal abrasion of the mandibular anterior teeth and loss of posterior occlusal stops.

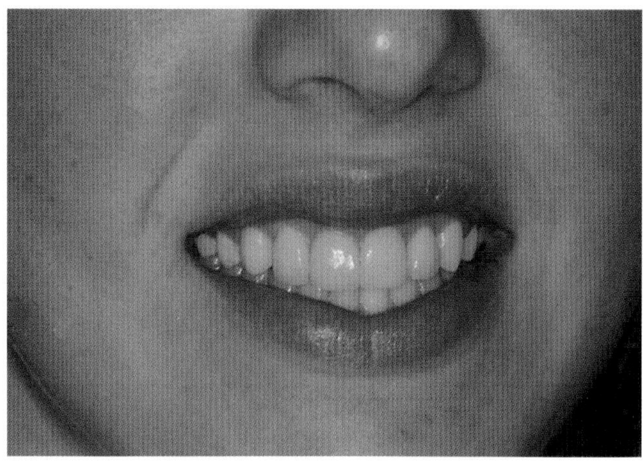

Figure 3.22. Photograph of a patient smiling with a high lip line. Note the amount of gingival tissues that are visible apical to the gingival two-thirds of the anterior teeth.

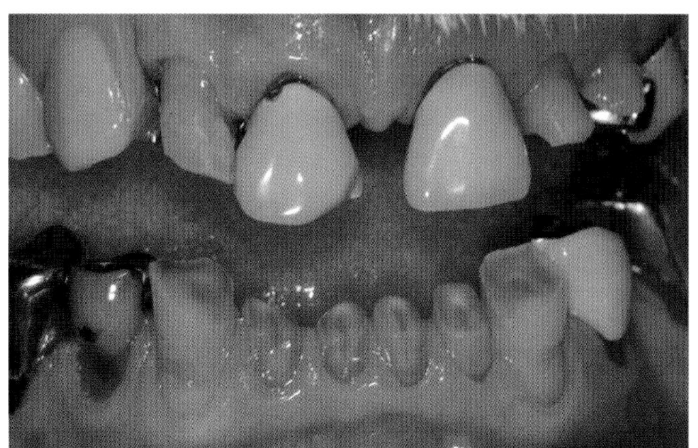

Figure 3.21. Intra-oral view of the patient in Figure 3.20 that demonstrates severe occlusal abrasion of the mandibular anterior teeth.

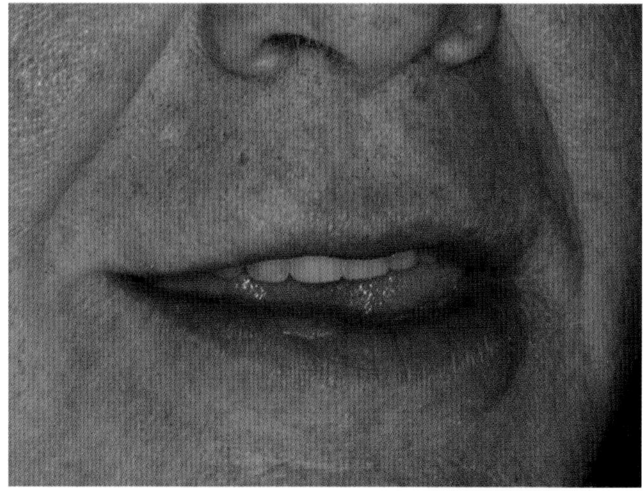

Figure 3.23. Photograph of a patient smiling with a low lip line. None of the maxillary anterior gingival tissues are visible with smiling.

provide clinicians with enough information to establish a diagnosis and formulate treatment options.

Extra-Oral Examination

The extra-oral portion of the examination should include evaluation of:

- Facial symmetry
- Vertical dimension of occlusion (Figures 3.20, 3.21)
- Smile line (amount of teeth and/or gingival displayed while smiling and speaking) (Figures 3.22, 3.23)
- Condition of the muscles of mastication
- Mandibular range of motion
- Amount/noise associated with condylar translation
- Soft tissue profile: Class I, II or III
- Soft tissue pathology

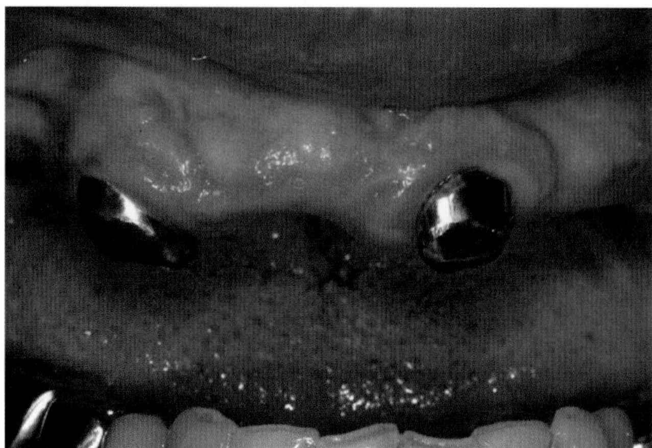

Figure 3.24. Clinical photograph of partially edentulous maxillae where the maxillary right canine and maxillary left central incisor were retained as overdenture abutment teeth. Note the minimal resorption that has occurred over the 10 years that the patient had been restored with the maxillary overdenture.

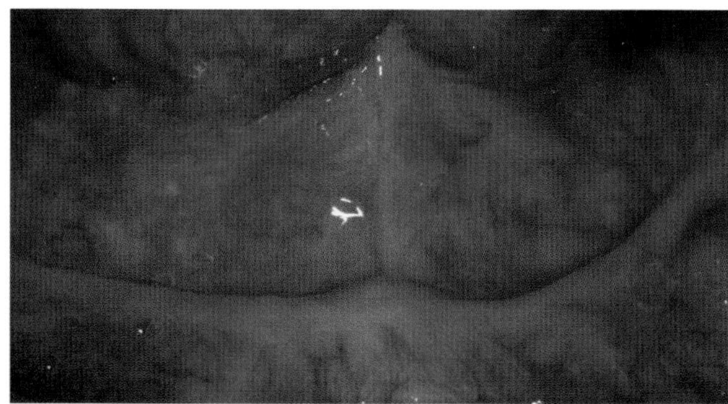

Figure 3.25. Clinical image of an edentulous mandible that has undergone severe resorption. This patient had been edentulous for 40 years.

Intra-Oral Examination

The intra-oral portion of an examination for an edentulous patient should include evaluation of:

- Amount of resorption of the edentulous ridges (Figure 3.24)
- Size and shape of the edentulous jaws (Figure 3.25)
- Quality of tissues: attached, keratinized, non-keratinized, loosely attached, mucosa
- Inter-occlusal space
- Jaw relationship: Class I, II or III
- Location and activity of the floor of the mouth
- Lateral throat form
- Anatomy of the hard and soft palates
- Soft tissue pathology

If the patient is partially edentulous, dental implants may represent only a portion of the potential treatment options. The intra-oral examination should also consist of:

- Identification of the remaining teeth—Periodontal charting: sulcus depths, mobility, furcation involvement, presence/absence of attached gingival, bleeding, suppuration
- Dental caries
- Defective restorations
- Malposed teeth
- Occlusal analysis
- Quality/quantity of saliva
- Soft tissue pathology

Diagnostic Articulator Mounting

Properly oriented diagnostic casts provide clinicians with three-dimensional views of dental and inter-arch relationships and allow assessment of the amount and location of resorption, inter-arch spacing, vertical dimension of occlusion, and so on. Articulator mounted diagnostic casts are called for in the presence of malocclusions, malposed and missing teeth, and debilitated dentitions. Diagnostic mountings may be made on various types of articulators: simple hinge, semi-adjustable, and fully adjustable. In "normal" cases, diagnostic casts may be mounted on simple hinge articulators (Figure 3.26). In cases in which the vertical dimension of occlusion will be altered or there are minimal posterior occlusal stops, semi- or fully adjustable articulators are generally warranted (Besimo and Rohner 2005) (Figure 3.27).

Diagnostic Wax Patterns

Diagnostic wax patterns that identify the optimal positions of missing teeth are critical to surgeons, restorative dentists, and dental laboratory technicians. It has been well established that diagnostic wax patterns serve as the basis for planning and treatment of patients with multiple missing teeth (Nyman and Lindhe 1979). The maxillary dental midline generally is in line with the facial midline (Chiche and Penault 1994). The diagnostic wax patterns or denture teeth should be constructed to develop pleasing proportions relative to the size of the missing teeth, location and shape of the gingival margins, and location of the upper and lower lip lines. Of course, other anatomical limitations must be taken into account prior to treatment (Figures 3.28 through 3.30).

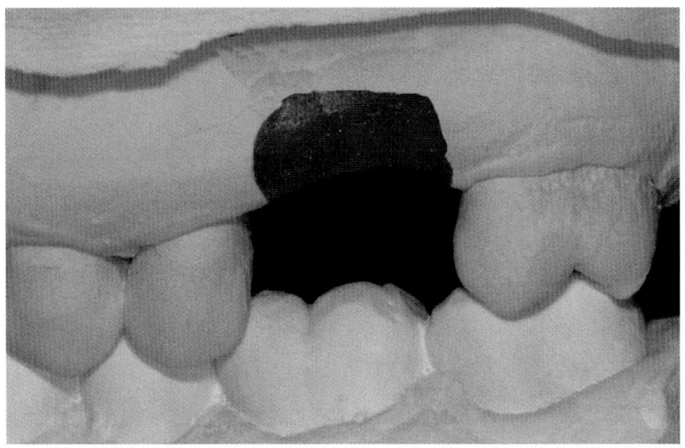

Figure 3.26. Laboratory view of a maxillary master cast mounted against a mandibular diagnostic cast on a simple hinge articulator. Natural teeth surround the implant. The natural teeth have maintained the vertical dimension of occlusion.

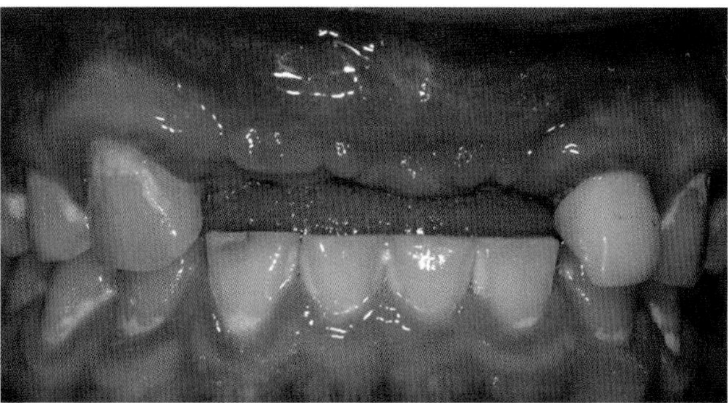

Figure 3.28. Clinical view of a patient who suffered the loss of several maxillary anterior teeth and portions of the maxillary alveolar process. Note the asymmetry in the level of the gingival margin across the anterior segment. The restorative volume available for the restorations decreases from right to left.

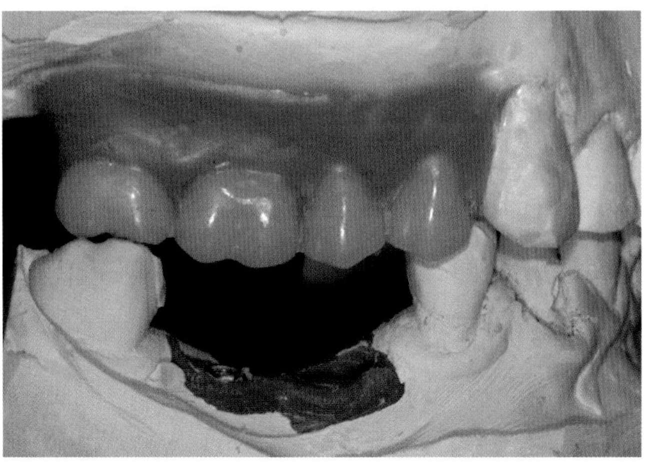

Figure 3.27. Laboratory view of a mandibular master cast mounted against a maxillary diagnostic cast. The denture teeth in the maxillary right posterior quadrant have been set into optimal positions in anticipation of the final occlusal relationships between the maxillary and mandibular prostheses.

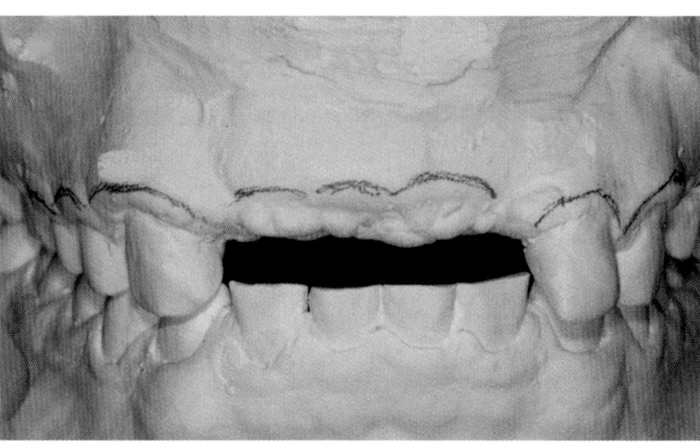

Figure 3.29. Laboratory view of diagnostic casts for the patient in Figure 3.28 mounted on a semi-adjustable articulator with an adjustable incisal guide table. The pencil lines represent the tentative location of the gingival margins of the planned restorations. This information was transferred to the implant surgeon via a surgical guide.

Surgical Guides

Surgical guides are useful in determining optimal implant positioning in both edentulous and partially edentulous patients (Garber 1995; Becker and Kaiser 2000). Surgical guides are more difficult to use in edentulous patients because once the soft tissue flaps have been reflected, the surgical guides will no longer fit as they did on the diagnostic casts due to the lack of rigid anatomical landmarks that can support the guides. Stability of surgical guides during surgery is a key element in accurate implant placement in edentulous patients. Transitional implants have been advocated for use in stabilizing surgical guides in

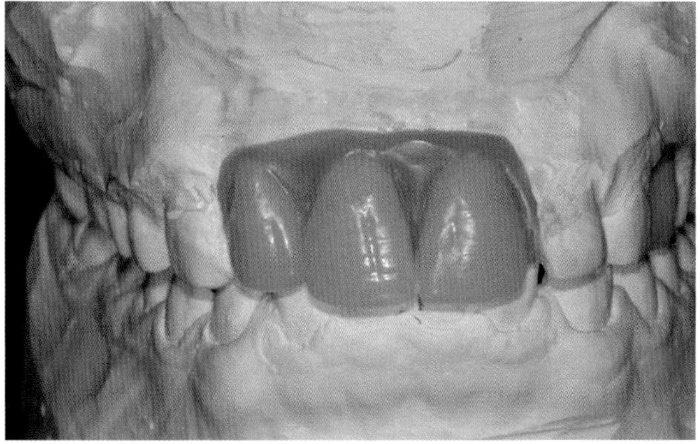

Figure 3.30. Laboratory view of diagnostic wax patterns for the patient in Figures 3.28 and 3.29. The dental midline has been placed to be consistent with the facial midline and relative symmetry has been established with the remaining natural teeth.

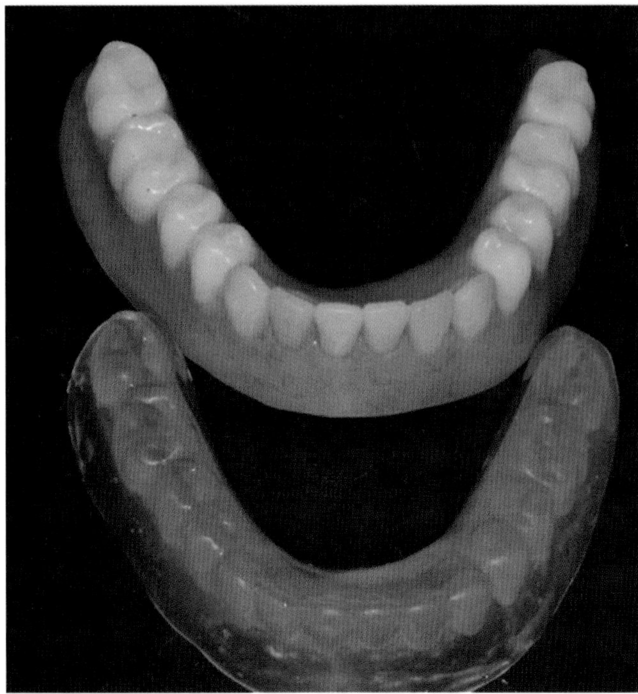

Figure 3.31. Laboratory view of a mandibular complete denture and acrylic resin surgical guide. The surgical guide was made as a duplicate complete denture with clear, autopolymerizing acrylic resin.

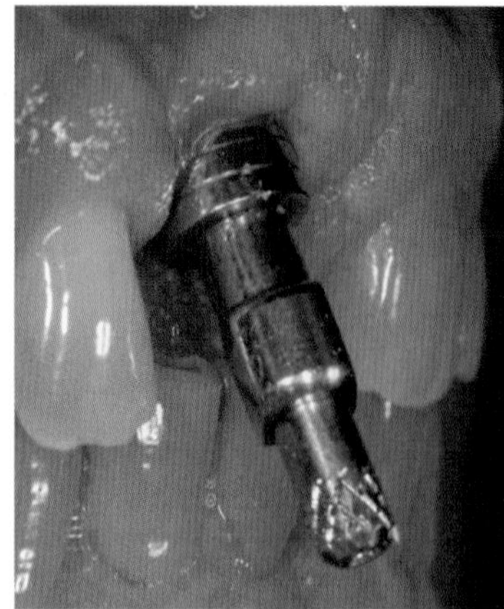

Figure 3.32. Clinical view of implant impression coping in place. Note the labial inclination and the location of the implant restorative platform approximately 5–6 mm above the cemento-enamel junctions of the adjacent teeth.

edentulous situations (Aalam and Reshad 2005). In edentulous cases, surgical guides can be made duplicating the dentures that have been made or that the patient presented with (Feldmann and Morrow 1970) (Figure 3.31).

The optimal placement of dental implants is dependent on the amount and quality of bone available at the implant sites and on the predetermined position of the implant retained restorations (Graver and Belser 1995). To avoid non-optimal implant placement, communication between the implant surgeon and restorative dentist is essential. The implant in Figure 3.32 was placed without the benefit of a surgical guide (Figure 3.32). It was placed 5–6 mm superior to the cemento-enamel junctions of the adjacent teeth, as well as with a significant labial inclination. This situation required the restorative dentist to use a custom abutment for the implant-retained crown. Surgical guides provide the surgeon with the requisite information relative to the three-dimensional placement of implants (Figure 3.33).

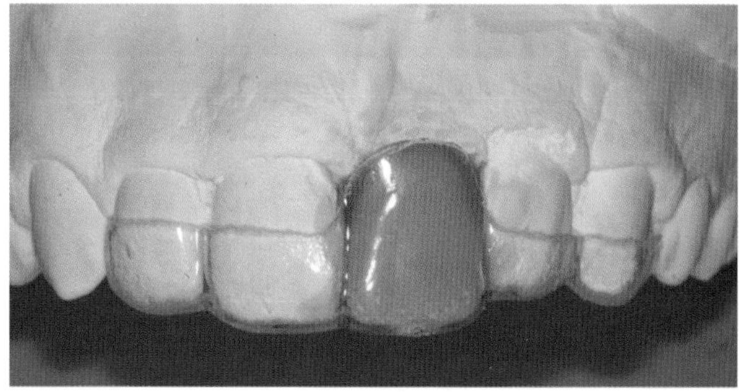

Figure 3.33. Laboratory view of surgical guide in place on a maxillary diagnostic cast. The surgical guide has been contoured and clearly identified the planned location of the cervical aspect of the implant-retained crown that will replace the maxillary left central incisor.

Surgical guides for both edentulous and partially edentulous situations may be made from multiple materials including autopolymerizing acrylic resin, heat-cured acrylic resin, and vacuum-formed materials (Sadan and Raigrodski 1997). The critical criterion for surgical guides is that they provide accurate information that identifies the predetermined position of the implant restoration(s) at the time of implant placement. If implants cannot be placed in appropriate positions to support/retain the implant restorations, consideration should be given to abandoning the implant portion of the procedure and attention be given to preparing the site for future implant placement with bone grafting.

Implant Bone Volume

One of the requirements for implant dentistry is that there has to be an adequate amount of bone available for implant placement. Long-term tooth loss is directly related to decreased bone volume in edentulous patients (Crum and Rooney 1978). Crum and Rooney used comparative cephalometric radiographs and found that the retention of mandibular canines led to preservation of alveolar bone when compared to edentulous patients over a five-year period. The vertical bone loss in the anterior mandible for edentulous patients averaged 5.2 mm; the vertical bone loss in the anterior mandible for overdenture patients aver-

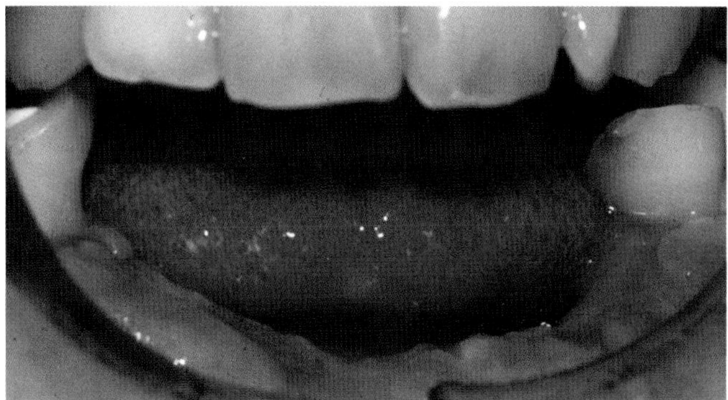

Figure 3.34. Clinical view of an anterior mandible several months after the patient experienced traumatic loss of the mandibular anterior teeth, first premolars, and a significant portion of the anterior alveolar process. A skin graft was performed as part of the reconstructive surgery in order to provide fixed, keratinized tissues in lieu of masticatory mucosa.

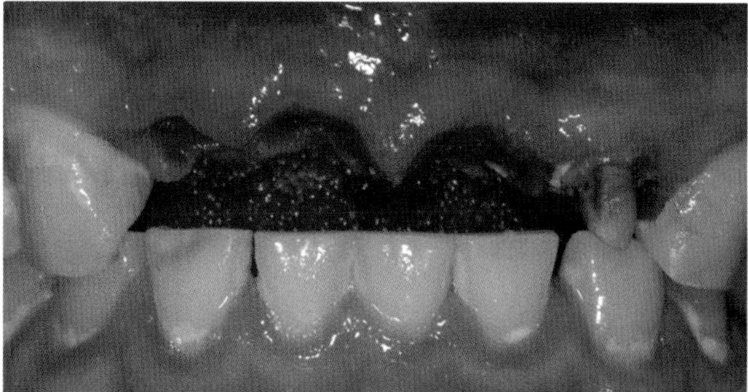

Figure 3.35. Clinical view of the anterior maxillae where three implants were placed to replace the missing central and right lateral incisors. Implant positioning was consistent with the original location of the missing teeth. Inter-dental papillae were reestablished secondary to optimal implant placement.

aged 0.6 mm. Edentulous mandibles resorb significantly faster than edentulous maxillae (Tallgren 1967, 1969).

Bone volume will also decrease secondary to traumatic loss of teeth (Figure 3.34). With appropriate treatment planning, the bone and peri-implant soft tissue anatomy can be reestablished to provide the support required for predictable and long-term function and aesthetics. If the bone and soft tissue contours are inadequate, attempts must be made to improve them prior to or during implant surgery. Restoration-driven implant treatment must include an understanding of the relationship between implants, the available bone, and surrounding soft tissue contours (Garber and Belser 1995).

Bone volume should be viewed in three dimensions to design implant placement for optimal aesthetics and function, with the appropriate implant length, diameter, restorative platform, and abutment connection (Figures 3.35 and 3.36). The supra-crestal gingival mucosa can be approximately 3 mm in depth for patients with thick periotypes and potentially 5 mm for patients with thin periotypes when the sulcus is measured adjacent to a natural tooth (Saadoun and Le Gall 2004). Sulcular depths can vary between 2.7 and 3 mm, respectively when measured in the mid-cervical area of the tooth for the 2 biotypes (Kois 1994). Implants should also ideally be surrounded by at least 2 mm of bone to minimize facial bone resorption and to develop appropriate contours to the peri-implant soft tissue (Saadoun and Le Gall 2004).

Ohrnell and Palmquist (1992) determined that at least 6.5 mm of space was needed to place a 4.0 mm diameter implant between teeth. Esposito and Ekestubbe (1993) have proposed 2 mm as the required space between the periphery of implants and adjacent natural teeth that will result in the development of acceptable inter-dental papillae. Hebel and Gajjar (1997) have suggested that a distance of 2 mm plus the radius of the implant should exist from the center of an implant to the curvature of the arch formed by the facial surfaces of the adjacent teeth.

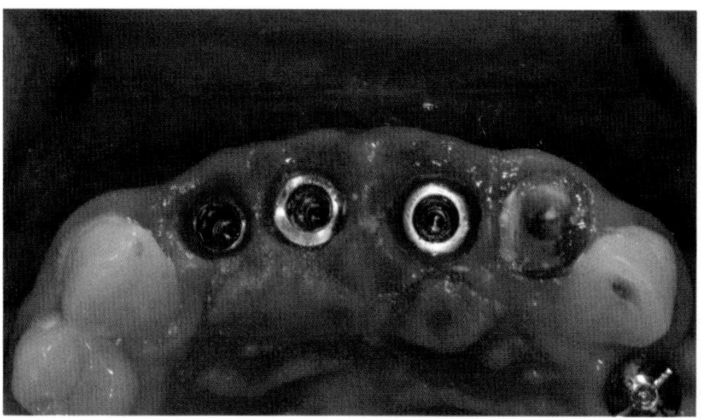

Figure 3.36. Clinical view of the implant restorative platforms of the patient in Figure 3.35. Inter-implant distance was determined at the time of the diagnostic wax patterns and transferred to the mouth via surgical guides. The implant sizes were selected based on the size of the missing teeth: 4.1 mm for the maxillary lateral incisor and 5.0 mm diameters for the maxillary central incisors.

Inter-implant distance is also a critical concern when clinicians are faced with multiple missing teeth. Tarnow and others (2000) have suggested that 3 mm of space exist between adjacent implants to prevent resorption cones around implants from fusing together. This parameter is critical if patients are to be restored with individual porcelain fused to metal crowns. Testori has recommended that 5 mm as the inter-implant distance in the aesthetic zone is safer than the 3 mm recommended above because 3 mm may cause the loss of the inter-proximal bone peak that support inter-dental papillae. (Testori and Bianchi 2005) However, in the presence of significant vertical resorption,

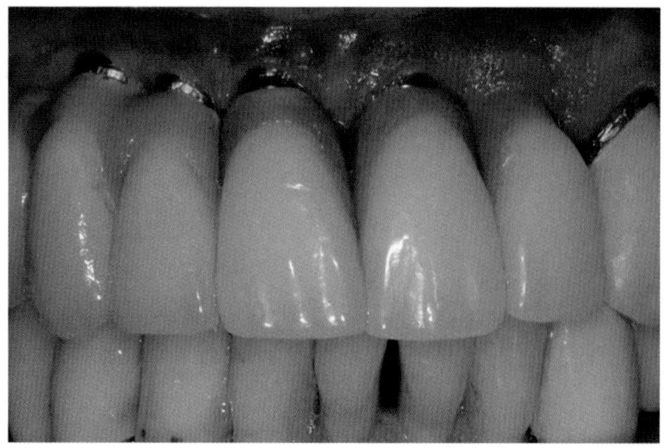

Figure 3.37. Clinical view of a patient missing multiple maxillary anterior teeth for 10 years prior to implant treatment. Vertical resorption with loss of alveolar bone and soft tissue was evident prior to implant placement and prosthetic replacement.

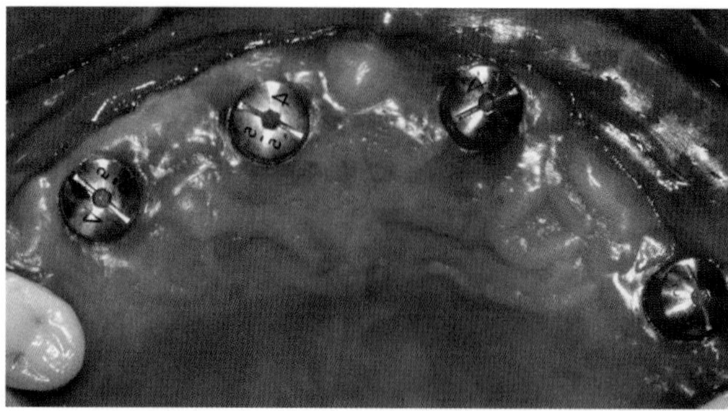

Figure 3.38. Maxillary occlusal view of a patient missing teeth from the right first premolar to the left second premolar. Implants were placed according to an edentulous criterion for a fixed, hybrid implant prosthesis.

this criterion alone will not guarantee optimal aesthetics (Figure 3.37). If a patient presents with multiple missing teeth in a large, continuous edentulous area, edentulous criteria (7–8 mm inter-implant distance) might be used for optimal implant placement (Figure 3.38, 3.39).

The height of the inter-dental papillae between natural teeth has been correlated with the distance between the inter-proximal height of bone and the dental inter-proximal contact area (Tarnow and Magner 1992) The height of the papillae between natural teeth and implants is correlated with the position of the inter-proximal height of bone adjacent to the natural teeth (Garber 1995; Saadoun 1999; Touati 2003) (Figure 3.40, 3.41). It has been demonstrated that the ideal condition for creating inter-dental papillae between natural teeth and implants is when the distance between the inter-proximal bone and the inter-proximal contact area is 3.4 mm (Choquet and Hermans 2001; Tarnow and Elian 2003).

Testori has also suggested that in the aesthetic zone, clinicians should not merely consider implant survival as the only success parameter (Testori 2005). Clinicians should also address the aesthetic results and long-term stability of the soft tissues (Kan and Rungcharassaeng 2003). Testori and others (2005) have developed an Implant Aesthetic Score based on the presence and stability of the inter-dental papillae; facial/palatal ridge stability; texture of the peri-implant soft tissue; color of the peri-implant soft tissue; and gingival contours. Perfect outcomes would yield an Implant Aesthetic Score of 9; acceptable outcome scores range from 4–8; and compromised outcomes range from 0–3.

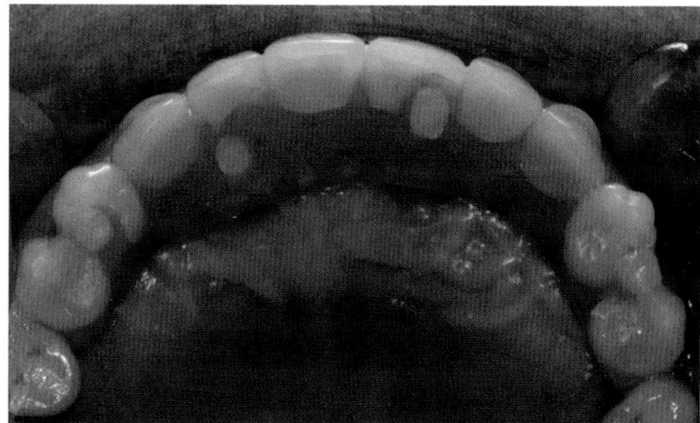

Figure 3.39. Occlusal view of maxillary fixed hybrid implant-retained prosthesis for the patient in Figure 3.38. This patient had minimal A/P resorption and required minimal lip support from the prosthesis.

Implant treatment, especially in the aesthetic zone, demands predictability and good long-term prognoses. An understanding of the biology of both the hard and soft tissues is necessary to generate optimal aesthetics. Biologic and restorative considerations must drive clinical implant treatment. Optimal treatment depends on the shape and density of the alveolar bone, the gingival biotype and thickness, and the presence of inter-proximal bone for the adjacent natural teeth. The preceding discussion has also illustrated that the three-dimensional position of the implant restorative platform, the horizontal distance between implants and adjacent teeth, the vertical distance between inter-proximal bone, and the apical inter-proximal contact areas also must be factored into implant surgical treatment.

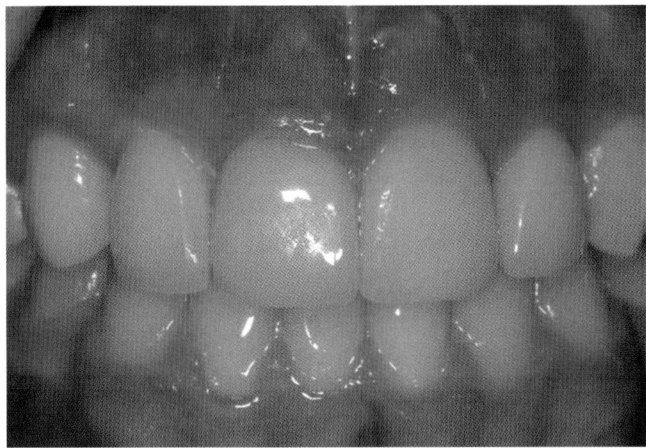

Figure 3.40. Anterior view of implant-retained crowns that replace the maxillary lateral incisors: inter-dental papillae completely fill the gingival embrasures.

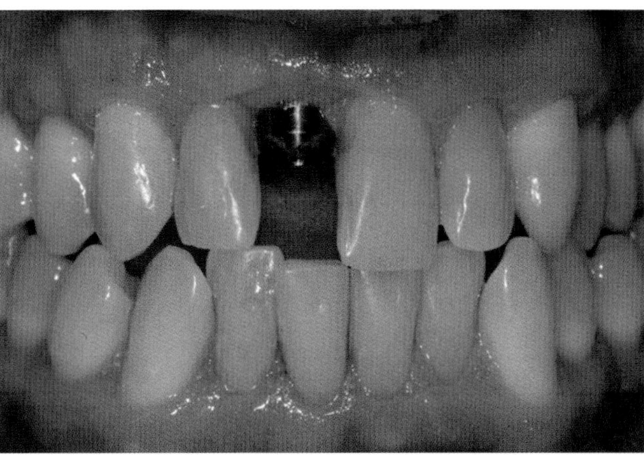

Figure 3.42. Clinical view of a healing abutment in place in the site of a missing maxillary right central incisor. The peripheral surfaces of the healing abutment were in contact with the interproximal surfaces of the adjacent teeth.

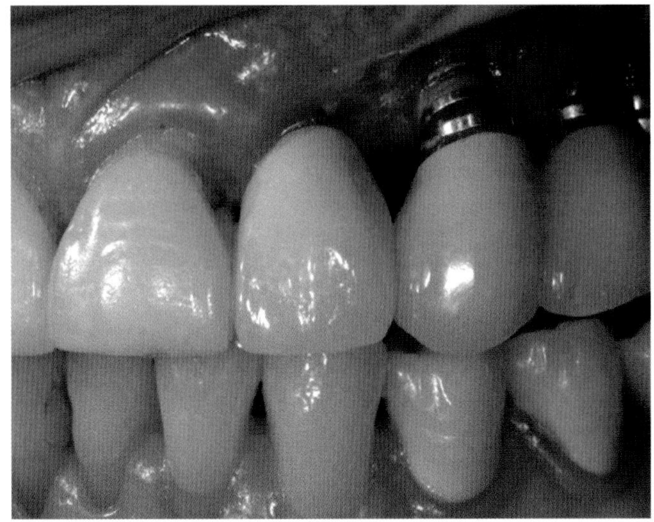

Figure 3.41. Anterior view of an implant-retained crown that replaced a maxillary lateral incisor 17 months post insertion. Note the differences in restorative volume associated with the adjacent natural tooth (maxillary central incisor) and adjacent implant restorations (maxillary canine and premolars).

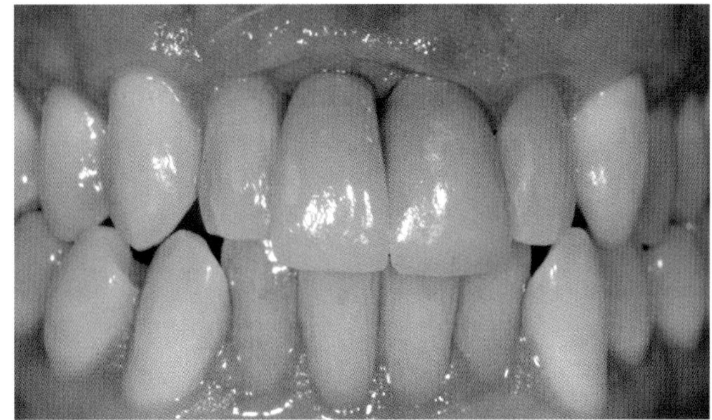

Figure 3.43. Clinical view of the implant-retained crown for the patient in Figure 3.42. Even with restoration of the left maxillary central incisor with a porcelain veneer, there was not enough restorative volume available for optimal symmetry between the two maxillary central incisors.

Implant Restorative Volume

Implant restorative volume refers to the amount of space available for the actual implant-retained restoration (Jansen and Weisgold 1995). It may refer to both removable and fixed restorations. Managing dental conditions related to premature tooth loss generally requires an interdisciplinary approach. The design of implant restorations is dependent on anatomic parameters, personal opinions, and financial data. One of the anatomic parameters involves the amount of space available for implant and prosthetic components. Too little space in any of the three dimensions for a given restoration is a contra-indication for implant surgery (Figures 3.42, 3.43). Optimal treatment in this case may have included orthodontics or inter-proximal stripping of the adjacent teeth prior to implant placement. Implant restorative volume must be viewed in conjunction with implant bone volume.

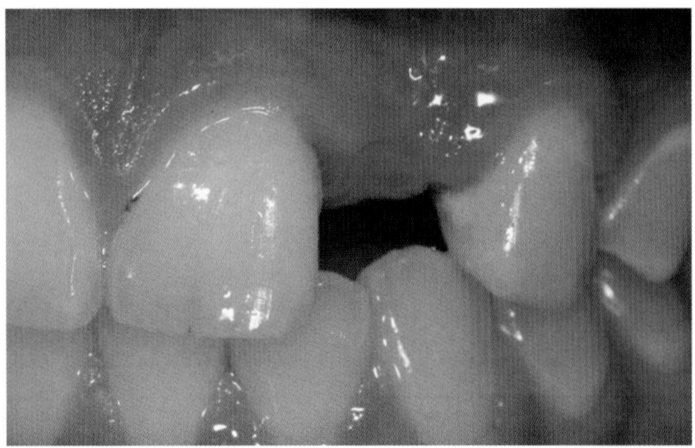

Figure 3.44. Clinical view of a patient with agenesis of the maxillary left lateral incisor. There appears to be adequate space available for an implant-retained crown.

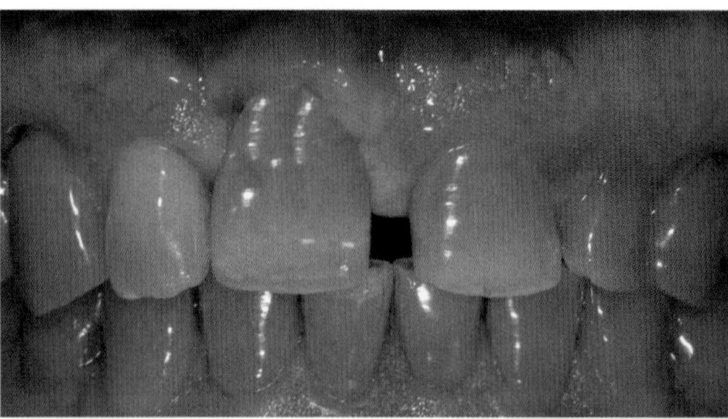

Figure 3.46. Clinical photograph of an implant-retained crown replacing a maxillary right central incisor. Due to a lack of vertical bone, the implant had to be placed approximately 5–6 mm apical to the CEJs of the adjacent natural teeth. The implant restorative volume was greater than normal and resulted in a longer implant restoration when compared to the adjacent natural teeth.

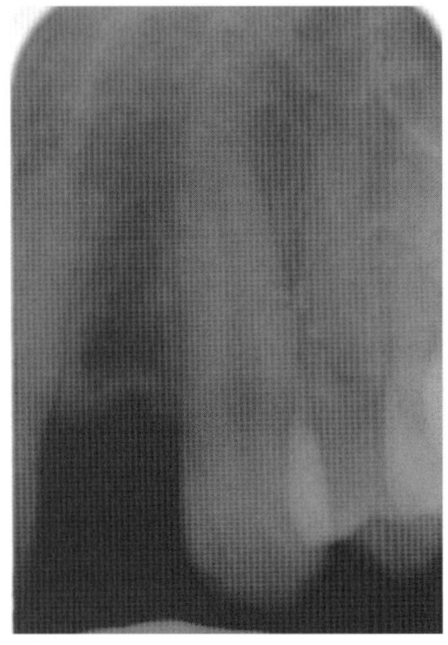

Figure 3.45. Radiograph of the patient in Figure 3.44 demonstrated that there was inadequate bone volume for implant placement in the area of the lateral incisor.

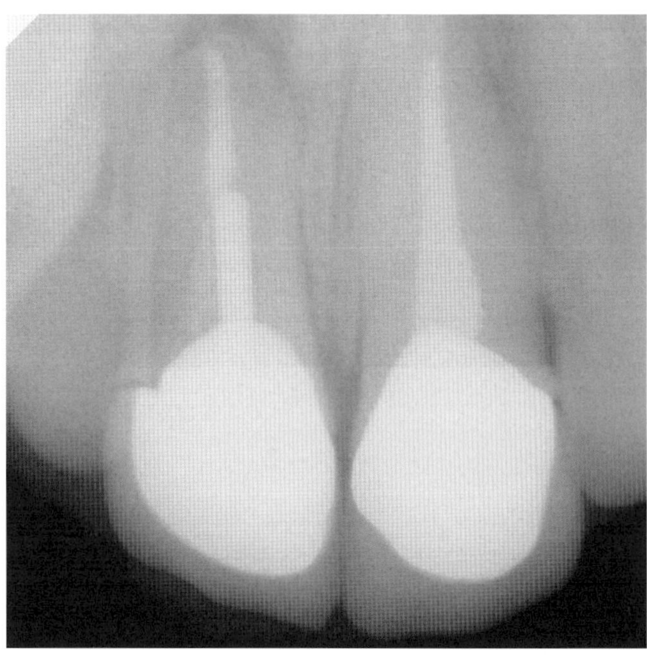

Figure 3.47. Radiograph of two maxillary central incisors. The left central incisor had a horizontal root fracture (not visible on the radiograph).

Clinicians should also not assume that edentulous spaces with adequate restorative volume always have enough bone available for implant placement (Figures 3.44, 3.45).

Implant restorative volume is also critical in the vertical plane and may be too great if the implant bone volume is deficient in the vertical plane (Figure 3.46). Kois (1994) has described variations in levels of the osseous crest based on the vertical distance of the osseous crest to the Free Gingival Margin (FGM) as normal, high and low. Kois stated that the greater the distance between the osseous crest and FGM of a natural tooth prior to extraction, the greater the risk of tissue loss post-operatively. If the depth of the gingival sulcus in the mid-facial area of a tooth is 3 mm, one may expect minimal gingival recession of 1 mm after extraction of a tooth with immediate implant placement. If the depth is significantly greater than 3 mm, there may be aesthetic compromises in the symmetry of the gingival margins (Figures 3.46–3.49).

The height of the inter-dental papillae is related to the vertical distance between the greatest height of inter-proximal bone of an adjacent tooth and the level of the inter-

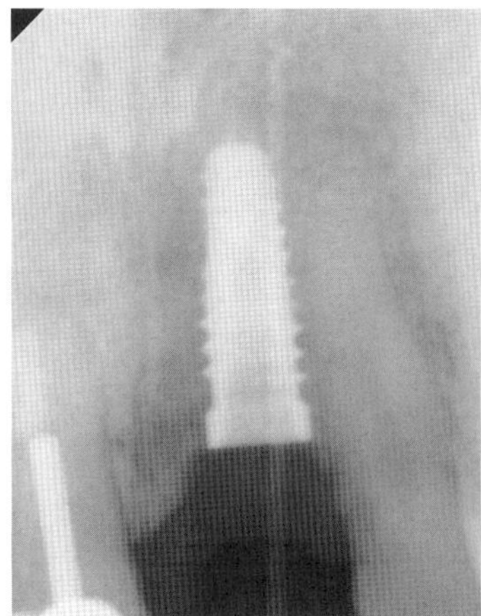

Figure 3.48. Radiograph of the implant that was placed immediately after the maxillary left central incisor in Figure 3.47 was extracted. Note the distance between the implant restorative platform and the location of the Cemento-Enamel Junctions of the adjacent teeth.

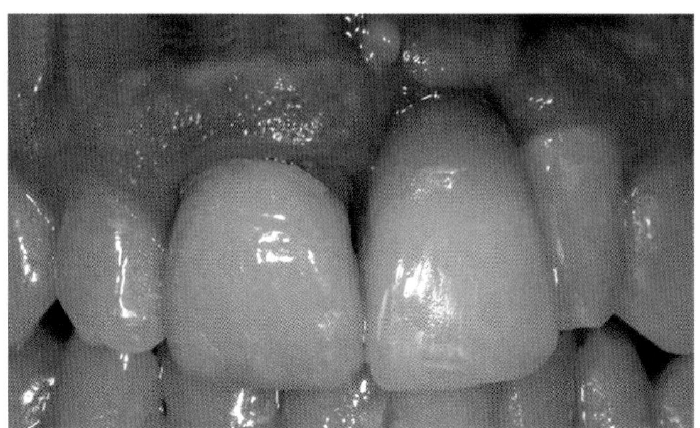

Figure 3.49. Clinical view of implant-retained crown from the patient in Figures 3.47 and 3.48. Note the length of the implant restoration relative to the lengths of the adjacent anterior teeth. Pink gingival porcelain was used to mask the height of the restoration.

proximal contact area between the natural tooth and the implant-retained crown (Tarnow and Elian 2003). If this distance is less than 4 mm, there is less risk for loss of the inter-dental papilla (Kois 2004) (Figures 3.50, 3.51).

Inadequate restorative volume can also be found in edentulous patients. The implant surgeon must be aware of the design of the planned prosthesis. In this instance, the restorative components were too large relative to the available space (Figure 3.52). This situation reduced the

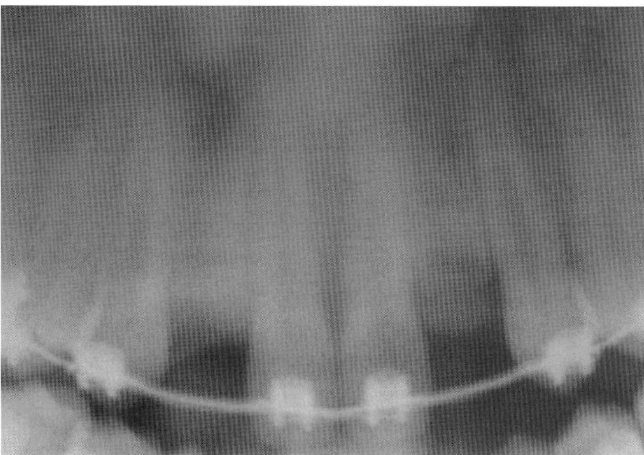

Figure 3.50. Panoramic radiograph of a patient with congenital absence of the maxillary lateral incisors. The vertical bone levels of the implant sites are within 1–2 mm of the CEJs of the adjacent natural teeth.

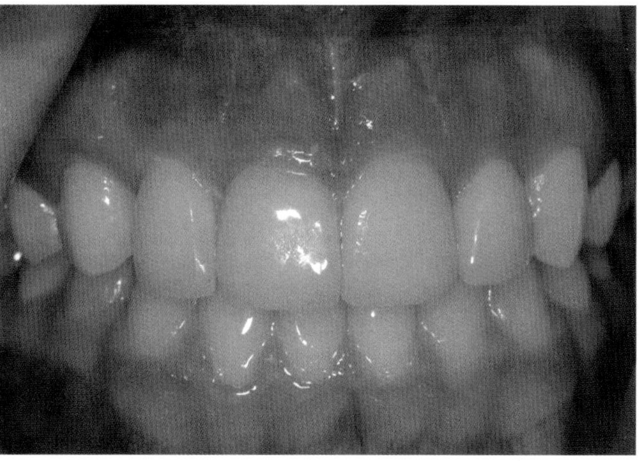

Figure 3.51. Clinical image of the implant-retained crowns replacing the missing maxillary lateral incisors of the patient in Figure 3.50. Note the presence of inter-dental papillae in the gingival embrasures surrounding the implant restorations.

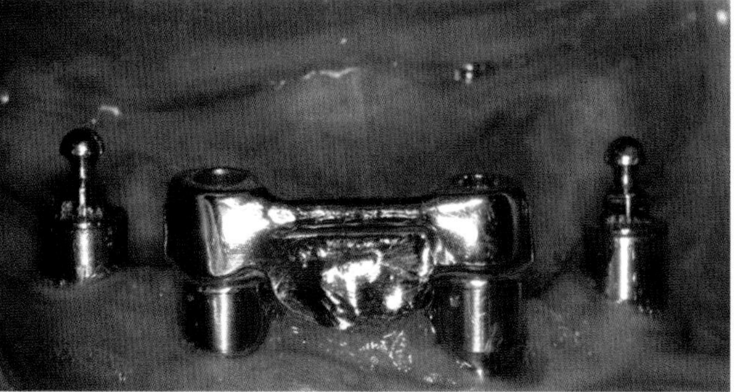

Figure 3.52. Clinical view of a cast framework and two O-ring abutments that were used to retain and support a mandibular overdenture. There was not enough restorative volume available to provide adequate thickness to the overdenture and these oversized implant restorative components.

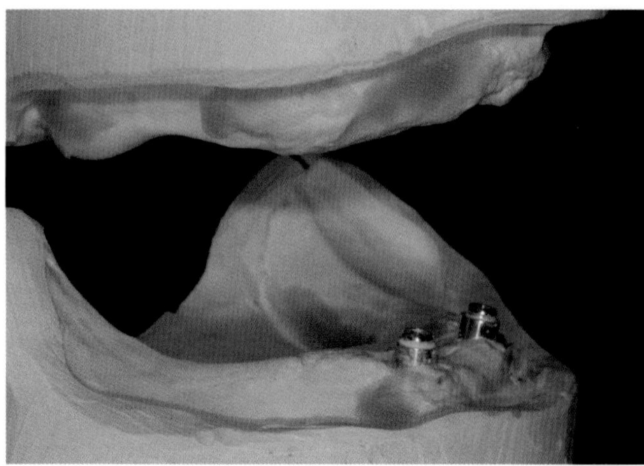

Figure 3.53. Laboratory view of mounted master casts for a patient who has been edentulous for 23 years. Note the significant amount of implant restorative volume available for implant restorative components, denture teeth, and denture bases.

restorative volume available for the removable prosthesis and caused the prosthesis to fracture. There is generally adequate implant restorative volume in patients who have been edentulous for extended lengths of time (Figure 3.53).

Treatment Planning

Treatment planning is essential for the efficient, timely treatment of patients. Dental treatment planning can be developed in the following fashion:

1. Relief of pain
2. Elimination of infection
3. Interim correction/treatment for aesthetics per patient request
4. Endodontic therapy
5. Periodontal therapy
6. Interim treatment related to significant functional impairment
7. Removal of hopeless, nonstrategic teeth
8. Occlusal treatment including occlusal adjustment and orthodontic therapy
9. Definitive treatment including surgical placement and restoration of implants

The final implant treatment plan must be deferred until the patient's condition is stabilized. At this time the oral conditions should be recharted and the patient's initial response to treatment should be reassessed. Consideration can then be given to the type of prosthesis required for a particular patient and the position and number of implants required to meet the functional and aesthetic requirements. This assessment must then be shared with the implant surgeon prior to implant surgery.

During the last 20 years, dental implants have become one of the first options that clinicians consider in the treatment of edentulous and partially edentulous patients. The advantages associated with dental implants have been presented in numerous studies and include, but are not limited to, increased chewing efficiency, improved retention and support for removable prostheses, and decreased bone loss. There are also several disadvantages associated with dental implants that include long treatment times, financial expense, multiple surgeries, and the potential to have to go without existing prostheses for several periods of time. Dentulous and edentulous patients present with different anatomical conditions and prosthetic requirements and are discussed separately.

Edentulous Patients

Patients who have lost all their natural teeth have generally been treated with complete dentures. Function, phonetics, aesthetics, and comfort are key elements of successful complete denture treatment (Terrel 1958). Edentulous patients cannot be classified as a single diagnostic group because of the significant variations among them and the different treatment modalities that may be used to treat them. McGarry and others (1999) have developed a graduated classification system that describes the varying levels of loss of denture-supporting structures. A complete discussion of this classification system is beyond the scope of this text. However several key points are addressed. (McGarry and others 2006)

The identification and measurement of residual mandibular ridge bone height is the most easily quantified objective criterion (Atwood 1962). Mandibular ridge height has been classified as Type I (most favorable: radiographic measurement of at least 21 mm of bone height at the shortest vertical height) through Type IV (least favorable: where the greatest residual height measured at the shortest level is 10 mm or less).

Residual ridge morphology is the most objective criterion for edentulous maxillae because measurement of the maxillary residual ridge height by radiography is not reliable (Davis 1997). The morphology is identified as Type A (most favorable) to Type D (least favorable). The system qualifies other anatomic conditions that include mandibular muscle attachments and maxillomandibular relationships. These classifications are then considered in the overall diagnostic classification of edentulism.

All the criteria are considered and patients are placed into a diagnostic classification system. Class I patients have residual mandibular bone heights of at least 21 mm; maxillary residual ridge morphology that will resist horizontal and vertical movement of denture bases; muscle attachments that are conducive to denture base stability and retention; and a Class I maxillomandibular relationship. Class IV patients have a mandibular residual bone height of 10 mm or less; maxillary edentulous ridges that offer no resistance to horizontal or vertical movement; muscle attachments that can be expected to have significant influence on denture base stability and retention; with Class I, II or III maxillomandibular relationships.

Experienced clinicians have noticed that clinical success in treating edentulous patients will not be guaranteed by simply making a diagnosis and performing impressions, jaw relation records, and so on. Achieving clinical success is a complex task; implant-retained or supported prostheses will not guarantee success.

Implants have proven to be successful for fixed and removable implant prostheses (Brånemark and Tolman 1998; Engquist and others 2005). In addition to anatomic considerations, clinicians also must identify existing problems that patients are experiencing and be aware of financial considerations in determining potential solutions to those problems. The prostheses can then be designed that will also include the number and location of dental implants required to support/retain the implant prostheses (Carpentieri 2004)

Overdentures

Bone remodeling is influenced by mechanical and biologic factors (Frost 1983). There has been significant discussion relative to the causes of residual ridge resorption; it is sufficient to say that residual ridge resorption occurs at varying rates for individuals and at different rates within the same individual (Atwood 1963; Tallgren 1972; Woelfel and others 1976). Due to continued residual ridge resorption, even patients with implants in the anterior mandible will need to have their overdentures relined or re-based, retentive clips changed, and resilient attachments replaced at timely intervals (Figure 3.54).

Maxillary and mandibular implant-supported/retained overdentures are significantly different from each other. This discussion concentrates on implant overdentures in the treatment of the edentulous mandible. A significant number of edentulous patients seek implant treatment that calls for multiple, splinted implants for fixed, nonremovable prostheses. However, in cases in which there has been significant resorption, a removable implant-supported overdenture may be the treatment of choice, because a flange is required to provide optimal lip support (Parel 1986) (Figures 3.55, 3.56).

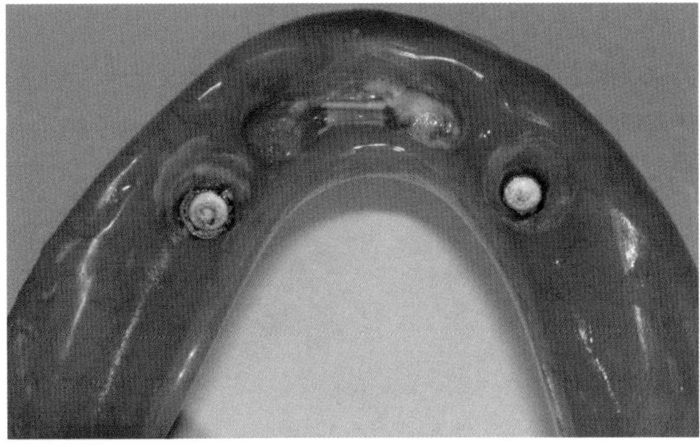

Figure 3.54. Intaglio surface of a mandibular implant-supported overdenture for which the patient did not return for recall appointments on a timely basis. Notice the damage to the O-rings and the plastic retentive clip.

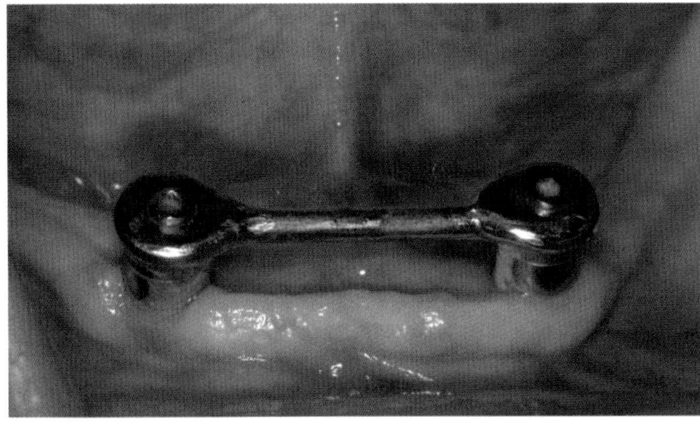

Figure 3.55. Intra-oral photograph of 2 mandibular implants splinted with a cast bar to support and retain a mandibular overdenture (10 years post insertion).

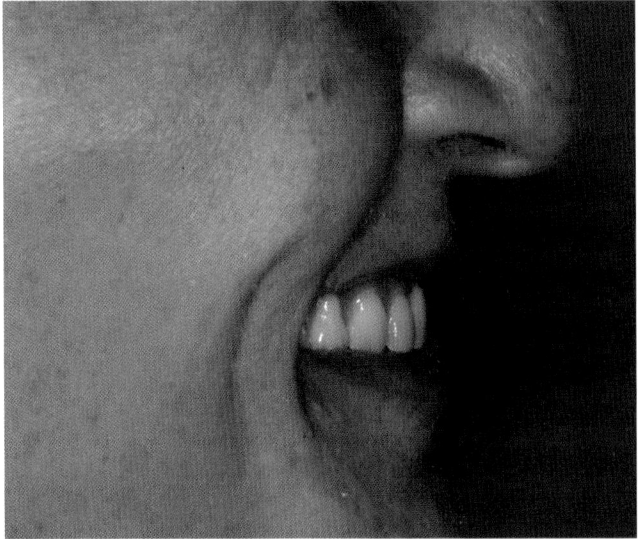

Figure 3.56. Extra-oral photograph of the patient in Figure 3.54 where due to the loss of the mandibular teeth and alveolar bone, the mandibular overdenture flange was required to support the lower lip, consistent with the patient's aesthetic requirements.

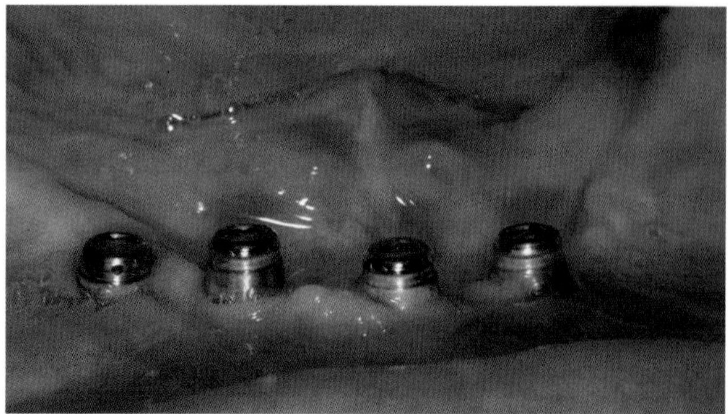

Figure 3.57. Clinical image of four unsplinted implants with resilient overdenture abutments in place. In the presence of severe resorption, lack of adequate space is rarely a clinical challenge.

Multiple mandibular implants can preserve and maintain more bone than two implants that have been placed in the anterior segments. Removable implant prostheses require less bone for implants than do their fixed prosthetic counterparts (Hobo 1989) and can be considerably less expensive to fabricate (Walton and MacEntee 1994). One of the more common methods used to treat edentulous patients was to place and splint the implants together with a cast bar. Attachments could be fabricated within the bars for additional retention (Naert, Quirynen, and others 1994). Alternatively, implants could be used and not splinted together.

Overdentures tend to be space sensitive, and therefore proper treatment planning and communication between the restorative dentist and implant surgeon is essential. Unsplinted mandibular implants generally require 5 to 7 mm of vertical restorative space and have to be placed within the dimensions of the denture base (Figure 3.57). Splinted implants generally require at least 9 to 11 mm of vertical restorative space, have to be placed within the denture base, and must allow adequate thickness for acrylic resin to withstand masticatory forces without fracturing (Figure 3.58).

The relative success of the two methods has been the subject of multiple studies (Naert, De Clercq, and others 1988; Engquist 1991). Kirsch (1991) reported that unsplinted implants were not successful over time. Mericske-Stern (1994) reported that there was no difference in clinical success between bar-clip and ball attachment-retained overdentures. In a one-year randomized clinical trial, Walton and others (2002) reported that fabrication time, number of appointments, and chair time were similar for prostheses made with bar/clip or ball attachment retentive elements. However, the ball attachment dentures required about eight times longer repair times than did repairs for bar/clip overdentures.

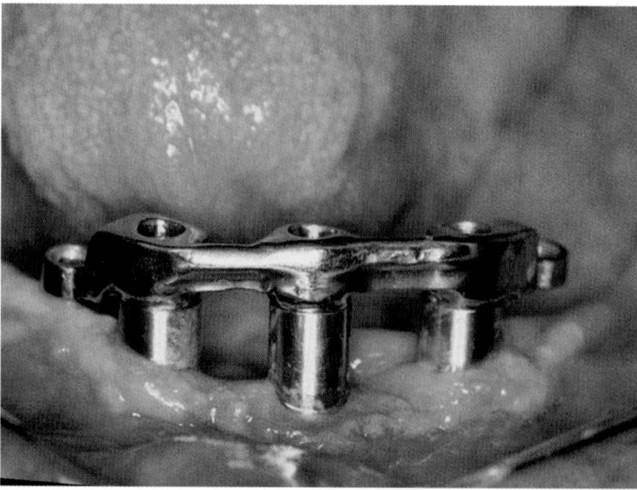

Figure 3.58. Intra-oral view of an implant-retained bar that splinted three mandibular implants. Note the significant height of the abutments and casting. The increased bulk of the casting required increased thickness in the lingual denture flange or an increased risk of denture fracture. Due to the limited inter-arch distance, this patient may have been better served with non-splinted overdenture attachments.

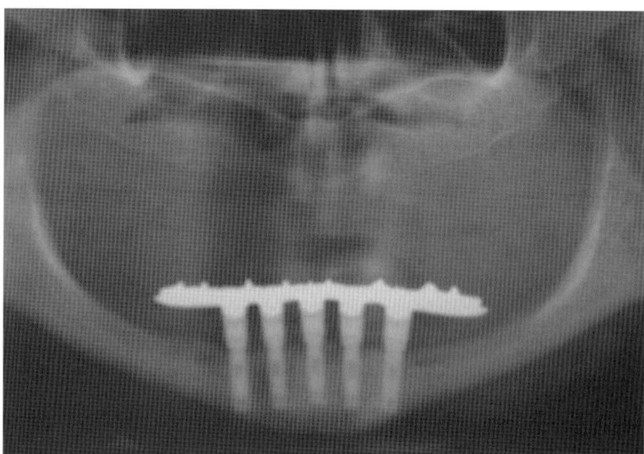

Figure 3.59. Panoramic radiograph of a patient at the 10-year recall appointment. Pre-operatively, this patient had experienced considerable bone resorption in the mandible. The patient did not wish to undergo bone grafting for the resorption in the posterior mandibular segments. However, the patient did have adequate bone volume between the mental foramen for implants and has successfully maintained the implants and anterior bone volume for 10 years.

Fixed Hybrid Implant-Retained Prostheses-Edentulous Mandible

The use of osseointegrated implants in the treatment of the edentulous mandible is the most documented type of dental implant therapy (Adell and others 1981). Placement of 4–6 endosseous implants between or distal to the mental foraminae with either single-stage or two-stage surgical

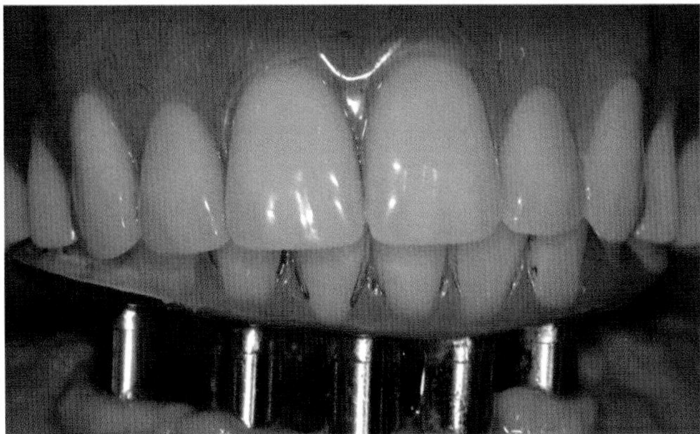

Figure 3.60. Intra-oral photograph of a patient with a maxillary complete denture and a mandibular fixed implant-retained prosthesis at the 12-year recall appointment.

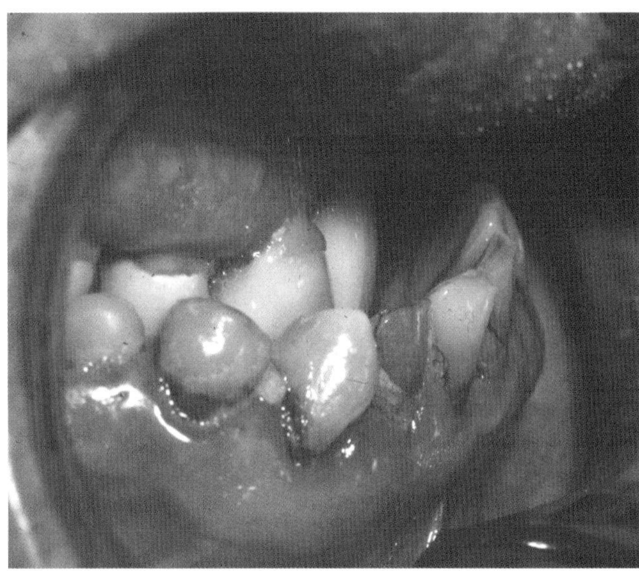

Figure 3.62. Clinical photograph of a patient with a severe Class III malocclusion. This patient would probably not do well with conventional complete dentures.

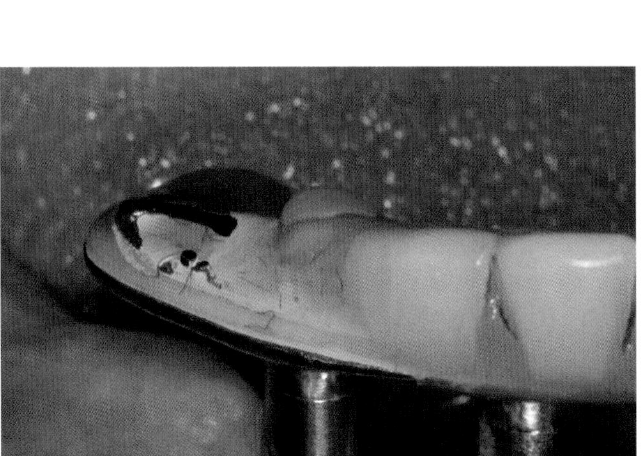

Figure 3.61. Intra-oral photograph of the right posterior segment of the patient in Figure 3.60 that demonstrates significant occlusal abrasion of the mandibular prosthesis. The amount of occlusal abrasion demonstrated by this edentulous patient was unusual, but illustrates how much force an edentulous patient can generate with osseointegrated implants.

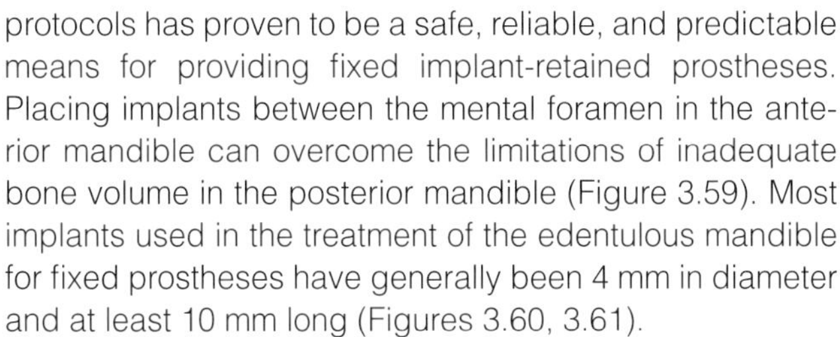

protocols has proven to be a safe, reliable, and predictable means for providing fixed implant-retained prostheses. Placing implants between the mental foramen in the anterior mandible can overcome the limitations of inadequate bone volume in the posterior mandible (Figure 3.59). Most implants used in the treatment of the edentulous mandible for fixed prostheses have generally been 4 mm in diameter and at least 10 mm long (Figures 3.60, 3.61).

Fixed implant-retained prostheses provide patients with the most stable and retentive prostheses. They have been particularly useful in patients who cannot manage conventional complete dentures secondary to severe resorption, trauma, severe malocclusions, or tumors (Figure 3.62). The patient illustrated in Figure 3.62 presented with a severe Class III malocclusion and periodontal disease. He decided to have his remaining teeth extracted and initially replaced them with complete dentures. He was unable to manage the complete dentures and proceeded with implant placement and construction of a fixed implant-retained prosthesis.

Fixed Hybrid Implant-Retained Prostheses-Edentulous Maxillae

Treatment of edentulous maxillae with dental implants is considered to be more challenging than treatment of edentulous mandibles (Adell and others 1970; Jemt 1993; Lekholm and Zarb 1983; Misch 1993). The upper jaw is actually composed of paired maxillary bones. The maxillary complex sustains and protects the organs associated with sight, smell, and taste. Each maxillary bone contains an air-filled sinus that is connected to the other sinuses of the face.

The maxillary alveolar ridge is also responsive to physical stimuli. Compressive forces can destroy the maxillary alveolus after the natural teeth have been lost (Atwood 1963). The maxillae generally resorb vertically and medially, whereas edentulous mandibles resorb anteriorly and

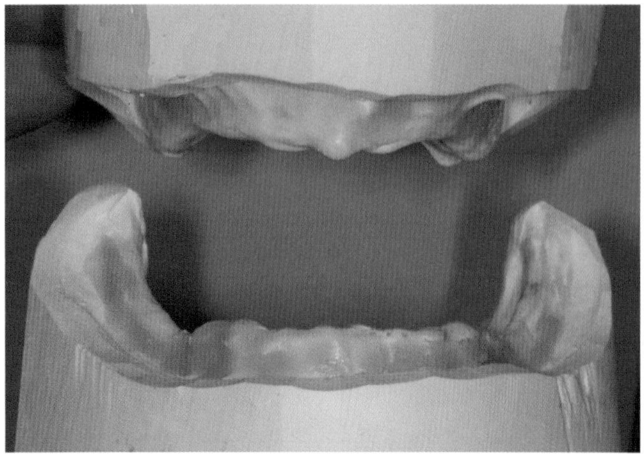

Figure 3.63. Laboratory mounting of edentulous master casts at the determined vertical dimension of occlusion. Note that the maxillary edentulous ridge is within the confines of the mandibular edentulous ridge.

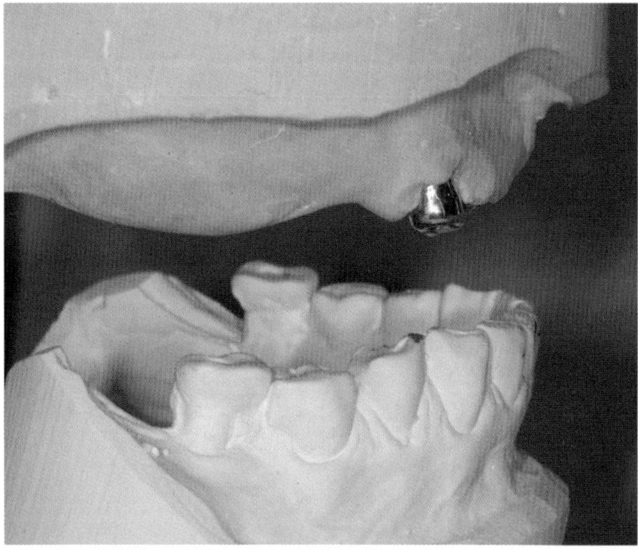

Figure 3.64. Laboratory mounting of an edentulous maxillary cast approximately 15 years post implant placement. Note the minimal anterior/posterior resorption that has occurred relative to the casts in Figure 3.63. This edentulous maxilla has been physiologically loaded by virtue of the endosseous implants and has undergone minimal resorption.

laterally (Figures 3.63, 3.64). This resorption pattern is partly responsible for the difficulties encountered in replacing the maxillary dentition with a fixed implant-retained prosthesis, because often a denture flange is required to provide lip support (Figures 3.65–3.68).

The loss of mechanical stimulation within the maxillary alveolus leads to resorption, and this needs to be anticipated for both surgical placement of implants and the prosthetic reconstruction. (Schnitman 1998) Long-term

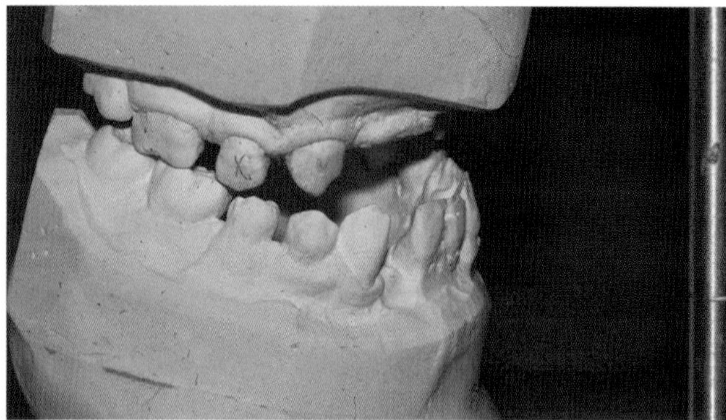

Figure 3.65. Laboratory articulator mounting of a patient with retrognathic maxillae associated with cleidocranial dysostosis. This type of jaw relationship would be a contra-indication for a fixed implant-retained prosthesis because a flange would be needed for lip support.

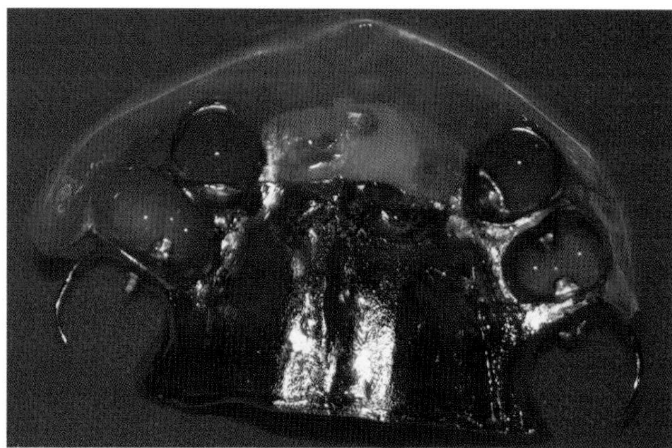

Figure 3.66. Laboratory view of the removable partial overdenture used to treat the patient in Figure 3.65. The labial flange was required to provide optimal support for the upper lip and compensated for the anterior/posterior skeletal deficiency of the maxillae relative to the mandible.

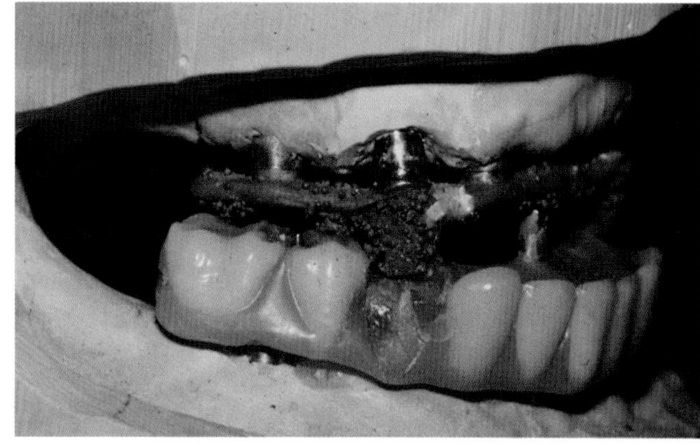

Figure 3.67. Laboratory view of articulated edentulous maxillary and mandibular casts. Note the anterior/posterior deficiency of the anterior maxillary ridge relative to the labial surface of the mandibular waxed denture. This patient wanted a fixed, implant-retained prosthesis. The initial prosthesis was designed with a labial flange for optimal lip support.

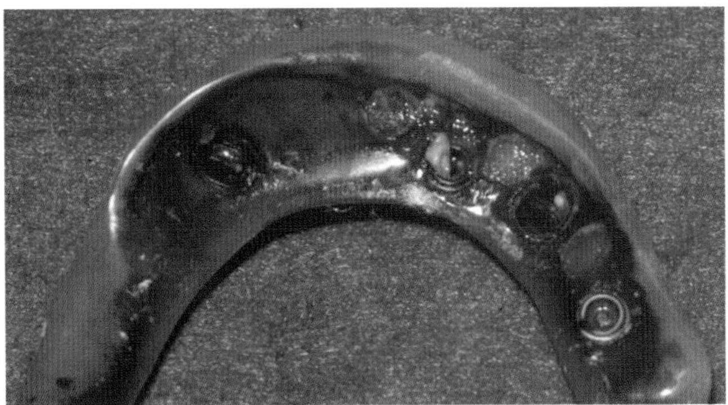

Figure 3.68. Intaglio surface of the maxillary fixed implant-retained prosthesis one month post insertion for the patient in Figure 3.67. The thickness and depth of the labial flange precluded oral hygiene procedures in and around the abutments. This resulted in significant plaque accumulation along with extrinsic staining of the intaglio surface of the fixed prosthesis. For this patient, a fixed implant-retained prosthesis was contra-indicated due to the amount of anterior/posterior maxillary resorption and the amount of lip support required to satisfy the patient's aesthetic requirements.

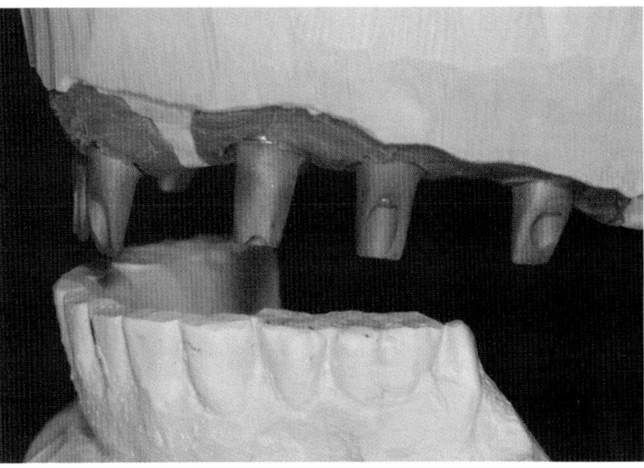

Figure 3.70. Laboratory articulator mounting of the edentulous maxillary cast with implant abutments for a porcelain fused to metal FPD from Figure 3.69. Note and contrast the relationship between the labial surfaces of the maxillary anterior abutments and the facial surfaces of the mandibular teeth in this figure with the relationship demonstrated in Figure 3.67. Minimal anterior/posterior resorption is correlated with less need for labial flanges in maxillary implant prostheses.

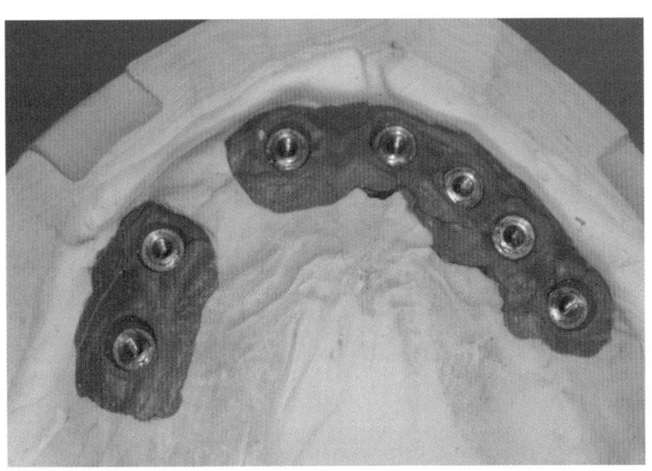

Figure 3.69. Laboratory view of an edentulous maxillary cast with seven implant analogs. These implants were restored with individual custom cast abutments and all of the teeth were replaced with three fixed partial dentures.

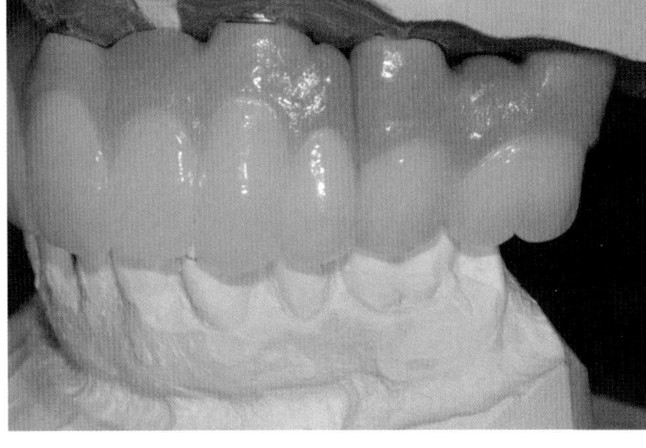

Figure 3.71. Laboratory view of the left maxillary FPD from Figures 3.69 and 3.70. This patient did not require a flange for lip support. The maxillary anterior FPD provided appropriate lip support with the contours of the metal/ceramic prosthesis.

success for fixed implant-retained maxillary prostheses has been achieved with 4–8 implants (Brånemark 1977); some authors have suggested that 8–12 implants are required (Scortecci 1999). In the case of minimal anterior/posterior maxillary resorption, a fixed implant-retained prosthesis can be utilized to replace a missing maxillary dentition (Figures 3.69–3.71).

Partially Edentulous Patients

Dental implants may also be used to successfully treat partially edentulous patients missing one or more teeth. The procedures associated with replacing single missing teeth with implant-supported restorations have high success rates, do not involve irreversible preparation of the adjacent natural teeth, typically yield high patient satisfaction, and have been documented in virtually all anatomic locations within either arch (Naert and others 2000; Haas and others 2002; Krennmair and others 2003; Vermylen and others 2003).

Treatment Goals

Sadan and others (2004) identified two treatment goals for replacing single missing teeth with dental implant restorations: restoration of occlusal stability with opposing and adjacent natural teeth; and creation of an illusion of a natural dento-gingival complex. In a perfect world, all the preceding goals should be accomplished in every clinical situation. However, the significance of each goal may be different for patients with missing teeth in different anatomic locations.

Sadan and others (2004) have recommended that the dental implant restoration must first achieve the treatment goals that are crucial to the location of the missing tooth and then achieve the remaining goals only if they can be accomplished in a practical manner. This approach may preclude additional surgeries and/or multiple procedures. They have classified implant restorations into anterior versus posterior. Posterior restorations should first satisfy occlusal function; anterior restorations may address aesthetics first (Figure 3.72, 3.73).

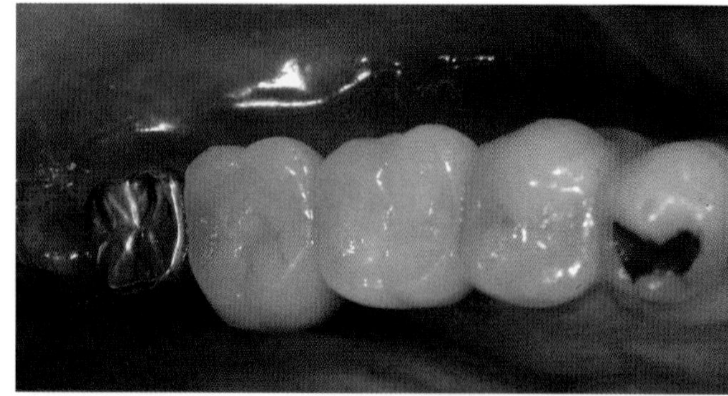

Figure 3.72. Occlusal view of three individual implant crown restorations replacing the mandibular left first and second molars and the left second premolar. Note the decreased occlusal table for the second molar restoration. This crown was supported by a 4.1 mm by 8.5 mm implant. The decreased occlusal table minimized the cantilevers that may have been evident if the crown was made with a normal occlusal table for a second molar.

Screw-Retained Restorations

Single-implant restorations may be either screw- or cement-retained. Both of these designs have benefits and limitations for restorative dentists and patients. The most advantageous design feature for screw-retained crowns involves the issue of retrievablility of implant restorations (Jemt and others 1991). The success or failure of implant restorations often depends on the success or failure of the abutment/implant connection (Figure 3.74). Screw-retained single unit implant restorations may have the advantage of using titanium trans-gingival cylindrical abutments that provide an optimal biologic seal (Figure 3.75). However, standard titanium abutments do not provide the emergence profile required of natural teeth (Figure 3.76).

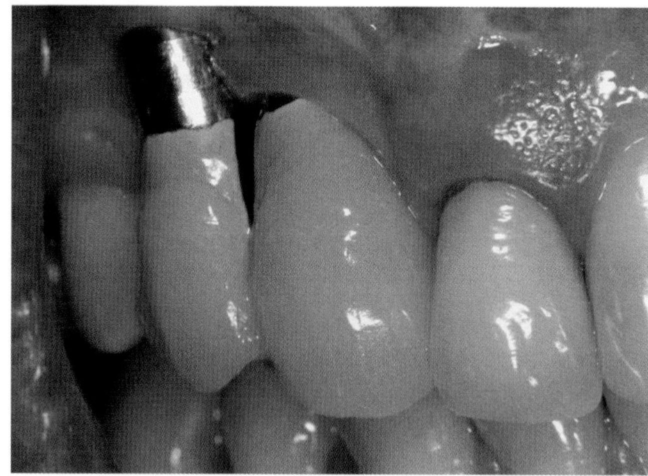

Figure 3.73. Clinical buccal view of individual implant restorations replacing the maxillary right first premolar and canine teeth 10 years post restoration. The peri-implant soft tissues surrounding the implant in the first premolar site apparently did not have an adequate blood supply to sustain the soft tissues around the implant abutment. The soft tissue receded and exposed the implant abutment. However, this patient had a low lip line and did not expose the implant restorations during speaking or smiling. The canine restoration was visible during speaking and smiling and satisfied the patient's aesthetic needs.

The most problematic characteristic associated with implant retained single-unit restorations involves the risk of screw loosening. There have been numerous reports of screw loosening and/or screw fracture in implant dentistry (Jemt and others 1992; Becker and Becker, 1995; Goodacre and others, 1999). Screw loosening of small cylinder retaining screws was encountered more frequently than abutment screw loosening. Screw-retained restorations that included abutments and cylinders required a significant amount of inter-occlusal clearance in order to provide sufficient space for all the implant restorative components. If vertical space was limited, the retaining screws were frequently exposed to the oral cavity, and occlusal morphology was sacrificed (Figure 3.77).

Screw retention may be the treatment of choice if the implant margin extends greater than 3 mm into the subgingival environment (Taylor and others 2000). This rationale has been explained as the limited capacity for removal of excess cement. With continued technological advances including precise machining, enhanced screw surfaces, and predictable application of appropriate torque, abutment screw loosening does not seem to be a significant clinical problem (Keith and others 1999; Drago 2003).

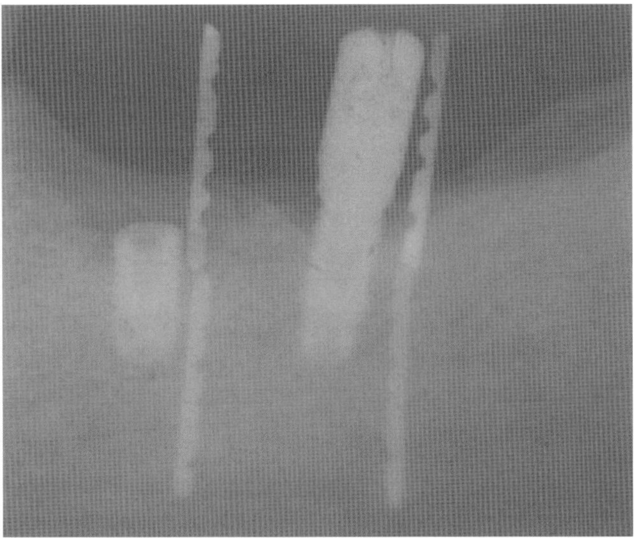

Figure 3.74. Radiograph of two implants in the left posterior mandible: the posterior, 4.1 mm by 10 mm implant fractured 18 months post insertion under occlusal loading and had to be removed.

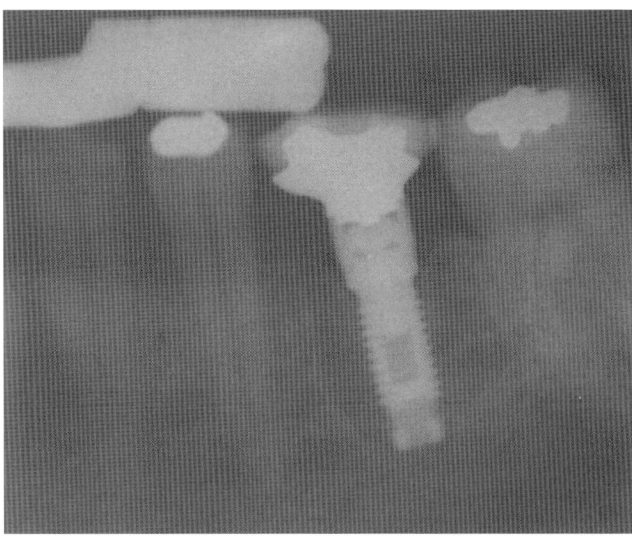

Figure 3.76. Radiograph of the abutment in Figure 3.75. Note the cylindrical, non-anatomic shape of the standard abutment.

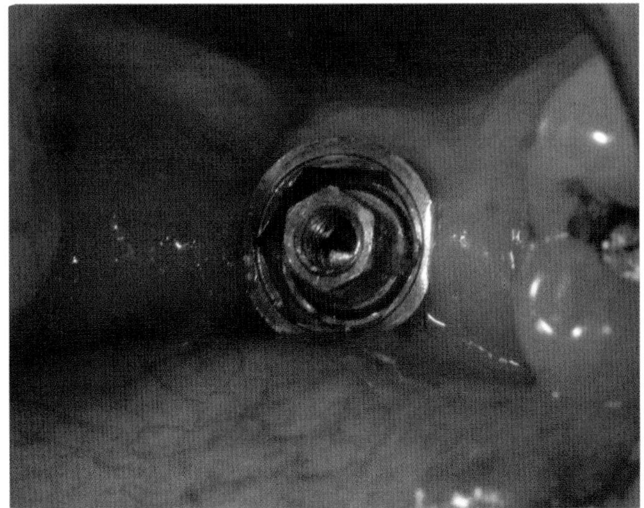

Figure 3.75. Occlusal surface of a standard abutment that had been used in conjunction with a gold cylinder for a screw-retained crown restoration replacing the mandibular left first molar. The gold retaining screw had fractured inside the channel of the abutment screw. Note the healthy appearance of the peri-implant tissues surrounding the titanium abutment.

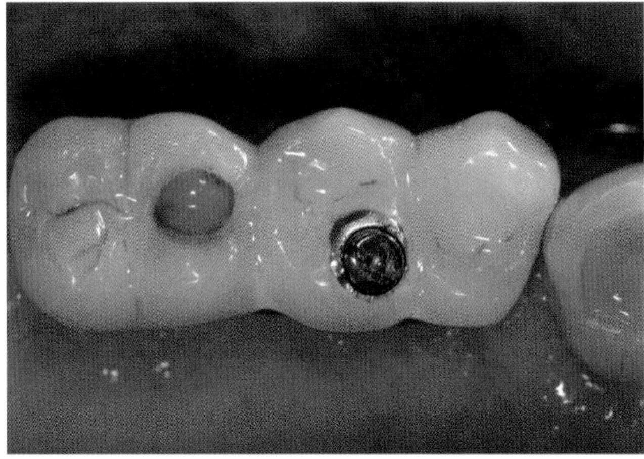

Figure 3.77. Occlusal view of a screw-retained implant prosthesis 10 years post insertion. The prosthesis was designed as two crowns, splinted together to replace two maxillary molars. The prosthesis was supported by two 4.1 mm diameter implants. In the event that one or more of the screws became loose, the prosthesis could be retightened.

Cement-Retained Restorations

The major limitation in using cement-retained single-unit implant restorations was the potential of an abutment screw becoming loose, while the cement-retained crown remained cemented to the abutment (Sadan and others 2004). This clinical situation would involve sectioning the cement-retained crown in order to get access to the abutment screw. A loose abutment screw might necessitate remaking the cement-retained crown.

Cement-retained single-unit implant restorations are indicated where angle correction is needed and the long axis of the implant would create a screw access opening in the facial or buccal surface of a screw-retained single-unit implant restoration. This is frequently seen in the anterior maxillae in which the orientation of the alveolus is not coincidental with the angulation of the teeth (Figures 3.78, 3.79).

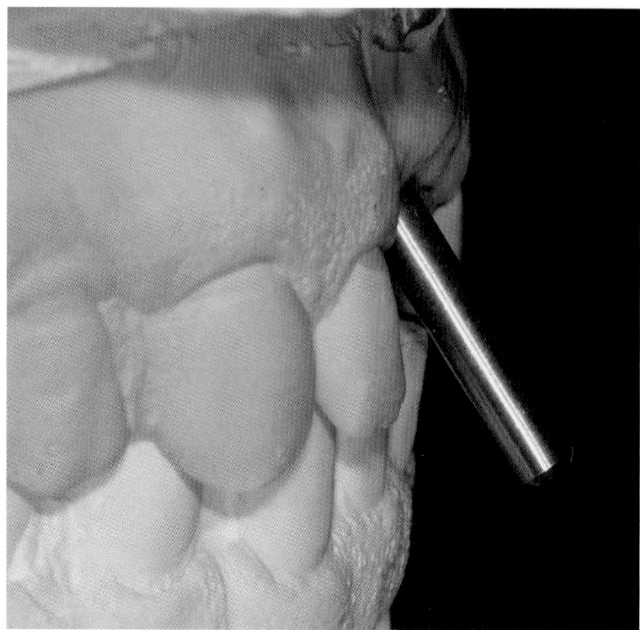

Figure 3.78. Lateral view of a laboratory abutment screw that was screwed into an implant laboratory analog. The implant was placed appropriately within the alveolus. For a screw-retained restoration, the screw access opening would have been located in the gingival third of the crown restoration. An abutment and cement-retained crown was the treatment of choice for optimal replacement of this missing tooth.

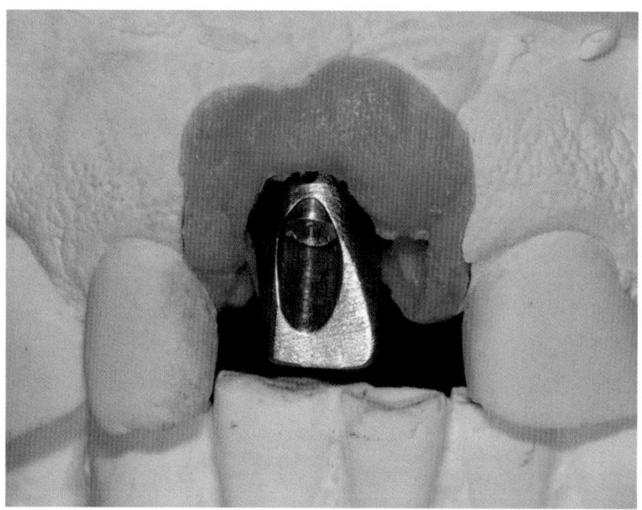

Figure 3.79. Facial view of the custom implant abutment in place on the master cast from Figure 3.78. Note the minimal vertical height of the facial surface of the abutment and the location of the screw access opening. The crown cemented to this abutment was retained by virtue of the retention and resistance form generated with the abutment design, similar to crown retention on natural teeth preparations.

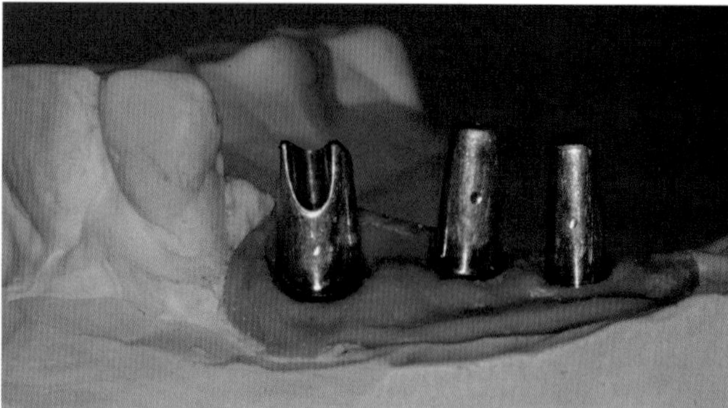

Figure 3.80. Three titanium alloy custom abutments in place on a master cast that will be used in conjunction with three individual cement-retained crowns.

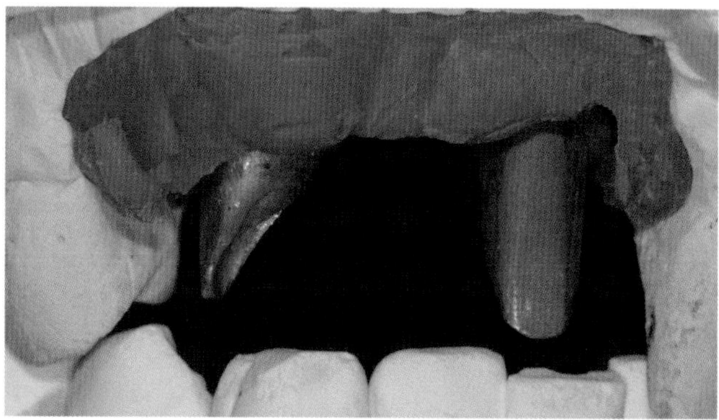

Figure 3.81. Laboratory view of a custom gold alloy cast UCLA Abutment (maxillary right cuspid) and a stock, pre-machined titanium alloy abutment (GingiHue® Post, maxillary right central incisor). The custom UCLA Abutment was needed because the distal implant was placed in a more mesial location than originally treatment planned. The axial walls of both abutments were prepared with minimal taper to provide retention and resistance form for retention for the 3-unit fixed partial denture.

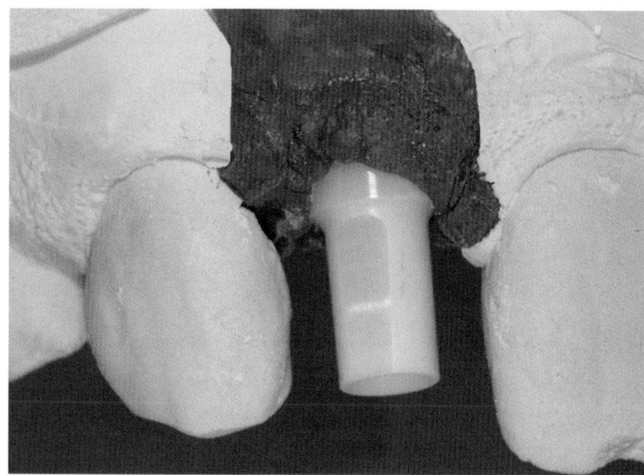

Figure 3.82. Laboratory facial view of zirconia abutment (ZiReal™ Post), as received from the manufacturer, in place on a master cast. The abutment will be prepared consistent with preparation guidelines for a natural tooth to be restored with an all-ceramic crown.

Cement-retained implant crowns require the use of abutments with configurations similar to those associated with preparation of natural teeth: 6° axial convergence, subgingival margin placement in aesthetic areas, and adequate reduction in preparation for appropriate thickness of restorative materials (Salinas and others 2004). Abutments may be made from titanium, cast gold alloys or high-strength ceramics (Figures 3.80–3.82). Each of these materials will be illustrated in the appropriate clinical chapters.

Implant Loading Protocols

Two-Stage Surgical Protocol

The concept of osseointegration of dental implants is based on research that began in 1952 with microscopic studies of bone marrow in rabbit's fibula (Brånemark 1959). Through animal and human controlled experimental studies, it was found that a titanium implant inserted into an osteotomy of a predetermined size, allowed to heal without macroscopic movement in an unloaded, nonfunctional environment, became surrounded by a layer of compact bone without soft tissue interposed between implant and bone (Brånemark 1983). The first edentulous patient was treated in 1965 using Brånemark's principles of osseointegration with a two-stage surgical protocol and unloaded healing.

With this protocol, a full thickness muco-periosteal flap was reflected and the edentulous ridge was exposed. Osteotomies were prepared into the bone at preselected sites, consistent with the design of the definitive implant-retained prosthesis. The osteotomies were gradually enlarged with a series of drills with increasing diameters until a certain diameter was reached, consistent with the size of the planned implants. The implants were placed into the osteotomies below the crest of bone, and cover screws were applied and hand tightened. The flap was primarily closed and the patient was dismissed. The implants were allowed to heal without occlusal function for a period of three to four months in mandibles and at least six months in maxillae (Brånemark and others 1977). Patients generally could not wear their preexisting dentures for the first several days after this first surgery. The dentures were then relieved and relined with a tissue conditioning material that would be changed periodically during osseous healing (Figures 3.83, 3.84). The implants were then uncovered and transmucosal abutments were placed in preparation for the prosthetic treatment (Figure 3.85).

The original purpose of osseointegration in clinical dentistry was to rehabilitate the edentulous or partially edentulous patient back to a state similar to a dentate condition. Adell and others (1981) published one of the initial long-term studies that reported on the success of osseointegrated implants in edentulous jaws. During a 15-year period, 2,768 implants were placed into 410 edentulous

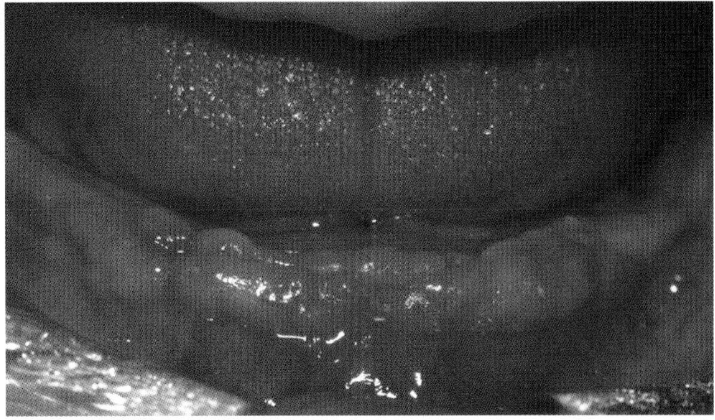

Figure 3.83. Clinical photograph of an edentulous mandible two weeks after four implants were placed with a two-stage surgical protocol.

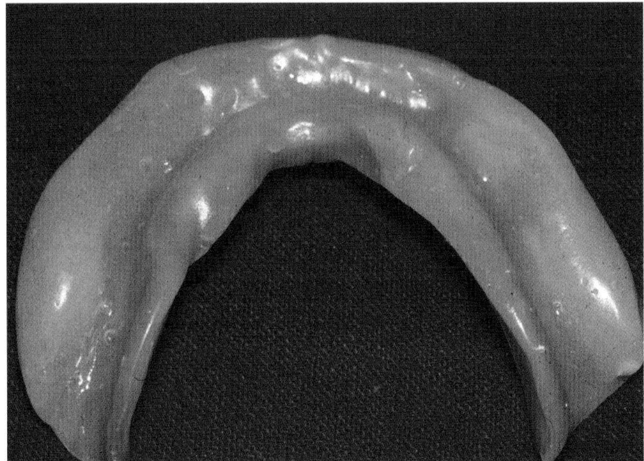

Figure 3.84. Intaglio surface of the complete denture for the patient in Figure 3.83 after it was relined with a tissue conditioning material.

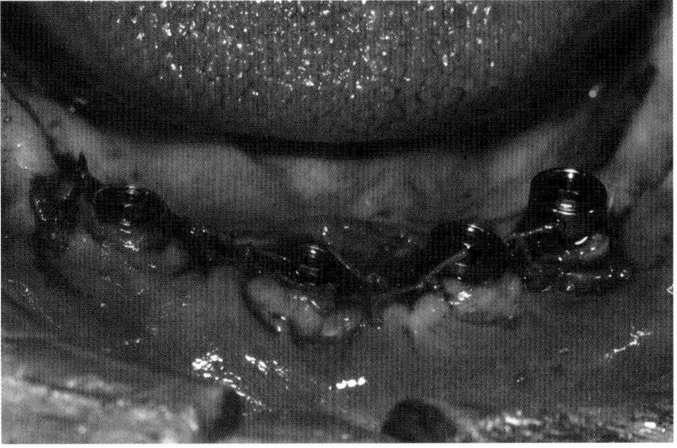

Figure 3.85. Transmucosal standard abutments in place after the second surgical procedure was performed for the patient in Figure 3.83.

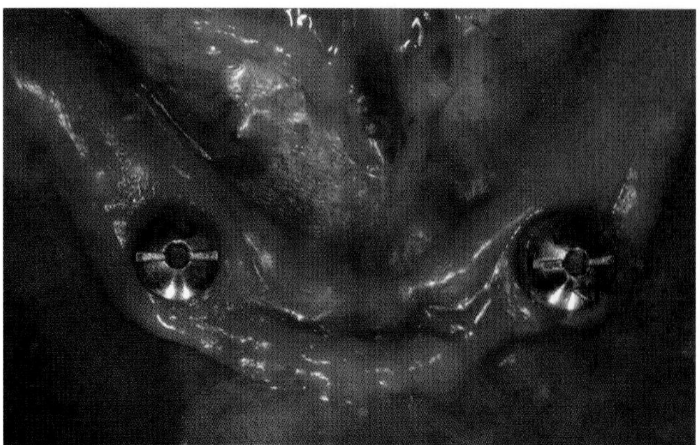

Figure 3.86. This patient had two implants placed three weeks prior to this photograph. Healing abutments were placed at the time of implant placement in a one-stage surgical protocol. The pre-existing denture was relieved and relined with a tissue conditioning material at the time of surgery.

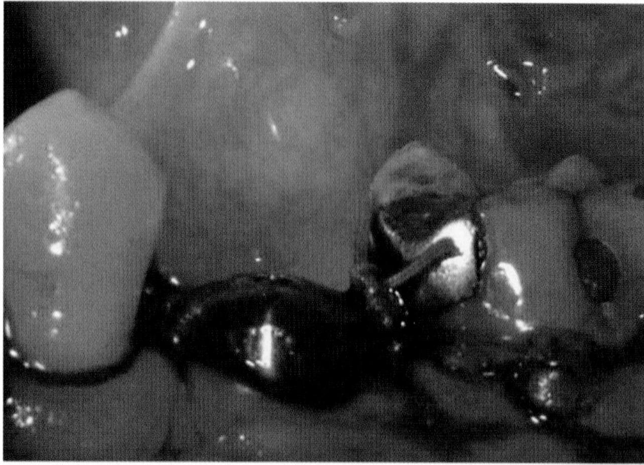

Figure 3.87. This patient had this implant and healing abutment placed at the same surgical appointment (single stage protocol). The healing abutment was selected to approximate the contours of the premolar that was congenitally missing.

jaws of 371 consecutive patients. Patients were followed between five and nine years. Patients with 895 implants in 130 jaws were followed with clinical and radiographic examinations. Eight-one percent of the maxillary implants and 91% of the mandibular implants were stable and continued to support the implant fixed prostheses. Eighty-nine percent of the maxillary prostheses and 100% of the mandibular prostheses were reported as stable and functional.

Numerous other studies have replicated or improved upon the above results (Lekholm and others 1994; Lekholm and others 1999; Friberg and others 1997; Testori and others 2001).

There are two major disadvantages associated with two-stage surgical protocols: patients are asked to go without their preexisting dentures for a period of time immediately after the first surgery; patients have to undergo a second surgical procedure to uncover the implants.

Single-Stage Surgical Protocol

In single-stage surgical protocols, implants are placed into osteotomies prepared similarly to osteotomies in two-stage surgical protocols. However, instead of placing cover screws and closing the surgical wound for unloaded healing, the implants are restored with healing abutments that are left exposed to the oral environment (Figure 3.86). Despite the differences in the preceding protocols, both single- and two-stage protocols have demonstrated highly predictable, favorable outcomes (Buser and others 1999; Adell and others 1990; Haas and others 1996; Bernard and others 1995). Single-stage surgical protocols have also been used with single implants replacing individual teeth (Figure 3.87).

Early Loading Protocol

The traditional loading protocol for machined titanium endosseous implants was initially established at four and six months for edentulous mandibles and maxillae, respectively. Testori and others (2002) reported the results of a three-year study in which OSSEOTITE®implants were placed and loaded with full functional occlusions eight weeks post implant placement. The study reported on the clinical success of implants and prostheses: 405 implants; 99 single tooth restorations; 119 short-span fixed partial dentures; and 11 full arch prostheses. The mean time interval from implant placement to provisional restoration with full occlusion was 2.0+/−0.7 months. Nine failures were reported with up to three years of follow-up. Four mandibular and two maxillary implants failed prior to occlusal function; three additional mandibular implants failed after loading. Testori and others reported a cumulative survival rate of 97.5% for mandibular implants, 98.9% for maxillary implants. The post occlusal loading cumulative survival rate was 98.9% for mandibular implants and 100% for maxillary implants. They concluded that OSSEOTITE® implants could be safely loaded two months post placement. Early loading of OSSEOTITE® implants may be safely prescribed in certain clinical situations. It may be important to note that this study reflected the success of straight walled implants. The results may not be applicable to tapered implants, which have decreased bone/implant contact because tapered implants have less surface areas than do straight wall implants.

However, there is still some controversy relative to early loading protocols (Szmukler-Moncler and others 2000). The aforementioned researchers raised a question in that most clinical studies report the success or failure of implants to become osseointegrated as the clinical absence of mobility. Szmukler-Moncler discussed the possibility that this alone is not enough to assess osseointegration. They postulated that a thin, fibrous layer can develop at the bone/implant interface and if this layer is thin enough, clinical immobility can still be ascertained in short or intermediate time frames. Readers are advised to carefully evaluate research papers relative to early loading of dental endosseous implants.

Immediate Occlusal Loading® Protocol

The original Brånemark implant protocol recommended multiple months of stress-free healing to achieve osseointegration of dental implants (Adell and others 1970; Adell and others 1981; Brånemark 1983; Brånemark and others 1973). There are now numerous studies that demonstrate that immediate loading of dental implants may lead to predictable osseointegration (Schnitman and others 1997; Tarnow and others 1997; Testori and others 2001).

In a comprehensive review of the literature, Szmukler-Moncler and others (2000) concluded that early loading is not responsible for the lack of osseointegration. Failure of implants to become osseointegrated is due to the presence of excessive micromotion during healing. There appears to be a tolerance of micromotion between 50 and 150 μm. They demonstrated that implant design, surface texture, loading, and prosthetic treatment dictate the type of bone response around implants before the traditional healing periods of at least three months. Implants should be at least 10 mm in length and bone densities of less than Type III should be avoided.

Immediate Occlusal Loading® in edentulous mandibles requires the presence of multiple, splinted implants with cross-arch stabilization. Primary stability is required of implants placed and restored with this protocol. This has been defined as insertional torque values of at least 32 Ncm (Nikellis and others 2004). The implants must be loaded within 72 hours of implant placement (Cooper and others 2002). Rough surface texture implants may demonstrate greater initial bone to implant contact and greater biomechanical interlocking of the implants to bone than machined surface implants (Cooper 2000).

Immediate Occlusal Loading® of dental implants has not been quite as successful in maxillae when compared to the successes noted in edentulous mandibles (Schnitman and others 1997; Balshi and Wolfinger 1997). Immediate Occlusal Loading® of dental implants requires a careful and precise process in which the primary goal is to provide patients with optimal treatment in a timely fashion. Long-term clinical follow-up studies are still required in order to assess the long-term efficacy of Immediate Occlusal Loading® of multiple, splinted implants in edentulous jaws.

Immediate Non-Occlusal Loading Protocol

Immediate Non-Occlusal Loading (INOL) of single dental implants is distinctly different from Immediate Occlusal Loading® of multiple, splinted implants. When Immediate Occlusal Loading® protocols were successfully applied in the treatment of partially edentulous patients, the implant restorations were taken out of direct occlusal contact (Wohrle 1998; Degidi and Piattelli 2003).

Testori and others (2003) reported the results of a clinical study that involved 32 patients and 101 implants. All of the implants were seated with at least 30 Ncm of insertional torque. Implants (17 tapered, 35 straight wall) were restored with provisional restorations on the same day or the next day and were kept out of occlusal contact. Implants (19 tapered, 30 straight wall) were also placed and loaded eight weeks after placement. The cumulative survival rate (CSR) for the INOL implants was 96.15%; the CSR for the implants restored eight weeks after placement was 97.96%. Other studies have replicated the results of this study with CSRs of over 96% (Drago and Lazzara 2004; Kan and Rungcharassaeng 2000; Malo and others 2000).

Testori concluded that a nonocclusal immediate loading protocol might be considered a viable approach in select clinical cases. The shortened treatment time can be beneficial for both clinicians and patients. Long-term evaluations are necessary to confirm the encouraging results of Testori's study before this protocol should be considered for everyday practice.

PATIENT CONSULTATION

Principles

Dental treatment, with or without implants, is dependent upon multiple factors: anatomy, systemic health, medications, patient wants and finances, and so on. Some edentulous patients consider a complete, fixed implant-supported prosthesis to be the ultimate solution to their dental/masticatory problems. This may also be the case for some dentulous patients who want to have their teeth extracted and have implants and fixed prostheses placed on the same day. However, there are also some patients for whom the loss of all their natural teeth represents a significant psychological trauma. Extraction and complete dentures treatments must be taken on with great care and respect for patients. Restorative dentists and implant surgeons must be sensitive to both the physical and psychological aspects of the proposed dental treatments.

Patient consultations can be held in the treatment room or in a separate consultation room. It is the author's opinion that the consultation should begin with a review of the patient's chief complaint and medical/dental history. This review should be followed by an explanation of the diagnoses involved in their particular situation. The level of the conversation should be tailored to each patient. Written treatment plans should be presented to patients and their significant others with the plan having the best prognosis presented first. A complete and frank discussion is vital to the overall success of treatment. The consultation should include a discussion of the treatments, fees, benefits, and limitations of the proposed treatment(s).

Informed Consent

Informed consent must be obtained prior to initiation of treatment. The primary function of informed consent is the protection of the patient's right to self-determination to accept the proposed treatment (Schloendorff 1914). The central premise of informed consent is the patient's freedom to decide what will be done to his/her body. The doctrine of informed consent has been divided into three areas (Graskemper 2005):

1. What information has been presented to the patient and how was it presented so that the patient was sufficiently informed?
2. When did the patient give consent to be treated or refuse treatment?
3. Did any misrepresentations and nondisclosures occur that may have affected the patient's decision?

Informed consent has been given when the risks and benefits of the recommended treatment, the anticipated outcome and the alternatives, along with their respective risks and benefits were explained (Canterbury 1972).

Patient consent for treatment is based on two conditions: the patient's willingness to have treatment rendered; and, regardless of the patient's actual consent, the patient, through his or her conduct, may be found to have granted consent for treatment (King 1986).

The most common method to obtain informed consent is written consent. Written consent can take many forms including multiple pages with small-font print or one or two lines in a patient chart. With written informed consent, Graskemper (2002) suggested that practitioners be careful of making a "laundry list" of risks for each procedure. He has advised putting the phrase "but not limited to" before any list to inform patients that other unforeseeable risks may occur.

For a more detailed discussion of informed consent and risk management, readers are advised to consult texts, peer-reviewed journals, and experts in medical/dental malpractice law.

Implant Coordinators

Implant coordinators have been defined as the right hand of the doctor (Beissel 1997). The implant coordinator should oversee, manage, and assist the clinician in implementing and achieving the practice goals relative to implant dentistry.

Implant coordinators should be identified by clinicians as key staff members in both surgical and restorative offices and should be responsible for the day-to-day operations of the implant portions of the practice, including inventory management, scheduling of implant cases, and coordination/communication between surgical offices, restorative offices, and commercial dental laboratories (Daniels 2005).

Surgical implant coordinators need to ensure that the required restorative components, including surgical guides, have been fabricated and delivered to the surgical offices in a timely manner. If a nontraditional implant loading protocol has been the treatment planned for a given patient, the surgical and restorative appointments must be coordinated for optimal treatment. Surgical implant coordinators should be proactive in informing the restorative implant coordinator on the day of implant surgery of the following information:

1. Patient name
2. Date of surgery
3. Procedures performed
    - **a.** Implant manufacturer
    - **b.** Implant sizes (implant restorative platforms)
    - **c.** Locations
    - **d.** Implant/abutment connection types (internal/external connections)
    - **e.** Surgical protocol followed (immediate loading, immediate non-occlusal loading, single stage or two stage protocols, grafting, membranes)
    - **f.** Patient wearing/not wearing provisional prosthesis
    - **g.** Healing abutments placed (height, emergence profile, implant restorative platform)
    - **h.** Recommended healing times
    - **i.** Patient response to surgery/complications
    - **j.** First surgical/restorative follow-up visit

For many restorative dentists, the surgical offices monitor patients during post-operative healing. In these cases, implant surgeons determine when patients are ready to proceed with the restorative treatment phase. The surgical implant coordinator should then communicate with the restorative implant coordinator that the patient is ready to proceed with restoration of the implants.

Surgical implant coordinators may communicate the following information to restorative implant coordinators at the time patients are discharged from the surgical offices:

1. Patient name
2. Implant site(s)
3. Implant manufacturer
4. Implant size: diameter, implant restorative platform, and implant/abutment connection
5. Healing abutment: emergence profile, height, and restorative platform
6. Suggested definitive abutment: emergence profile, height, restorative platform, and stock or custom abutment
7. Recommended abutment screw
8. Driver
9. Recommended torque of abutment screw
10. Impression coping: type (transfer/pick-up); emergence profile; implant/abutment connection
11. Implant analog
12. Laboratory abutment holder

SUMMARY

In summary, the first three chapters of this text provide readers with an overview of implant dentistry. Diagnosis, treatment planning, implants, implant restorative components, drivers, laboratory components, implant loading protocols, and informed consent are discussed in these chapters in detail. References are provided for readers to more completely explore areas of specific interest to them. This text is not intended to be an all-inclusive text on implant dentistry. It is intended to provide insight to clinicians with limited experience in implant dentistry on the logistics of implant treatment on an appointment-by-appointment basis.

The following chapters illustrate specific clinical situations. Physical evaluations, diagnosis and treatment planning, and clinical/laboratory treatments are illustrated on an appointment-by-appointment basis. Costs and fees associated with these treatments are also described.

The author has chosen to illustrate all the treatments using components manufactured by ***3i*®**, Implant Innovations, Inc.®, Palm Beach Gardens, Florida. The specifics of implant treatment are unique to specific implant components, which differ with each manufacturer. However, the principles of implant treatment are more generic in nature. It is the author's intent that restorative dentists who choose to use implant components manufactured by other manufacturers will still be able to apply the principles illustrated in this text.

BIBLIOGRAPHY

Aalam, A, Reshad, M, Chee, W, Nowzari, H, 2005. Surgical template stabilization with transitional implants in the treatment of the edentulous mandible: a technical note. *Int J Oral Maxillofac Implants* 20:462–465.

Adell, R, Hansson, B, Brånemark, P-I, Breine, U, 1970. Intraosseous anchorage of dental prostheses II. Review of clinical approaches. *Scand J Plast Reconstr Surg* 4:19–34.

Adell, R, Lekholm, U, Rockler, B, Brånemark, P-I, 1981. A 15-year study of osseointegrated implants in the treatment of the edentulous jaw. *Int J Oral Surg* 10(6):387–416.

Adell, R, Eriksson, B, Lekholm, U, Brånemark, P-I, Jemt, T, 1990. Long-term follow-up study of osseointegrated implants in the treatment of totally edentulous jaws. *Int J Oral Maxillofac Implants* 5:347–359.

American Academy of Oral and Maxillofacial Surgeons, 2001. Parameters and Pathways: Clinical Practice Guidelines for Oral and Maxillofacial Surgery. Version 3.0 Supplement, Rosemont, IL.

Atwood, D, 1962. Some clinical factors related to rate of resorption of residual ridges. *J Prosthet Dent* 12:441–448.

Atwood, D, 1963. The reduction of residual ridges. A major oral disease entity. *J Prosthet Dent* 26:266–279.

Balshi, T, Wolfinger, G, 1997. Immediate loading of Brånemark implants in edentulous mandibles: a preliminary report. *Implant Dentistry* 6:83–88.

Becker, W, Becker, B, 1995. Replacement of maxillary and mandibular molars with single endosseous implant restorations: a retrospective study. *J Prosthet Dent* 74:51–55.

Becker, C, Kaiser, D, 2000. Surgical guide for dental implant placement. *J Prosthet Dent* 83:248–251.

Beissel, D, 1997. Practice management: formula for a successful implant practice. *Acad Osseointegration Newsletter* 8:1–4.

Bellaiche, N, 1997. Indications des techniques d'imagerie en implantologie oral. *J Prosthet Dent* 129:23–30.

Bellaiche, Norbert, 2001. "Imaging in Oral Implantology." In *Implants and Restorative Dentistry*, edited by Gerard Scortecci, Carl Misch, Klaus-U Benner, p. 178–196. New York, NY: Thieme.

Bernard, J, Belser, U, Martinet, J, Borgis, S, 1995. Osseointegration of Brånemark fixtures using a single-step operating technique. A preliminary prospective one-year study in the edentulous mandible. *Clin Oral Implants Res* 6:122–129.

Besimo, C, Rohner, HR, 2005. Three-dimensional treatment planning for prosthetic rehabilitation. *Int J Perio Rest Dent* 25:81–87.

Brånemark, P-I and Tolman, Daniel, eds., 1998. *Osseointegration in Craniofacial Reconstruction*. Chicago: Quintessence.

Brånemark, P-I, 1959. Vital microscopy of bone marrow in rabbit. *Scand J Lab Invest* 11(Suppl 38):1–82.

Brånemark, P-I, 1983. Osseointegration and its experimental background. *J Prosthet Dent* 50:399–410.

Brånemark, P-I, Hansson, B, Adell, R, Breine, U, Lindstrom, J, Hallen, O, Ohman, H, 1977. Osseointegrated implants in the treatment of the edentulous jaw. Experience from a 10-year period. *Scand J Plast Reconstr Surg* 16:1–132.

Buser, D, Mericske-Stern, R, Dula, K, Lang, N, 1999. Clinical experience with one-stage, nonsubmerged dental implants. *Adv Dent Res* 13:153–161.

Canterbury v Spence, 1972. 464 F2d 772, 783 (DC Cir).

Carpentieri, J, 2004. Clinical protocol for an overdenture bar prosthesis fabricated with CAD/CAM technology. *Pract Proced Aesthet Dent* 16:755–757.

Chiche, G, Penault, A, 1994. "Replacement of deficient crowns." In *Esthetics of Anterior Fixed Prosthodontics*. G. Chiche and A Penault, eds. Chicago: Quintessence, p. 53–74.

Choquet, V, Hermans, M, Adriaenssens, P, 2001. Clinical and radiographic evaluation of the papilla level adjacent to single-tooth dental implants. A retrospective study in the maxillary anterior region. *J Periodontol* 72(10):1364–1371.

Cooper, L, 2000. A role for surface topography in creating and maintaining bone at titanium endosseous implants. *J Prosthet Dent* 84:522–534.

Cooper, L, Rahman, A, Moriarty, J, Chaffee, N, Sacco, D, 2002. Immediate mandibular rehabilitation with endosseous implants: simultaneous extraction, implant placement and loading. *Int J Oral Maxillofac Implants* 17:517–525.

Crum, R, Rooney, G, 1978. Alveolar bone loss in overdentures: a 5-year study. *J Prosthet Dent* 40:610–613.

Daniels, A, 2005. Personal communication.

Davis, D M, 1997. "Developing An Analogue/Substitute for the Maxillary Denture-Bearing Area." In *Prosthodontic Treatment for Edentulous Patients,* 11th Ed., George Zarb and Gunnar Carlsson, eds. p. 141–149. St. Louis, MO: Mosby-Year Book.

Degidi, M, Piattelli, A, 2003. Immediate functional and non-functional loading of dental implants: a 2- to 60-month follow-up study of 646 titanium implants. *J Periodontol* 74:225–241.

Drago, C, 2003. A clinical study of the efficacy of gold-tite square abutment screws in cement-retained implant restorations. *Int J Oral Maxillofac Implants* 18:273–278.

Drago, C, Lazzara, R, 2004. Immediate provisional restoration of Osseotite implants: a clinical report of 18-month results. *Int J Oral Maxillofac Implants* 19:534–541.

Engquist, B, 1991. "Six Years Experience of Splinted and Non-Splinted Implants Supporting Overdentures in Upper and Lower Jaws." In *Overdentures on Oral Implants*, E Schepers, I Naert, and G Theuniers, eds. Leuven: Leuven University Press, p. 27–41.

Engquist, B, Astrand, P, Anzen, B, Dahlgren, S, Engquist, E, Feldmann, H, Karlsson, U, Nord, P, Sahlholm, S, Svardstrom, P, 2005. Simplified methods of implant treatment in the edentulous lower jaw: a 3-year follow-up report of a controlled prospective study of one-stage versus two-stage surgery and early loading. *Clin Implant Dent Relat Res* 7:95–104.

Esposito, M, Edestubbe, A, Grondahl, K, 1993. Radiological evaluation of marginal bone loss at tooth surfaces facing single Brånemark implants. *Clin Oral Impl Res* 4:151–157.

Feldmann, E, Morrow, R, Jameson, W, 1970. Relining complete dentures with an oral cure silicone elastomer and a duplicate denture. *J Prosthet Dent* 23(4):387–393.

Frederiksen, N, 1995. Diagnostic imaging in dental implantology. *Oral Surg Oral Med Oral Pathol Oral Radiol Endod* 80:540–554.

Friberg, N, Nilson, H, Olsson, M, Palmquist, C, 1997. MkII: The self-tapping Brånemark implant: 5-year results of a prospective 3-center study. *Clin Oral Implants Res* 8:279–285.

Friedland, B, 2005. Risk-benefit analysis of the radiographic standards of care. *Int J Perio and Restor Dent* 25(1):6–7.

Frost, H, 1983. A determinant of bone architecture. *Clin Orthopaed Rel Res* 175:286–292.

Garber, D, 1995. The esthetic dental implant: letting restoration be the guide. *J Am Dent Assoc* 126:319–325.

Garber, D, Belser, U, 1995. Restoration driven implant placement with restoration generated site development. *Compend Contin Educ Dent* 16:796–799.

Garlini, G, Bianchi, C, Chierichetti, V, 2003. Retrospective clinical study of Osseotite implants: zero- to 5-year results. *Int J Oral Maxillofac Implants* 18:589–593.

Givol, N, Taicher, S, Halamish-Shani, T, Chaushu, G. 2002. Risk management aspects of implant dentistry. *Int J Oral Maxillofac Implants* 17:258–262.

Goodacre, C, Kan, J, Rungcharassaeng, K, 1999. Clinical complications of osseointegrated implants. *J Prosthet Dent* 81:537–552.

Graskemper, J, 2002. A new perspective on dental malpractice: practice enhancement through risk management. *J Am Dent Assoc* 133:752–757.

Graskemper, J, 2005. Informed consent: a stepping stone in risk management. *Compend Contin Dent Ed* 26:286–290.

Guerra, Louis and Finger, Israel, 1995. "Restorative Procedures for Dental Implants." In *Endosseous Implants for Maxillofacial Reconstruction*, M Block and J Kent, eds. Philadelphia: Saunders, p. 135–150.

Haas, R, Mensdorff, P, Mailath, G, Watzek, G, 1996. Survival of 1920 IMZ implants followed for up to 100 months. *Int J Oral Maxillofac Implants* 11:581–588.

Haas, R, Polak, C, Furhauser, R, 2002. A long-term follow-up of 76 Brånemark single-tooth implants. *Clin Oral Implants Res* 13:38–45.

Hebel, K, Gajjar, R, 1997. Achieving superior aesthetic results: parameters for implant and abutment selection. *Int J Dent Symp* 4(1):42–47.

Hobo, S, Ichida, E, Garcia, L, 1989. *Osseointegration and Occlusal Rehabilitation.* Tokyo: Quintessence.

Jansen, C, Weisgold, A. 1995. Presurgical treatment planning for the anterior single tooth implant restoration. *Compend Contin Dental Ed* 16(8):746–761.

Jemt, T, Linden, B, Lekholm, U, 1992. Failures and complications in 127 consecutively placed fixed partial prostheses supported by Brånemark implants: from prosthetic treatment to first annual checkup. *Int J Oral Maxillofac Implants* 7:40–44.

Jemt, T, 1993. Implant treatment in resorbed edentulous upper jaws. A three-year follow-up study on 70 patients. *Clin Oral Implant Res* 4:187–194.

Kan, J, Rungcharassaeng, K, Lozada, J, 2003. Immediate placement and provisionalization of maxillary anterior single implants: 1-year prospective study. *Int J Oral Maxillofac Implants* 18:31–39.

Kassebaum, K, Nummikoski, P, Triplett, R, Langlais, R, 1990. Cross-sectional radiography for implant site assessment. *Oral Surg Oral Med Oral Pathol* 70:674–678.

Keith, S, Miller, B, Woody, R, 1999. Marginal discrepancy of screw-retained and cemented metal-ceramic crowns on implant abutments. *Int J Oral Maxillofac Implants* 14:369–378.

King, J Jr. 1986. *The Law of Medical Malpractice in a Nutshell,* 2nd Ed. Eagan, MN: West Publishing.

Kirsch, A, 1991. "Overdentures on IMZ Implants: Modalities and Long-Term Results." In *Overdentures on Oral Implants,* E Schepers, I Naert, and G Theuniers, eds. Leuven: Leuven University Press, p. 15–17.

Kois, J, 1994. Altering gingival levels: the restorative connection. Part I: biologic variables. *J Esthet Dent* 6:3–9.

Kois, J, 2004. Predictable single-tooth peri-implant esthetics: five diagnostic keys. *Comp Contin Dent Ed* 25:895–905.

Krennmair, G, Piehslinger, E, Wagner, H, 2003. Status of teeth adjacent to single-tooth implants. *Int J Prosthodont* 16:524–531.

Laney, W, Jemt, T, Harris, D, 1994. Osseointegrated implants for single tooth replacement: progress report from a multi-center prospective study after 3 years. *Int J Oral Maxillofac Implants* 9:49–54.

Lekholm, Ulf and Zarb, George, 1985. "Patient Selection and Preparation." In *Tissue-Integrated Prostheses. Osseointegration in Clinical Dentistry,* P-I Brånemark, George Zarb, and Tomas Albrektsson, eds. Chicago: Quintessence, p. 199–210.

Lekholm, U, van Steenberghe, D, Herrmann, I, 1994. Osseointegrated implants in the treatment of partially edentulous jaws: a prospective 5-year multicenter study. *Int J Oral Maxillofac Implants* 9:627–635.

Lekholm, U, Gunne, J, Henry, P, 1999. Survival of the Brånemark implant in partially edentulous jaws: a 10-year prospective multicenter study. *Int J Oral Maxillofac Implants* 14:639–645.

Malo, P, Ranger, B, Dvarsater, L, 2000. Immediate function of Brånemark implant in the esthetic zone: a retrospective clinical study with 6 months to 4 years of follow-up. *Clin Implant Dent Relat Res* 2:138–146.

McGarry, T, Edge, M, Gillis, R, Jr, Hilsen, K, Jones, R, Shipman, B, Tupac, R, Wiens, J, 2006. Parameters of care for the specialty of prosthodontics. *J Prosthod* 14: (supplement 1) 1–103.

McGarry, T, Nimmo, A, Skiba, J, Ahlstrom, R, Smith, C, Koumjian, J, 1999. Classification system of complete edentulism. *J Prosthod* 8:27–39.

Mericske-Stern, R, 1994. Overdentures with roots or implants for elderly patients: a comparison. *J Prosthet Dent* 72:543–550.

Misch, Carl, 1993. "Implant Success or Failure: Clinical Assessment in Implant Dentistry." In *Contemporary Implant Dentistry,* Carl Misch, ed., p. 29–42. St. Louis: Mosby.

Naert, I, De Clercq, M, Theuniers, G, Schepers, D, 1988. Overdentures supported by osseointegrated fixtures for the edentulous mandible: a 2.5-year report. *Int J Oral Maxillofac Implants* 3:191–196.

Naert, I, Quirynen, M, Hooghe, M, van Steenberghe, D, 1994. A comparative prospective study of splinted and unsplinted Brånemark implants in mandibular overdenture therapy: a preliminary report. *J Prosthet Dent* 71:486–492.

National Institutes of Health Consensus Development Conference Statement, 1988. *Dental Implants,* U.S. Department of Health and Human Services 7:108.

Naert, I, Koutsikakis, G, Duyck, J, 2000. Biologic outcome of single-implant restorations as tooth replacements: a long-term follow-up study. *Clin Implant Dent Relat Res* 2:209–215.

Nikellis, I, Levi, A, Nicolopoulos, C, 2004. Immediate loading of 190 endosseous dental implants: a prospective observational study of 40 patient treatments with up to 2-year data. *Int J Oral Maxillofac Implants* 19:116–123.

Nyman, S, Lindhe, J, 1979. A longitudinal study of combined periodontal and prosthetic treatment of patients with advanced periodontal disease. *J Periodontol* 50:163–169.

Ohrnell, L, Palmquist, J, Brånemark, P-I, 1992. "Single Tooth Replacement." In *Advanced Osseointegration Surgery Applications in the Maxillofacial Region,* P Worthington and P-I Brånemark, eds., p. 211–232.

Parel, S, 1986. Implants and overdentures: the osseointegrated approach with conventional and compromised applications. *Int J Oral Maxillofac Implants* 1:93–99.

Peterson, Larry J, 1998. *Contemporary Oral and Maxillofacial Surgery,* 3rd Ed. St Louis: Mosby.

Rosenfeld, A, McCall, R, 1996. The use of interactive computed tomography to predict the esthetic and functional demands of implant-supported prostheses. *Compend Cont Dent Ed* 17:1125–1144.

Saadoun, A, Le Gall, M, Touati, B, 1999. Selection and ideal tridimensional implant position for soft tissue aesthetics. *Pract Periodont Aesthet Dent* 11:1063–1072.

Saadoun, A, Le Gall, M, Touati, B, 2004. Current trends in Implantology: Part II-treatment planning, aesthetic considerations, and tissue regeneration. *Pract Proced Aesthet Dent* 16:707–714.

Sadan, A, Raigrodski, A, Salinas, T, 1997. Prosthetic considerations in the fabrication of surgical stents for implant placement. *Pract Periodont Aesthet Dent* 9:1003–1011.

Sadan, A, Blatz, M, Salinas, T, Block, M, 2004. Single-implant restorations: a contemporary approach for achieving a predictable outcome. *J Oral Maxillofac Surg* 62:73–81, Suppl 2.

Salinas, T, Block, M, Sadan, A, 2004. Fixed partial denture or single-tooth implant restorations? Statistical considerations for sequencing and treatment. *J Oral Maxillofac Surg* 62:2–16, Suppl 2.

Santos, LL, 2002. Treatment planning in the presence of congenitally absent second premolars: a review of the literature. *J Clin Ped Dent* 27:13–17.

Schloendorff v Society of NY Hospital, 1914. 211 NY 125, 129, 105 NE 92, 93.

Schnitman, P, 1998. The profile prosthesis: an aesthetic fixed implant supported restoration for the resorbed maxillae. *Pract Perio Aesthet Dent* 11:143–151.

Schnitman, P, Wohrle, P, Rubenstein, J, DaSilva, J, Wang, N, 1997. Ten-year results for Brånemark implants immediately loaded with fixed prostheses at implant placement. *Int J Oral Maxillofac Implants* 12:495–503.

Scortecci, G, Garcias, D. 2001. "Dental implant treatment planning." In *Implants and Restorative Dentistry*, Gerard Scortecci, Carl Misch, and Klaus-U Benner, eds. New York, NY: Thieme, p. 166–177.

Scortecci, G, 1999. Immediate function of cortically anchored disc-design implants without bone augmentation in moderately to severely resorbed completely edentulous maxillae. *Oral Implantol* 25:70–79.

Szmukler-Moncler, S, Piattelli, A, Favero, G, Dubruille, J, 2000. Considerations preliminary to the application of early and immediate loading protocols in dental Implantology. *Clin Oral Impl Res* 11:12–25.

Tallgren, A, 1967. The effect of denture wearing on facial morphology. *Acta Odont Scand* 25:563–592.

Tallgren, A, 1969. Positional changes of complete dentures—a 7 year longitudinal study. *Acta Odont Scand* 27:539–561.

Tallgren, A. 1972. The continuing reduction of the residual alveolar ridges in complete denture wearers: a mixed longitudinal study covering 25 years. *J Prosthet Dent* 27:120–132.

Tarnow, D, Cho, S, Wallace, S, 2000. The effect of interimplant distance on the height of interimplant bone crest. *J Periodontol* 71(4):546–549.

Tarnow, D, Elian, N, Fletcher, P, 2003. Vertical distance from the crest of bone to the height of the interproximal papilla between adjacent implants. *J Periodontol* 74:1785–1788.

Tarnow, D, Emtiaz, D, Classi, A, 1997. Immediate loading of threaded implants at stage 1 surgery in edentulous arches: Ten consecutive case reports with 1- to 5-year data. *Int J Oral Maxillofac Implants* 12:319–324.

Tarnow, D, Magner, A, Fletcher, P, 1992. The effect of the distance from the contact point to the crest of bone on the presence or absence of the interproximal dental papilla. *J Periodontol* 63:995–996.

Taylor, T, Belser, U, Mericske-Stern, R, 2000. Prosthodontic considerations. *Clin Oral Implants Res* 11:101–110 (Suppl).

Terrell, W, 1958. Fundamentals important to good complete denture construction. *J Prosthet Dent* 8:740–753.

Testori, T, Bianchi, F, Del Fabbro, M, Capelli, M, Zuffetti, F, Berlucchi, I, Taschieri, S, Francetti, L, Weinstein, R, 2005. Implant aesthetic score for evaluating the outcome: immediate loading in the aesthetic zone. *Pract Proced Aesthet Dent* 17:123–130.

Testori, T, Bianchi, F, Del Fabbro, M, Szmukler-Moncler, S, Francetti, L, Weinstein, R, 2003. *Pract Proced Aesthet Dent* 15:787–794.

Testori, T, Szmukler-Moncler, S, Francetti, L, Del Fabbro, M, Scarano, A, Piattelli, A, Weinstein, R, 2001. *Int J Perio Rest Dent* 21:451–459.

Testori, T, Del Fabbro, M, Feldman, S, Vincenzi, G, Sullivan, D, Rossi, R, Jr, Anitua, E, Bianchi, F, Francetti, L, Weinstein, R, 2002. A multicenter prospective evaluation of 2-months loaded Osseotite implants placed in the posterior jaws: 3-year follow-up results. *Clin Oral Implants Res* 13:154–161.

Testori, T, Wiseman, L, Woolfe, S, Porter, S, 2001. A prospective multicenter clinical study of the Osseotite implant: 4-year interim report. *Int J Oral Maxillofac Implants* 16:193–200.

Touati, B, 2003. Biologically driven implant treatment. *Pract Proced Aesthet Dent* 15:734–737.

Tyndall, D, Brooks, S. 2000. Selection criteria for dental implant site imaging: a position paper of the American Academy of Oral and Maxillofacial Radiology. *Oral Surg Oral Med Oral Pathol Oral Radiol Endod* 89:630–637.

Vermylen, K, Collaert, B, Linden, U, 2003. Patient satisfaction and quality of single-tooth restorations. *Clin Oral Implants Res* 14:119–123.

Walton, J, MacEntee, M, 1994. Problems with prostheses on implants—a retrospective study. *J Prosthet Dent* 71:283–288.

Walton, J, MacEntee, M, Glick, N, 2002. One-year prosthetic outcomes with implant overdentures: a randomized clinical trial. *Int J Oral Maxillofac Implants* 17:391–398.

Woelfel, J, Winter, C, Igarashi, T, 1976. Five year cephalometric study of mandibular ridge resorption with different posterior occlusal forms. Part I: denture construction and initial comparison. *J Prosthet Dent* 36:602–623.

Wohrle, P, 1998. Single-tooth replacement in the aesthetic zone with immediate provisionalization: fourteen consecutive case reports. *Pract Periodont Aesthet Dent* 10:1107–1114.

Chapter 4: Treatment of an Edentulous Mandible with an Implant-Retained Overdenture and Resilient Attachments

LITERATURE REVIEW

Traditionally, complete dentures have been the standard of care for edentulous patients in the United States. Despite advances in periodontics and restorative dentistry, the number of edentulous and partially edentulous people is expected to increase in the first part of the twenty-first century (Douglass, Shih, and Ostry 2002; Douglass and Watson 2002). One-third of Americans over the age of 65 are thought to be edentulous (Oral Health in Americans 2000). Edentulism is considered to be a major health problem by virtue of the physical impairments and disabilities associated with this condition by the World Health Organization (World Health Organization 2001). A significant number of patients who wear maxillary and mandibular complete dentures are dissatisfied with the lack of retention and stability in their complete dentures (Bourgeois and others 1998).

Numerous studies have demonstrated that mandibular two-implant overdentures can simply and effectively solve many of the problems experienced by patients with mandibular complete dentures (Schmitt and Zarb 1998; Gotfredsen and Holm 2000; Awad and others 2003; Cune and others 2005). An international group of scientists, researchers, and clinicians developed and published the McGill consensus on the standard of care for edentulous mandibles (McGill 2002). The consensus included a statement that mandibular 2-unit overdentures should be considered as a first choice standard of care for edentulous patients. The McGill Consensus does not preclude other types of implant-retained overdentures such as cast bars with attachments, primary and secondary castings, fixed implant-retained prostheses, and so on (Figures 4.1, 4.2).

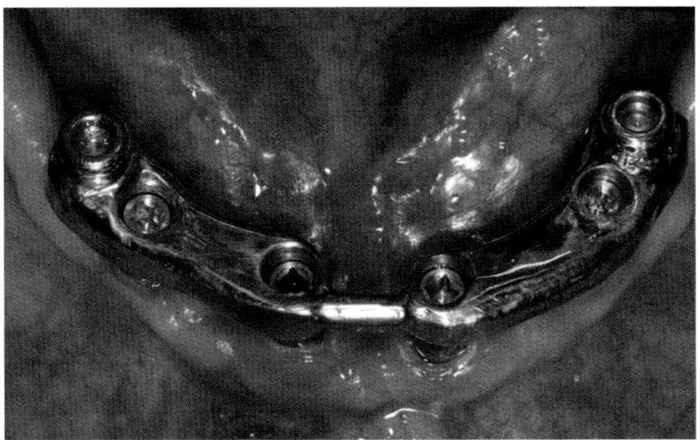

Figure 4.1. Facial view of implant-retained bar splinting four mandibular implants.

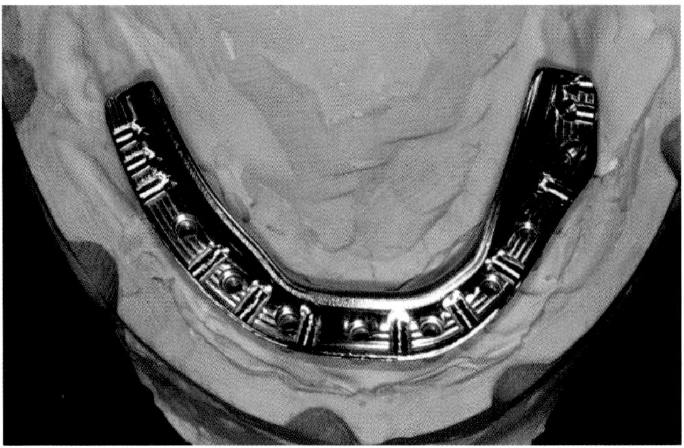

Figure 4.2. Casting that was designed for a full arch, fixed, screw-retained prosthesis.

Edentulous patients may experience reduction in height of alveolar ridges of up to 0.4 mm per year (Tallgren 1972) (Figure 4.3). Mandibular resorption can occur four times greater than maxillary resorption. However, this process does not have to occur. If the roots of mandibular cuspids are maintained as overdenture abutments, there is a significant reduction of alveolar bone loss (Morrow and Brewer 1980) (Figure 4.4). Patients with less bone loss generally have more positive experiences with overdentures than do edentulous patients with mandibular complete dentures. However, there are potential concerns with recurrent caries and periodontal disease around the retained natural teeth (Figure 4.5).

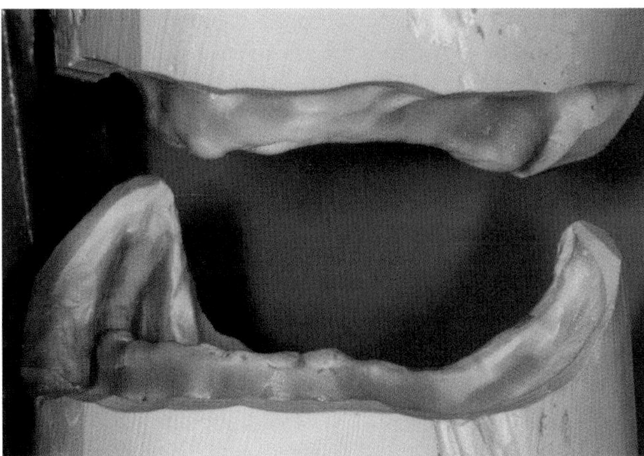

Figure 4.3. Articulator mounting of an edentulous patient 10 years post extraction of the natural teeth. Note the amount of inter-occlusal clearance secondary to resorption of both edentulous jaws.

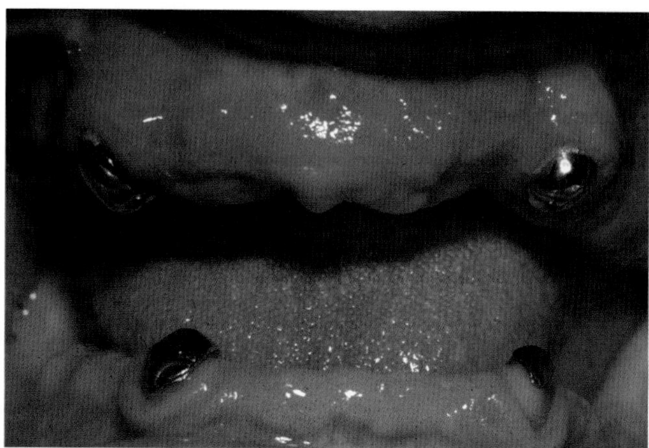

Figure 4.4. Clinical anterior view of a partially edentulous patient who chose to retain two anterior teeth in both jaws for use as overdenture abutments 10 years prior to this photograph. Note that the bone volume of both jaws has been maintained.

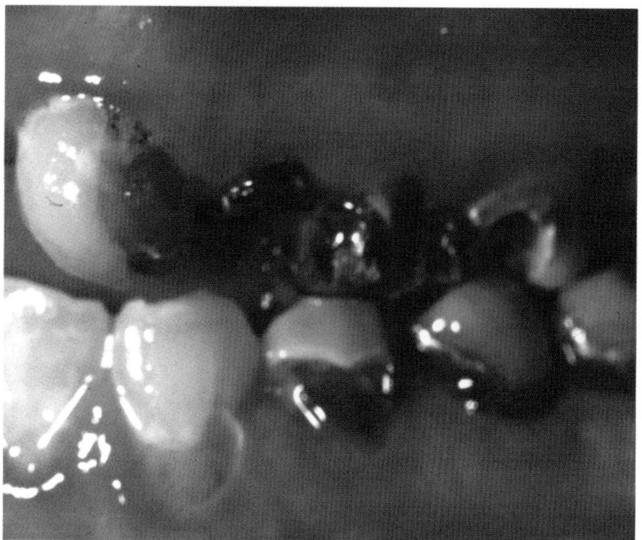

Figure 4.5. Clinical photograph of a 17-year-old patient with severe dental caries. Though overdentures would be the ideal treatment to maintain bone on a long-term basis, this patient would not be good candidate for overdentures unless the caries were controlled.

Cune and others (2005) performed a clinical study with 18 edentulous patients to determine patient satisfaction with implant-supported mandibular overdentures using magnet, bar-clip, and ball-socket attachments and also to determine a correlation between maximum bite force and patient satisfaction. New mandibular and maxillary dentures were fabricated for all of the patients in this study. Initially, the patients functioned only with the new complete dentures. After three months, the mandibular dentures were fitted with overdenture attachments in a random fashion. The attachments were switched again after three months of function. Patients were asked to express their overall satisfaction of their dentures using a Visual Analog Scale. Mean scale and VAS scores were compared at five times during the study. Mandibular implant-supported overdentures consistently reduced traditional denture complaints such as sore spots that required adjustments. The patients in this study strongly preferred bar-clip attachments (10/18) and ball-socket attachments (7/18) over magnetic attachments. Maximum bite forces were not correlated with VAS scores. The authors concluded that patients with higher bite forces were not necessarily more satisfied with their dentures than patients with lower bite forces.

Awad and others (2003) performed a randomized clinical study to compare elderly patients' satisfaction and oral-health-related quality of life with mandibular two-implant supported overdentures and conventional dentures. Sixty patients were divided into experimental and control groups: edentulous patients and patients with two implants and ball attachments for overdentures. Subjects were asked to rate their general satisfaction, comfort, stability, ability to chew, speech, aesthetics, and cleaning ability. The outcomes were better for the implant group, and the authors further stated that mandibular two-implant overdentures with maxillary complete dentures provided better function and oral-health-related quality of life than conventional dentures.

There are two basic ways to treat patients with dental implants in edentulous mandibles: fixed or removable prostheses. There are benefits and limitations with both prosthetic options. Prior to selecting a treatment option (fixed or removable), the restorative dentist and patient must first discuss the overall treatment objectives and expectations. Aesthetics and function are probably the two key points that restorative dentists and patients must agree on (Table 4.1). The final aesthetics and tooth arrangement of the prostheses need to be determined as much as possible, prior to sending the patient to an implant surgeon. This may be as

TABLE 4.1. Intra-oral Diagnostic Guidelines for Fixed/ Removable Implant Prostheses

	Fixed	**Removable**
Ridge Shape	Thin, knife-edged	Broad, U-Shaped
Inter-occlusal clearance	10mm	>15 mm
Jaw Relationship	Class I	Class II, III
Biotype	Thick	Thin

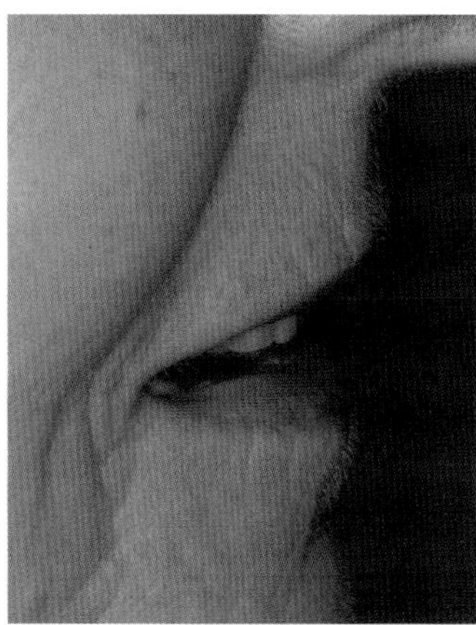

Figure 4.6. Profile view of a patient who presented with a request for increased retention and stability of her preexisting mandibular denture. These dentures were judged to be satisfactory; the mandibular denture was duplicated for use as a surgical guide.

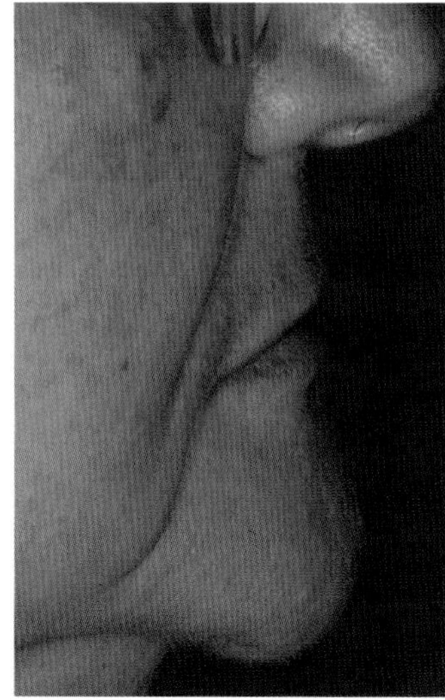

Figure 4.7. Profile view of a patient who presented with a request for increased retention and stability of her preexisting mandibular denture. The dentures were judged to be unacceptable: poor lip support, decreased vertical dimension of occlusion. New dentures were needed to identify the location of the teeth prior to referring the patient to an implant surgeon for implant placement.

simple as recognizing that the existing prostheses are acceptable relative to aesthetics, lip support, and occlusal relationships (Figure 4.6). If the existing dentures are unacceptable, new dentures need to be considered prior to treatment planning implant placement (Figure 4.7).

It has been the author's experience that patients rarely ask for removable implant-retained overdentures. It is critical for restorative dentists to discuss the merits of this type of treatment and how an implant-retained overdenture will function. Carpentieri (2004) discussed common misconceptions among clinicians that all rigid prostheses must be fixed and nonrigid prostheses must be removable. Rigid prostheses are not always fixed prostheses. With bar-retained overdentures, removable options may now be nonrigid (resilient) or rigid.

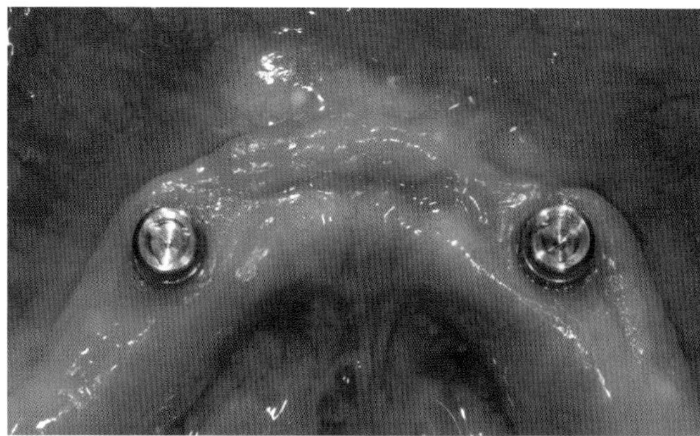

Figure 4.8. Occlusal view of two unsplinted mandibular implants with resilient attachments.

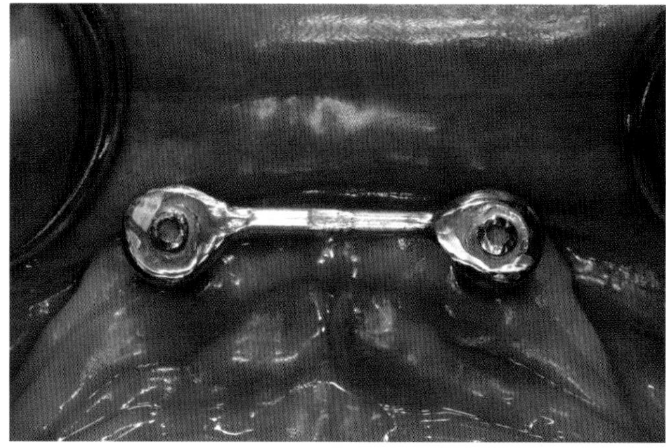

Figure 4.9. Occlusal view of a casting 10 years post insertion that splinted two mandibular implants. A rotation component was built into the casting between the two implants.

Implant-retained overdentures need to be designed to be consistent with removable prosthodontic principles (buccal shelf and retromolar pad coverage with adequate vestibular extensions) along with implant attachments. This type of prosthesis can be made with nonsplinted retainers/attachments that allow rotation (Figure 4.8) or with a framework that splints two or more implants with a casting and allows rotation around the bar (Figure 4.9).

Resilient attachments are easier for clinicians to use and vary in how they may be incorporated into the mandibular prostheses. With each treatment option, there will be varying amounts of clinical time and laboratory costs involved

TABLE 4.2. Cost Comparisons of Treatment Options of Mandibular Overdentures with Resilient Attachments

	Chair Side Pick-Up LOCATOR® Abutments	Reline Impression	New Overdenture
Component Cost (2)	$300	$300	$300
Clinical Overhead	(1/2 hr @ $400 per hour) $200	(3/4 hr @ $400 per hour) $300	(4 hrs @ $400 per hour) $1600
Laboratory Cost	0	$100	$330
Total Costs	$500	$700	$2230
Fee	$750	$1100	$3000
Profit	$250	$400	$770
Profit per Hr	$500	$300	$195

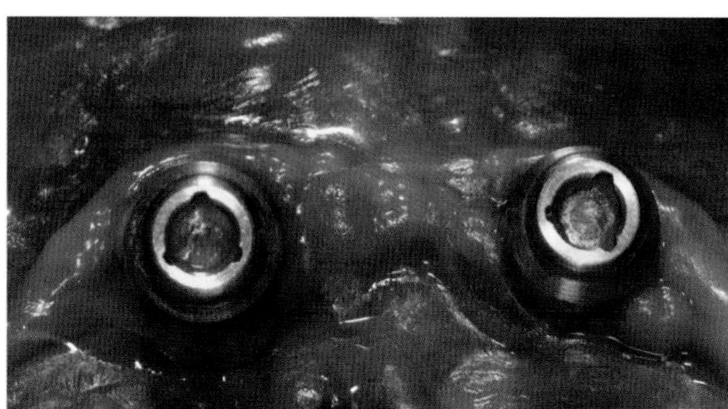

Figure 4.10. Occlusal view of 2 LOCATOR® Abutments in place on two unsplinted mandibular implants.

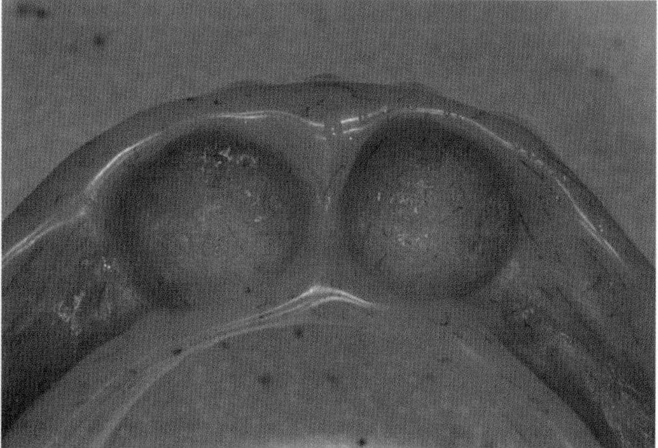

Figure 4.11. The intaglio surface of the denture base in the areas of the attachments was thoroughly relieved to ensure that the denture was completely seated. The keepers should not touch the denture base.

(Table 4.2). The simplest method using resilient attachments (LOCATOR® Abutments, Zest Anchors, Inc) is to place them intra-orally, relieve the denture, and attach the stainless steel keepers to the dentures with autopolymerizing acrylic resin (Figures 4.10, 4.11, 4.12). The major limitation with this technique is the potential to lock the acrylic resin into undercuts in and around the implants and/or alveolar process. This approach would make it very difficult to remove the denture without causing abrasion to the soft tissues or dislodging the keeper from the denture base.

Mandibular overdentures that incorporate a bar splinting multiple implants may or may not have the same number of implants as a fixed, screw-retained implant prosthesis. This type of prosthesis usually includes multiple retentive elements (Figure 4.13).

Mandibular implant-retained overdentures need to be treatment planned relative to patient desires, expectations, anatomy, and finances. Implant-retained overdentures made on four or more implants will be significantly more rigid and exhibit less movement than overdentures made

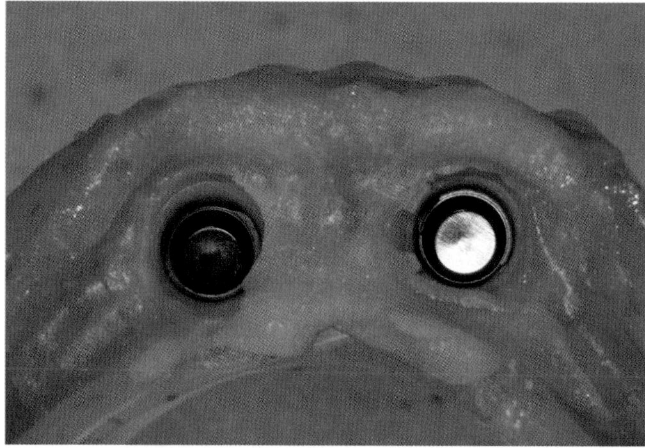

Figure 4.12. The intaglio surface of the mandibular overdenture after the resin had completely set. The black keepers were removed and replaced with retentive elements consistent with the patient's need for retention.

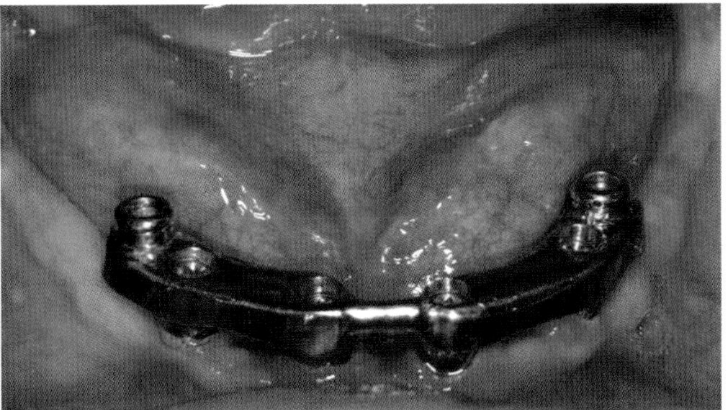

Figure 4.13. Occlusal view of four mandibular implants that were splinted with a casting that incorporated a clip in the anterior position that allowed rotation of the denture around the bar in an A/P direction. Resilient attachments were incorporated into the distal portions of the framework to provide retention and support for the overdenture.

on two nonsplinted implants with resilient attachments. Overdentures may actually be the treatment of choice if implants cannot be placed with an acceptable A/P spread (Rangert and others 1989). This is not to say that one of these designs is better than the other. Oral hygiene is also easier to accomplish on two unsplinted implants than on implants splinted with a complex casting.

Treatment planning must strike a balance between the factors noted above. Indications for two implant-supported overdentures generally include patients unable to adapt to conventional mandibular dentures or patients who desire increased retention and stability for their mandibular dentures. Clinicians must understand what it is that a particular patient wants: increased retention, stability, function, cleansability, and so on. Restorative dentists must therefore present a range of treatment options that will satisfy a particular patient's concerns.

Multiple, splinted implants with bars and attachments are generally indicated in patients who desire rigid prostheses but who present with significant bone loss (great intermaxillary distance). Flanges are generally required in order to provide optimal lip support and appropriate incisal display. This type of restoration may also be indicated in patients with natural or implant-retained, nonremovable prostheses in the opposing jaw (maxillae). Patients with four implants and rigidly attached overdentures will probably generate large occlusal forces that may fracture an all-acrylic resin denture base. An additional design feature for this latter type of patient would include a secondary bar within the denture base or a metal mini-base. Nonparallel implants may also be indications for splinting because resilient attachments have limitations in the amount of angle correction (Figure 4.14).

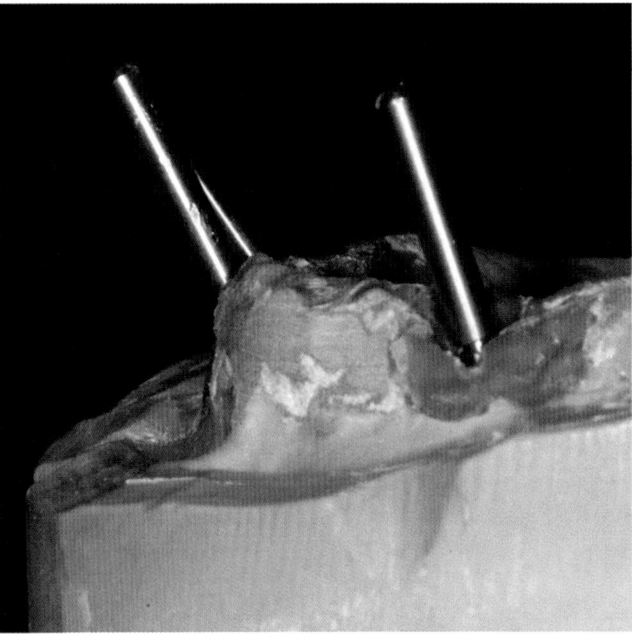

Figure 4.14. These three maxillary implants are non-parallel and warrant a bar to re-orient the path of insertion of the overdenture.

Both types of implant prostheses (splinted/nonsplinted implants) have proven to be clinically successful (MacEntee and others 2005; Walton and others 2002). Clinicians must carefully evaluate each patient's individual desires, needs, anatomy, and so on in developing treatment plans that include implants and removable prostheses.

CLINICAL CASE PRESENTATION

Appointment 1. Initial Examination (3/4 Hour)

A 64-year-old female patient presented to the author with a chief complaint, "My lower denture is too loose for me to wear" (Figures 4.15, 4.16).

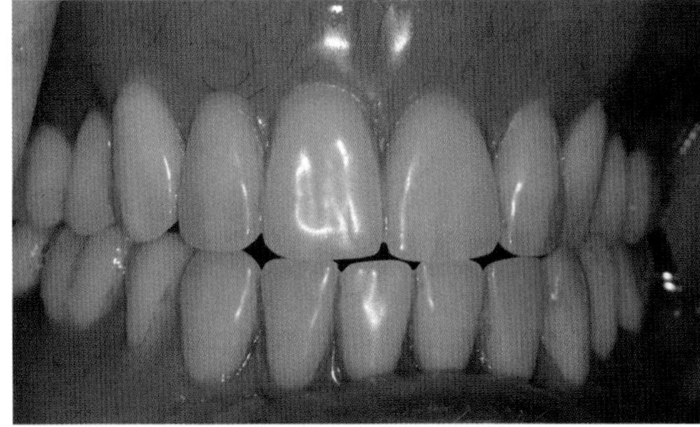

Figure 4.15. Anterior view of the maxillary and mandibular dentures as the patient originally presented.

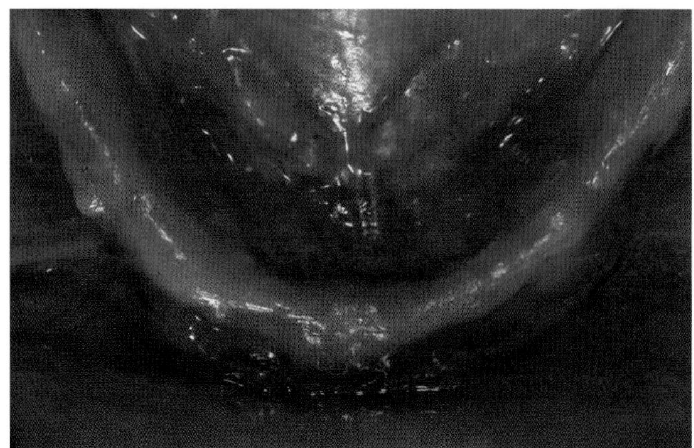

Figure 4.16. Intra-oral occlusal view of the edentulous mandible. There has been moderate buccal/lingual and vertical resorption of the edentulous jaw, high muscle attachments, and also a high and active floor of the mouth.

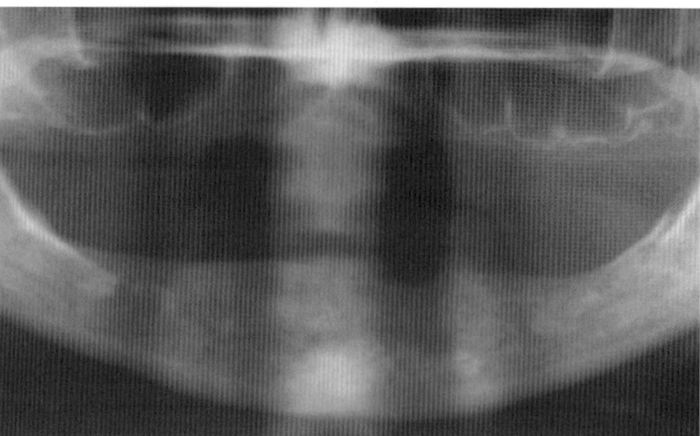

Figure 4.18. Panoramic radiograph two years post extraction of the mandibular dentition. Bone resorption has occurred, but the mandible still has adequate bone volume for implant placement.

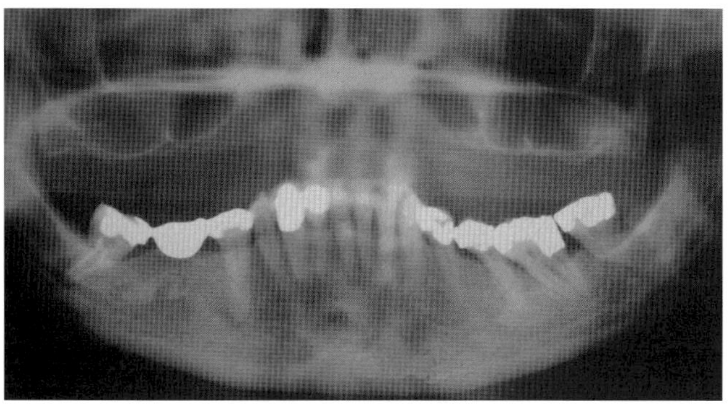

Figure 4.17. Original pre-operative panoramic radiograph that demonstrated severe resorption of the edentulous maxillae, an altered occlusal plane, moderate bone loss, and periapical disease.

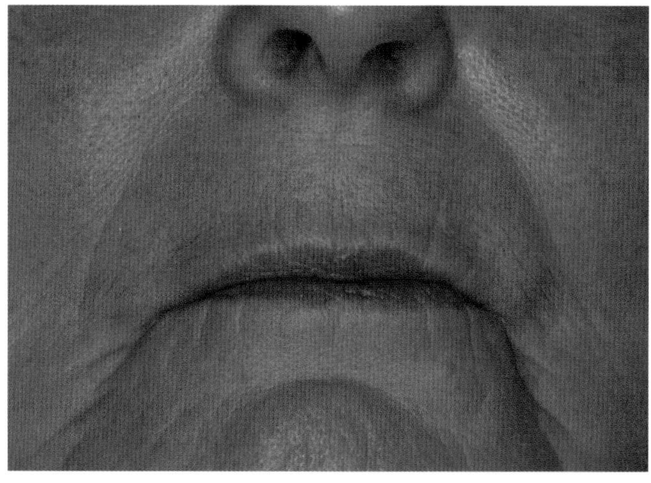

Figure 4.19. Extra-oral view of the patient in centric occlusion.

This patient had undergone full extractions approximately two years previous (Figure 4.17). Immediate dentures were constructed and laboratory relines were accomplished approximately five months later. The patient presented with difficulties associated with eating and comfort and was not adapting to the mandibular denture. She was getting along well with the maxillary denture. The patient reported that she was basically pleased with the aesthetic and phonetic results of her dentures. She wanted improved function. Her medical history was noncontributory.

Radiographs

The initial diagnostics included a panoramic radiograph, clinical examination, and diagnostic impressions (Figure 4.18). The panoramic radiograph demonstrated adequate bone volume for placement of two implants in the anterior mandible.

Physical Examination

The physical examination consisted of a detailed evaluation of the existing dentures relative to lip support, vertical dimension of occlusion, vertical dimension of rest position, closest speaking space, freeway space, status of the oral tissues, ridge height and width, presence or absence of keratinized tissues, and location of muscle attachments (Figure 4.19).

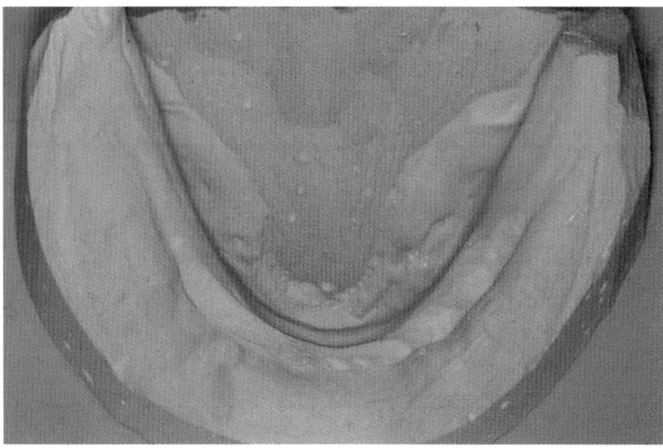

Figure 4.20. Occlusal laboratory view of mandibular diagnostic cast.

Diagnostic Cast

A mandibular diagnostic cast was made from an alginate impression. The anterior ridge was thin and knife-edged. There were adequate buccal shelves with good disto-lingual extensions (Figure 4.20).

Diagnoses

The following diagnoses were made:

1. Edentulous maxillae with moderate resorption
2. Edentulous mandible with moderate resorption
3. Relatively well-fitting dentures
4. Class I occlusion
5. Decreased vertical dimension of occlusion
6. Adequate bone volume for implant placement

Appointment 2. Consultation Restorative Dentist/Patient (1/2 Hour)

A definitive consultation appointment was scheduled as the patient left the office from the first visit. The time between the first and second appointments allowed for development of the treatment options for this particular patient.

Treatment Options

The first treatment option described placement of two 4.1 mm diameter implants in the areas of the mandibular right and left cuspids areas, preferably with a single-stage protocol. New dentures were not required because the preexisting dentures were clinically acceptable in terms of retention, stability, lip support, centric jaw relationships, aesthetics, and phonetics. The vertical dimension of occlusion was decreased, but the author thought that it could be corrected during the processed reline procedure associated with an implant-retained overdenture (Table 4.3). The second treatment option described the protocol for a processed laboratory reline of the mandibular denture (Table 4.4).

Benefits and limitations of each treatment option were described in detail on the written treatment plans. The prosthodontic fees, or ranges of fees for each procedure, were also listed on each treatment plan. The patient was given copies of the treatment plans. The patient agreed to proceed with the first treatment plan including implant placement and was referred to a periodontist for the surgical diagnostic work up.

Appointment 3. Consultation Restorative Dentist/Surgeon (1/2 Hour)

This appointment generally takes place before or after normal business hours and should precede the surgeon's examination appointment. It may occur at lunch, at either practitioner's office, or at another convenient location. This consultation is critical for the long-term functional and aesthetic success of implant treatment. It is essential that the restorative dentist explain to the surgeon the physical and radiographic findings, the diagnoses, and the treatment options that were explained to the patient. This particular case presentation was not technically demanding and the consultation between restorative dentist and the surgeon was completed within 30 minutes. Other, more complex treatment options are discussed in later chapters.

Type/Number/Size of Implants

In this case, the patient was edentulous in both jaws. She had adapted well to the maxillary denture but was having difficulty managing the mandibular denture. The author suggested that 4.1 mm diameter implants with internal connections be placed (OSSEOTITE® Certain® Implant System). The surgeon would determine the shape of the implant body. In this case, the surgeon preselected tapered implants.

Abutment/Prosthesis Design

The author planned to use resilient overdenture attachments (LOCATOR® Abutments) (Figure 4.21). The actual abutment height would not be determined until after osseointegration and soft tissue healing.

Implant/Abutment Connection

The ***3i***® internal connection implant was designed with a 4 mm-long implant/abutment connection.

TABLE 4.3. Treatment Plan #1. (Implant-Retained Overdenture with Resilient Attachments)

Diagnoses:

1. Edentulous maxillae with moderate resorption
2. Edentulous mandible with moderate resorption
3. Relatively well–fitting dentures
4. Class I occlusion
5. Decreased vertical dimension of occlusion
6. Adequate bone volume for implant placement

Restorative Services	**ADA #**	**Fee**
Comprehensive oral evaluation	D0150	
Diagnostic casts	D0470	
Panoramic radiograph	D0330	
Surgical guide	D6190	

Referral to Oral Surgical Office:

1. Evaluate and treat for placement of two OSSEOTITE® Certain® implants (4.1 mm diameter) in the areas of the mandibular cuspid teeth.
2. Single-stage surgical protocol, if possible.
3. Healing abutments should have the following profiles: 4.1 mm restorative platforms, 5 mm emergence profiles. Occlusal surfaces should be 1 mm supra-gingival.
4. Post-operative instructions.
5. Schedule a denture tissue conditioning appointment 10 days post implant surgery.
6. Discharge to prosthodontist for prosthetic care.

Fees and services will be determined by the oral surgeon.

	ADA #	**Fees**
Healing/osseointegration		
Tissue conditioning of preexisting mandibular denture, per time	D5851	
Prosthodontic reevaluation	D0140	
Placement of LOCATOR® Abutments	D6199	
Laboratory processed reline of preexisting mandibular denture	D5751	
Yearly recall appointment	D0120	
Periapical radiographs	D0220	

Benefits of Treatment Plan #1

With osseointegration of the implants, the lower denture should have significantly more retention, which should improve the patient's function. The denture occlusion (bite) will be improved; facial aesthetics should be improved. The patient should enjoy a good, long-term prognosis. Bone loss will be minimized in the front part of the lower jaw.

Limitations of Treatment Plan #1

Cost, complexity, and length of treatment (3–6 months). Implants are generally successful in the front part of the lower jaw approximately 96–99% of the time. The implants have to be placed optimally for the above treatments to be accomplished. If the implants cannot be placed optimally, changes in the treatments (surgical and prosthetic), fees, and designs will be likely. The upper denture will move. Bone loss will continue in the upper jaw without implants. If the denture/implant experience is unsatisfactory, additional implants may be placed in one or both jaws, at additional cost. The patient will be asked to take the dentures out during nighttime sleep. The patient needs to return to this office at least once per year for follow up, which will include radiographs (x-rays) to assess osseointegration of the implants, fit and occlusion of the dentures, health of the soft tissues, and the integrity of the implant/abutment connections. This treatment plan itemizes only the prosthetic phase of treatment.

Patient signature ______________________

Date ______________________

Witness ______________________

Date ______________________

TABLE 4.4. Treatment Plan #2 (Processed Laboratory Reline Existing Mandibular Denture)

Diagnoses:

1. Edentulous maxillae with moderate resorption
2. Edentulous mandible with moderate resorption
3. Relatively well-fitting dentures
4. Class I occlusion
5. Decreased vertical dimension of occlusion
6. Adequate bone volume for implant placement

Restorative Services	**ADA #**	**Fee**
Comprehensive oral evaluation	D0150	
Tissue conditioning of preexisting mandibular denture, per time	D5851	
Laboratory processed reline of preexisting mandibular denture	D5751	
Yearly recall appointment	D0120	
Periapical radiographs	D0220	

Benefits of Treatment Plan #2

The denture occlusion (bite) will be made optimal; facial aesthetics should be improved. The fit of the lower denture should be improved.

Limitations of Treatment Plan #2

Cost, complexity, and length of treatment (1–3 months). Facial aesthetics may not be acceptable with this denture reline procedure. The patient will have to go without the lower denture for one working day when the laboratory reline procedure is accomplished. If the aesthetics are not satisfactory, a new mandibular denture will be needed (at additional cost). Both dentures will move. Bone loss will continue in jaws without implants. If the denture experience is unsatisfactory, implants may be placed in one or both jaws, at additional cost. The patient will be asked to take the dentures out during nighttime sleep. The patient needs to return to this office at least once per year for follow-up, which will include radiographs (x-rays) to assess the fit and occlusion of the dentures and health of the soft tissues. This treatment plan itemizes only the prosthetic phase of treatment.

Patient signature ______________________

Date ______________________

Witness ______________________

Date ______________________

ADA #'s, CDT 2005 Current Dental Terminology, Council on Dental Benefit Programs, American Dental Association, 211 East Chicago Avenue, Chicago, IL 60611

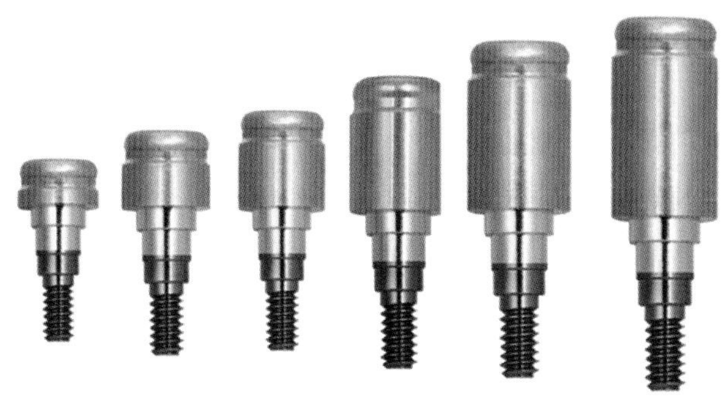

Figure 4.21. LOCATOR® Abutments for the OSSEOTITE® Certain® implant system are available with six different collar heights: 1–6 mm, left to right.

Surgical Guide

A surgical guide was fabricated on the mandibular diagnostic cast (Figure 4.22). Holes, in anticipation of optimal implant placement, were placed in the areas of the mandibular cuspid teeth. This placement was designed for maximum overdenture retention.

Surgical Protocol

The author also suggested that if possible, a one-stage surgical protocol be followed. Published reports have indicated that single-stage surgical protocols have been as efficacious as the traditional two-stage surgical protocols (Testori and others 2002). However, the surgeon always has the final decision relative to the surgical protocol.

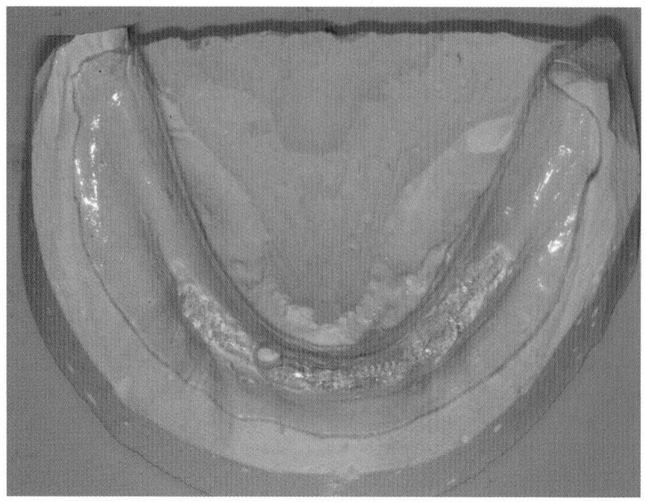

Figure 4.22. Laboratory occlusal view of the surgical guide in place on the mandibular diagnostic cast. A guide hole has been placed for the right implant. A contra-lateral hole was to be placed for the left implant.

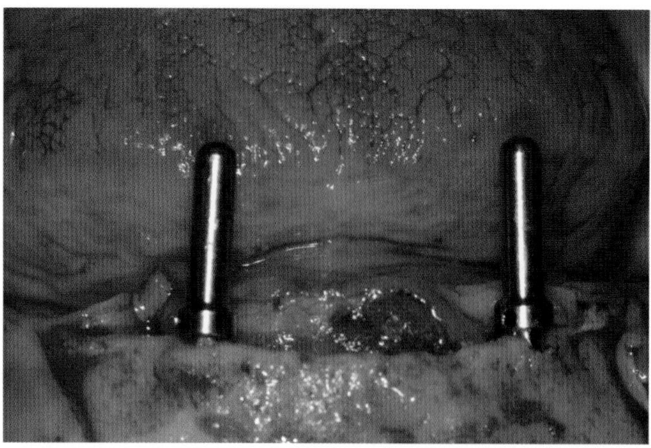

Figure 4.23. Direction indicators (NTDI411) in place just prior to implant placement. The osteotomies were prepared consistent with the surgical guide.

TABLE 4.5. The Implant Restorative Wish List

Mandibular Implant Retained Overdenture	
Type of Implant	OSSEOTITE® Certain®
Implant Restorative Platform	4.1 mm
Surgical Protocol	Single stage
Implant/Abutment Connection	Internal (Certain)
Healing Abutment	5 mm × 5 mm × 2, 3, or 4 mm (supra-gingival occlusal surface)
Occlusal Loading Protocol	8–10 weeks

Healing Abutment Selection

If a single-stage surgical protocol was followed, the predetermined healing abutment size would be 4.1 mm restorative platforms, 5 mm emergence profiles, and the occlusal surfaces should be slightly supra gingival at the time of implant placement (2, 3, or 4 mm). If a two-stage surgical protocol was followed, cover screws would be placed prior to closure of the surgical wound. The above healing abutments would be placed at the time of second stage surgery.

Implant Restorative Wish List

The preceding concepts have proven to be an excellent starting point for discussions between the author and surgeon. A form was developed that incorporated all of the concepts noted above and is called the Implant Restorative Wish List (Table 4.5). It is now completed for each patient and sent to the implant surgeon prior to patient treatment.

Appointment 4. Implant Placement

Two-Stage Surgical Protocol

In this instance, the surgeon prepared the osteotomies as discussed in the restorative dentist/surgeon consultation appointment (Figure 4.23). The surgeon was not comfortable placing these implants with a single-stage surgical protocol and therefore placed cover screws and closed the wound over the implants (Figures 4.24 and 4.25).

Postoperative Instructions

The patient was instructed by the surgeon not to wear the mandibular denture until the first postoperative visit. She was given analgesics, antibiotics, and 0.12% chlorhexidine mouthwash. She was instructed to eat a soft diet and return in 10 days for two clinical appointments: suture removal and the first application of tissue conditioning material to the intaglio surface of the mandibular denture.

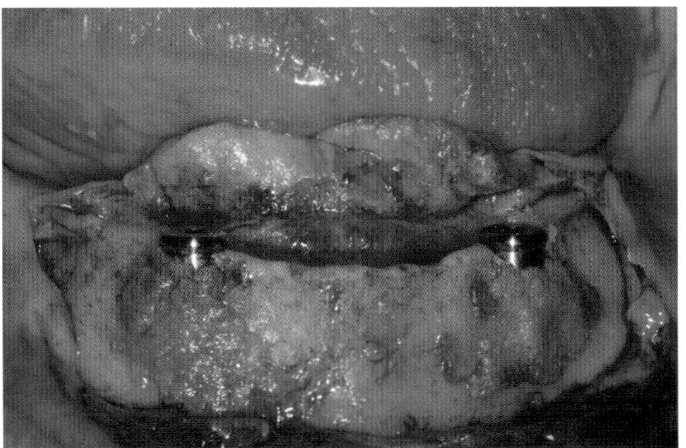

Figure 4.24. The surgeon decided to place these implants with a two-stage surgical protocol. Cover screws were placed into the occlusal aspects of the implants in preparation for closure of the wound.

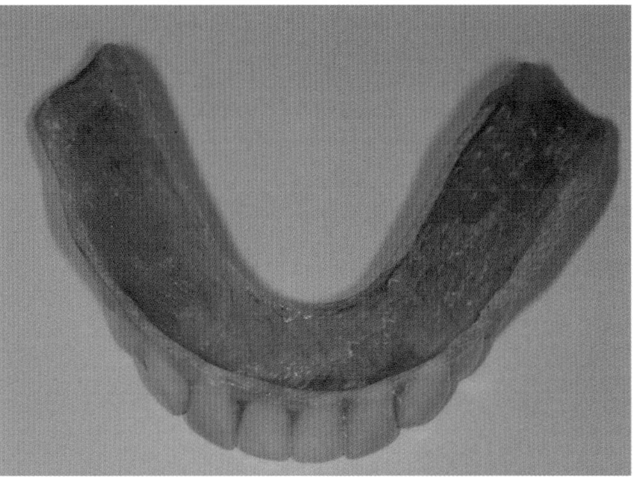

Figure 4.26. The intaglio surface of the mandibular denture was thoroughly relieved prior to the application of tissue conditioning material.

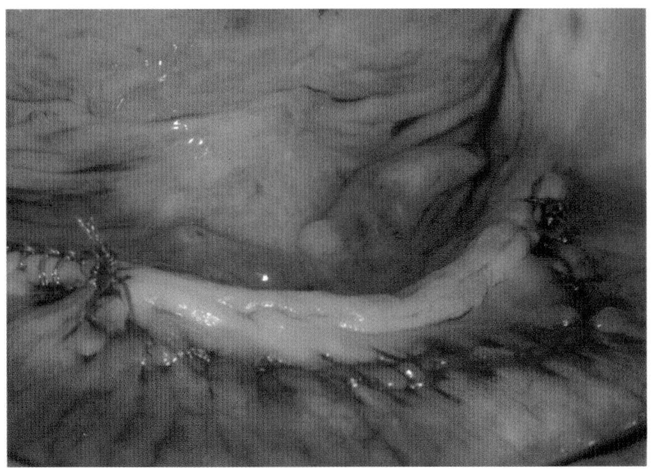

Figure 4.25. The full thickness flap was closed primarily. The patient was instructed not to wear the mandibular denture until she returned in 10 days for suture removal.

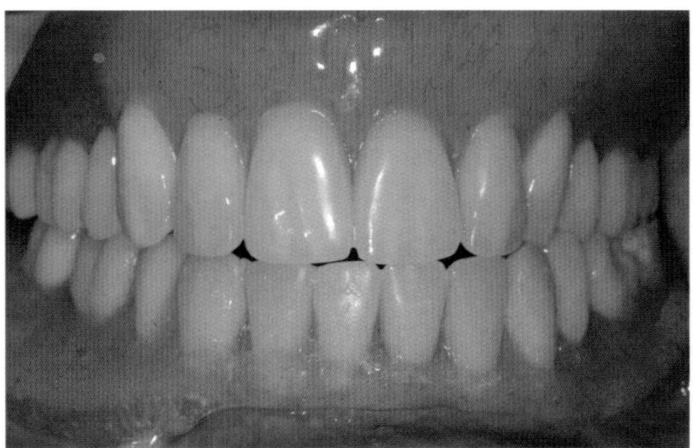

Figure 4.27. Intra-oral, anterior view of the patient in centric occlusion after the tissue conditioning material had set. The mandibular midline is off to the left approximately 2 mm.

Appointment 5. Follow Up Appointments (1/2 Hour)

Suture Removal

This patient returned 10 days post surgery and reported no ill effects from the surgery. The surgeon removed the sutures and the patient was transferred to the author's office for relief of the denture and the first application of tissue-conditioning material.

Tissue Conditioning

The mandibular denture was thoroughly relieved, especially in the anterior segment (Figure 4.26). The tissue conditioning material (Visgo-gel, Dentsply International, York, PA) was mixed so that the material was thick and viscous and applied to the intaglio surface of the denture. The patient was guided into centric occlusion, at an appropriate vertical dimension of occlusion (Figure 4.27). The material set intra-orally for five minutes and was removed.

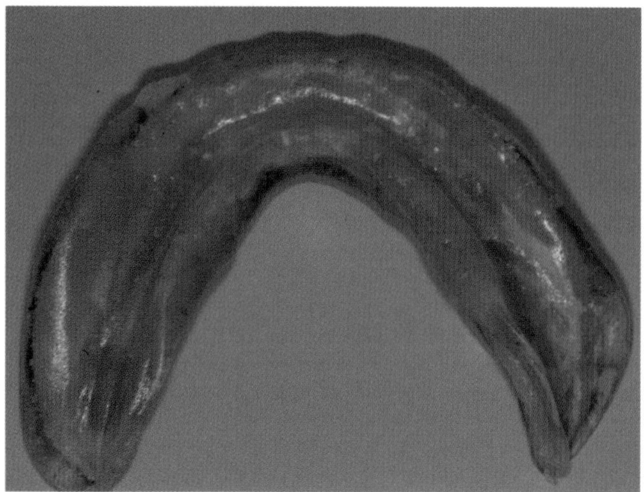

Figure 4.28. The intaglio surface of the denture after the tissue conditioning material had set. This material usually remains resilient and serviceable for between six and 10 weeks.

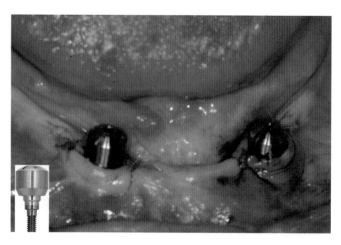

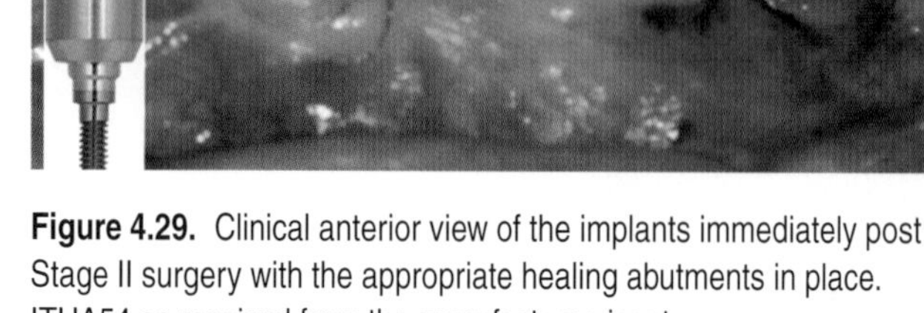

Figure 4.29. Clinical anterior view of the implants immediately post Stage II surgery with the appropriate healing abutments in place. ITHA54 as received from the manufacturer, inset.

It was placed into a pressure pot with 120° water under 10 psi and allowed to cure for 10 minutes. The excess was trimmed and re-inserted into the mouth (Figure 4.28).

This procedure was repeated eight weeks post implant placement and the patient was scheduled for Stage II surgery.

Appointment 6. Stage II Surgery

The implants were uncovered 10 weeks after they were placed. As soon as the patient was seated in the surgical office, one of the surgical assistants brought the denture with the tissue conditioning material in place to the prosthodontic laboratory for removal of the soft liner.

Healing Abutments (1/2 Hour)

Healing abutments were placed with 5 mm emergence profile diameters and were 4 mm tall (ITHA54) (Figures 4.29, 4.30). The peri-implant soft tissues would then heal in a manner consistent with the shape of the healing abutments. This would make the LOCATOR® Abutment insertion procedure simple and predictable because the soft tissue profiles would be larger than the abutments. The surgeon torqued the healing abutments to 10 Ncm and discharged the patient to the author.

Tissue Conditioning

Healing abutments take up a significant amount of restorative volume and extra relief is therefore required in the anterior segment of the mandibular denture. The location of the healing abutments was identified with indelible pencil (Dr. Thompson's Sanitary Color Transfer Applicators, Great Plains Dental Products Co., Inc., Kingman, KS) and

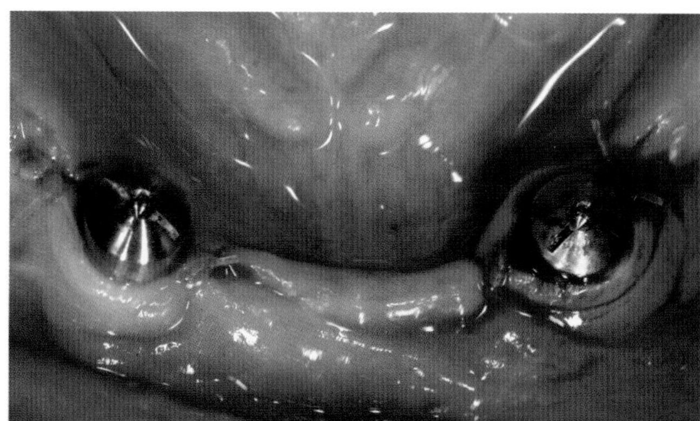

Figure 4.30. Occlusal view of healing abutments in place immediately after Stage II surgery. The implants were in positions consistent with the pre-operative planning.

the marks were transferred to the intaglio surface of the mandibular denture (Figures 4.31, 4.32). The mandibular denture was relieved so that it fit onto the denture-bearing tissues with the patient in centric occlusion at an appropriate vertical dimension of occlusion. The denture was relined with tissue conditioning material as described previously. The denture now functioned as an overdenture with the healing abutments providing increased stability and support to the prosthesis. They did not provide additional retention (Figure 4.33).

The patient was instructed to massage and cleanse the surgical sites with a soft toothbrush and 2 × 2 gauze. She was urged to continue with 0.12% chlorhexidine after the hygiene procedures were accomplished at night. The patient was reappointed for the laboratory-processed reline procedures in three weeks.

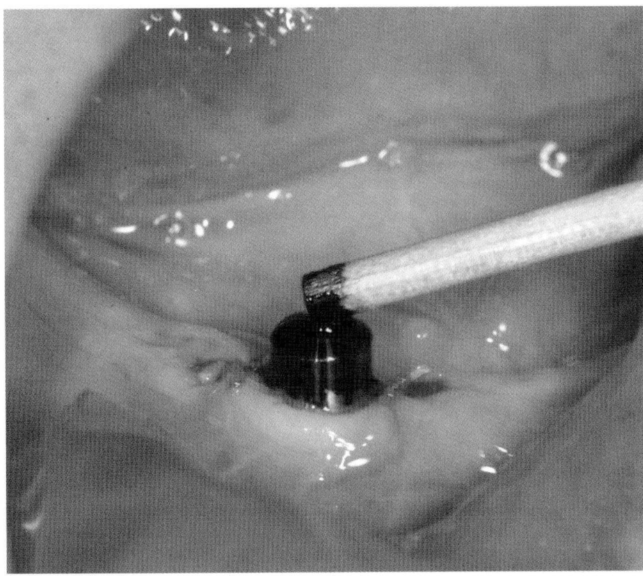

Figure 4.31. Indelible pencil was applied to the healing abutments to identify their locations within the denture base.

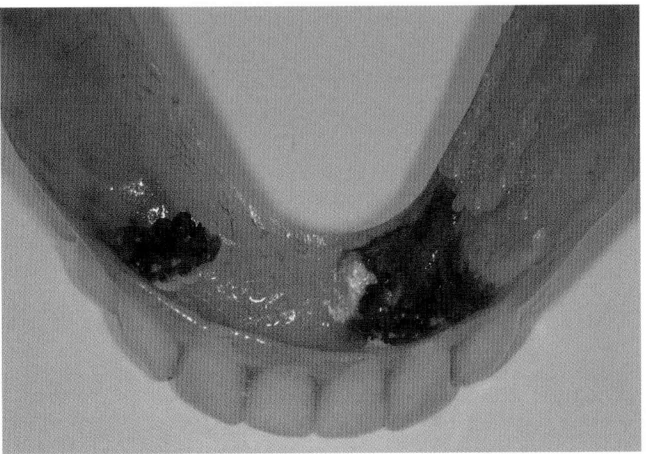

Figure 4.32. The marks were transferred to the intaglio surface of the denture base so that the relief was accomplished accurately.

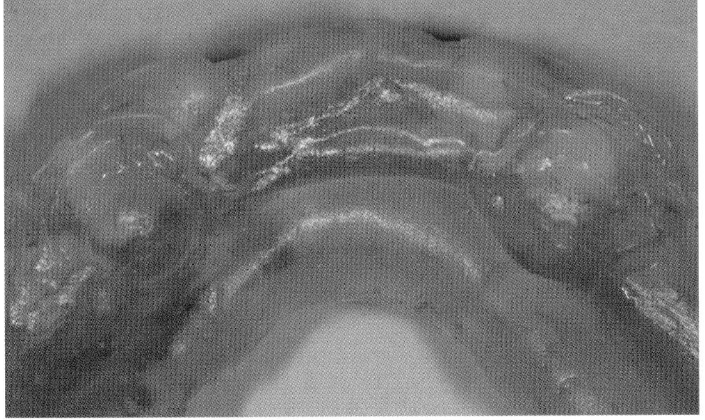

Figure 4.33. The intaglio surface of the soft liner inside the mandibular denture after Stage II surgery. The indentations in the liner corresponded to the locations of the healing abutments and provided increased support for the patient.

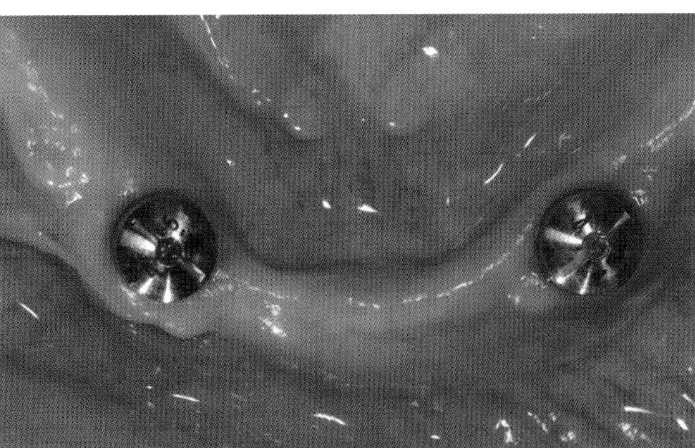

Figure 4.34. Occlusal view of the healing abutments three weeks after the implants were uncovered. The patient's oral hygiene was excellent, the healing abutments were highly polished, and the peri-implant soft tissues were firm, pink, and non-inflamed.

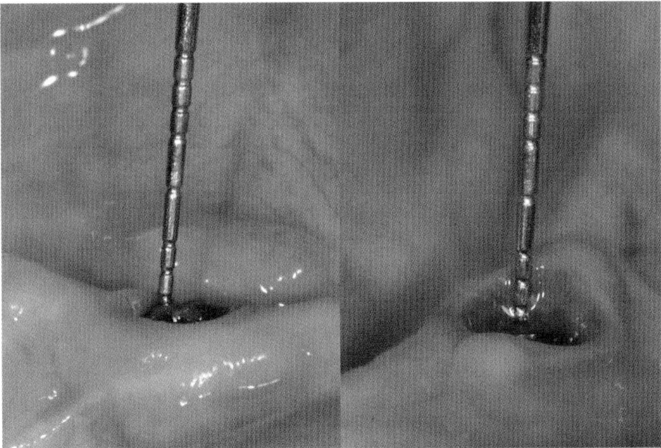

Figure 4.35. Labial views of the implant restorative platforms 10 weeks post implant placement. Periodontal probes were placed on the implant restorative platforms and the heights of the sulcus were measured. The left sulcus measured 2+ mm; the right sulcus measured approximately 1+ mm.

Appointment 7. Abutment Connection and Reline Impression (3/4 Hour)

The patient was seen in the first morning appointment (Figure 4.34). The healing abutments were removed and a periodontal probe was used to measure the sulcular depths. The left sulcus measured 2+ mm at its greatest depth. The right sulcus measured 1+ mm at its greatest depth. A periodontal probe was placed at the soft tissue margin for both healing abutments (Figure 4.35). Three and 2 mm LOCATOR® Abutments were used for the respective implants, left and right (ILOA003 and ILOA002, respectively).

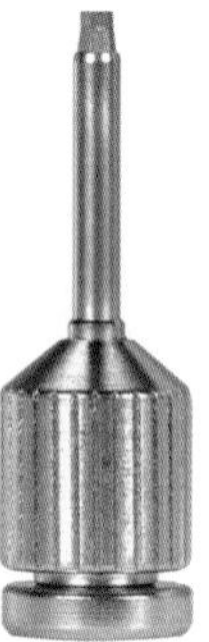

Figure 4.36. This driver (PHD03N) was used to remove the healing abutments from the implants.

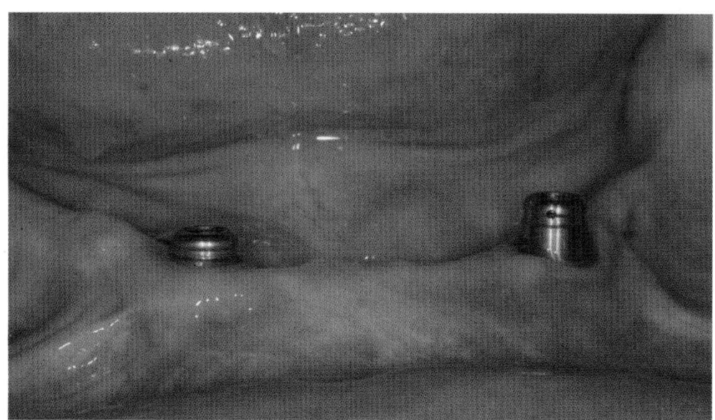

Figure 4.37. LOCATOR® Abutments (ILOA003 and ILOA002, left, right respectively) in place.

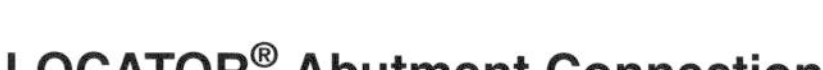

LOCATOR® Abutment Connection

The healing abutments were removed with the large hex driver (PHDO2) (Figure 4.36). The LOCATOR® Abutments were placed and tightened by hand (Figure 4.37).

Torque

They were torqued to 20 Ncm with the Restorative Torque Indicator (RTI2035) and the Driver Tip (LOADT4) (Figure 4.38).

Impression Copings

Impression copings (LAIC1) were placed onto the abutments (Figure 4.39). In the areas in and around the healing abutment, impressions within the denture base, windows were drilled completely through the mandibular denture, and all of the tissue-conditioning material was removed (Figure 4.40). The denture fit around the abutments and impression copings and the patient was able to close into centric occlusion at the predetermined vertical dimension of occlusion (Figure 4.41).

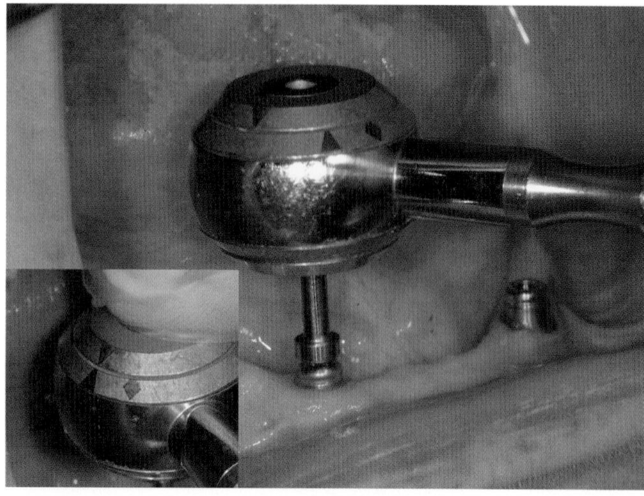

Figure 4.38. The abutments were torqued to 20 Ncm with the torque driver and driver tip (RTI2035 at 20 Ncm inset).

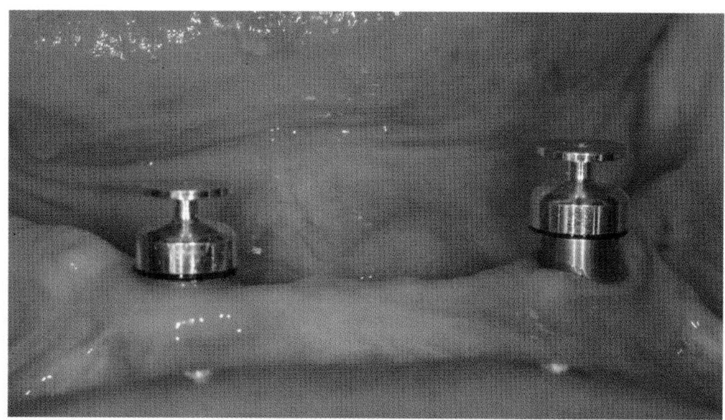

Figure 4.39. Impression copings (LAIC1) in place on the LOCATOR® Abutments.

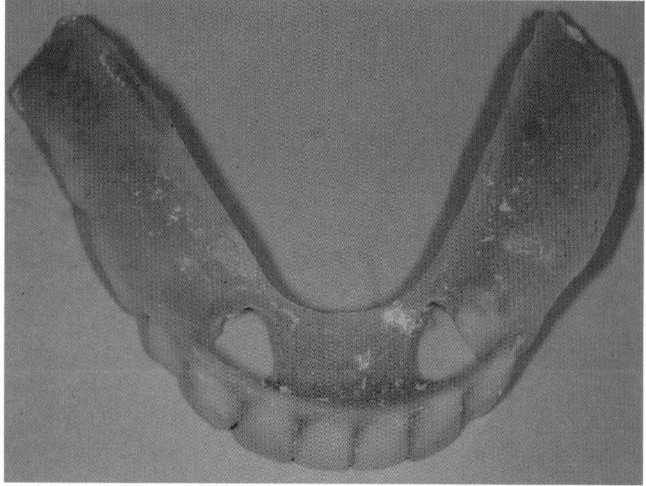

Figure 4.40. Windows were prepared completely through the denture base so as to prevent interferences between the implant restorative components and the denture base.

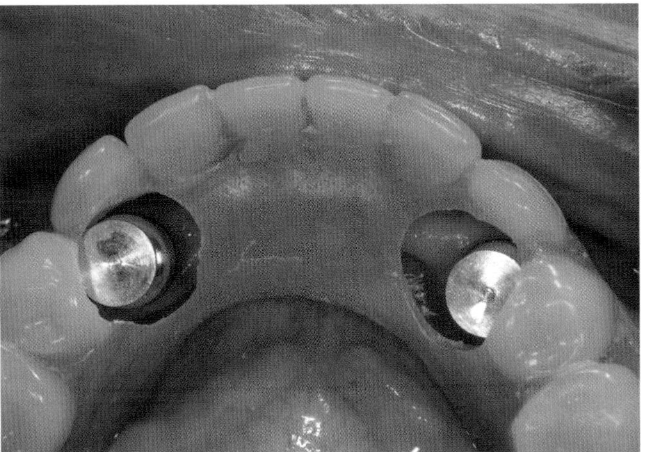

Figure 4.41. Occlusal view of the mandibular denture completely seated around the impression copings and abutments.

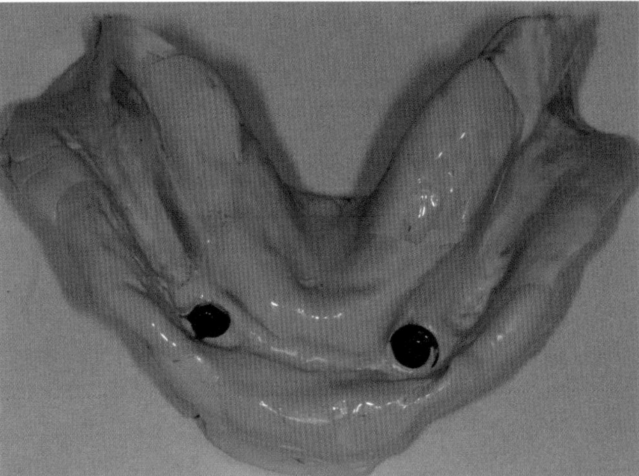

Figure 4.43. The intaglio surface of the reline impression: The impression copings remained inside the impression.

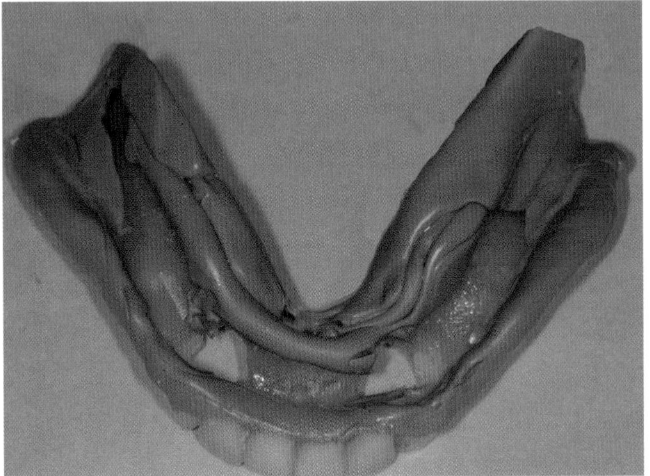

Figure 4.42. The mandibular denture border molded with heavy body poly vinylsiloxane impression material.

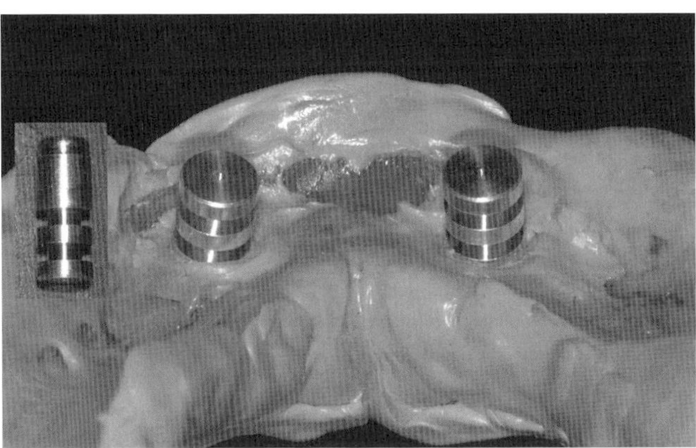

Figure 4.44. Analogs (LALA1) attached to the impression copings within the impression. Analog as received from the manufacturer, inset.

Reline Impression

The borders of the denture were adjusted to be approximately 2 mm short of the reflections and were reestablished with heavy body poly vinylsiloxane impression material (Extrude® Extra, Kerr Corporation, Romulus, MI) (Figure 4.42). Multi-purpose viscosity poly vinylsiloxane impression material (Extrude® MPV, Kerr Corporation, Romulus, MI) was injected around the impression copings intraorally. The author has found that light-body poly vinylsiloxane impression material is not consistently strong enough to remove the impression copings with removal of the impression from the mouth. Light-body poly vinylsiloxane impression material was used to fill the denture and the denture was inserted.

The patient was guided into centric occlusion at the predetermined vertical dimension of occlusion and the material was allowed to set. The denture was removed; the impression copings were contained within the impression (Figure 4.43). The patient was discharged to return the next day for insertion of the relined denture.

Laboratory Work Order/Procedures

The author routinely accomplishes denture reline procedures within his own office. However, these procedures may also be sent to commercial dental laboratories. The laboratory procedures are illustrated in the following paragraphs. Laboratory work orders for the procedures are identified in Table 4.6.

LOCATOR® Abutment analogs (LALA1) were placed into the apical ends of the impression copings within the impression (Figure 4.44). The reline impression was boxed and poured in dental stone. The denture was placed into a reline denture jig in conventional fashion. The denture was removed from the cast and the analogs were visualized (Figure 4.45).

TABLE 4.6. Laboratory Work Orders For Mandibular Denture Reline/LOCATOR® Abutments

Enclosed:

1. Mandibular denture reline impression with two LOCATOR® Abutment impression copings.
2. Place LOCATOR® Abutment analogs (LALA1) into impression copings.
3. Box and pour impression in dental stone for denture reline procedures.
4. Place in reline jig.
5. Remove impression material.
6. Place LOCATOR® Abutment housings and black males onto the analogs.
7. Block the housings out with a 50/50 mixture of plaster and pumice.
8. Reline the denture with heat processed acrylic resin.
9. Do not remove the denture from the cast.
10. Identify the locations of the housings and remove the acrylic resin surrounding them.
11. Remove all of the plaster/pumice mixture.
12. Use autopolymerizing acrylic resin and attach the housings to the acrylic resin denture.
13. Place into pressure pot with 120° water and 20 psi for 10 minutes.
14. Remove denture from cast, finish, and polish.
15. Remove black processing males from the housings and place light retention males (pink).

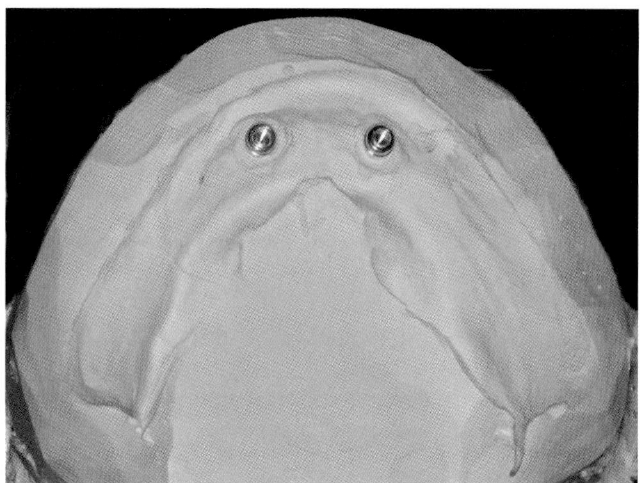

Figure 4.45. The cast after the reline impression was removed.

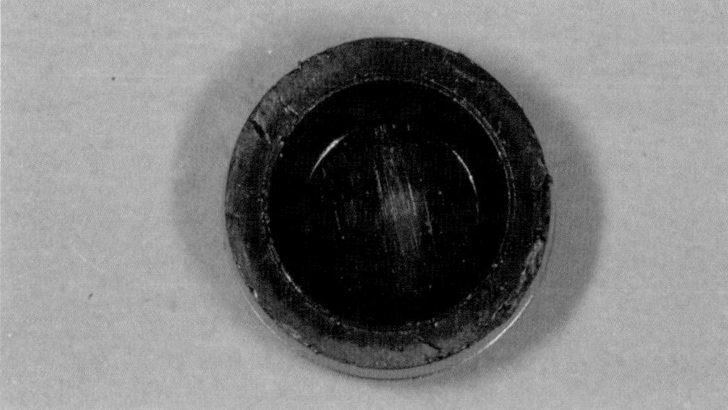

Figure 4.46. Housing and black processing male (LORHK).

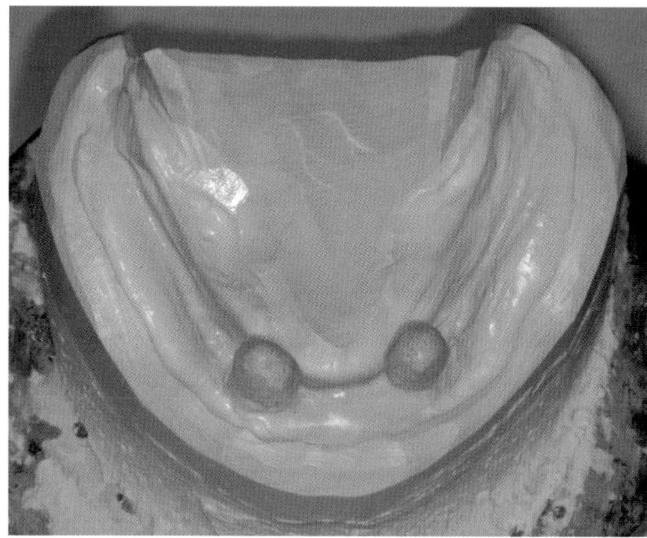

Figure 4.47. The housings were blocked out with a 50/50 plaster and pumice mixture.

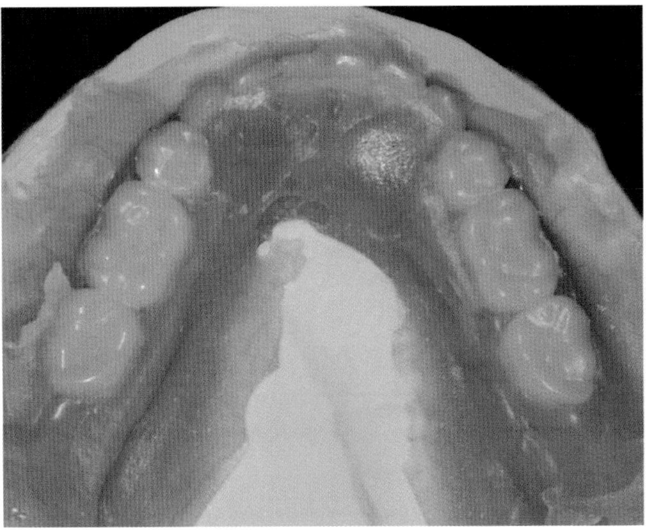

Figure 4.48. Occlusal view of the processed denture after it was relined with autopolymerizing acrylic resin. It was not removed from the cast.

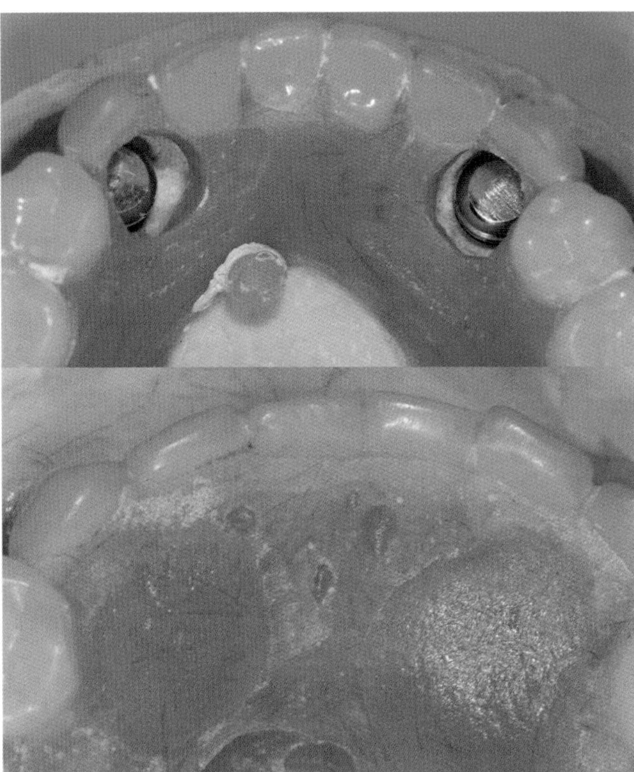

Figure 4.50. The housings were placed onto the analogs (top) and autopolymerizing acrylic resin was injected into these areas to attach the housings to the denture base (bottom).

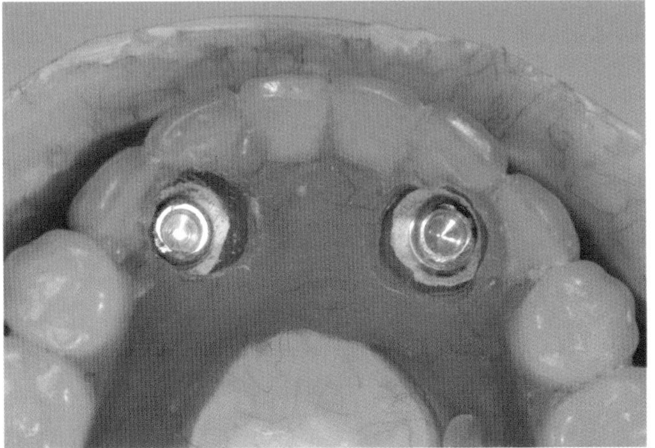

Figure 4.49. Resin was removed from the areas of the abutments, completely exposing the abutment analogs.

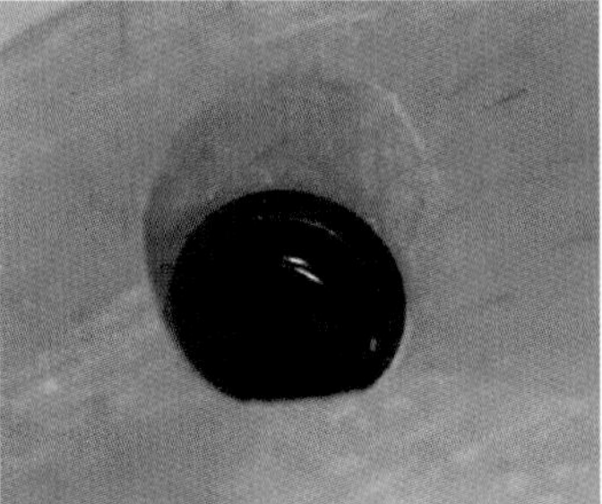

Figure 4.51. Intaglio surface of the relined dentures with one black processing male inside the housing.

The housings and black processing males were placed onto the analogs and blocked out with a 50/50 mixture of plaster and pumice (Figures 4.46, 4.47). The reline impression material was removed and the denture was relined with autopolymerizing acrylic resin (Figure 4.48).

After polymerization, the locations of the analogs and housings were identified and the resin was removed in these areas (Figure 4.49). The housings were removed. The analogs were completely exposed and the housings were placed back onto the analogs. Additional acrylic resin was placed around the housings and the housings were attached to the denture (Figure 4.50). The denture was placed into a pressure pot with 120° water under 20 psi for 10 minutes. It was removed, finished, and polished (Figure 4.51).

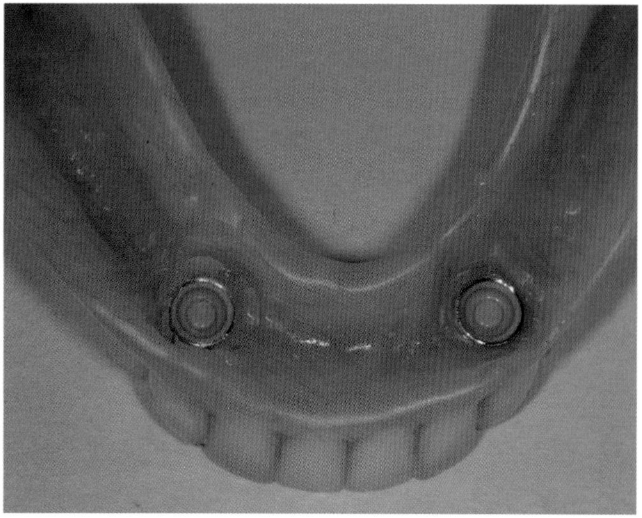

Figure 4.52. Intaglio surface of the mandibular relined denture with light pink retentive male attachments in place.

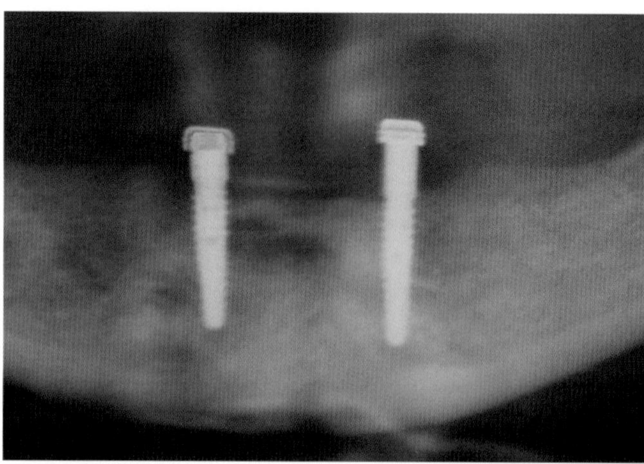

Figure 4.54. Panoramic radiograph one-year post loading was taken with the denture in place and demonstrated less than 1 mm bone loss at the occlusal aspects of both mandibular implants.

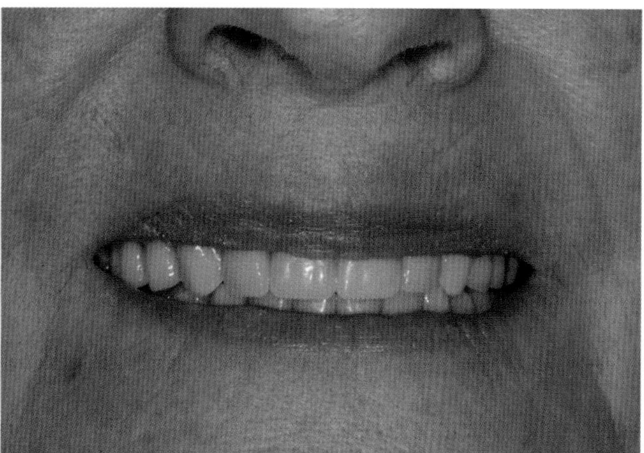

Figure 4.53. Clinical anterior view of maxillary complete denture and mandibular implant-retained overdenture in place.

TABLE 4.7. Restorative Costs/Fees/Profitability

Implant Components, Lab Fees and Overhead Costs	Costs
LOCATOR Abutments	$212
Impression Copings	$24
Analogs	$36
Denture Lab Processing	$100
Clinical Overhead (¾ hour) @400 per hour	$300
Total Costs	$672
Professional Fee	$1100
Profit	$428
Profit per hour	$321

The black processing males were removed and replaced with light retention males (pink attachments with 3 lbs of retention) (Figure 4.52). The denture was ready for insertion. This technique provides dental laboratory technicians and restorative dentists with improved accuracy and decreased processing error in reline procedures (Drago and Gingrasso 2005).

Appointment 8. Insertion Relined Denture (1/2 Hour)

The patient presented the next day for the insertion of the relined denture. The denture went to place without incident. Both attachments were engaged. The flanges and occlusion were adjusted as needed (Figure 4.53). Oral hygiene was reviewed and the patient was dismissed.

Appointment 9. Follow-Up Appointments (1/2 Hour)

Two Weeks

The patient returned for the two-week follow-up appointment and was thrilled with the retention, stability, comfort, and function of the mandibular implant-retained overdenture. She had no soreness and related minimal problems adapting to the new overdenture. Her oral hygiene was excellent. Her prognosis for successful adaptation was also excellent.

One-Year Recall Clinical and Radiographic Evaluations

The patient returned approximately one year post insertion of the mandibular implant-retained overdenture and continued to do well. Her occlusion was stable, the dentures and abutments were clean, and there was minimal attachment wear. The panoramic radiograph demonstrated satisfactory bone/implant adaptations and approximately 1 mm of bone loss (Figure 4.54).

Costs/Fees/Profitability

The following discussion (Table 4.7) relative to fees is reflective of late 2006 in the Midwest United States. The costs of the implant components are retail prices from Implant Innovations, Inc., Palm Beach Gardens, Florida. The costs, fees, and profitability for this procedure are shown in Table 4.7.

Surgeon: Michael Banasik, DDS, Gundersen Lutheran Medical Center, LaCrosse, WI

Dental Laboratory Technician: Andrew Gingrasso, Gundersen Lutheran Medical Center, LaCrosse, WI

BIBLIOGRAPHY

Awad, M, Lund, J, Shapiro, S, Locker, D, Klemetti, E, Chehade, A, Savard, A, Feine, J, 2003. Oral health status and treatment satisfaction with mandibular implant overdentures and conventional dentures: a randomized clinical trial in a senior population. *Int J Prosthodont* 16:390–396.

Bourgeois, D, Nihtila, A, Mersel, A, 1998. Prevalence of caries and edentulousness among 65–74 year olds in Europe. *Bull World Health Organ* 76:413–441.

Carpentieri, J, 2004. Treatment options for the edentulous mandible: clinical application of the two-implant overdenture. *Pract Proced Aesthet Dent* 16:105–112.

Cune, M, van Kampen F, van der Bilt, A, Bosman, F, 2005. Patient satisfaction and preference with magnet, bar-clip and ball-socket retained mandibular implant overdentures: a cross-over clinical trial. *J Prosthet Dent* 18:99–105.

Douglass, C, Shih, A, Ostry, L, 2002. Will there be a need for complete dentures in the United States in 2020? *J Prosthet Dent* 87:5–8.

Douglass, C, Watson, A, 2002. Future needs for fixed and removable partial dentures in the United States. *J Prosthet Dent* 87:9–14.

Drago, C, Gingrasso, A, 2005. Simplified laboratory procedures for processing Locator abutments into mandibular implant supported overdentures. *J Dent Tech* 22:40–46.

Gotfredsen, K, Holm, B, 2000. Implant-supported mandibular overdentures retained with ball or bar attachments: a randomized prospective 5-year study. *Int J Prosthodont* 13:125–130.

MacEntee, M, Walton, J, Glick, N, 2005. A clinical trial of patient satisfaction and prosthodontic needs with ball and bar attachments for implant-retained complete dentures: three-year results. *J Prosthet Dent* 93:28–37.

McGill Consensus Statement on Overdentures, 2002. *Int J Prosthodont* 15(4):413–414.

Morrow, Robert and Brewer, Allen. 1980. *Overdentures*, 2nd ed. St. Louis: The CV Mosby Company.

Oral Health in Americans. A Report of the Surgeon General, 2000. Rockville, MD: US Department of Health and Human Services. National Institute of Dental and Craniofacial Research.

Pavlatos, J, 1998. Root-supported overdentures. *Chicago Dental Society Rev* 91:20–25.

Rangert, B, Jemt, T, Jorneus, L, 1989. Forces and moments on Brånemark implants. *Int J Oral Maxillofac Implants* 4:241–247.

Schmitt, A, Zarb, G, 1998. The notion of implant-supported overdentures. *J Prosthet Dent* 79:60–65.

Tallgren, A, 1972. The continuing reduction of the alveolar ridges in complete denture wearers: a mixed longitudinal study covering 25 years. *J Prosthet Dent* 27:120–132.

Testori, T, Del Fabbro, M, Feldman, S, Vincenzi, G, Sullivan, D, Rossi, Jr, R, Anitua, E, Bianchi, F, Francetti, L, Weinstein, R. 2002. A multicenter prospective evaluation of 2-months loaded Osseotite implants placed in the posterior jaws: 3-year follow-up results. *Clin Oral Implants Res* 13:154–161.

Walton, J, MacEntee, M, Glick, N, 2002. One-year prosthetic outcomes with implant overdentures: a randomized clinical trial. *Int J Oral Maxillofac Implants* 17:391–398.

World Health Organization, 2001. International classification of functioning, disability and health. Geneva, Switzerland.

Chapter 5: Treatment of a Partially Edentulous Mandible with a Pre-Machined Titanium Abutment and Single-Unit Porcelain Fused to Metal Crown

LITERATURE REVIEW

Endosseous implants have become an integral part of prosthodontic treatment for edentulous and partially edentulous patients. This fact has come about for multiple reasons, among them, excellent long-term success rates published in multiple refereed journals around the world; improvements in implant and restorative component designs and machining; and decreased surgical morbidity and increased consumer demand for non-invasive tooth replacements (O'Neal and Butler 2000).

Dental implants were originally developed to restore compromised edentulous patients to normal function (Brånemark and others 1985). Aesthetics and phonetics were of lesser importance. Implant restorations are now expected to predictably restore function, aesthetics, and phonetics. In edentulous patients, dental implants were originally placed into sites where there was adequate bone for implants. Precise implant placement relative to tooth positions was not required because implants could be placed between artificial teeth of the implant prosthesis without aesthetic compromise (Figure 5.1). Implants placed into embrasure spaces in partially edentulous patients may result in aesthetic and phonetic compromises (Figure 5.2).

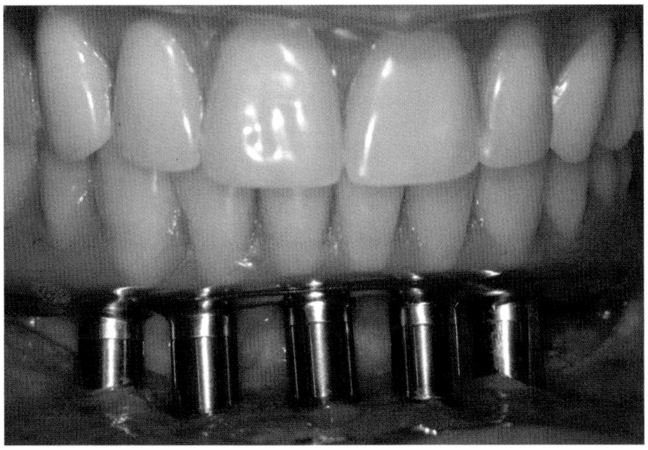

Figure 5.1. Anterior view of a maxillary complete denture and mandibular fixed implant prosthesis 14 years after placement. Note that the implants were not placed directly behind any of the anterior teeth. This implant placement was based on the location of available bone and was independent of the position of the artificial anterior teeth.

If dental implants are to succeed in solving the functional, aesthetic, and phonetic needs of partially edentulous patients, they must satisfy the same demands that patients have for natural teeth or conventional restorations (Garber 1995) (Figure 5.3).

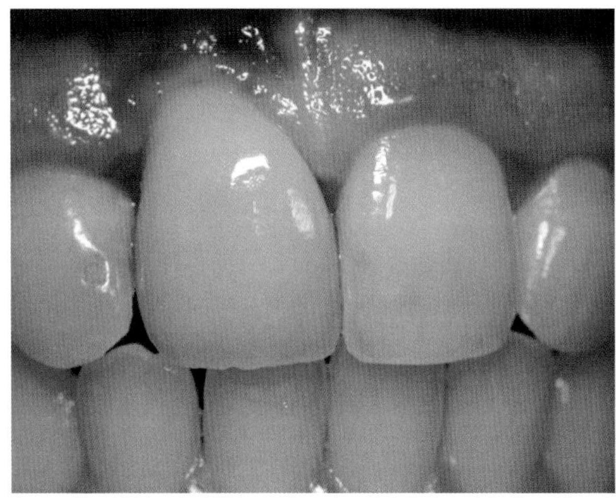

Figure 5.2. Anterior view of an implant-retained crown replacing the maxillary right central incisor. The implant was not placed relative to the center of the edentulous space; it was placed where the bone was most favorable. The emergence profiles of the crown and abutment as they exited the gingival sulcus were distorted and resulted in a non-anatomic restoration.

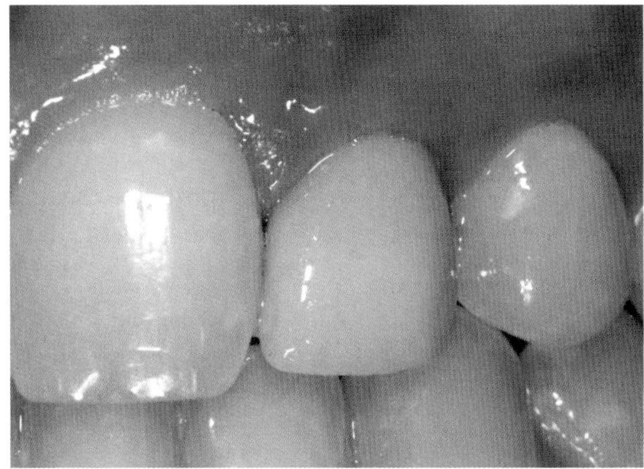

Figure 5.3. Implant-retained crown that replaced a congenitally missing left maxillary lateral incisor. Initially, there was not enough bone for optimal implant placement. The surgeon grafted bone and allowed the site to heal. The implant was then placed into an optimal position for an aesthetic and functional restoration.

Single missing teeth may be replaced with fixed partial dentures or single implant-retained crown restorations. Priest (1996) performed a comprehensive review of failure rates for conventional fixed partial dentures (FPDs), resin-bonded FPDs and single-unit implant-retained crown restorations. Priest acknowledged the difficulties in obtaining data on FPD failures due to nonstandardized methods of reporting and recording failures. Schwartz and others (1970) reported that a mean life for 3-, 4-, and 5-unit FPDs was 12.3 years. Authors had identified the most frequent cause of failures for FPDs as recurrent caries and endodontic problems post prosthesis insertion (Schwartz and others 1970; Reuter and Brose 1984; Walton and others 1986).

Single-unit implant restorations were initially reported as having more mechanical problems than full arch implant restorations. The success of single-unit implant restorations was dependent upon two distinct entities: osseointegration of the implants and biomechanical success of the restorations (Priest 1996). The long-term effectiveness (osseointegration) of dental implants has been well documented and is thought to be predictable in clinical practice (Adell and others 1981; Lazzara and others 1996; Testori and others 2002).

The biomechanical success and failure of single-unit implant restorations have been the subject of multiple reports (Jemt and others 1990; Lindh and others 1998; Andersson and others 1998) (Figure 5.4). Eckert and Wollan (1998) reviewed 1,170 dental implants in partially edentulous patients that had been qualified into placement into the anterior/posterior maxillary and mandibular quadrants. They reported Cumulative Survival Rates (CSR) at 10 years in the mid to high 90 percents, except for the posterior mandible. They noted cement-retained crown failures (biomechanical) at five years to be 22.5%. Eckert and Wollan also noted a significant difference in biomechanical success after June 1, 1991. Prosthetic components were reengineered and improved for the system that they reviewed after this date. They determined that the relative risk for implants placed and restored prior to June 1991 was 2.096 times greater than for implants placed and restored after this date. They also noted a reduction in screw loosening from more than 46% to 3.2% after the abutment screws were redesigned.

Dental endosseous implants have demonstrated high CSRs in numerous prospective and retrospective studies around the world. Dental implant manufacturers have continued to improve the machining of implant components and made improvements in the biologic designs to make dental implant treatment for edentulous and partially edentulous patients predictable and practical for patients and practitioners alike.

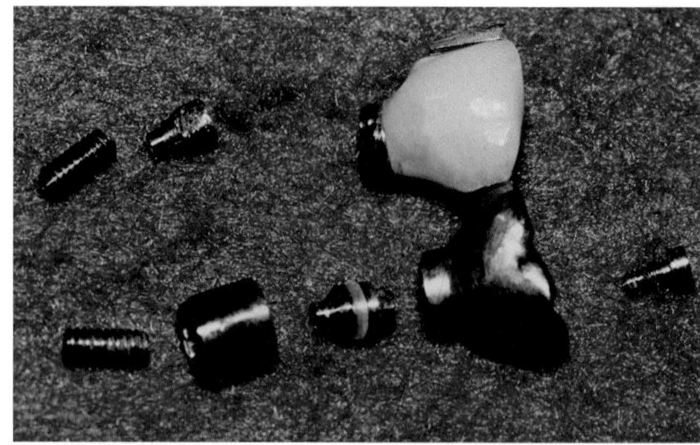

Figure 5.4. Laboratory view of broken implant restorative components. This prosthesis was inserted in 1989. There was micro movement among the implant restorative components that was below the consciousness of the patient. The movement continued until such time that the abutment screws fractured.

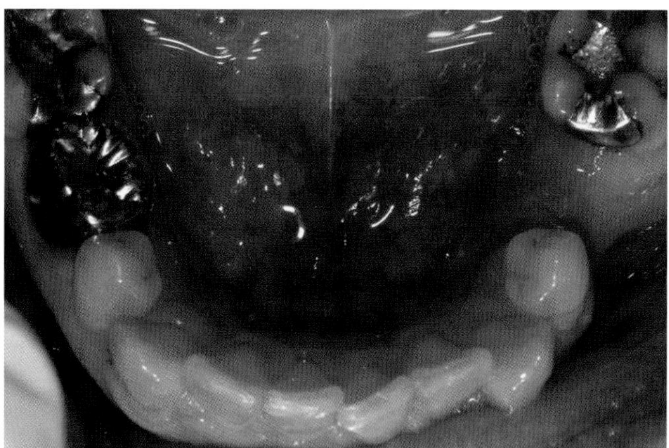

Figure 5.5. Clinical occlusal view of the patient at her initial presentation.

CLINICAL CASE PRESENTATION

Appointment 1. Initial Examination (3/4 Hour)

A 45-year-old female patient presented to the author's office with a chief complaint: "I am missing a lower back tooth and want it replaced with an implant" (Figure 5.5).

This patient was congenitally missing the mandibular second premolar and lost the second primary molar three months previous to the above visit. Her medical history was noncontributory.

The initial diagnostics included panoramic and bitewing radiographs, and clinical examination including periodontal pocket measurements and diagnostic impressions (Figures 5.6, 5.7).

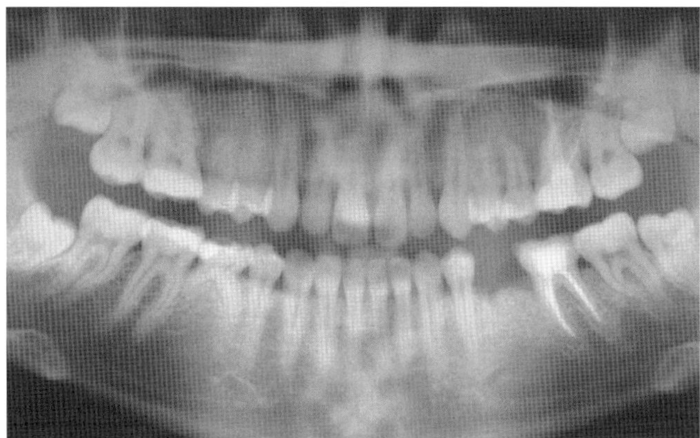

Figure 5.6. Initial panoramic radiograph demonstrated adequate bone in two dimensions for implant placement.

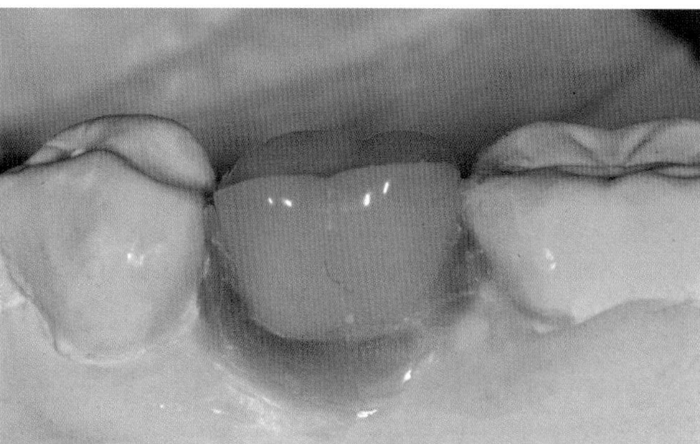

Figure 5.8. Denture tooth set into the edentulous space.

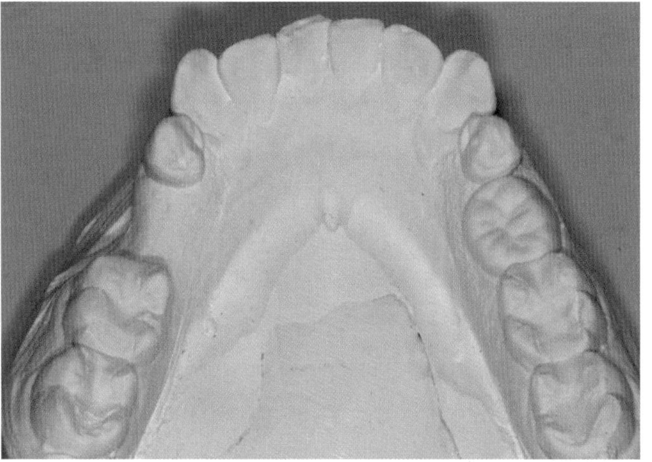

Figure 5.7. Mandibular diagnostic cast made from an alginate impression.

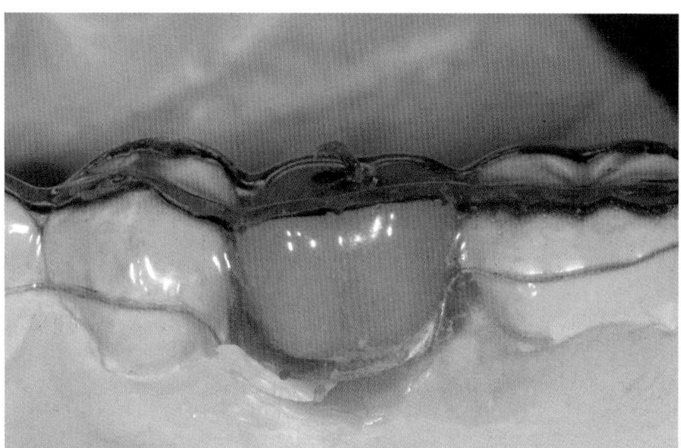

Figure 5.9. Surgical guide was made from a rigid plastic to identify the planned location of the implant restoration.

Diagnostic Casts

Diagnostic casts were poured in dental stone. A denture tooth was selected that fit into the edentulous space in the mandibular left posterior quadrant (Figure 5.8). A surgical guide (Biocryl [2 mm × 125 mm square], Great Lakes, Buffalo, NY) was made using a heat/vacuum machine (Biostar, Great Lakes, Buffalo, NY) (Figure 5.9). A 2 mm circular hole was drilled into the central fossa of the surgical guide as a starting point for the implant surgeon (Figure 5.10).

Diagnoses

The following diagnoses were made:

1. Congenital absence of mandibular left second premolar
2. Adequate bone volume for placement of a 5 mm diameter implant
3. Adequate restorative volume for an implant-retained crown
4. Type I, mild gingivitis

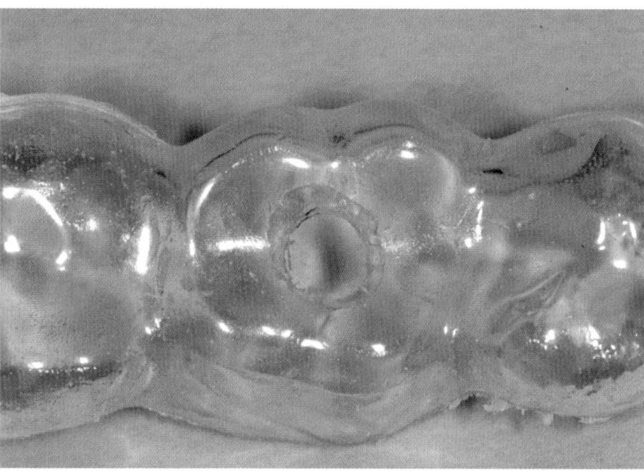

Figure 5.10 Occlusal view of the surgical guide with a 2 mm circular hole in the central fossa. The hole identified the planned location of the implant restoration. The hole allowed for the first bur in the sequence for development of the implant osteotomy.

TABLE 5.1. Treatment Plan #1 (Implant Restoration)

Diagnosis: Congenital absence of mandibular left second premolar

Restorative Services	**ADA #**	**Fee**
Comprehensive oral evaluation	D0150	
Diagnostic casts	D0470	
Panoramic radiograph	D0330	
Diagnostic wax pattern (#20)	D9999	
Surgical guide	D5988	

Referral to periodontal office:

1. Evaluate and treat for replacement of the missing mandibular left second premolar
2. Place a 4 mm diameter, internal connection implant with a single-stage protocol, if possible.
3. Healing abutment should have the following profiles: 5 mm restorative platform, 6 mm emergence profile. Occlusal surface should be 1 mm supra-gingival
4. Post-operative instructions
5. Post-operative follow-up appointments until soft tissues and osseointegration have occurred
6. Discharge to restorative dentist

Fees and services will be determined by the periodontist.

	ADA #	**Fee**
Restorative re-evaluation	D0140	
Pre-machined implant abutment	D6056	
Or		
Custom implant abutment	D6057	
Abutment supported porcelain fused to metal crown (noble metal)	D6061	
Yearly recall appointment	D0120	
Periapical radiograph	D0220	

Benefits of Treatment Plan #1

The missing tooth in the lower left quadrant will be replaced with an implant restoration that will not be removable by the patient. Occlusion (bite) will be optimized. Patient should enjoy improved function with good aesthetics on a long-term basis. Some of the services may be eligible for payment under your medical insurance policy because you never developed this permanent tooth. The teeth adjacent to the missing tooth will not have to be prepared for crowns (caps).

Limitations of Treatment Plan #1

Cost, complexity and length of treatment (4–12 months). Implants are generally successful in the back part of the lower jaw approximately 96–99% of the time. The implant has to be placed optimally for the above treatments to be accomplished. If the implant cannot be placed optimally, changes in the treatments (surgical and prosthetic), fees, and designs will be likely. The patient needs to return to this office at least once per year (may be in conjunction with planned recall appointments) for follow-up, which will include radiographs (x-rays) to assess osseointegration of the implant, status of the occlusion, health of the soft tissues, and the integrity of the implant/abutment connection. This treatment plan itemizes only the prosthetic phase of treatment.

Patient signature ______________________________

Date ______________________________

Witness ______________________________

Date ______________________________

ADA #'s, CDT 2005 Current Dental Terminology, Council on Dental Benefit Programs, American Dental Association, 211 East Chicago Avenue, Chicago, IL 60611

TABLE 5.2. Treatment Plan #2 (Fixed Bridge)

Diagnosis: Congenital absence of mandibular left second premolar

Restorative Services	**ADA #**	**Fee**
Comprehensive oral evaluation	D0150	
Diagnostic casts	D0470	
Panoramic radiograph	D0330	
Diagnostic wax pattern (#20)	D9999	
Tooth #19 (first molar)		
Porcelain Fused to Metal Retainer	D6752	
Tooth #20 (missing second premolar)		
Porcelain Fused to Metal Pontic	D6242	
Tooth #21 (first premolar)		
Porcelain Fused to Metal Retainer	D6752	
Yearly recall appointment	D0120	
Periapical radiograph	D0220	

Benefits of Treatment Plan #2

The missing tooth in the lower-left quadrant will be replaced with a fixed prosthesis that will not be removable by the patient. Occlusion (bite) will be optimized. Patient should enjoy improved function with good aesthetics on an intermediate term basis (10 years).

Limitations of Treatment Plan #2

Cost, complexity, and length of treatment (1–2 months). The teeth in front and behind the missing tooth will have to be prepared (ground down) for crowns, even though neither one of them warrant such treatment. Local anesthesia will have to be used during the preparation appointment. The pulps (nerves) in one or both teeth may become irritated during the preparation procedures. The worst-case scenario would be that one or both of the teeth may warrant endodontic therapy (root canal treatment) during or after completion of the prosthesis. It may be slightly more difficult for you to accomplish satisfactory levels of oral hygiene in and around the prosthesis. One or both of the abutment teeth may be more likely to experience decay and/or periodontal (gum) disease. The patient needs to return to this office at least once per year (may be in conjunction with planned recall appointments) for follow-up, which will include radiographs (x-rays) to assess the integrity of the fit between the crowns and the abutment teeth, status of the occlusion, and health of the soft tissues. Fixed bridges generally have life expectancies of 5–12 years.

Patient signature ______________________

Date ______________________

Witness ______________________

Date ______________________

ADA #'s, CDT 2005 Current Dental Terminology, Council on Dental Benefit Programs, American Dental Association, 211 East Chicago Avenue, Chicago, IL 60611.

Appointment 2. Consultation Restorative Dentist/Patient (1/2 Hour)

A definitive consultation appointment was scheduled as the patient left the office from the first visit. The time between the first and second appointments allowed for development of the treatment options for this particular patient.

Treatment Options

The first treatment option described placement of a 4 mm diameter implant, and osseointegration and fabrication of an implant-retained crown (Table 5.1). The second treatment option described the replacement of the mandibular left second premolar with a 3-unit fixed partial denture (Table 5.2). The third treatment option deferred prosthetic treatment at this time (Table 5.3).

TABLE 5.3. Treatment Plan #3 (No Definitive Treatment)

Diagnosis: Congenital absence of mandibular left second premolar

Restorative Services	**ADA #**	**Fee**
Yearly recall appointment	D0120	
Bitewing radiographs	D0274	

Benefits of Treatment Plan #3

No invasive procedures will be performed in conjunction with the missing tooth in the lower left quadrant.

Limitations of Treatment Plan #3

Both of the back, left quadrants (upper and lower jaws) may be unstable and the teeth subject to drifting into the space of the missing tooth. Long-term function may be compromised by nonreplacement of the second premolar. If the teeth in the quadrants drift and then the patient decides to proceed with prosthetic treatment, orthodontics may be needed to put the teeth back into optimal positions prior to proceeding with definitive treatment.

Patient signature ______________________

Date ______________________

Witness ______________________

Date ______________________

ADA #'s, CDT 4 Current Dental Terminology, Council on Dental Benefit Programs, American Dental Association, 211 East Chicago Avenue, Chicago, IL 60611.

Benefits and limitations of each treatment option were described in detail on the written treatment plans. The prosthodontic fees, or ranges of fees for each procedure, were also listed on each treatment plan. The patient was given copies of the treatment plans. The patient agreed to proceed with the first treatment plan including implant placement and was referred to a periodontist for the surgical diagnostic work up. Surgical costs were not discussed because they would be the obligation of the surgical office to define.

Appointment 3. Consultation Restorative Dentist/Surgeon (1/2 Hour)

This appointment generally takes place before or after normal business hours and should precede the surgeon's examination appointment. It may occur at lunch, at either practitioner's office, or at another convenient location. This consultation is critical for the long-term functional and aesthetic success of implant treatment. It is essential that the restorative dentist explain to the surgeon the physical and radiographic findings, the diagnosis, and the treatment options that were explained to the patient. This particular case presentation was not technically demanding, and the consultation between restorative dentist and the periodontist was completed within 30 minutes. Other, more complex treatment options are discussed in later chapters.

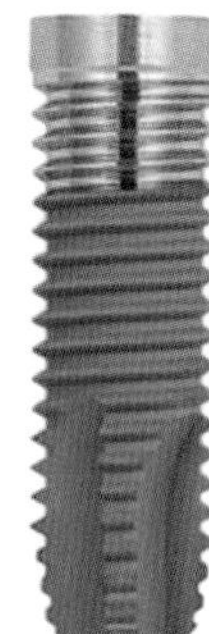

Figure 5.11. A parallel walled, internal connection implant (OSSEOTITE® Certain IOSS411) was preselected by the periodontist for use in the mandibular left posterior quadrant prior to implant surgery.

Type/Number/Size of Implants

In this case, the patient was missing a single tooth and had adequate space for both the surgical and prosthetic phases of implant treatment. The author suggested that a 4 mm diameter implant be placed because this size implant most closely approximated the size of the missing tooth. The shape of the implant body would be determined by the periodontist at the time of implant placement. In this case, the periodontist preselected a parallel walled implant (OSSEOTITE® Certain IOSS411) (Figure 5.11).

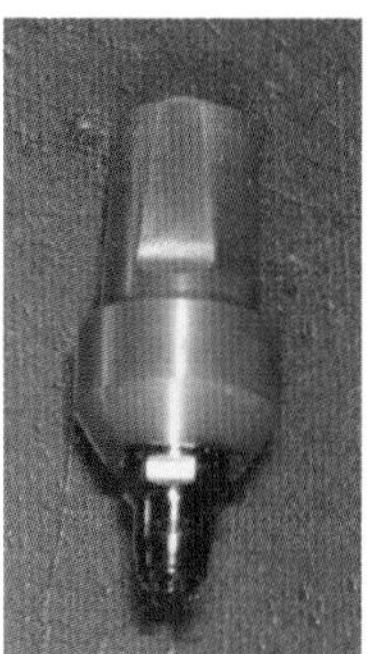

Figure 5.12. Pre-machined titanium abutment as received from the manufacturer. This GingiHue® Post (IAPP454G) was made for a 4.1 mm diameter, internal connection implant. It has a 5 mm emergence profile and a 4 mm collar height.

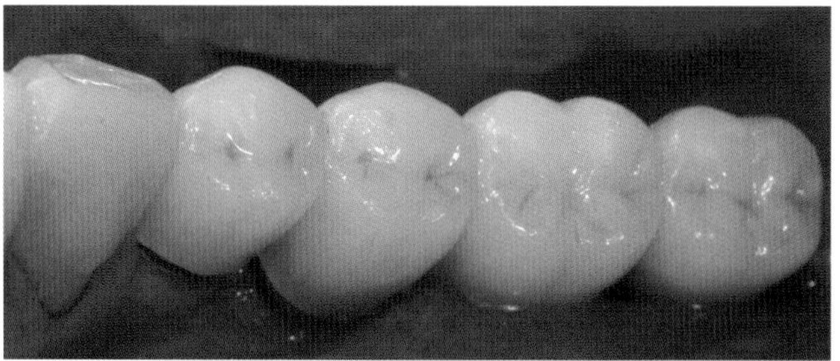

Figure 5.13. Occlusal view of four implant-retained cemented crowns replacing the mandibular right posterior teeth.

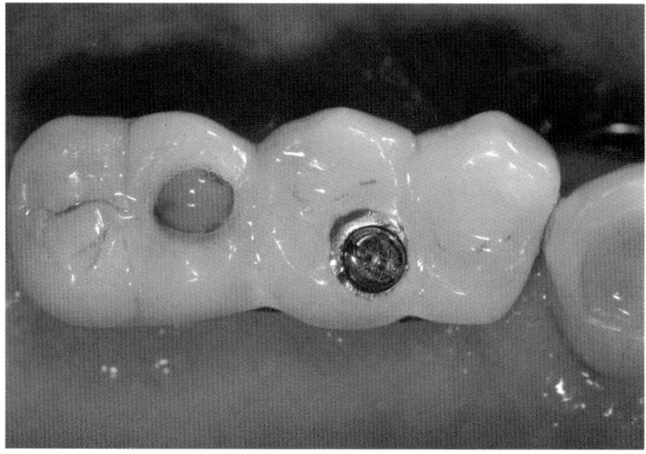

Figure 5.14. Occlusal view of an implant screw-retained fixed partial denture replacing maxillary posterior teeth 10 years post insertion. The occlusal anatomy was distorted secondary to the location of the screw access openings.

Abutment/Prosthesis Design

The author planned to use a pre-machined titanium abutment (GingiHue® Post, IAPP454G) with a cement-retained crown (Figure 5.12). Cement-retained crowns generally allow restorative dentists to develop optimal occlusal anatomy and function (Figure 5.13). Screw-retained crowns

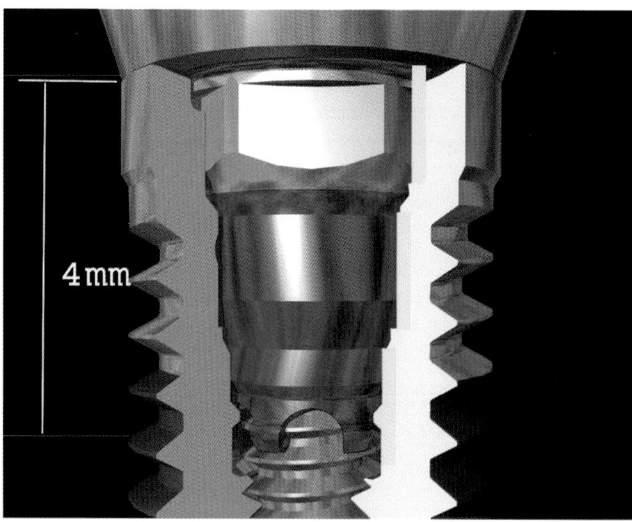

Figure 5.15. Profile view of a diagram of the 4 mm long internal connection of OSSEOTITE® Certain® implants.

may distort occlusal anatomy based on the angulation of the implant and how it relates to the occlusal anatomy of the tooth (Figure 5.14).

Implant/Abutment Connection

The ***3i***® internal connection implant was designed with a 4 mm long implant/abutment connection (Figure 5.15).

Internal implant/abutment connections, from various manufacturers, have proven to be successful in clinical practice. ***3i***® introduced their internal connection implant (OSSEOTITE® Certain®) in 2003. The clamping forces between implants and abutments in this system are significantly greater than some clamping forces that have been reported for external implant/abutment connections (***3i***® 2003).

This is not to say that external hex implant/abutment connections are not clinically acceptable (Figures 5.16, 5.17). The author reported on the clinical success of external hex implant/abutment connections in 2003 (Drago 2003). Seventy-three patients were treated with OSSEOTITE® implants (external hex implant/abutment connections) and were followed for one year. All of the abutments were attached to the implants with square abutment screws that were torqued to 35 Ncm with a torque instrument. All of the abutments were designed with the Gold Standard ZR™ (Zero Rotation) feature. One abutment screw was found to be loose at the end of the 12-month study; the CSR for the implant/abutment connections was 99%.

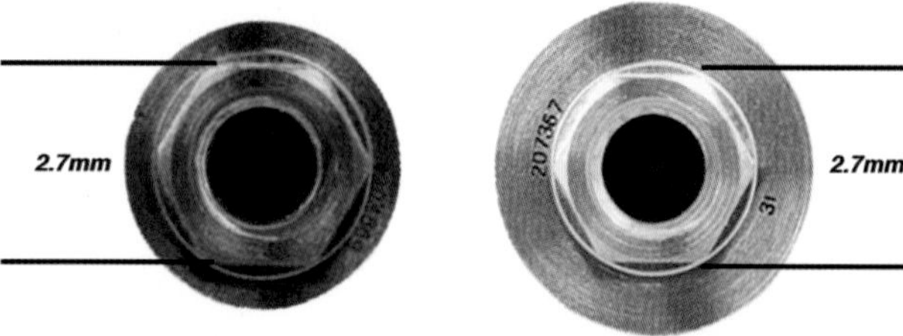

Figure 5.16. Occlusal view of the implant restorative platform implant/abutment external hex connections for the 4.1 and 5.0 mm diameter OSSEOTITE® implant system (left, right, respectively).

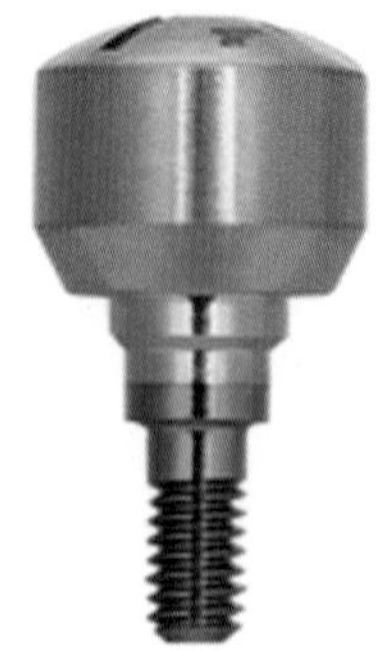

Figure 5.18. Profile view of a healing abutment for a 4.1 mm implant restorative platform, 6 mm emergence profile, and 4 mm collar height for the OSSEOTITE® Certain® implant system (ITHA464).

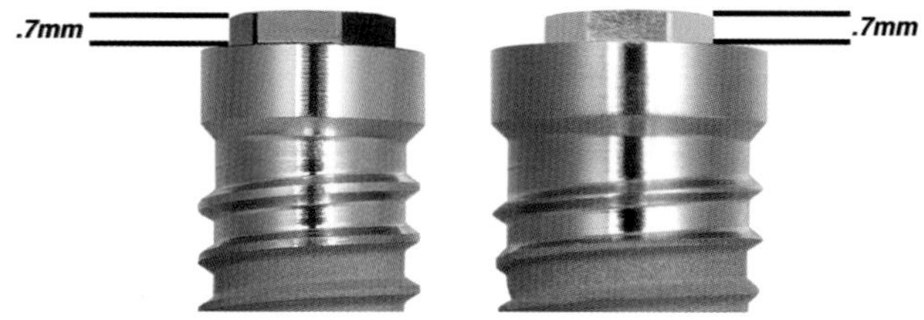

Figure 5.17. Profile view of the heights of the implant/abutment external hex connections for the 4.1 and 5.0 mm diameter OSSEOTITE® implant system (left, right, respectively).

TABLE 5.4. The Implant Restorative Wish List

Tooth # 20 (Left Mandibular Second Premolar)	
Type of Implant	OSSEOTITE® Certain®
Implant Restorative Platform	4.1 mm
Surgical Protocol	Single stage
Implant/Abutment Connection	Internal (Certain)
Healing Abutment	6 mm X 2, 3, or 4 mm (supra-gingival occlusal surface)
Occlusal Loading Protocol	8–10 weeks

Surgical Protocol

The author also suggested that, if possible, a one-stage surgical protocol be followed. Published reports have indicated that single-stage surgical protocols have been as efficacious as the traditional two-stage surgical protocols (Testori and others 2002).

Healing Abutment Selection

In this case, a single-stage surgical protocol was followed. The predetermined healing abutment size was 4.1 mm restorative platform and 6 mm emergence profile, and the occlusal surface should be slightly supra-gingival (2, 3, or 4 mm) (ITHA464, Figure 5.18).

Implant Restorative Wish List

The above concepts have proven to be an excellent starting point for discussions between the author and implant surgeons. A form was developed that incorporated all of the concepts noted above and is called the Implant Restorative Wish List (Table 5.4). It is now completed for each patient and sent to the implant surgeon prior to patient treatment.

Appointment 4. Implant Placement (1 Hour)

In this instance, the surgeon was able to place a 4 mm diameter implant with a single-stage protocol (Figures 5.19 and 5.20). A two-piece healing abutment was placed and the patient was discharged with postoperative instructions. She was to return for a clinical reevaluation 10 days post operatively. The abutment screw for this type of healing abutment may be torqued to 20 Ncm.

Appointment 5. Restorative Follow-Up Appointments (1/4 to 1/2 Hour)

Either the implant surgeon or restorative dentist may schedule follow-up appointments. It is important to coordinate the follow-up appointments so as to not duplicate the efforts of either office and to minimize inconvenience to patients. For single-stage surgical protocols in nonaesthetic zones, the author generally appoints patients at 10 days, four weeks, and eight weeks (Figures 5.21 and 5.22).

The patient's surgical site was examined for inflammation, infection, drainage, and plaque control. In this case, these appointments were scheduled for 15–30 minutes.

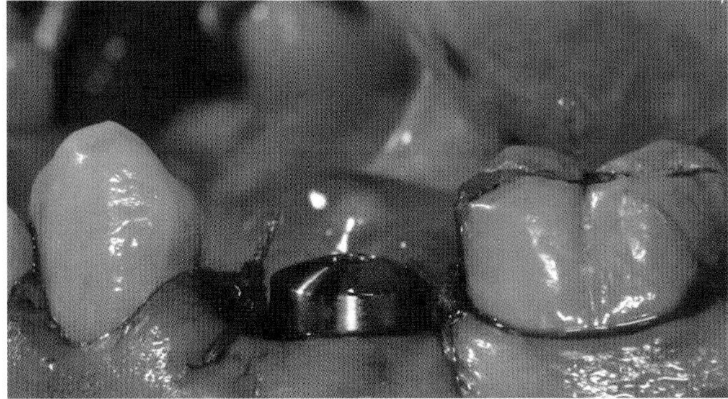

Figure 5.19. Buccal view of implant and healing abutment in place at the time of implant placement. In single-stage surgical protocols, the occlusal surfaces of the healing abutments should be supra-gingival.

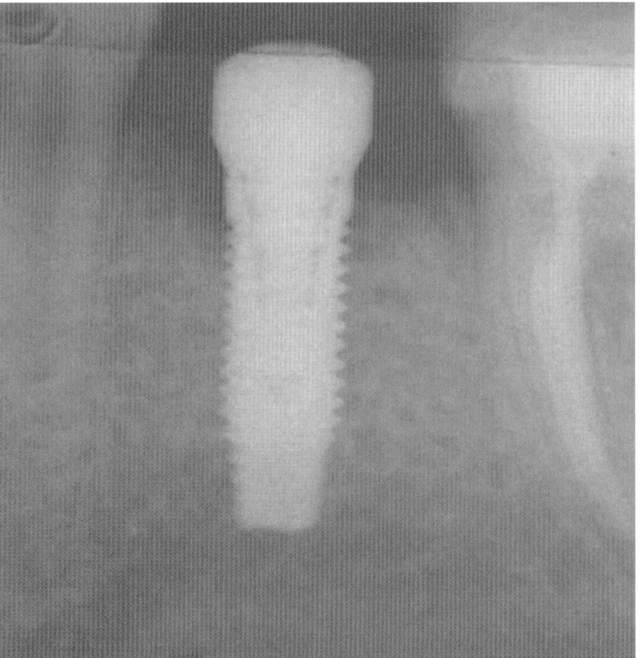

Figure 5.20. Radiograph of parallel wall internal connection implant and healing abutment at the time of implant placement.

Appointment 6. Reevaluation and Determination of Implant Impression Date (1/2 Hour)

The implant surgeon had informed the author that the bone in the area of this implant was probably Type II in hardness. He recommended that the implant remain undisturbed for at least eight weeks post implant placement. The reevaluation appointment occurred approximately eight weeks after implant surgery (Figure 5.23). The soft tissues had healed

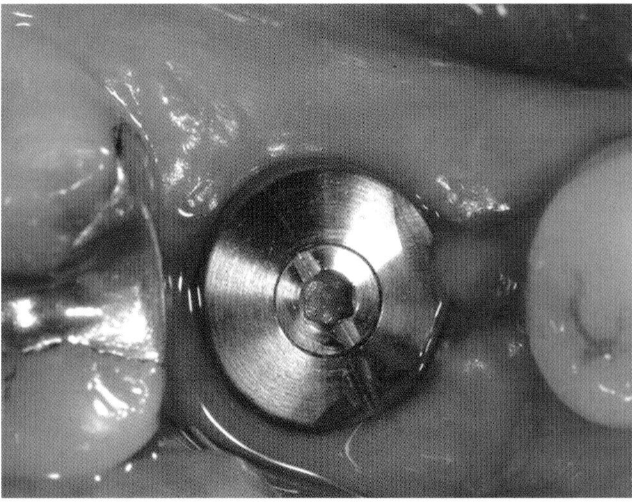

Figure 5.21. Occlusal view of two-piece healing abutment 10 days post implant placement.

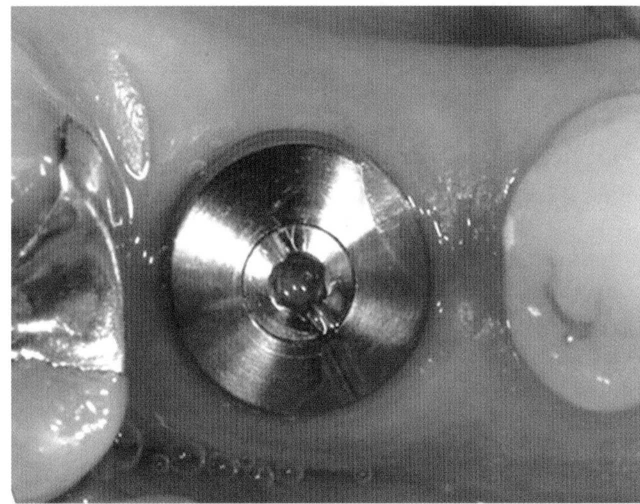

Figure 5.22. Occlusal view of healing abutment four weeks post implant placement.

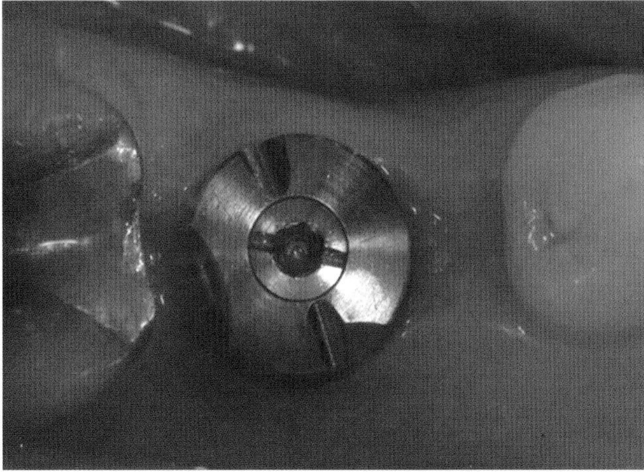

Figure 5.23. Occlusal view of healing abutment eight weeks post implant placement.

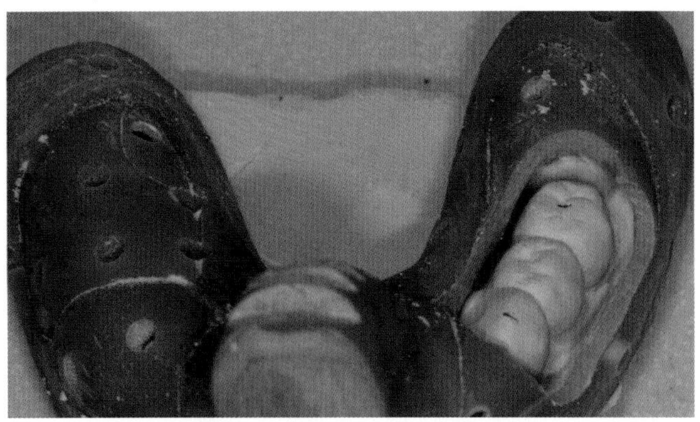

Figure 5.24. Custom open face impression tray in place on the diagnostic cast. A window was prepared in the tray in the mandibular premolar area.

in a manner consistent with the shape of the healing abutment, the healing abutment was stable, and no macroscopic movement was visualized between the implant and healing abutment. Diagnostic impressions were not needed because the implant was placed according to the surgical guide. If the implant was not placed optimally, a new diagnostic cast would be required if a custom impression tray was to be made. The patient was reappointed for an implant level impression in two weeks.

Laboratory Procedures

Custom Open Face Impression Tray

It is the author's preference to make implant level impressions with implant pick-up impression copings. This protocol required an open face tray. Custom impression trays may be made from light cured or autopolymerizing acrylic resin. In this case, light cure resin (Triad® Visible Custom Tray Material, DENTSPLY International, Inc., York, PA) was used to fabricate the custom impression tray (Figure 5.24). If there are significant undercuts in or around the teeth, they should be blocked out with wax prior to fabricating the tray.

Tentative Abutment Selection

The implant abutment for this case was selected according to the following criteria:

1. Implant/abutment connection
2. Implant restorative platform size
3. Diameter of healing abutment
4. Peri-implant sulcular depth
5. Implant angulation
6. Inter-occlusal clearance

Based on the above criteria, the author tentatively selected a pre-machined titanium alloy abutment: GingiHue® Post (Catalog # IAPP464G) (Figure 5.25).

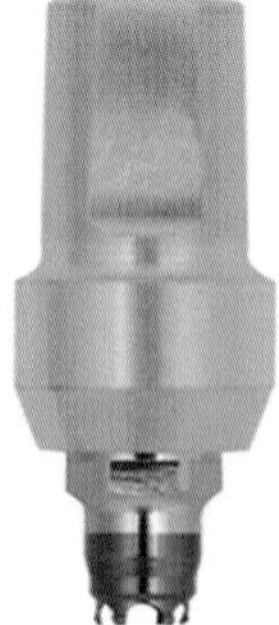

Figure 5.25. The GingiHue® Post as received from the manufacturer for a 4.1 mm diameter, internal connection implant (OSSEOTITE® Certain®); 6 mm emergence profile; 4 mm collar height (Catalog #IAPP464G).

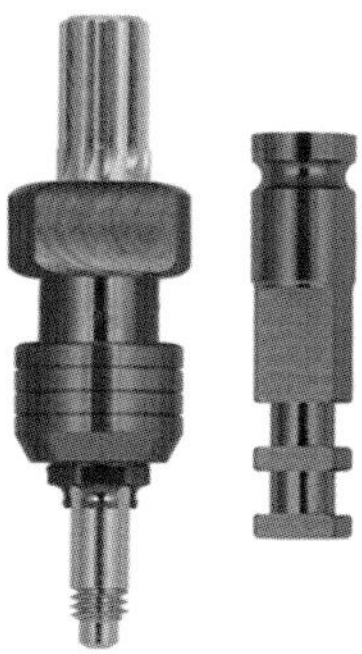

Figure 5.26. Implant impression coping (IIIC60) for the implant in Figure 5.25 (left); implant lab analog (Catalog #IILA20) that replicated the implant used in this case presentation.

Furthermore, the appropriate implant impression coping and implant lab analog were also preselected and placed into the laboratory case pan (Catalog #IIIC60, IILA20, respectively) (Figure 5.26). By preselecting the impression components, the restorative team was assured of having the correct components on hand for the impression appointment.

Appointment 7. Implant Level Impression (1/2 Hour)

Clinical Procedures

The healing abutment was removed with a driver (PHD02N) by placing the tip of the driver into the hex on the occlusal surface of the healing abutment (Figure 5.27). The implant restorative platform of the 4.1 mm diameter implant was completely visualized (Figure 5.28). In a single-stage protocol it is not unusual to visualize some hemorrhage, because this will be the first time the healing abutment has been removed after implant placement. The hemorrhage will generally stop on its own without the need for hemostatic agents.

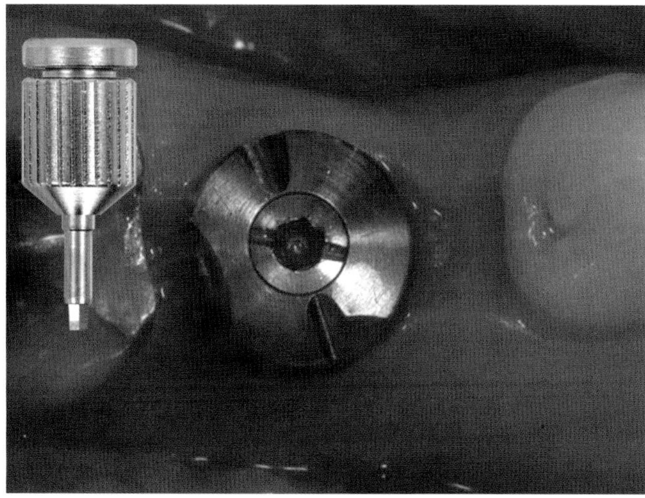

Figure 5.27. At 10 weeks, the PHD02N driver (inset) was used to remove the two-piece healing abutment from the implant.

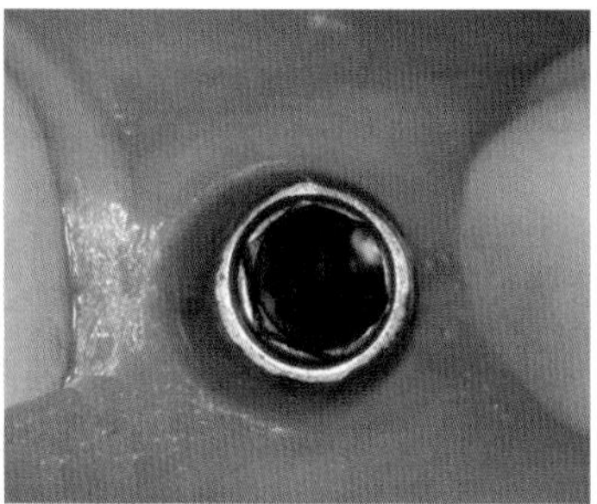

Figure 5.28. The implant restorative platform of the 4.1 mm OSSEOTITE® Certain® implant, color coded blue, after the healing abutment was removed.

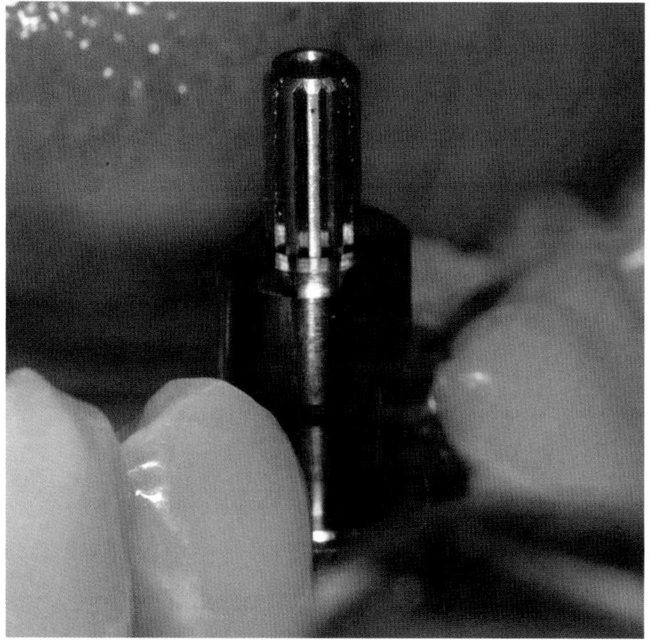

Figure 5.29. The implant impression coping, 4.1 mm implant restorative platform, 6 mm emergence profile (Catalog # IIIC60) that replicated the size of the healing abutment in place.

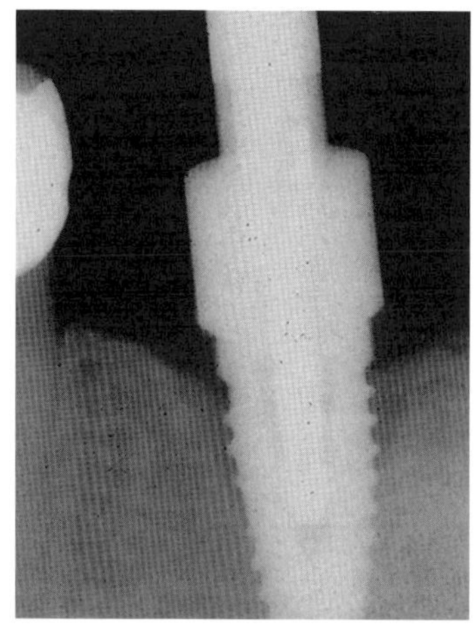

Figure 5.30. This radiograph verified that the implant impression coping was completely seated into the implant internal connection.

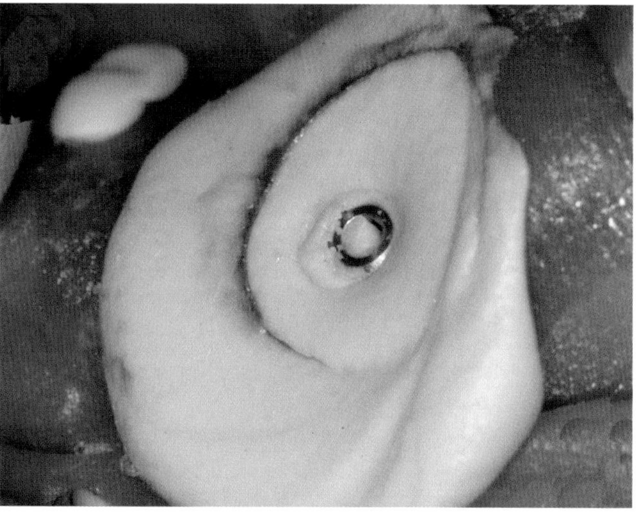

Figure 5.31. Clinical image of impression tray in place. Impression material must be cleared from the impression coping screw prior to polymerization of the impression material. In order for this technique to be successful, clinicians must have access to the impression coping screw and unscrew it from the implant prior to removing the impression tray from the mouth.

The implant impression coping was placed into the implant internal connection (Figure 5.29). Clinicians will feel and hear a "click" when the impression coping is properly seated. A verification radiograph was taken that verified an accurate implant/impression coping connection (Figure 5.30).

The impression tray was tried in to ensure that the impression coping did not interfere with complete seating of the tray. The definitive impression was made with a putty/injection poly vinylsiloxane impression material (Exafast™, GC America Inc., Alsip, IL) per the manufacturer's instructions (Figure 5.31).

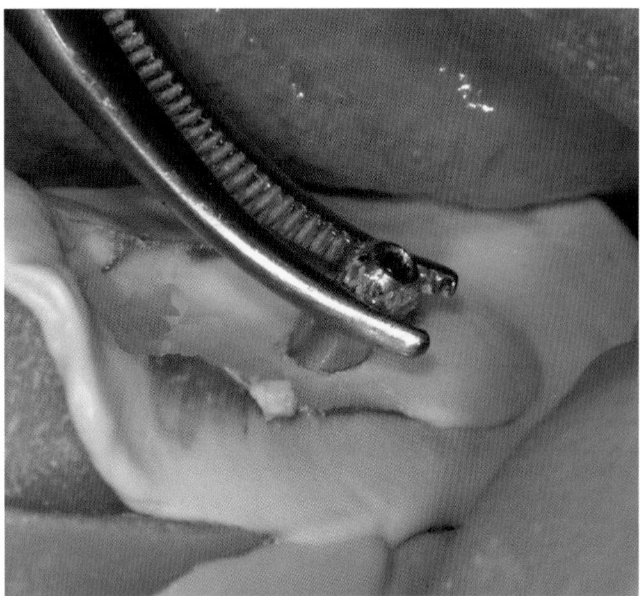

Figure 5.32. A hemostat was used to ensure that the impression coping screw was completely disengaged from the implant.

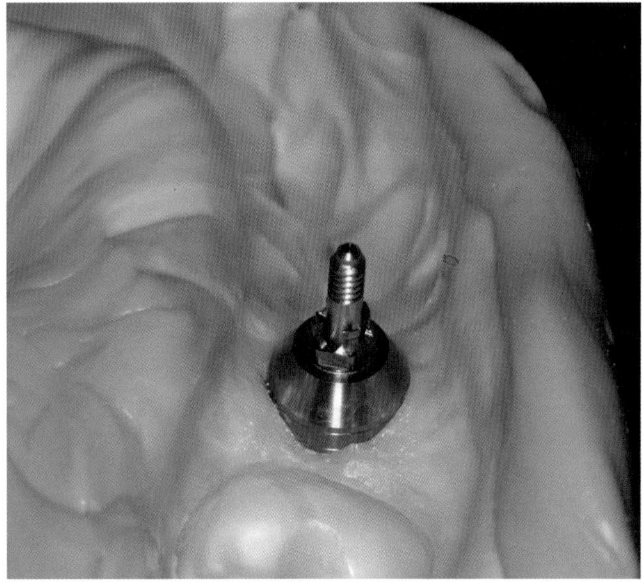

Figure 5.33. The intaglio surface of the definitive impression with the implant impression coping inside the impression material.

After the impression material polymerized, the impression coping screw was unscrewed and a hemostat was used to verify that the screw was completely disengaged from the implant (Figure 5.32). The impression tray was removed. With the pick-up impression protocol, the impression coping remains inside the impression (Figure 5.33). The healing abutment was replaced and hand tightened. A porcelain shade was selected and recorded, and the patient was discharged.

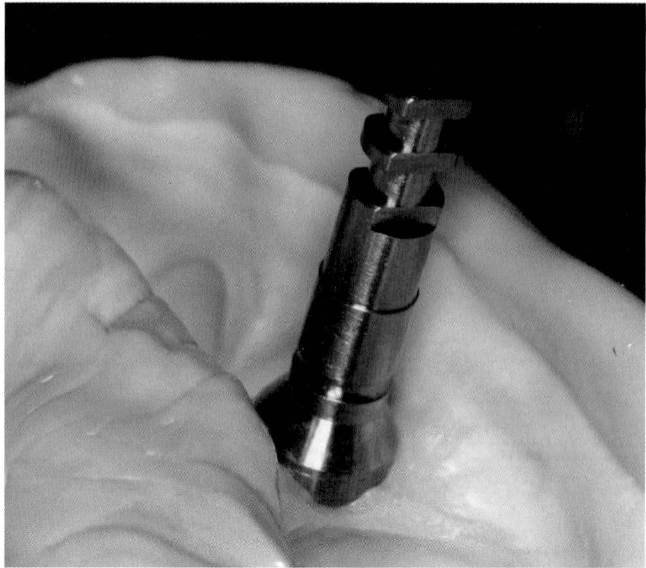

Figure 5.34. OSSEOTITE® Certain® laboratory analog (IILA20) for 4.1 mm implant seated onto the impression coping in Figure 5.33. Note the metal-to-metal contact between the implant restorative components.

Laboratory Procedures

Master Cast

The appropriate implant lab analog (Catalog # IILA20) was attached to the intaglio surface of the implant impression coping (Figure 5.34). A tactile and audible click was appreciated. Metal-to-metal contact between the implant lab analog and the impression coping was visualized, indicating that the components were correctly attached.

A polyether impression material (Impregum®, 3M Espe, Minneapolis, MN) was injected around the implant lab analog/impression coping interface, taking care not to let any of the material drift into either inter-proximal contact area mesial or distal to the implant (Drago 1994) (Figure 5.35). This material was allowed to polymerize and Type IV dental stone was mixed per the manufacturer's instructions and vibrated into the impression to fabricate the master cast (Figure 5.36). The master cast was mounted on a simple hinge articulator.

Laboratory Work Order for Abutment Preparation and Crown Fabrication

The abutment was selected based on the abutment selection criteria above (IAPP464G). Restorative clinicians may elect to have dental laboratory technicians select the abutments. In those cases, restorative clinicians should provide the technicians with the information described in the previous section.

In this instance, the tentative abutment selection was found to be accurate. The GingiHue® Post was sent along with

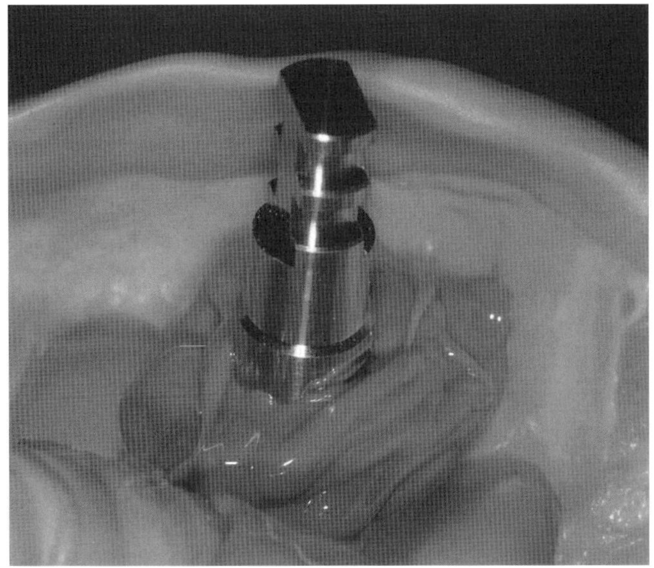

Figure 5.35. The polyether impression material was injected to cover the implant impression coping/implant lab analog junction.

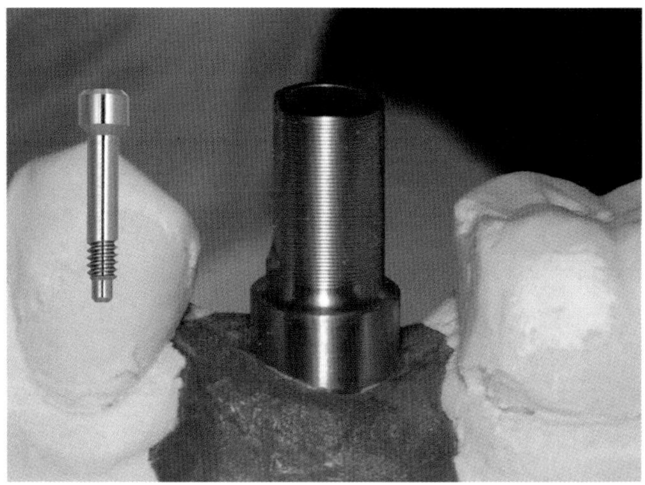

Figure 5.37. The pre-machined titanium alloy abutment (Catalog # IAPP464G) as received from the manufacturer in place on the master cast. The flat surface may be placed on any of the axial walls. The author prefers that it be placed on the longest axial wall as opposed to always placing it on the facial walls. Laboratory hexed screws should be used in the laboratory (IUNITS, inset).

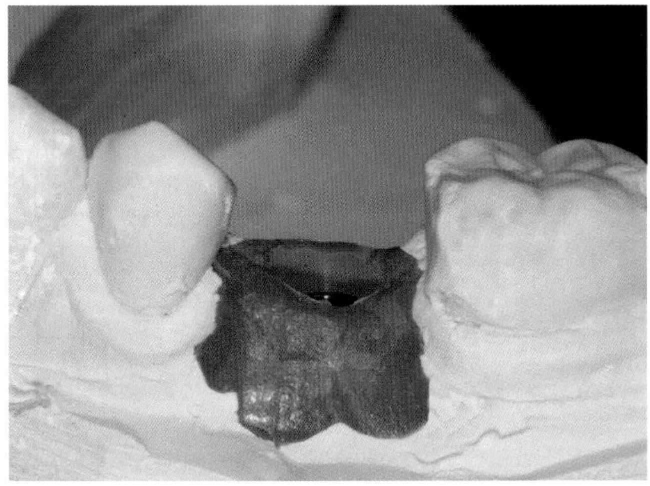

Figure 5.36. The mandibular master cast ready to be sent to commercial dental laboratory.

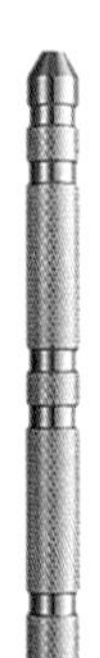

Figure 5.38. The Laboratory Abutment Holder for OSSEOTITE® Certain® implants (Catalog #ILTAH57).

the case to a commercial dental laboratory (Paramount Dental Lab, Menomonee Falls, Wisconsin). The hexed laboratory screw was also enclosed (IUNITS). The following work order was completed relative to abutment preparation (Drago 2003):

1. Place enclosed abutment (Catalog #IAPP464G) on implant in the mandibular left posterior quadrant with the flat side on the mesial surface (Figure 5.37). Use the enclosed Hexed Try-In Screw (IUNITS).
2. Identify the location of the facial gingival margin by scribing a line into the gold titanium nitride coating.
3. Remove the abutment from the cast and place it onto a Laboratory Abutment Holder (ILTAH57) for OSSEOTITE® Certain® implants (Figure 5.38).

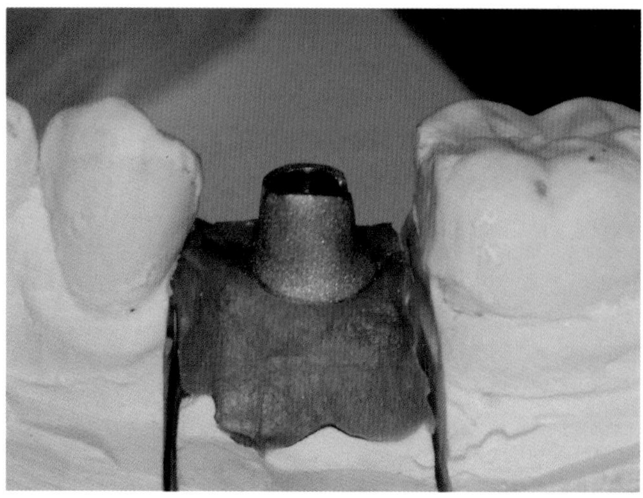

Figure 5.39. Titanium abutment after it was prepared per the laboratory work order in place on the master cast.

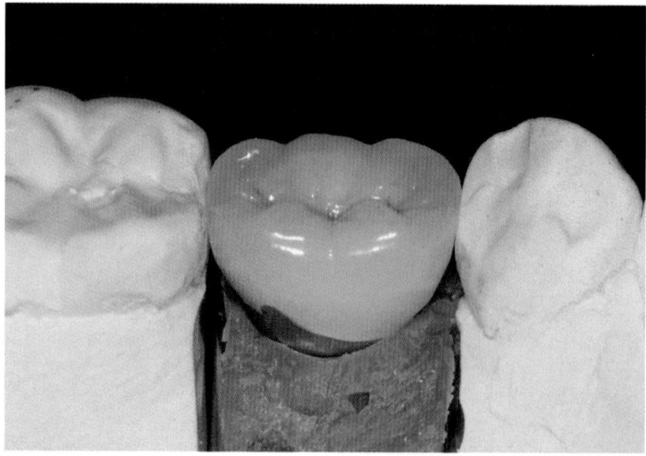

Figure 5.40. Lingual view of porcelain fused to metal crown in place on the prepared abutment, on the master cast. Note the optimal emergence profiles that were initially developed with the selection of the appropriate healing abutment.

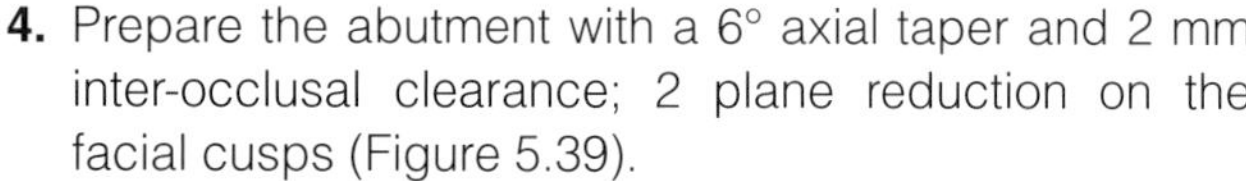

4. Prepare the abutment with a 6° axial taper and 2 mm inter-occlusal clearance; 2 plane reduction on the facial cusps (Figure 5.39).
5. Refine the facial and mesial inter-proximal margins so that they are 1 mm sub-gingival.
6. Leave the axial walls coarse; do not polish.
7. Apply two layers of die spacer.
8. Develop a wax pattern for porcelain fused to metal crown restoration by waxing the pattern to full contour and cut back for porcelain.
   a. Cusp/fossa occlusion
   b. No balancing interferences
   c. Optimal emergence profiles
   d. Standard inter-proximal contacts
9. Cast the wax pattern in a noble alloy (Olympia, JF Jelenko and Co.).
10. Finish the casting and apply porcelain (Figures 5.40, 5.41).
11. Return restoration by ________.

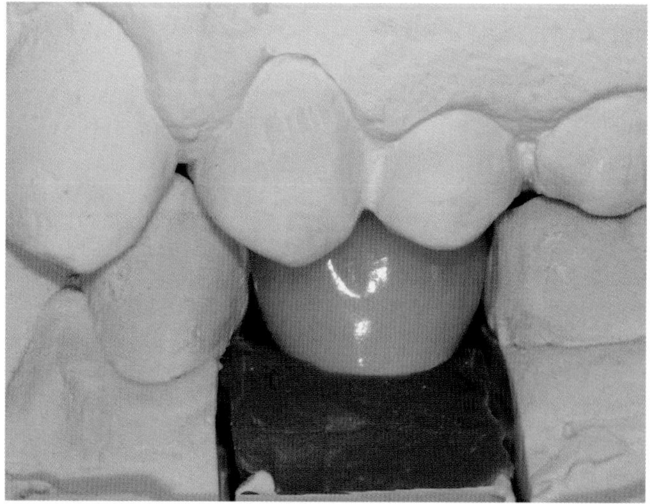

Figure 5.41. The porcelain fused to metal crown restoration in occlusion with the opposing diagnostic cast.

Appointment 8. Abutment and Crown Insertion Appointment (3/4 Hour)

Abutment Placement

The healing abutment was removed and the entire implant restorative platform was visualized. The prepared titanium alloy abutment was placed with a Hexed Try-In Screw (Catalog #IUNITS). A tactile and audible click were appreciated and indicated that the abutment was completely seated into the implant (Figure 5.42).

Radiographic Verification and Crown Try-In

A radiograph was taken to ensure that the abutment was completely seated (Figure 5.43). The porcelain fused to metal crown was tried in by adjusting the inter-proximal contacts until the crown margins fit the abutment margins. A periapical radiograph was taken to ensure that the crown was seated onto the abutment (Figure 5.44). The occlusion was adjusted to achieve occlusal contacts consistent with the patient's pre-operative occlusion; there were no balancing or lateral working contacts.

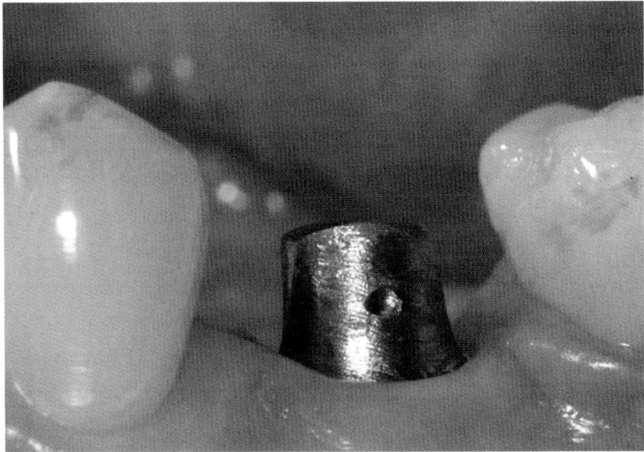

Figure 5.42. The prepared abutment in place at the abutment and crown try-in appointment.

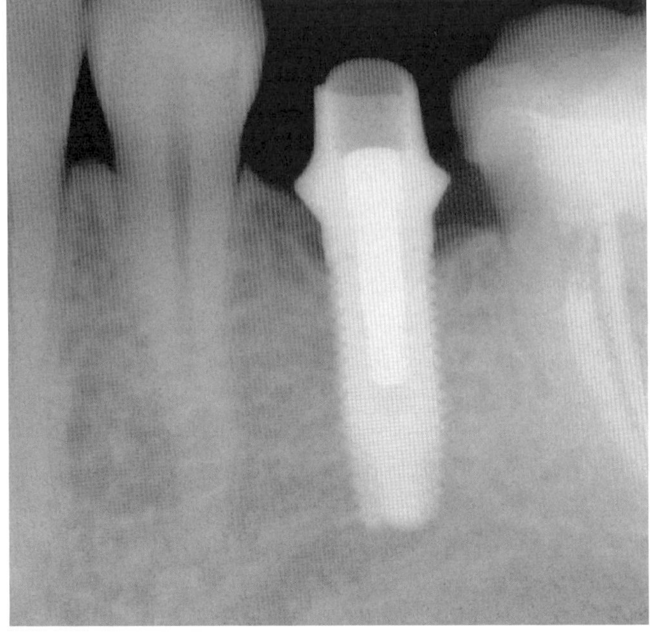

Figure 5.43. A periapical radiograph was taken that verified that the abutment was seated correctly onto the implant.

Torque

The crown and abutment were removed and the crown was polished. A Gold-Tite™ Hexed Screw (Catalog #IUNIHG) was used to attach the abutment to the implant (Figure 5.45). To verify that the abutment was in the correct position, the practitioner tried in the crown and fit it in the same fashion it did during the try-in procedures. The abutment screw was torqued to 20 Ncm with the Restorative Torque Indicator (Catalog #RTI2035) (Figure 5.46).

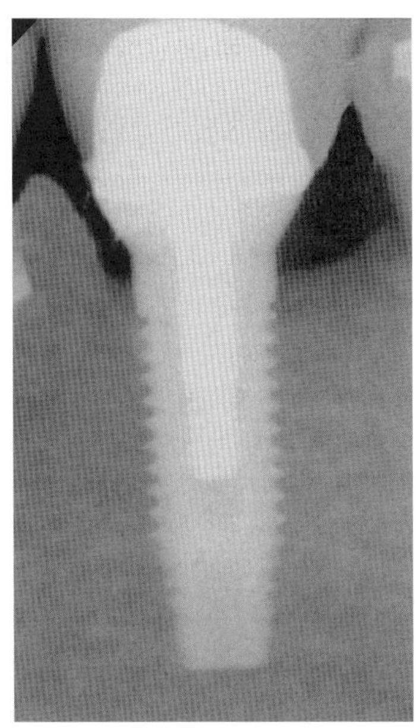

Figure 5.44. A periapical radiograph was taken that verified that the crown was seated correctly onto the abutment.

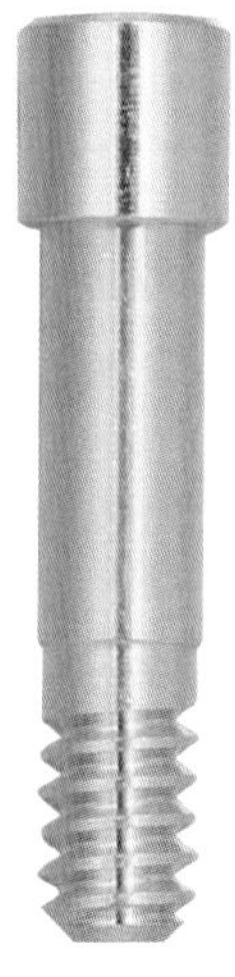

Figure 5.45. A Gold-Tite™ Hexed Abutment Screw (Catalog #IUNIHG) as received from the manufacturer.

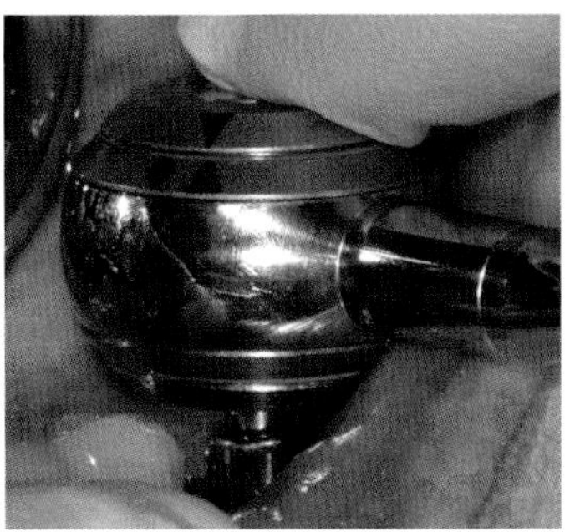

Figure 5.46. A Restorative Torque Indicator (Catalog #RTI2035) was used to torque the abutment screw in Figure 5.45 to 20 Ncm. (Triangle to triangle on the face of the RTI2035.)

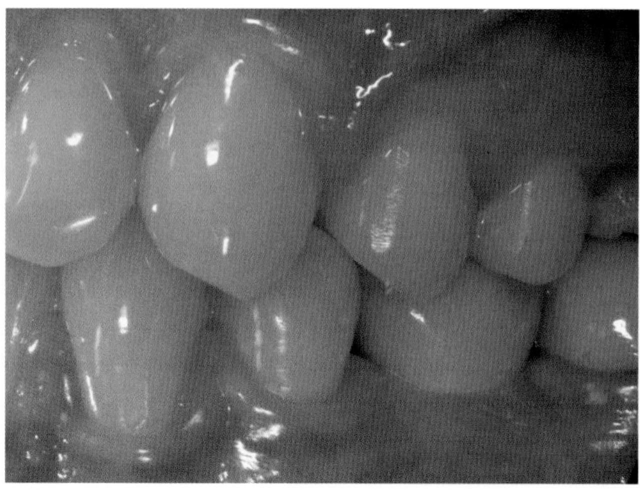

Figure 5.47. Clinical buccal image of the porcelain fused to metal in place after cementation to the titanium alloy abutment.

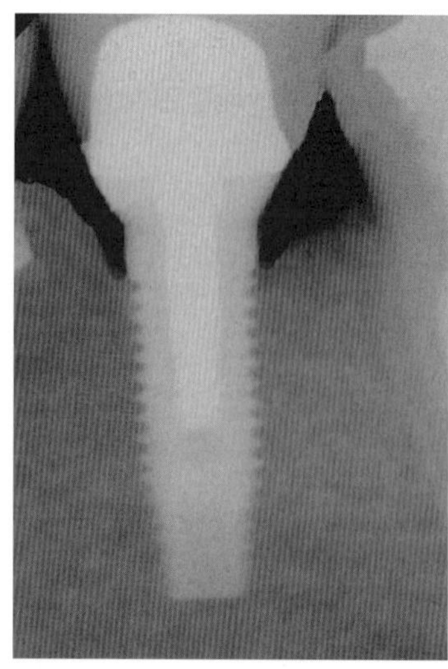

Figure 5.48. Radiograph that was taken one year post implant restoration and occlusal function. There was less than 1 mm of bone loss when compared to the bone levels at the time of implant abutment and crown restoration.

TABLE 5.5. Lab Fees, Component Costs, Overhead, Fees, and Profits for an Implant-Retained Crown

Fixed			
Chair Time	**Overhead**	**Laboratory Expenses**	
		Casts	$ 45
Impression		Articulation	$ 15
		PFM crown	$275
		Milling abutment	$ 75
.5 hours	$350/hr = $175	**Sub Total**	**$410**
		Implant Components	
		Healing abutment	$36
		Impression Coping	$45
		Analog	$21
		Pre-machined abutment	$90
		Lab screw	$14
		Abutment screw	$54
		Sub Total	**$260**
Crown Insertion			
.5 hours	$350/hr = $175		
TOTALS	**($350)**		**($670)**
Professional Fee			$1400
Costs (fixed overhead and laboratory expenses)			$1020
Profit (fees less costs)			$ 380
Profit per hour ($380/1 hr)			**$ 380**

Healing abutments, impression copings, and lab screws may be used multiple times, therefore costs will be decreased for each succeeding case and profits will be increased. Analogs should not be re-used.

Cementation

The crown was cemented to the abutment with permanent crown and bridge cement (GC Fuji Plus, GC America) (Figure 5.47). It has been the author's experience that this protocol ensures stable implant/abutment connections, and due to the precise fit between implant abutments and crowns fabricated in this fashion, even with temporary cement, implant crowns cannot be easily removed from abutments if needed (Drago 2005).

Appointment 9. Follow-Up Appointments

Two Weeks/Six Months

This patient was followed up at two weeks, six months and one year post implant crown insertion. The clinical appointments included an evaluation of the occlusion in both centric and eccentric movements; health of the soft tissues, plaque control, and so on. This patient adapted well to this restoration and no further treatment was needed.

One-Year Recall Clinical and Radiographic Evaluation

At the one-year recall appointment, a radiograph was taken to compare bone levels from the abutment insertion appointment to the bone levels one-year post occlusal loading. There was approximately 1 mm of crestal bone loss mesial/distally. There was satisfactory adaptation of the bone to the threads of the implant and there were no radiolucencies. The implant was considered to be osseointegrated (Figure 5.48).

Costs/Fees/Profitability

The following discussion (Table 5.5) relative to fees is reflective of late 2005 in the Midwest United States. The costs of the implant components are retail prices from Implant Innovations, Inc., Palm Beach Gardens, Florida.

Surgeon: Garry O'Connor, DDS, MS, Gundersen Lutheran Medical Center, LaCrosse, WI

Dental Laboratory Technician: Tom Dirks, CDT, Paramount Dental Laboratory, Menomonee Falls, WI

BIBLIOGRAPHY

Adell, R, Lekholm, U, Rockler, B, Brånemark, P-I. 1981. A 15-year study of osseointegrated implants in the treatment of the edentulous jaw. *Int J Oral Surg* 10:387–416.

Andersson, B, Odman, P, Lindvall, A. 1998. Cemented single crowns on osseointegrated implants after 5 years: results from a prospective study on CeraOne. *Int J Prosthodont* 11:212–221.

Brånemark, P-I, Zarb, George, and Albrektsson, Tomas, eds., 1985. *Tissue-Integrated Prostheses: Osseointegration in Clinical Dentistry.* Carol Stream, IL: Quintessence.

Drago, C, 1994. A laboratory technique for fabricating single tooth implant restorations with optimal subgingival contours. *Trends and Techniques* 11:39–43.

Drago, C, 2002. Prepable titanium abutments: principles and techniques for the dental laboratory technician. *J Dent Tech* 19:22–28.

Drago, C, 2003. A clinical study of the efficacy of gold-tite square abutment screws in cement-retained implant restorations. *Int J Oral Maxillofac Implants* 18:273–278.

Drago, C, 2005. A clinical report on the 18-month cumulative survival rates of implants and implant prostheses with an internal connection implant system. Accepted for publication, *The Compendium of Continuing Dental Education.*

Eckert, S, Wollan, P, 1998. Retrospective review of 1170 endosseous implants placed in partially edentulous jaws. *J Prosthet Dent* 79:415–423.

Garber, D, 1995. The esthetic dental implant: letting restoration be the guide. *J Am Dent Assoc* 126:319–325.

Jemt, T, Lekholm, U, Grondahl, K, 1990. 3-year followup study of early single implant restorations ad modum Brånemark. *Int J Periodont Rest Dent* 10:340–339.

Lazzara, R, Siddiqui, A, Binon, P, Feldman, S, Weiner, R, Phillips, R, 1996. Retrospective multicenter analysis of ***3i®*** endosseous dental implants placed over a five-year period. *Clin Oral Implants Res* 7:73–83.

Lindh, T, Gunne, J, Tillberg, A, 1998. A meta-analysis of implants in partial edentulism. *Clin Oral Implants Res* 9:80–91.

O'Neal, R, Butler, R, 2000. Restoration or implant placement: a growing treatment planning quandary. *J Periodont* 30:111–122.

Priest, G, 1996. Failure rates of restorations for single-tooth replacement. *Int J Prosthod* 9(1):38–45.

Reuter, J, Brose, M, 1984. Failures in full crown retained dental bridges. *Br Dent J* 157:61–63.

Schwartz, N, Whitsett, L, Berry, T, Stewart, J, 1970. Unserviceable crowns and fixed partial dentures: life-span and causes for loss of serviceability. *J Am Dent Assoc* 81:1395–1401.

Testori, T, Del Fabbro, M, Feldman, S, Vincenzi, G, Sullivan, D, Rossi, Jr, R, Anitua, E, Bianchi, F, Francetti, L, Weinstein, R. 2002. A multicenter prospective evaluation of 2-months loaded Osseotite implants placed in the posterior jaws: 3-year follow-up results. *Clin Oral Implants Res* 13:154–161.

Walton, J, Gardner, F, Agar, J. 1986. A survey of crown and fixed partial denture failures: length of service and reasons for replacement. *J Prosthet Dent* 56:416–421.

Chapter 6: Re-Treatment of a Fractured Implant Fixed Partial Denture in the Posterior Maxilla with CAD/CAM Abutments and a New Fixed Partial Denture

LITERATURE REVIEW

Dental implant restorations placed in the 1980s had challenges associated with the biology of osseointegration, as well as biomechanics of prosthesis survival (Adell and others 1981; Kallus and Bessing 1994). Implant prostheses were designed with screw retention to facilitate removal and repair, while sacrificing aesthetics and occlusion (Zarb and Schmitt 1990).

As the treatment modality changed from edentulous patients to include partially edentulous patients, there were reports of prosthetic complications that could have a negative impact on overall success rates in implant treatment. Zarb and Schmitt (1990) reported on 274 implants placed in 46 consecutive patients who were followed for up to nine years. The success rate for the implants was 89.05%; the success rate for the prosthetic treatment was 100%. They recorded complications and problems during the surgical, restorative, and follow-up phases of treatment. Zarb and Schmitt concluded that safe retrievable techniques would result in negligible morbidity.

Hemmings and others (1994) studied and compared the maintenance requirements for fixed prostheses and overdentures in edentulous mandibles. Post insertion adjustments were more common in the first year in the overdenture population, but thereafter, the fixed prostheses had more complications and required more maintenance. The average number of recalls for the first year was 2.27 and 1.57, respectively.

Attard and Zarb (2002) reported on the long-term success of implant-supported posterior zone prostheses in the first 35 consecutive, partially edentulous patients treated at the University of Toronto. They reported that the overall survival of the posterior implants was 94%. They concluded that Brånemark dental implants were highly effective in the rehabilitation of partially edentulous patients missing multiple posterior teeth.

The hexagonal extension on the coronal aspect of external hex implants was originally designed as a rotational torque transfer mechanism used during the surgical placement of implants. With the initiation of single unit implant restorations, the external hex was used as an anti-rotation component (Beaty 1994) (Figures 6.1 and 6.2). The precision fit between implants and abutments is one of the key elements in long-term prosthetic success of implant restorations. (Jemt 1986; Asavant and others, 1988). Binon (1995) contended that if the rotation between implants and abutments can be minimized, more stable and predictable screw joints will result and rotation of less than 5° is desirable for implant joint stability.

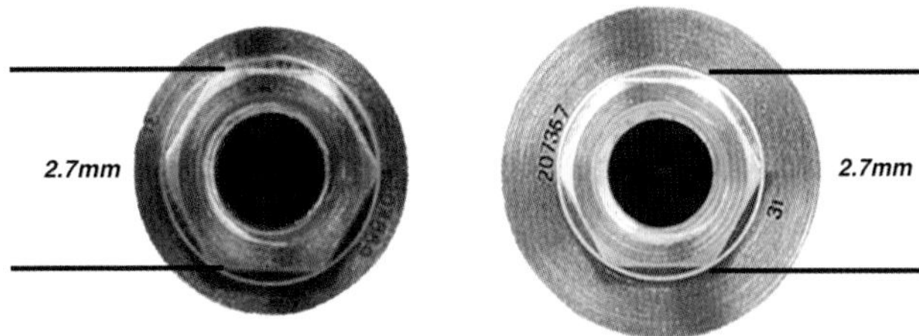

Figure 6.1. Occlusal view of 4.1 mm and 5.0 mm implant restorative platforms (left, right, respectively) that identifies the flat-to-flat surface configurations at 2.7 mm.

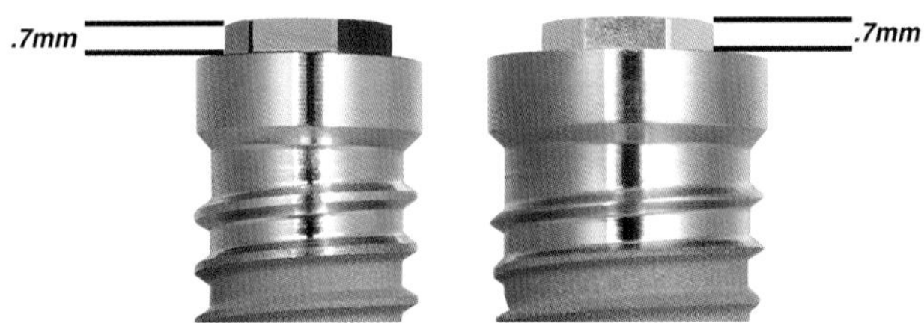

Figure 6.2. Profile view of 4.1 mm and 5.0 mm diameter implants that identifies the hexagonal height of 0.7 mm for both implants.

The implant/abutment interface determines joint strength, stability, and lateral/rotational stability. As implant design evolved, so did implant/abutment connections. One of the first internally hexed implant/abutment designs incorporated a 1.7 mm deep hex below a 0.5 mm wide, 45° bevel (Niznick 1983). Internal connection implants were intended to distribute masticatory forces deeper within implants, which would protect the abutment screw from excessive loading forces. For increased strength, internal connection implants were made from titanium alloy instead of commercially pure titanium, which provided superior strength to the implant/abutment connection (Norton 2000; Mollersten and others 1998).

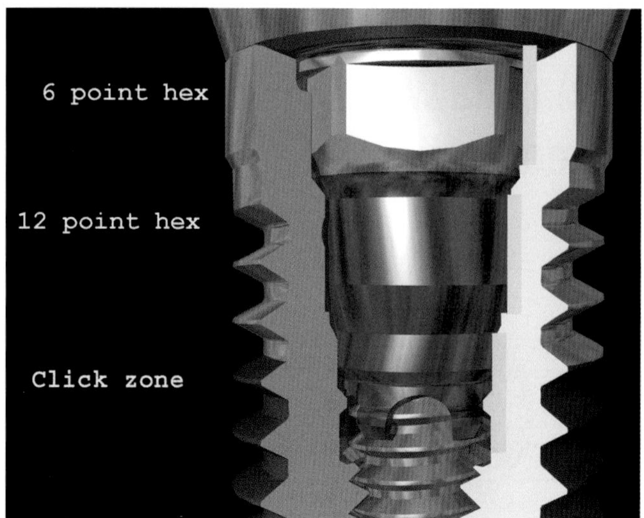

Figure 6.3. Cross sectional view of ***3i***®'s internal connection implant/abutment connection. There are three distinct zones within the implant/abutment connection: the occlusal most portion is specific for a 6-point hex; the middle portion for a 12-point hex; the lower portion for the audible "click" with complete insertion of the restorative component.

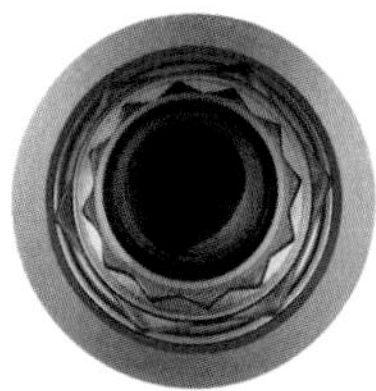

Figure 6.4. An occlusal view of the 6/12 point connection of ***3i***®'s internal connection implant.

There have been further design changes in attempts to improve stability and predictability of the implant/abutment interface. The design changes have included variations in joint designs, or the numbers of hexes present within the connection system (Sutter and others 1993; Perriard and others 2002).

Implant Innovations, Inc.® introduced their internal connection implant (OSSEOTITE® Certain®) in 2003 (Figures 6.3, 6.4). This internal connection provides 4 mm of internal engagement that provides lateral stability for off-axis masticatory forces (Niznick 1991; Norton 2000; Mollersten 1997). Mollersten and others (1997) performed a laboratory study in which they studied the depths of the joints in implant/abutment connections and found that the strength and failure modes varied significantly between the implant systems and deep joints, in contrast to shallow joints. They concluded that joint depth should be one of the considerations that should be taken into account in selecting predictable dental implant systems.

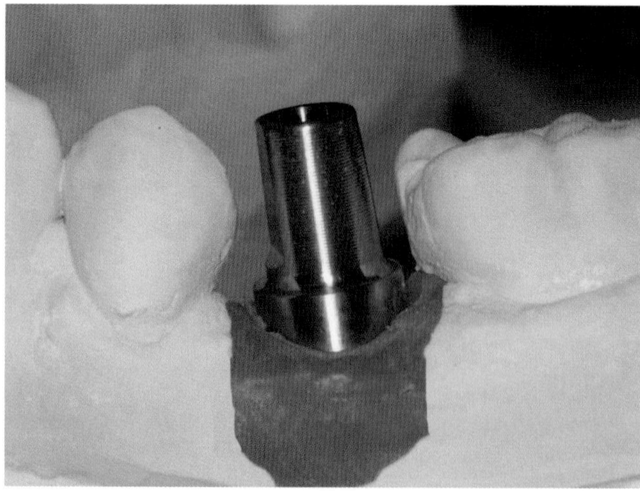

Figure 6.5. GingiHue® Post (IAPP454G) as received from the manufacturer in place.

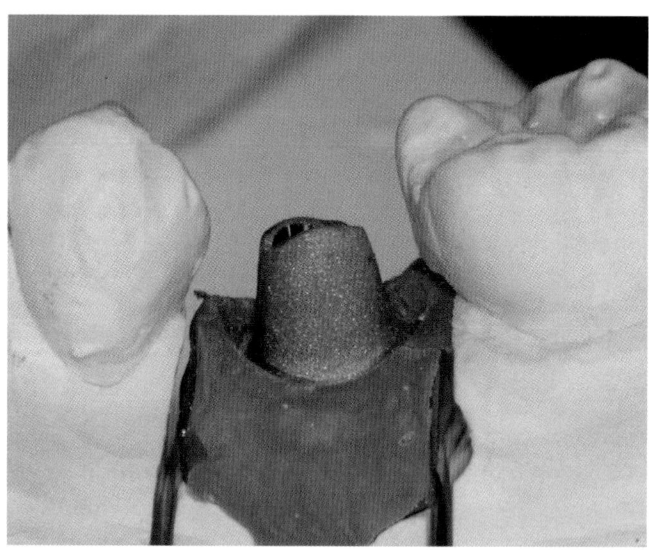

Figure 6.6. The above GingiHue® Post after it was prepared by a dental laboratory technician for use as an abutment for a cement-retained crown.

The height of the abutment screw is only 1.95 mm from the top of the screw to the seating surface. This allows greater flexibility in the amount of abutment preparation without risk of damaging the head of the screw (Figures 6.5, 6.6).

This internal connection system incorporates a 6-point hex design for use with straight abutments and a 12-point, double hex design for use with pre-angled abutments. Stock abutments are less expensive than custom abutments and therefore result in decreased costs for restorative dentists.

Abutment screws with ***3i***®'s internal connection have to be torqued only to 20 Ncm. Rodkey (1977) discussed that the type of finish present on abutment screws can have a considerable effect on the tension induced by a given torque.

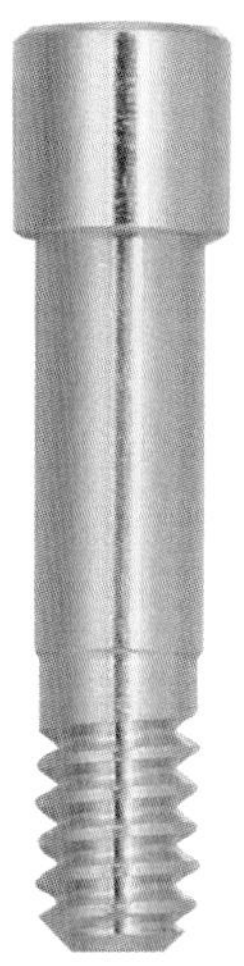

Figure 6.7. Profile view of a Gold-Tite™ hexed abutment screw for *3i*®'s internal connection implant.

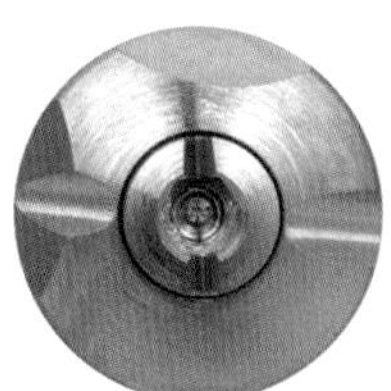

Figure 6.8. Occlusal view of an Encode™ Healing Abutment with a 5 mm emergence profile.

Sakaguchi and Borgersen (1995) reported that the actual preload developed within a screw joint system is dependent upon the finish of the interfaces, friction between the components, geometry, and properties of the materials in the system. Martin and others (2001) performed an extensive laboratory study in which they tested four commercially available abutment screws and their ability to generate preloads in dental implant (external hex)/abutment connections. The greatest preload values were calculated for Gold-Tite™ abutment screws at 20 and 32 Ncm levels. Enhanced screw surfaces were shown to generate less friction between screws and implants than non-enhanced screws (Figure 6.7).

CAD/CAM technology is an exciting new method for producing implant restorations for single, multiple, and full arch restorations. The protocol involves generating digital information relative to implant analogs, adjacent and opposing teeth, and the contours of the planned restoration in a computer. The information may be obtained with images or tactile probes. With the Encode™ Restorative System (***3i*®,** Palm Beach Gardens, FL), special healing abutments (Figure 6.8) are scanned and via a sophisticated computer software program, patient specific abutments are developed (Figure 6.9). This information is sent to a milling machine and abutments are milled from blanks of titanium alloy (Figure 6.10).

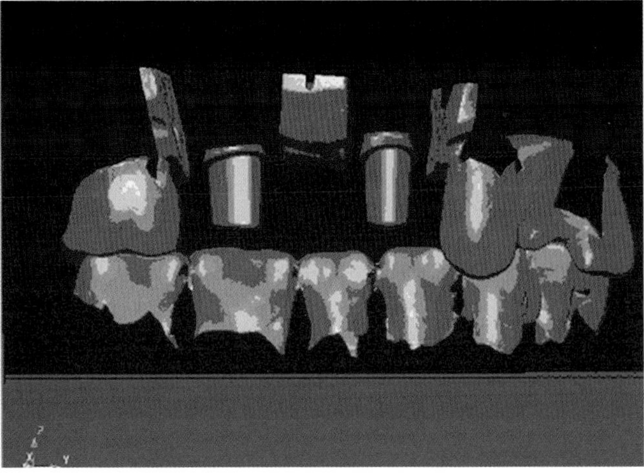

Figure 6.9. CAD/CAM design of two abutments for a 3-unit FPD.

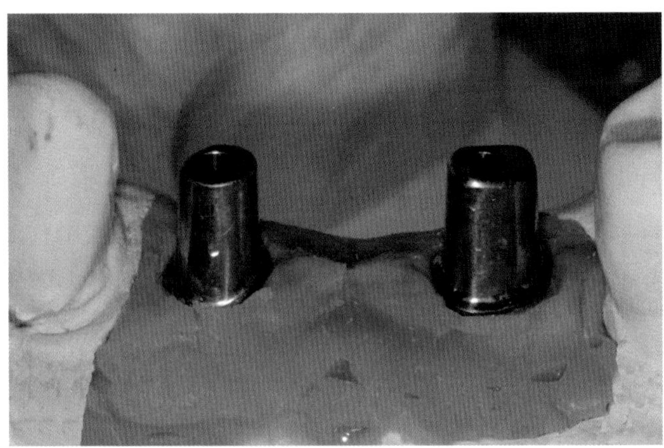

Figure 6.10. Facial laboratory view of two Encode Abutments on a master cast.

Milled titanium abutments fabricated with CAD/CAM technology provide clinicians and dental laboratory technicians significant advantages over custom cast abutments made with conventional casting technology. Waxing, casting, and finishing procedures associated with conventional cast abutments have been eliminated. Generally speaking, there are significant time savings with this process because the commercial dental laboratory will have to provide only the definitive porcelain fused to metal crown for implant restoration. This system actually has decreased the overall costs of implant treatment for laboratories, restorative dentists, and patients. There are clinical reports concerning this technology, but it should be noted that no laboratory studies on the precision of fit with this system have been published (Drago 2005).

The following clinical case presentation illustrates the use of CAD/CAM custom abutments and a 3-unit fixed partial denture to replace a screw-retained 3-unit FPD that failed after 10 years of function.

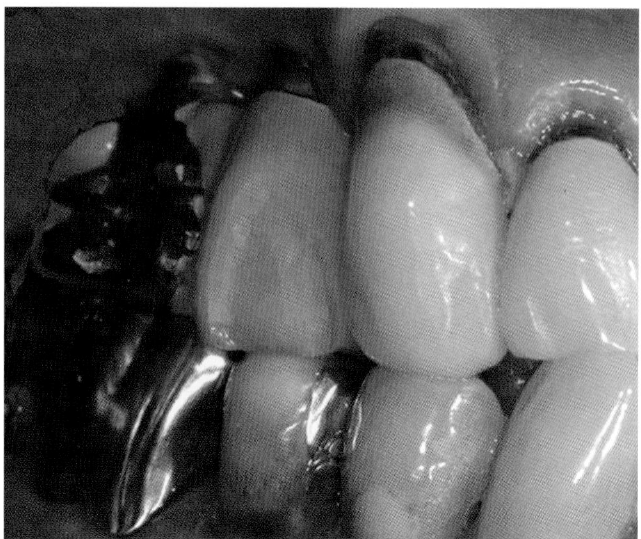

Figure 6.11. Pre-operative clinical appearance of the fractured implant-retained 3-unit fixed partial denture.

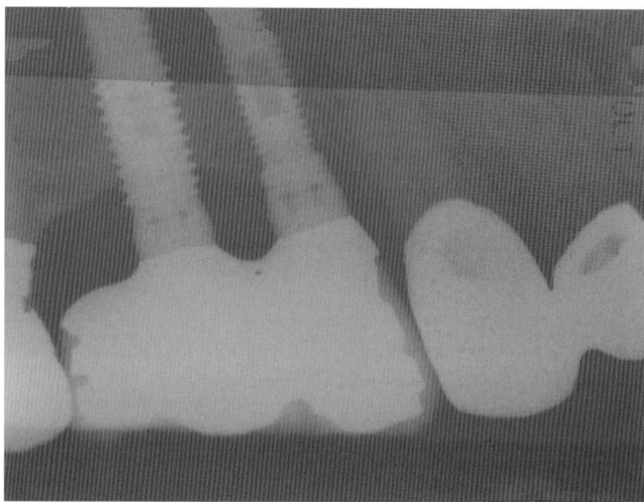

Figure 6.12. Pre-operative radiograph that demonstrated approximately 1–2 mm of bone loss around the osseointegrated implants in the right posterior maxilla.

CLINICAL CASE PRESENTATION

Appointment 1. Initial Examination (3/4 Hour)

A 62-year-old man presented to the author with a chief complaint: "I have a broken bridge" (Figure 6.11). His history included placement of two 4.1 mm diameter implants (external hex) approximately 10 years previous to this first visit. The implants had been placed by an oral surgeon and restored by a general dentist in Iowa. The patient had retired to LaCrosse, Wisconsin. The aesthetic veneer material had fractured. The patient was not sure which implant components had been placed (Figure 6.12).

The physical examination revealed an end-to-end occlusion, Type I gingivitis, a normal range of motion, and a dentition in good repair. The implant-retained fixed partial denture was screw-retained and appeared to be consistent with the original Brånemark implant system.

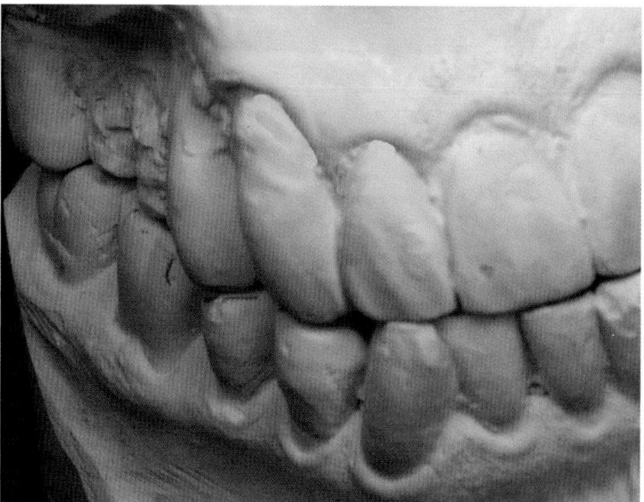

Figure 6.13. Diagnostic casts mounted in centric occlusion demonstrated an end-to-end occlusion. This occlusal relationship was probably implicated in the fracture of the aesthetic veneer material.

Diagnostic Casts

Diagnostic casts were made from alginate impressions (Figure 6.13). They were mounted in centric occlusion and the occlusal relationships were evaluated in preparation for a new fixed partial denture.

Diagnosis

The following diagnoses were developed:

1. Fractured aesthetic veneer, 3-unit fixed partial denture replacing teeth numbers 3–5
2. 4.1 mm diameter, external hex, osseointegrated implants, maxillary right posterior quadrant
3. Class III malocclusion with end-to-end occlusion, right posterior quadrants, minimal anterior guidance
4. Chronic, moderate gingivitis

This patient's condition was classified as patient type Class II per the American College of Prosthodontist's Classification system: moderately compromised based on the skeletal and dental malocclusion, missing three or fewer teeth in a given quadrant, and minimal periodontal involvement (McGarry and others 2002).

TABLE 6.1. Treatment Plan #1 (Implant Restoration)

Diagnosis: Fractured, pre-existing implant-retained fixed partial denture		
Restorative Services	**ADA #**	**Fee**
Comprehensive oral evaluation	D0150	
Diagnostic casts	D0470	
Panoramic radiograph	D0330	
Removal of preexisting FPD and abutments		
Assessment of implant position		
Assessment of peri-implant contours	D9999	
Implant level impression and fabrication of master cast		
Articulator mounting		
Abutment selection		
If implants are in optimal positions,		
Stock abutments	D6056	
If implants are not in optimal positions		
Custom abutments	D6057	
3-unit implant-retained FPD		
#3 Porcelain fused to noble alloy pontic	D6240	
#4 Abutment supported porcelain fused To metal crown (noble metal)	D6061	
#5 Abutment supported porcelain fused To metal crown (noble metal)	D6061	
Yearly recall appointment	D0120	
Periapical radiograph	D0220	

Benefits of Treatment Plan #1

The fractured, preexisting bridge will be replaced with a fixed prosthesis that will not be removable by the patient. The patient should enjoy improved aesthetics and function on a long-term basis. The malocclusion will be made optimal.

Limitations of Treatment Plan #1

Cost, complexity, and length of treatment (1–2 months). The basic malocclusion will remain. The preexisting implant prosthesis will have to be remade. There is a chance that the new prosthesis may fracture due to the malocclusion and alignment of the implants. The patient will continue to need to use additional techniques (floss threader) for hygiene procedures around the implant abutments and prosthesis. The patient needs to return to this office at least once per year for follow-up, which will include radiographs (x-rays) to assess osseointegration of the implants, status of the occlusion, health of the soft tissues, and the integrity of the implant/abutment connections.

Patient signature ______________________

Date ______________________

Witness ______________________

Date ______________________

ADA #'s, CDT 2005 Current Dental Terminology, Council on Dental Benefit Programs, American Dental Association, 211 East Chicago Avenue, Chicago, IL 60611

TABLE 6.2. Treatment Plan #2 (No Treatment)

Diagnosis: Fractured, preexisting implant-retained fixed partial denture		
Restorative Services	**ADA #**	**Fee**
Comprehensive oral evaluation	D0150	
Diagnostic casts	D0470	
Panoramic radiograph	D0330	

Benefits of Treatment Plan #2
No additional expenses will be incurred for a new prosthesis.

Limitations of Treatment Plan #2
The preexisting prosthesis may continue to fracture with potential damage to the implant/abutment connections and/or the abutment and/or retaining screws. The aesthetic and possibly the functional results may be adversely affected, including but not limited to loosening of implant screws, uneven wear of some or all of the components, and fracture of implants or restorative components. If there are fractures of the restorative and/or implant components, the situation may not be fixable without additional surgery to remove or replace an implant(s).

Patient signature ____________________
Date ____________________
Witness ____________________
Date ____________________

ADA #'s, CDT 2005 Current Dental Terminology, Council on Dental Benefit Programs, American Dental Association, 211 East Chicago Avenue, Chicago, IL 60611

Appointment 2. Consultation Restorative Dentist/Patient (1/2 Hour)

A definitive consultation appointment was scheduled as the patient left the office from the first visit. The time between the first and second appointments allowed the author to contact the oral surgeon who placed the implants and identify the type and size of the implants. It also allowed for development of the treatment options for this particular patient.

Treatment Options

The first treatment option involved removing the preexisting fixed partial denture and assessing the condition of the soft tissues surrounding the abutments, as well as identifying the three-dimensional location of the implants relative to the positions of the adjacent and opposing teeth (Table 6.1). The second treatment option described an option for which the patient elected not to proceed with treatment (Table 6.2).

Benefits and limitations of each treatment option were described in detail on the written treatment plans. The prosthodontic fees, or ranges of fees for each procedure, were also listed on each treatment plan. The patient was given copies of the treatment plans. The patient agreed to proceed with the first treatment plan for making a new implant-retained fixed partial denture on new abutments.

Laboratory Procedures

After the patient decided to proceed with treatment, several tasks had to be performed in anticipation of the prosthetic treatment.

Custom Impression Tray

The author prefers to use a pick-up impression technique. This warrants an impression tray with a window that provides access to the impression coping screws (Figure 6.14).

The implant surgeon had provided the author with the size and type of implants placed (4.1 mm diameter, external hex Brånemark implants). In order to make a prosthesis with optimal emergence profiles, implant level impressions with impression copings of the proper emergence profiles needed to be selected and on hand for the impression appointment. Because the missing teeth were premolars and the preexisting prosthesis replicated the anatomy of the missing teeth, implant impression copings for 4.1 mm

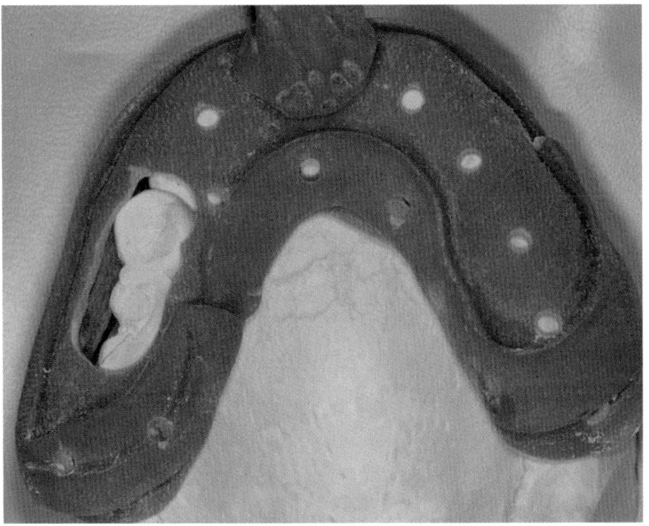

Figure 6.14. Laboratory occlusal view of open face custom impression tray in place on the maxillary diagnostic cast.

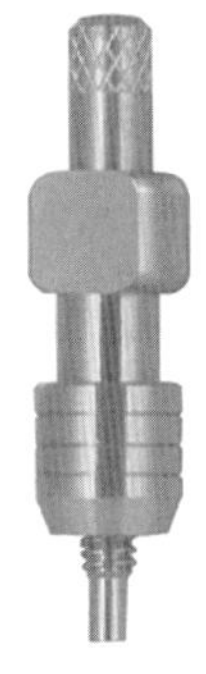

Figure 6.15. Implant impression coping with 4.1 mm restorative platform and 5 mm emergence profile (IIC12).

restorative platforms and 5 mm emergence profiles were preselected (IIC12) (Figure 6.15).

Appointment 3. Removal of Existing Prosthesis/Abutments; Implant Impression (1 Hour)

The pre-existing FPD was removed with a slotted driver (Figure 6.16). The two conical abutments were visualized (SCA003) and were removed with a conical abutment driver (PAD00) (Figure 6.17). The 4.1 mm implant restorative platforms were completely exposed (Figure 6.18).

Implant Level Impression

Implant impression copings (IIC12) were placed onto the external hexes of the implants. The screws were tightened with the posterior large hex driver (PHD02N). The definitive

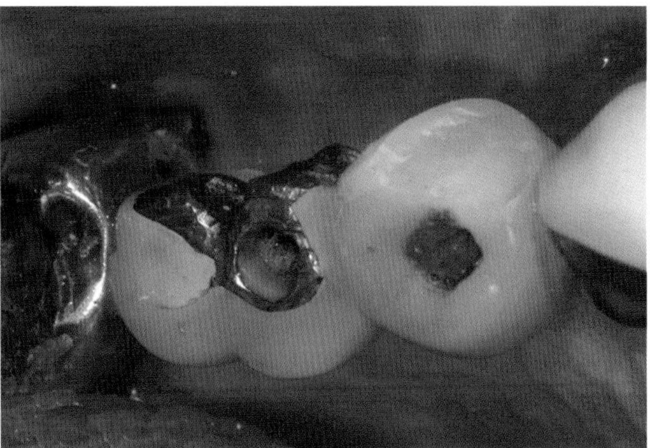

Figure 6.16. Occlusal view of preexisting 3-unit FPD.

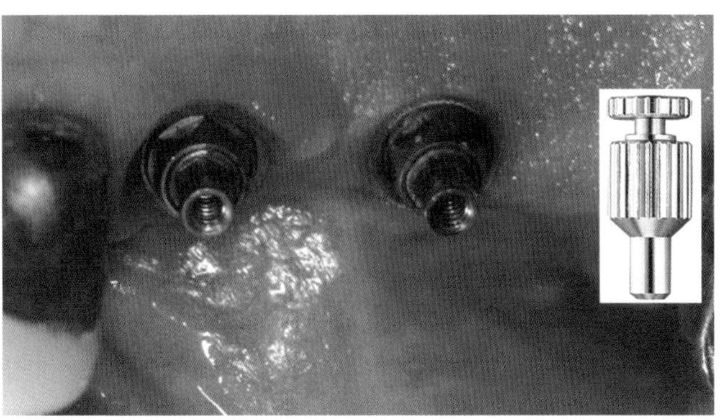

Figure 6.17. Palatal/occlusal view of conical abutments in place after the prosthesis in Figure 6.16 was removed. Abutment driver inset (PAD00).

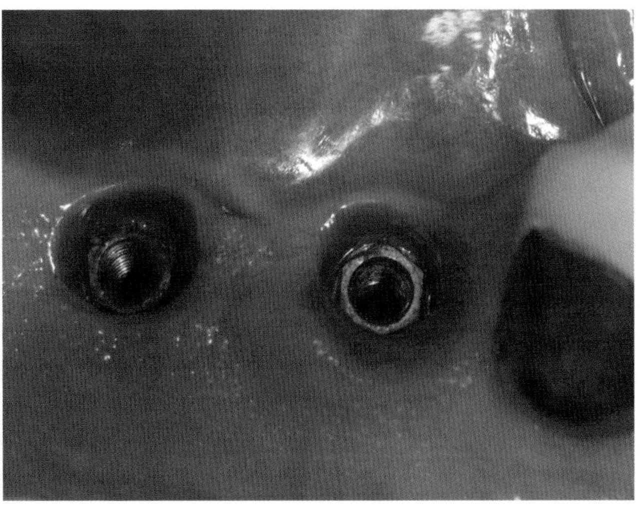

Figure 6.18. Implant restorative platforms (4.1 mm diameter) were completely exposed after removal of the conical abutments.

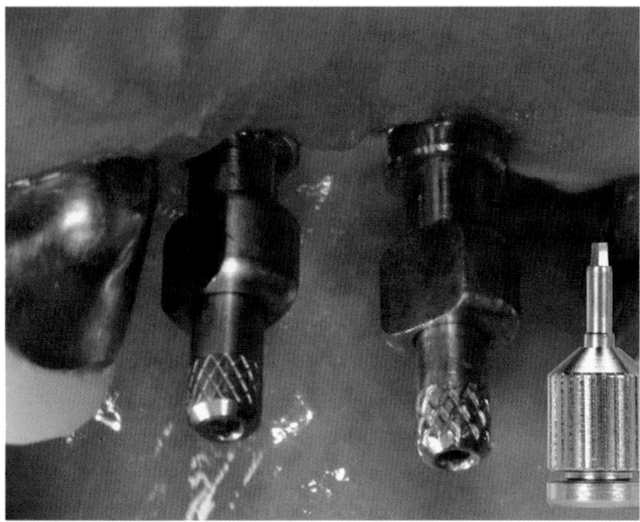

Figure 6.19. Palatal view of pick up implant impression copings in place. Large hex posterior driver (PHD02N) inset.

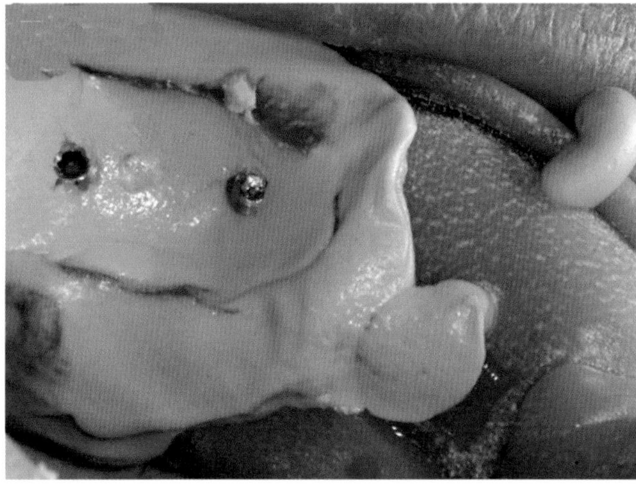

Figure 6.20. An open face tray was used for the pick-up impression technique. The window provided access to the impression coping screws, which had to be loosened prior to removal of the impression with PHD02N.

impression was made with injection and putty vinyl polysiloxane impression material (Figures 6.19 and 6.20).

Laboratory Procedures/Work Orders

Fabrication of Master Cast (Implant Analogs)

After the impression material polymerized, the impression coping screws were unscrewed with the large posterior hex driver (PHDO2N) and the impression was removed. The pick up implant impression copings remained inside the impression (Figure 6.21). Implant lab analogs for 4.1 mm diameter external hex implants were selected, attached to the apical surfaces of the pick-up implant impression copings, and screwed into place from the occlusal aspect of the impression tray (Figures 6.22, 6.23).

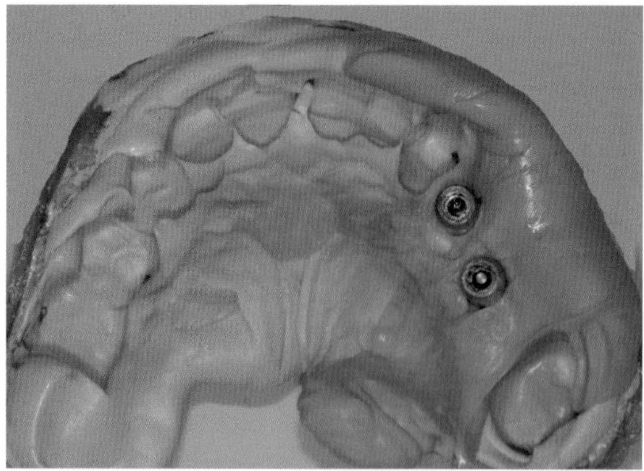

Figure 6.21. The pick-up implant impression copings remained inside the definitive impression after the impression was removed from the mouth.

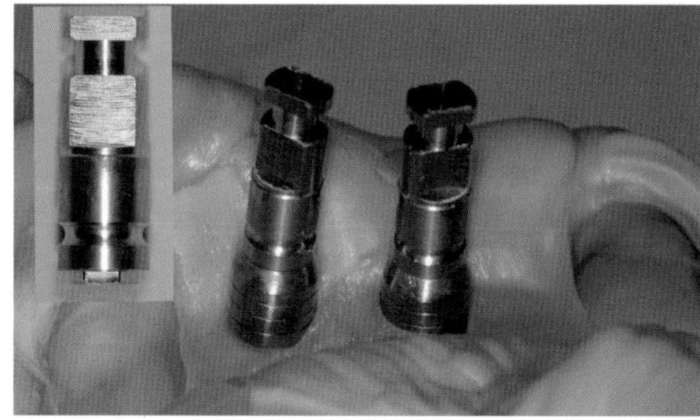

Figure 6.22. Implant lab analogs (ILA20), inset, were attached to the apical surfaces of the pick up implant impression copings. Metal-to-metal contact was visualized between the analogs and the impression copings.

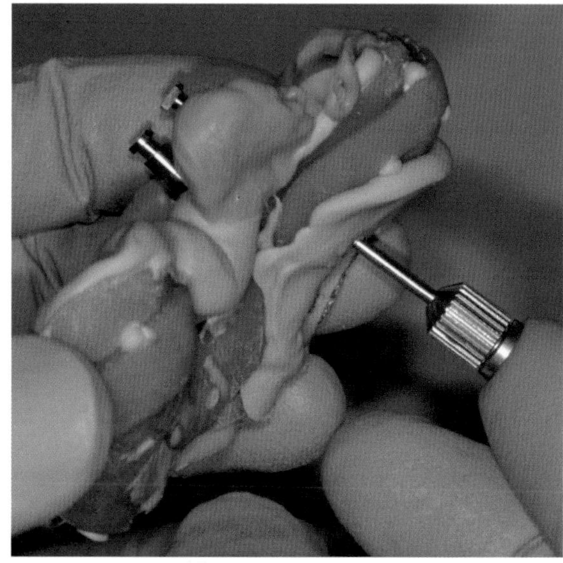

Figure 6.23. The PHD02N was used to screw the implant impression coping screws into the implant lab analogs. Care was taken not to over-tighten the screws because doing so may alter the positions of the impression copings within the impression.

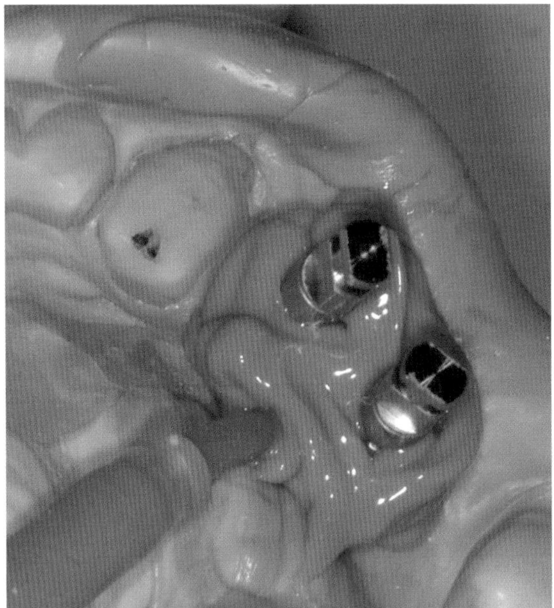

Figure 6.24. Poly vinylsiloxane impression material was injected in and around the impression coping/implant analog connections.

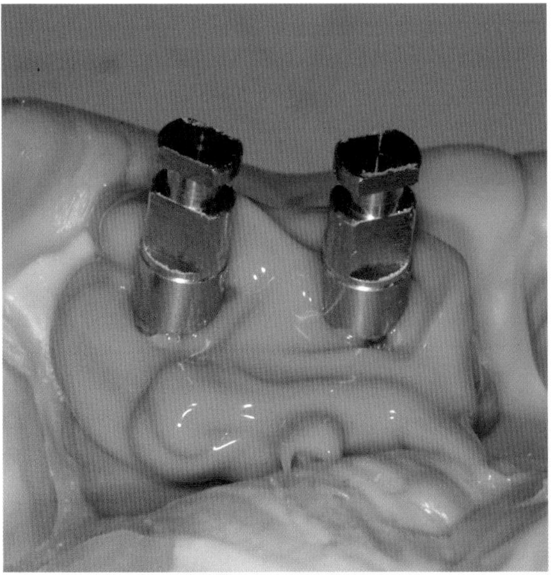

Figure 6.25. The impression was now ready to be poured in Type IV dental stone.

Because the implant restorative platforms were sub-gingival, the peri-implant soft tissues around the implant lab analogs in the master cast were made with a resilient material. In this case, a separator was placed around the impression copings/implant analogs prior to injecting poly vinylsiloxane impression material in and around the implant analog/impression coping connections (Figure 6.24, 6.25). Care was taken not to allow any of the impression material into the interproximal contact areas. The impression was now ready to be poured in Type IV dental stone to fabricate the master cast (Figure 6.26).

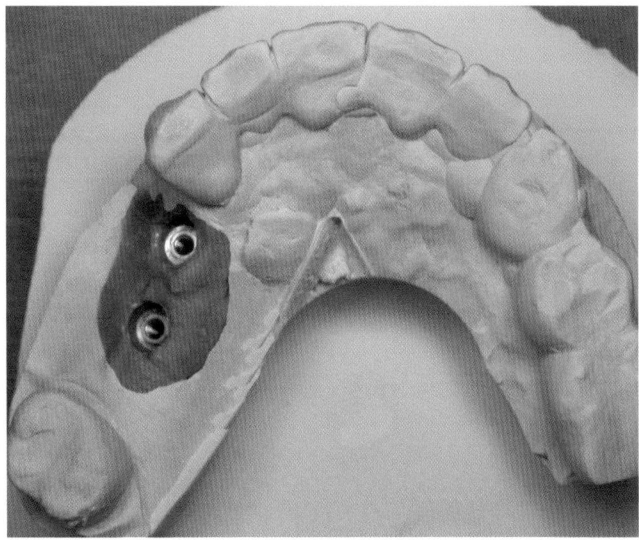

Figure 6.26. Occlusal view of the master cast with implant analogs in place.

TABLE 6.3. Laboratory Work Order for Fabrication of a Master Cast from an Implant Level Impression

Patient name	______________________
Doctor name	______________________
Doctor address	______________________
Phone number	______________________
Date	______________________

Treatment: Two custom abutments (Encode Abutments), 3-unit fixed partial denture (#3 is a pontic)

1. Enclosed is a poly vinylsiloxane implant impression for teeth #'s 3, 4, and 5.
2. The impression copings have 5 mm emergence profiles for 4.1 mm implant restorative platforms (external hex).
3. Place lab analogs (***3i***® ILA20) onto the impression copings.
4. Please make sure that you see metal-to-metal contact between the copings and the analogs.
5. Inject a resilient material around the impression coping/implant analog connections. Take care not to let any soft material into any interproximal contact areas.
6. Pour in Type IV die stone per the manufacturer's instructions.
7. Allow to set.
8. Pin, section as needed.
9. Mount on Stratos 100 articulator in preparation for fabrication of Encode Abutments and 3-unit FPD.

The preceding procedures describe fabrication of a master cast in the dental office. A laboratory work order for the above procedures is illustrated in Table 6.3.

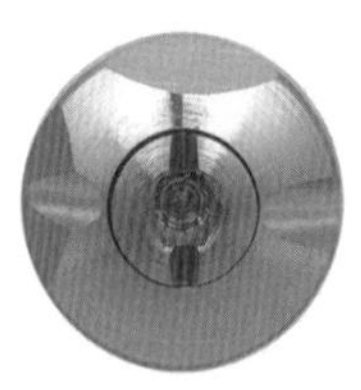 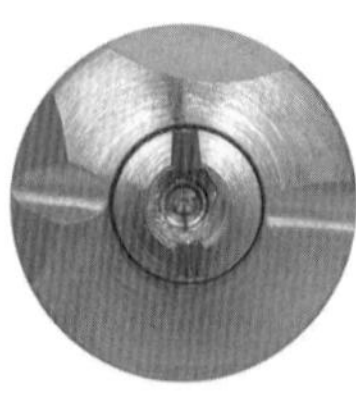 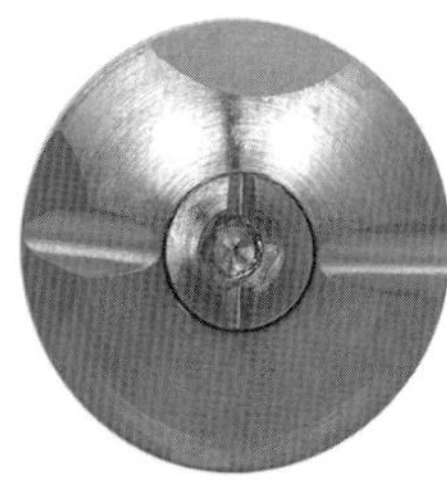

Figure 6.28. Encode Healing Abutments: 5 mm, 6 mm, 7.5 mm, left to right. (EHA454, EHA464, EHA474, respectively).

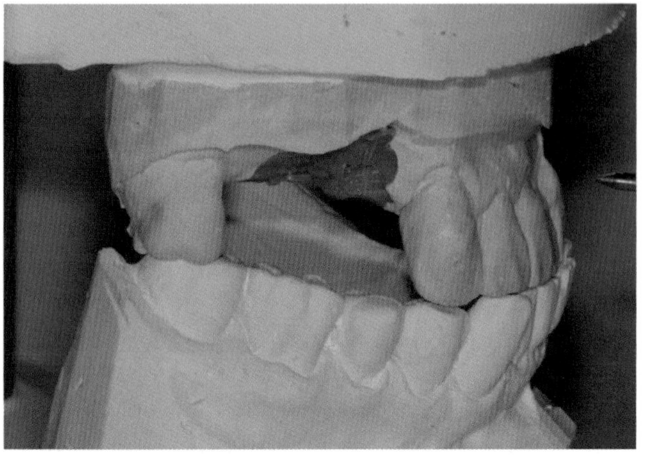

Figure 6.27. Maxillary master cast and mandibular cast were mounted on a semi-adjustable articulator in preparation for fabrication of the CAD/CAM abutments and definitive 3-unit FPD.

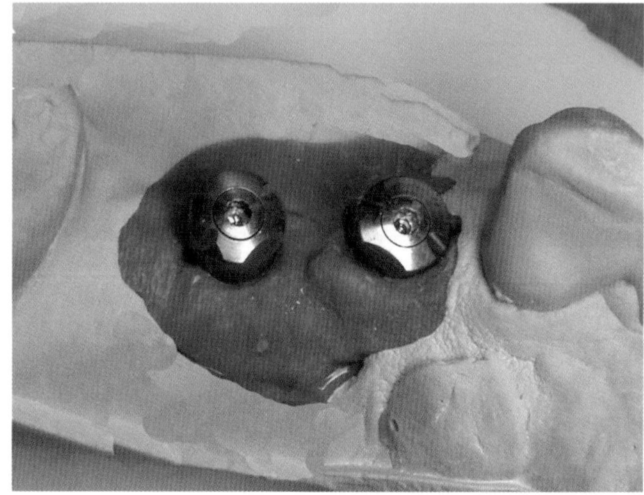

Figure 6.29. Encode Healing Abutments in place on master cast (EHA454).

A centric occlusal jaw relation record was made with Blu Mousse (Parkell Bio-Materials Division, Farmingdale, NY). Shades were selected and the casts were mounted on a Stratos 100 articulator (***3i®*** Package, Ivoclar Vivadent, Inc., Technical Division, Amherst, NY) (Figure 6.27).

The preexisting abutments were placed back onto the implants along with the preexisting 3-unit FPD, and the patient was discharged.

CAD/CAM Protocol

The CAD/CAM protocol for The Encode™ Restorative System is predicated on a digital scan of Encode™ Healing Abutments. These special healing abutments have codes embedded into their occlusal surfaces, and these codes provide the information required for the ideal anatomical design of final Encode Abutments (Figure 6.28).

In this case, the contours of the preexisting abutments were similar to 5 mm emergence profiles. Therefore, Encode Healing Abutments (EHA454) emergence profiles and 4 mm collar heights were placed onto the implant lab analogs in the master cast (Figure 6.29). The occlusal surfaces of Encode Healing Abutments must be supragingival to enable the scanner to accurately scan all of the codes within the occlusal surfaces.

The base of the cast was soaked in slurry water and an alginate impression was made. This cast was poured in Type IV die stone (GC FujiRock® EP Golden Brown, GC Europe, Leuven, Belgium) (Figure 6.30). This cast was pinned per conventional fixed prosthodontic protocols and sectioned. The gingival margins were not trimmed, because the scanner needs to identify the location of the gingival margins in conjunction with abutment margin design (Table 6.4).

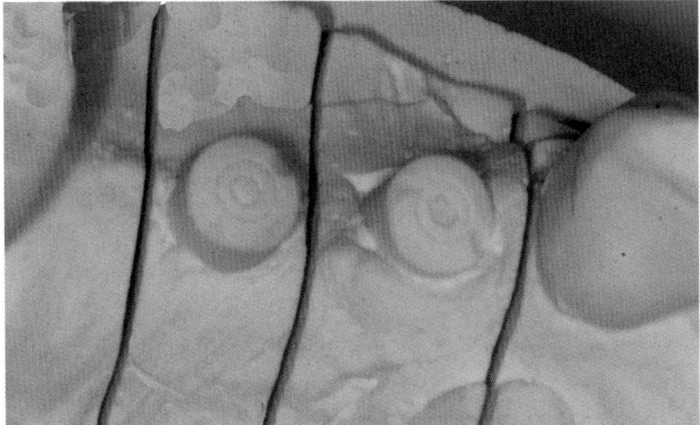

Figure 6.30. Occlusal view of die stone cast of Encode Healing Abutments.

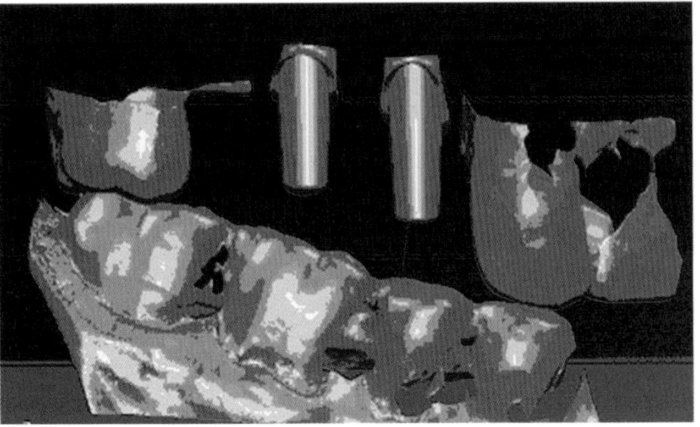

Figure 6.31. CAD design of abutments that will be used in conjunction with the planned 3-unit FPD.

TABLE 6.4. Laboratory Work Order for Fabrication of a Master Cast for Encode Abutments

Patient name	__________
Doctor name	__________
Doctor address	__________
Phone number	__________
Date	__________

Treatment: Two custom abutments (Encode Abutments), 3-unit fixed partial denture (#3 is a pontic)

1. Select 2 Encode Healing Abutments (IEHA454) and place them onto the implant lab analogs in the master cast.
2. Make sure that the occlusal surfaces of the Encode Healing Abutments are supra-gingival.
3. Make an alginate impression of the master cast.
4. Pour the alginate impression in FujiRock.
5. Mount this cast on a Stratos 100 articulator.
6. Complete the work order for two final Encode Abutments.
7. Send to ***3i***® ARCHITECH PSRY™, Palm Beach Gardens, FL.
8. Keep the master cast with the implant analogs in your laboratory for fabrication of the 3-unit FPD.

Articulator Mounting

This cast was mounted on the Stratos® 100 articulator in the same relationship as the original master cast (with implant analogs). A work order (Tables 6.5, 6.6) for final Encode Abutments was completed and, along with the casts, was sent to the ARCHITECH PSR™ Center in Palm Beach Gardens, FL.

CAD Design of Abutments

Using sophisticated computer software programs, a dental laboratory technician designed the abutment contours for the 3-unit FPD. In this case, the facial margins were placed 1 mm sub-gingival, and the interproximal and palatal margins were placed at the gingival crest. The axial contours were designed with 6° taper and a common path of insertion; the occlusal surfaces were reduced for 2 mm interocclusal clearance. The emergence profiles were made consistent with the anatomic contours of maxillary premolars (Figure 6.31).

TABLE 6.5. Blank Work Order for Final Encode Abutments

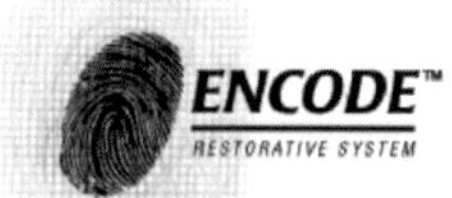

Work Order

* 1. Account Information

* Lab Name:________________

3i Account#:________________

* Contact:________________

* Phone:________________

Fax:________________

* Email:________________

* Patient ID:________________

* Ship To:________________

Bill To:________________

* 2. Preparing Your Case For Shipment

- *Use only **yellow** die stone for the Encode Casts.*
- *Verify that all of the codes on each healing abutment are completely visible on the cast.*
- *Section and pin the Encode Die Cast **(Please do not trim the Encode Die).***
- *Mount casts on Adesso Split Plates Articulator **only** (Stratos® or Baumann) and verify the vertical pin is set at zero and meets the occlusal table.*
- *Following mounting on the designated articulator please include the following in the shipment to **3i**:*
  - ❑ Pinned & Sectioned Encode Die Cast
  - ❑ Opposing Cast
  - ❑ Copy of the Completed Work Order
- *All un-articulated or mis-articulated casts will be returned to the lab*
- *Please **do not** send the articulator*

* 3. Case Information

Tooth Position	Connection Type		Gold Colored TiN** (Titanium Nitride) Yes or No
	Certain®	Ex-Hex	

** NOTE: TiN Coating will add two working days to the processing of your abutment. If a box is not checked the abutment will not be TiN coated.

* 4. Design Guidelines

Margin Style – Select One
❑ Shoulder
❑ Chamfer (Default)

Interocclusal Distance: _____mm

NOTE: Default on all margins = 1mm Subgingival

Buccal Margin Location
❑ Subgingival _____mm
❑ Flush with Gingiva

Lingual Margin Location
❑ Subgingival _____mm
❑ Flush with Gingiva
❑ Supragingival _____mm

* REQUIRED FIELD

5. Contour Guidelines

Please draw the approximate contour desired over the default images below. Note margin style. Please draw in tissue contour.
(Minimum abutment height = 4mm and minimum collar height = .5mm)

	Buccal	Interproximal
Anterior		
Posterior		

6. Special Instructions

❑ Polish entire abutment (Default)   ❑ Only polish the subgingival collar

____

____

____

❑ See back or attached page for additional instructions.

7. Screw Ordering

❑ I would not like to order screws at this time.

External Hex Abutment Screws	Qty.
Gold-Tite™ Square (UNISG)	____
Gold-Tite Hexed (UNIHG)	____
Titanium Hexed (UNIHT)	____
Laboratory Square Try-in Screw - 5 pack (UNITS)	____
Microminiplant™ Square Try-in Screw - 5 pack (MUNITS)	____

Certain Abutment Screws	Qty.
Gold-Tite Hexed (IUNIHG)	____
Titanium Hexed (IUNIHT)	____
Laboratory Hexed Try-in Screw - 5 pack (IUNITS)	____

* 8. Certification — must be signed

I certify that the stated information is correct and that the submitted materials are accurate. All items that have contacted the oral environment have been disinfected. This form authorizes *3i* to fabricate the patient specific abutment(s) using and consistent with the information provided on this work order.

Technician Signature ________________

Date ________________

Internal Use Only

Job #: ________________

Signature: ________________

3i®

Implant Innovations, Inc.
4555 Riverside Drive
Palm Beach Gardens, FL 33410
800.443.8166

ART881
REV E 10/05

TABLE 6.6. Work Order for Final Encode Abutments.

Tooth Number	Connection Type	Gold Titanium Nitride
4	Ext hex	No
5	Ext hex	No

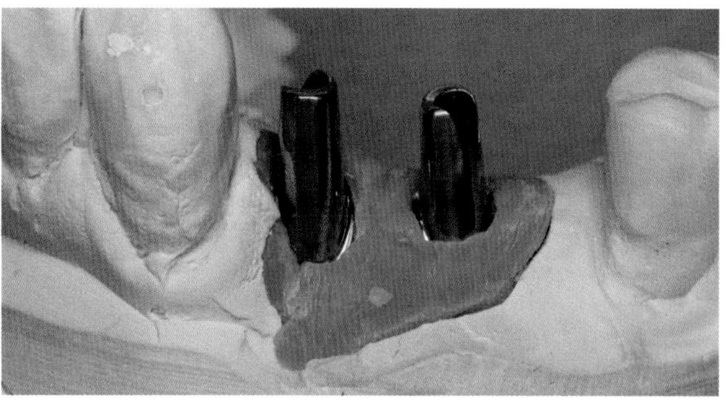

Figure 6.34. Laboratory facial view of the master cast with the 2 CAD/CAM abutments in place.

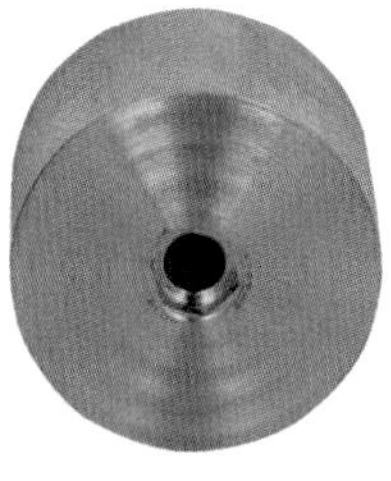

Figure 6.32. External hex blank of titanium alloy prior to milling the CAD/CAM abutments.

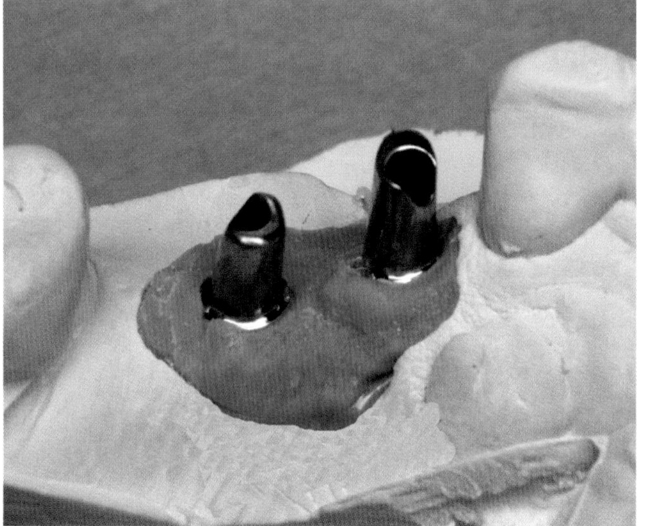

Figure 6.35. Laboratory palatal view of the master cast with the two CAD/CAM abutments in place.

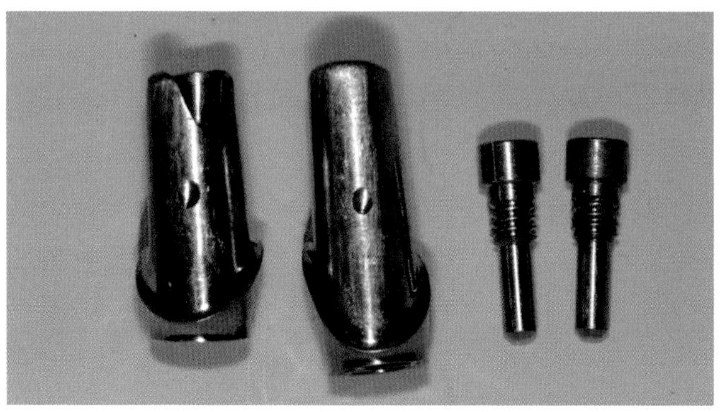

Figure 6.33. The CAD/CAM abutments after milling. Square try-in screws (UNITS) were included for use during fabrication of the FPD and also for the clinical try-in appointment.

CAM Milling of Abutments

The abutments were milled from blanks of titanium alloy. These blanks were already pre-machined with the external hex implant/abutment connection (Gold Standard ZR™) (Figure 6.32). The abutments were milled to precise tolerances and shipped to the commercial dental laboratory for fabrication of the 3-unit FPD (Figure 6.33).

Fabrication of 3-Unit Fixed Partial Denture

At the commercial dental laboratory, the final Encode Abutments were placed onto the implant lab analogs in the master cast (Figures 6.34 and 6.35). An abutment placement index was fabricated directly on the abutments while they were in their correct positions (Figures 6.36, 6.37, 6.38, 6.39).

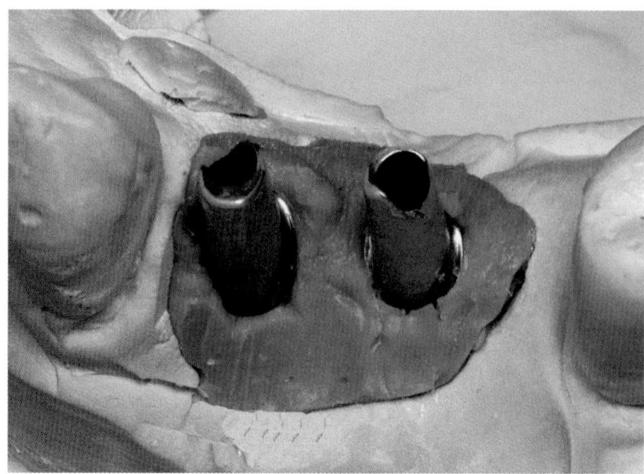

Figure 6.36. Two layers of die spacer were placed directly onto the abutments prior to waxing and fabricating the abutment placement index.

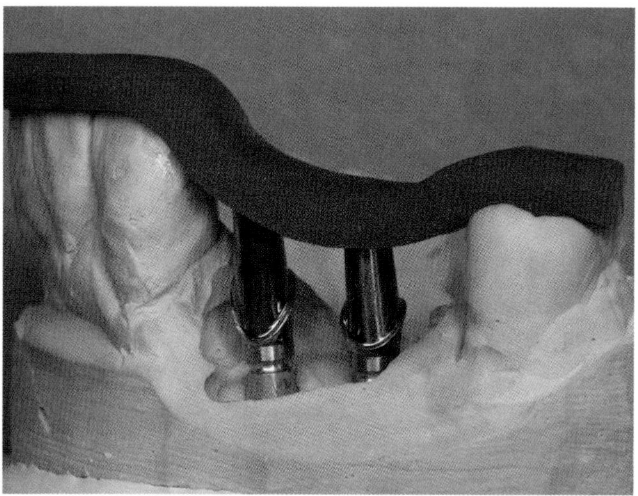

Figure 6.37. Light cured resin was adapted to the occlusal surfaces of the adjacent teeth, without engaging any undercuts. Autopolymerizing acrylic resin was used to make copings directly onto the abutments.

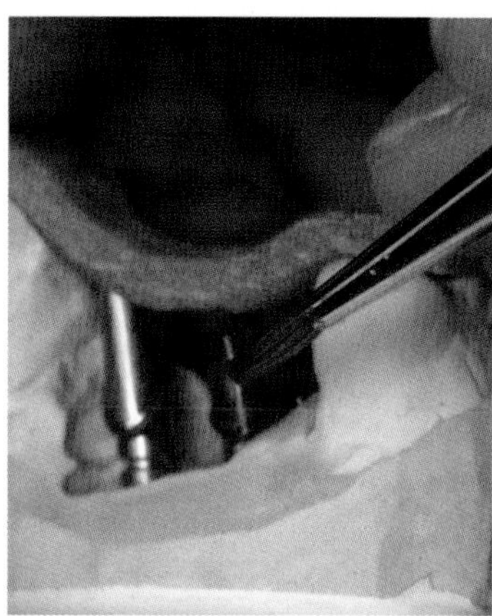

Figure 6.38. The resin copings were luted to the light cured resin strip for completion of the abutment placement index.

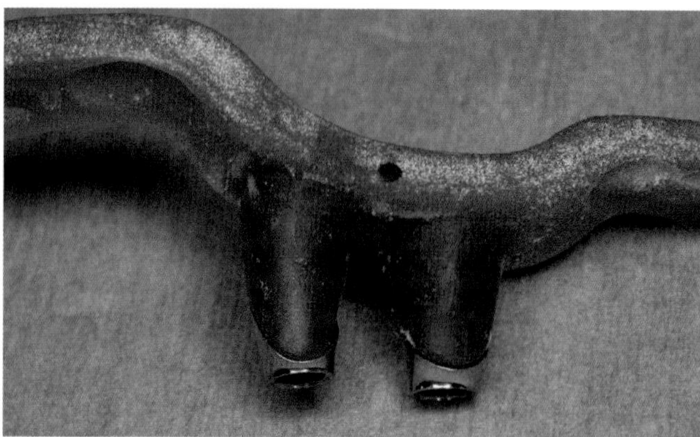

Figure 6.39. The abutments were contained within the abutment placement index. The index simplified insertion and removal of the abutments in the laboratory and intra-orally.

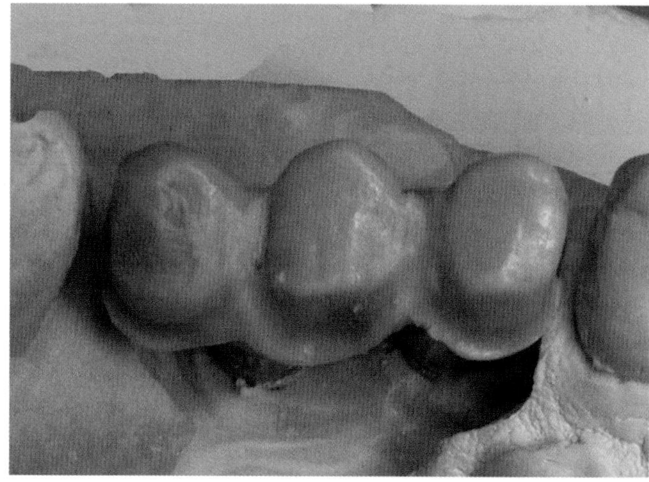

Figure 6.40. The wax pattern was waxed to full contour and cut back for porcelain.

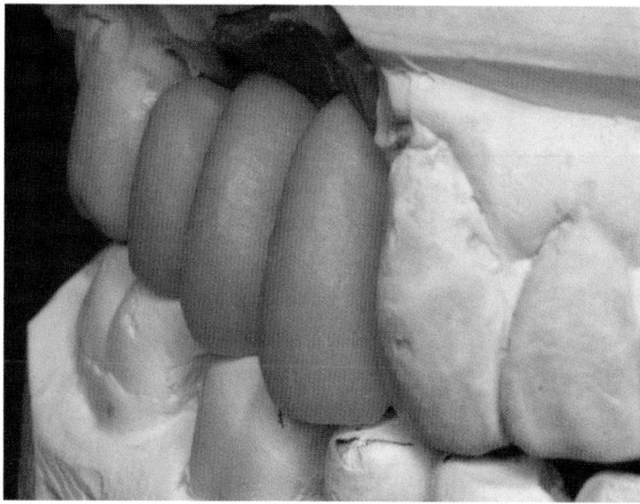

Figure 6.41. The 3-unit FPD was returned to the author for a clinical bisque bake try-in.

TABLE 6.7. Work Order for Fabrication of 3-Unit Fixed Partial Denture

Patient name	__________
Doctor name	__________
Doctor address	__________
Phone number	__________
Date	__________

Treatment: Two custom abutments (Encode Abutments), 3-unit fixed partial denture (#'s 3 to 5; #3 is a pontic)

1. Master cast with implant analogs mounted on Stratos 100 articulator
2. Place Encode Abutments onto their respective analogs. Each abutment package is marked with the respective tooth number. Square try-in screws enclosed.
3. Place two layers of die spacer on each abutment within 1 mm of the abutment margins.
4. Wax the 3-unit fixed partial denture to full contour. #3 is a pontic. Diagnostic cast enclosed.
   a. Occlusion
      i. Develop a normal Class I buccal/lingual relationship between the prosthesis and the opposing mandibular teeth.
      ii. Right working occlusion to be Group Function occlusion.
      iii. Eliminate/minimize balancing interferences.
      iv. Narrow the buccal/lingual dimensions of the occlusal tables.
   b. Emergence Profiles
      i. The abutments have been contoured for optimal emergence profiles. The margins of the FPD should flow into the abutment contours without overhangs.
   c. Cut back for porcelain.
   d. Cast in gold noble alloy (IPS d.SIGN®91, Ivoclar Vivadent-Au 60%, Pd 30.6%, In 8.4%).
   e. Finish the casting
   f. Apply porcelain
   g. Return in bisque bake for try-in.

The 3-unit FPD was fabricated per the work order in Table 6.7. and was returned for a bisque bake try-in (Figures 6.40, 6.41).

Appointment 4. Bisque Bake Try-In (3/4 Hour)

Removal of Preexisting Prosthesis and Abutments

The patient returned for the fourth appointment. The preexisting FPD and abutments were removed.

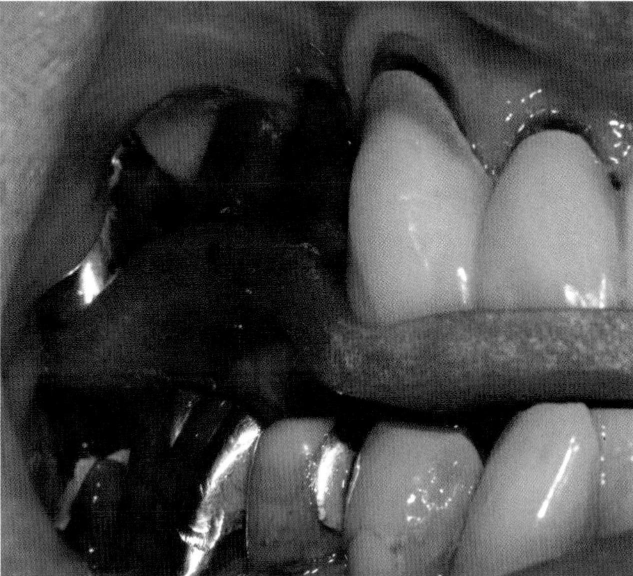

Figure 6.42. Abutment placement index in place. Abutments were contained within the index.

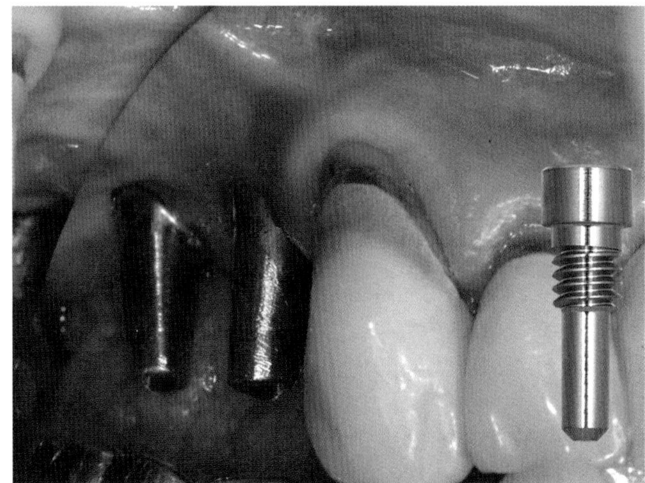

Figure 6.43. Square try-in screws were used to retain the abutments to the implants (UNITS, inset).

Try-In CAD/CAM Abutments

The Encode Abutments were tried in using the abutment placement index to facilitate abutment insertion (Figures 6.42, 6.43). Square try-in screws for external hex implants were used (UNITS).

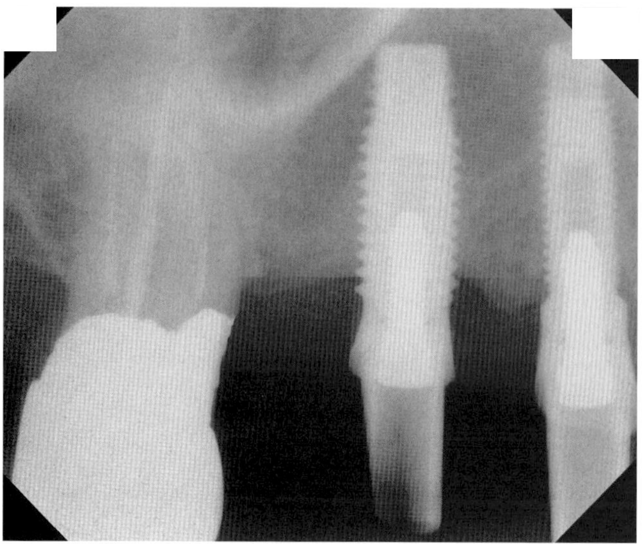

Figure 6.44. Periapical radiograph demonstrated an intimate metal-to-metal fit between the abutments and implants. The sub-gingival emergence profiles were fabricated by the CAD computer software program and milled by the CAM milling unit.

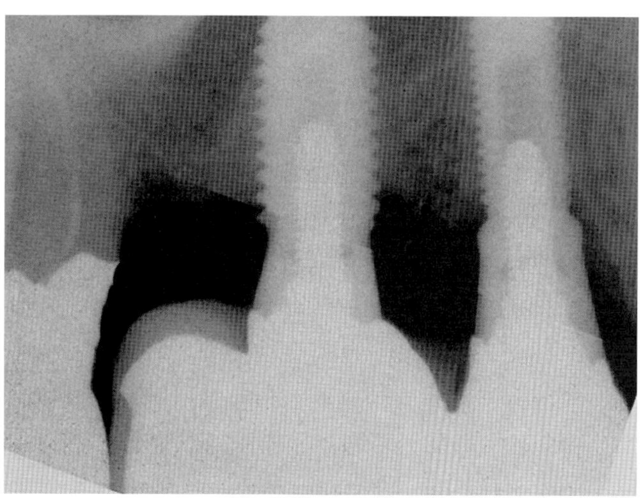

Figure 6.45. Periapical radiograph demonstrated metal-to-metal contact between the retainers of the FPD and the abutments.

Verification Radiograph (Abutments)

A radiograph was taken to verify that the abutments were seated (Figure 6.44).

Try-In Bisque Bake FPD

The 3-unit FPD was tried in by adjusting the interproximal contacts until floss could be passed between the prosthesis and the adjacent teeth easily.

Verification Radiograph (FPD)

Another radiograph was taken to verify complete seating of the prosthesis onto the abutments (Figure 6.45).

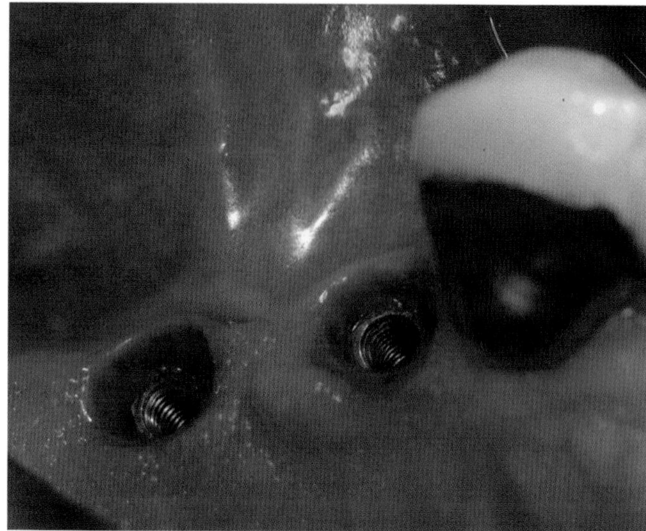

Figure 6.46. The implant restorative platforms for the external hex implants in the maxillary right posterior quadrant at the time of CAD/CAM abutment insertion.

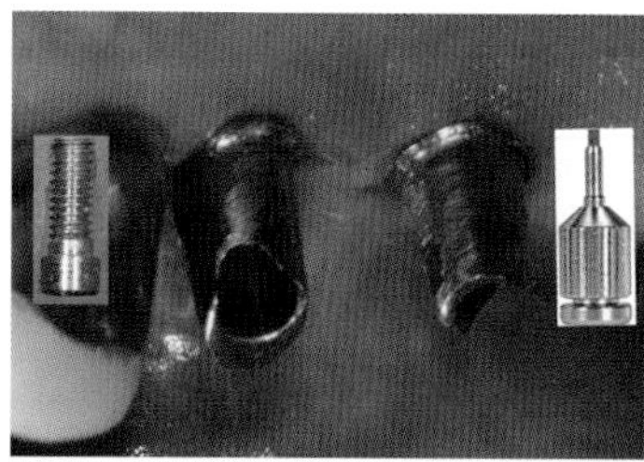

Figure 6.47. Final Encode Abutments were placed into the implants with definitive Gold-Tite™ abutment screws (UNISG, left inset). The abutment screw was tightened with the Posterior Square Driver (PSQD0N, right inset).

The occlusion was adjusted for stable centric contacts, right group function occlusion, and no balancing interferences. The porcelain shades were acceptable.

The prosthesis and abutments were removed and returned to the commercial dental laboratory for finishing procedures. The preexisting abutments and fixed partial denture were placed back onto the abutments, and the patient was discharged.

Appointment 5. Insertion Appointment (3/4 Hour)

The patient returned for insertion of the definitive CAD/CAM abutments and fixed partial denture.

Removal of Preexisting Abutments and Fixed Partial Denture

The preexisting prosthesis and conical abutments were removed. The peri-implant soft tissues duplicated the size and shape of the conical abutments. The implant restorative platforms were completely visualized (Figure 6.46).

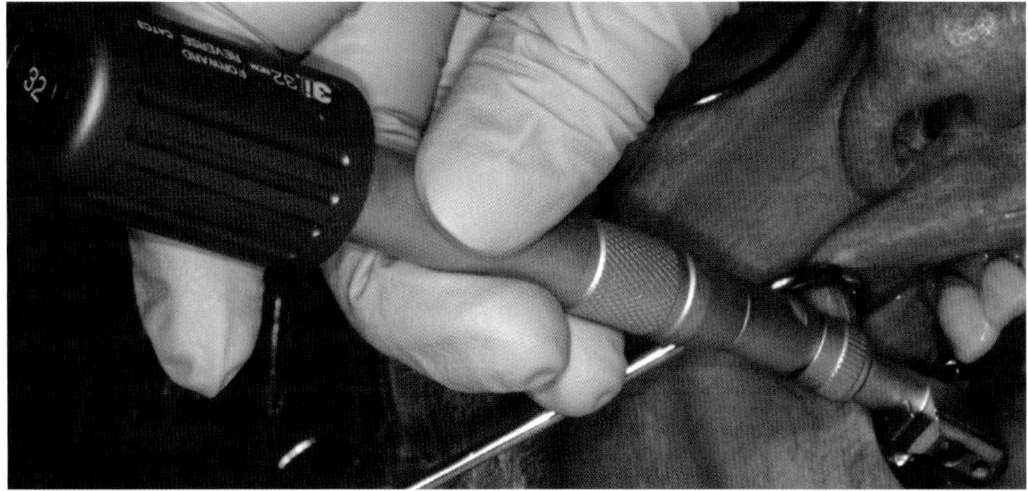

Figure 6.48. The Contra Angle Torque Driver Body (CADTB) and 32 Ncm torque controller (CATC3) in place.

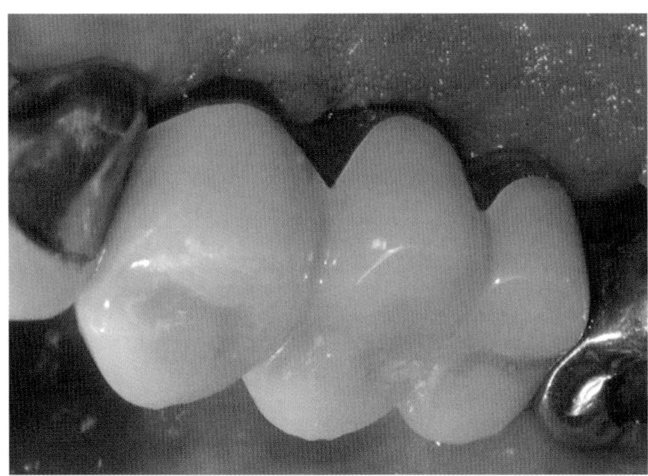

Figure 6.49. Palatal contours of the 3-unit fixed partial denture at the insertion appointment.

CAD/CAM Abutment Placement

The CAD/CAM abutments were put into place with the abutment placement index as per the procedures for the bisque bake try-in (Figure 6.47). Because the author knew that the abutments and FPD fit, the definitive abutment screws were used (UNISG). The Posterior Square Driver, 17 mm (PSQDON) was used to initially tighten the abutment screws.

Torque

The abutment screws were torqued to 32 Ncm with the Contra Angle Torque Driver (CATDB) and 32 Ncm torque controller (CATC3) (Figure 6.48). This was accomplished without pain or tenderness and generally represents a positive sign as to osseointegration of the implants.

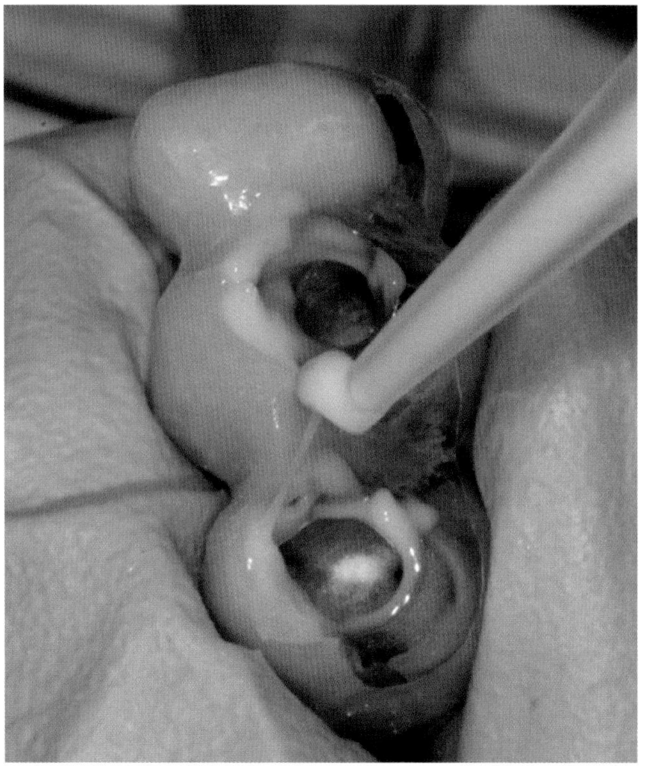

Figure 6.50. The margins of the retainers were rimmed with dental cement. Care should be taken to minimize the amount and placement of the cement so as to minimize changes in the fit between the retainers and the abutments.

Fixed Partial Denture Cementation

The fixed partial denture was tried in again for interproximal and occlusal contacts; pontic/tissue adaptation, and overall aesthetics (Figure 6.49). The FPD was polished, air abraded with 50 μm aluminum oxide, and steam cleaned. The FPD was cemented with reinforced glass ionomer luting cement (GC Fuji Plus, GC America Inc., Alsip, Il) (Figure 6.50). The cement was placed in and around the apical

2 mm of the retainers and seated into place. The cement was allowed to set for 2.5 minutes and the excess was removed.

Appointment 6. Follow-Up Appointments (1/2 Hour)

Two Weeks/Six Months

The patient was scheduled for two-week and six-month follow-up appointments. The patient reported no adverse effects and was quite pleased with the aesthetic, functional, and phonetic results.

One-Year Recall Clinical and Radiographic Evaluations

One year following abutment and prosthesis insertion, the patient returned for clinical and radiographic examina-

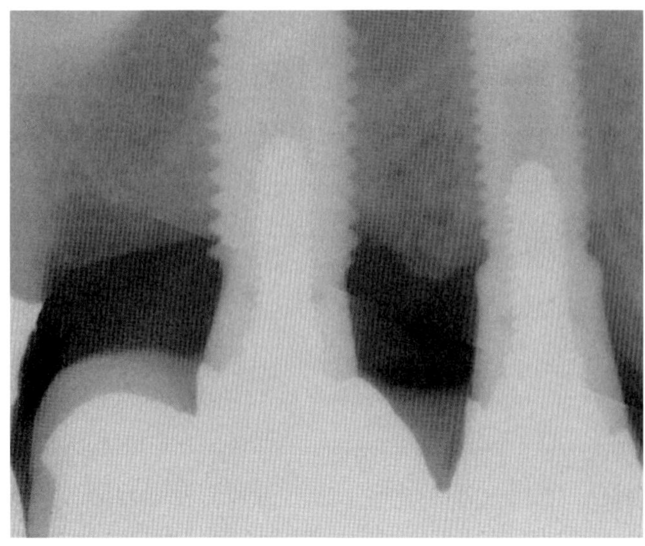

Figure 6.51. Periapical radiograph that was taken at the one-year post insertion recall appointment demonstrated bone levels consistent with the initial pre-operative radiograph.

TABLE 6.8. Lab Fees, Component Costs, Overhead, Fees, and Profits

	Fixed		
Chair Time	**Overhead**	**Laboratory Expenses**	
		Casts	$60
Impression		Articulation	$50
		3 unit FPD	$900
1 hour	**$350/hr = $350**	**Sub Total**	**$1,010**
		Implant Components	
		Healing abutments	$120
		Impression Copings	$90
		Analogs	$42
		Encode Abutments	$500
		Lab screws	$ 25
		Abutment Screws	$110
		Encode Cast	$ 50
		Sub Total	**$937**
Bisque Bake Try-In			
1 hour	$350/hr 5 $350		
Abutment and FPD Insertion			
1 hour	$350/hr 5 $350		
TOTALS	**$1,050**		**$1,947**
Professional Fee			**$5,000**
Costs (fixed overhead and laboratory expenses)			**$2,997**
Profit (fees less costs)			**$2,003**
Profit per hour ($2,003/3 hr)			**$ 667**

Healing abutments, impression copings, and lab screws may be used multiple times, therefore costs will be decreased for each succeeding case and profits will be increased. Analogs should not be re-used.

tions. He again reported that there were no problems and was quite pleased with the results of treatment. Clinically, the prosthesis was evaluated for marginal discrepancies between retainers and their respective abutments, soft tissue marginal adaptation, and occlusal relationships in centric and eccentric excursions.

A periapical radiograph was taken to assess the relationship between the interproximal heights of bone and the implant/abutment interfaces (Figure 6.51). There was no additional bone loss when the initial radiographs were compared to the one-year recall radiographs.

Costs/Fees/Profitability

The following discussion (Table 6.8) relative to fees is reflective of 2006 in the Midwestern United States. The costs of the implant components are retail prices from Implant Innovations, Inc., Palm Beach Gardens, Florida.

Surgeon: Ken Kempf, DDS, Iowa City, Iowa

Dental Laboratory Technicians: Tom Peterson, MDT, CDT, Northshore Dental Laboratories, Lynn, Massachusetts; Andrew Gingrasso, Gundersen Lutheran Medical Center, LaCrosse, Wisconsin

BIBLIOGRAPHY

Asavant, S, Jameson, L, Hesby, B, 1988. Single osseointegrated prostheses. *Int J Prosthodont* 1:291–296.

Adell, R, Lekholm, U, Rockler, B, Brånemark, P-I, 1981. A 15-year study of osseointegrated implants in the treatment of the edentulous jaw. *Int J Oral Surg* 10:387–416.

Attard, N, Zarb, G, 2002. Implant prosthodontic management of posterior partial edentulism: long-term follow-up of a prospective study. *J Can Dent Assoc* 68:118–124.

Beaty, K, 1994. The role of screws in implant systems. *Int J Oral Maxillofac Implants* 9(Special Suppl):52–54.

Binon, P, 1995. Evaluation of machining accuracy and consistency of selected implants, standard abutments and laboratory analogs. *Int J Prosthodont* 8:162–178.

Drago, C, 2005. An overview of CAD/CAM restorations: 2 clinical/laboratory protocols. Submitted to *J Am Dent Assoc*, November 2005.

Hemmings, K, Schmitt, A, Zarb, G, 1994. Complications and maintenance requirements for fixed prostheses and overdentures in the edentulous mandible: a 5-year report. *Int J Oral Maxillofac Implants* 9:191–196.

Jemt, T, 1986. Modified single and short span restorations supported by osseointegrated fixtures in the partially edentulous jaw. *J Prosthet Dent* 55:243–247.

Kallus, T, Bessing, C, 1994. Loose gold screws frequently occur in full-arch fixed prostheses supported by osseointegrated implants after 5 years. *Int J Oral Maxillofac Implants* 9:169–178.

McGarry, T, Nimmo, A, Skiba, J, Ahlstrom, R, Smith, C, Koumjian, J, Arbree, N, 2002. Classification system for partial edentulism. *J Prosthodont* 11:181–193.

Mollersten, L, Lockowandt, P, Linden, L, 1997. Comparison of strength and failure mode of seven implant systems: an in vitro test. *J Prosthet Dent* 78:582–591.

Niznick, G, 1983. The Core-Vent™ implant system. The evolution of the osseointegrated implant. *Oral Health* 73:13–17.

Niznick, G, 1991. The implant abutment connection: the key to prosthetic success. *Compend Cont Educ Dent* 12:932–937.

Norton, M, 2000. In vitro evaluation of the strength of the conical implant to abutment joint in two commercially available implant systems. *J Prosthet Dent* 83:567–571.

Perriard, J, Wisckott, W, Mellal, A, 2002. Fatigue resistance of ITI implant-abutment connectors—a comparison of the standard cone with a novel internally keyed design. *Clin Oral Impl Res* 13:542–549.

Rodkey, E, 1977. Making fastened joints reliable. . .ways to keep'em tight. *Assembly Eng* 3:24–27.

Sakaguchi, R, Borgersen, S, 1995. Nonlinear contact analysis of preload in dental implant screws. *Int J Oral Maxillofac Implants* 10:295–302.

Sutter, F, Weber, H, Sorenson, J, Belser, U, 1993. The new restorative concept of the ITI dental implant system: design and engineering. *Int J Periodont Rest Dent* 13:409–431.

Zarb, G, Schmitt, A, 1990. The longitudinal clinical effectiveness of osseointegrated dental implants: the Toronto study. Part III: Problems and complications encountered. *J Prosthet Dent* 64:185–194.

Chapter 7: Treatment of an Edentulous Mandible with a CAD/CAM Titanium Framework/Fixed Hybrid Prosthesis

Multiple prosthetic options exist for rehabilitation of edentulous mandibles: conventional complete dentures; implant-retained/supported overdentures; and fixed implant-retained full arch prostheses. These treatments all have benefits and limitations associated with them: cost, complexity, length of treatment, prognosis, function, and aesthetics (Morin and others 1998; Allen and others 1999; Adell and others 1981; Wright and others 2002).

Patients treated with complete dentures often express dissatisfaction with function, aesthetics, and phonetics (Carlsson and others 1967; Awaad and Feine 1998). In these situations, dental implants may provide significant improvements in terms of increased retention, stability, comfort, and decreased bone resorption (Melas and others 2001; Awad and others 2003; Lindquist and others 1988).

Prosthetic/implant treatment options should be carefully evaluated early in the planning process because the options will have different requirements relative to anatomical constraints, surgical morbidity, patient expectations, patient function, and costs (Zitzmann and Marinello 2002; DeBoer 1993; Feine and others 1998). The fixed mandibular implant-retained prosthesis supported by commercially pure titanium implants represents one of the earliest, most predictable treatments on a long-term basis, for edentulous patients (Adell and others 1981). This implant treatment protocol took advantage of large amounts of residual bone in edentulous mandibles (anterior, between the mental foraminae) and avoided areas that exhibited more resorption (posterior) (Figures 7.1 and 7.2). Some of the posterior teeth were replaced on cantilevered segments.

Numerous studies have demonstrated excellent long-term results for edentulous patients treated with dental implants per the Brånemark protocol (Albrektsson and others 1986; Lindquist and others 1996). Age does not seem to be an absolute contra indication for dental implants. In a retrospective study, Engfors and others (2004) studied 133 edentulous patients who were 80 or more years of age and who were consecutively treated with fixed implant-retained prostheses. Seven hundred and sixty-one Brånemark type implants were placed in 139 edentulous jaws. The five-year Cumulative Survival Rate (CSR) for the above group for both jaws was 93%. A control group of patients younger than 80 years of age was 92.6%. The corresponding CSRs

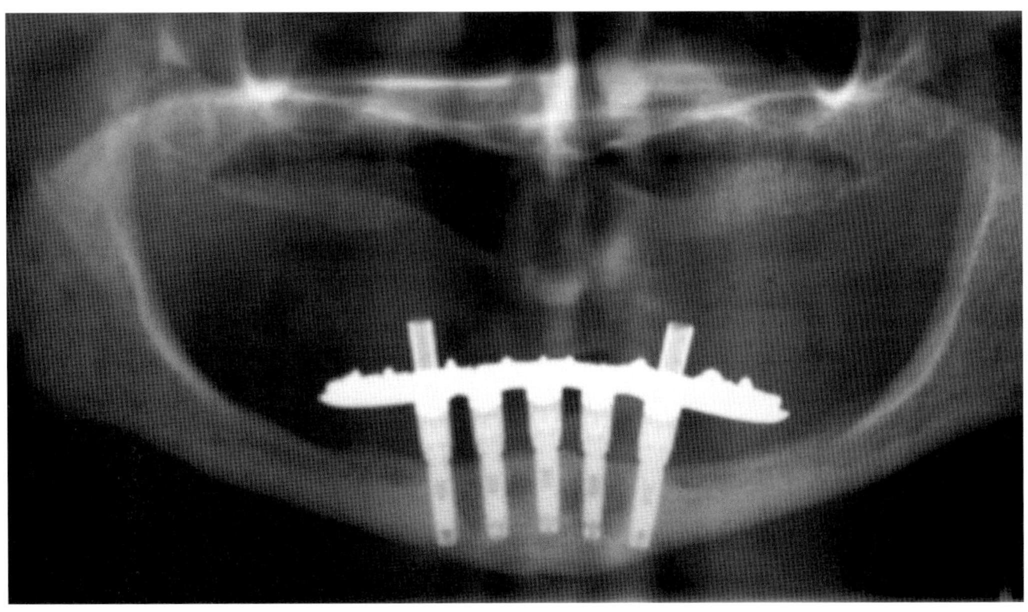

Figure 7.1. Radiograph of an edentulous mandible with five implants between the mental foraminae. Some of the posterior teeth have been replaced on the cantilevered segments of the prosthesis.

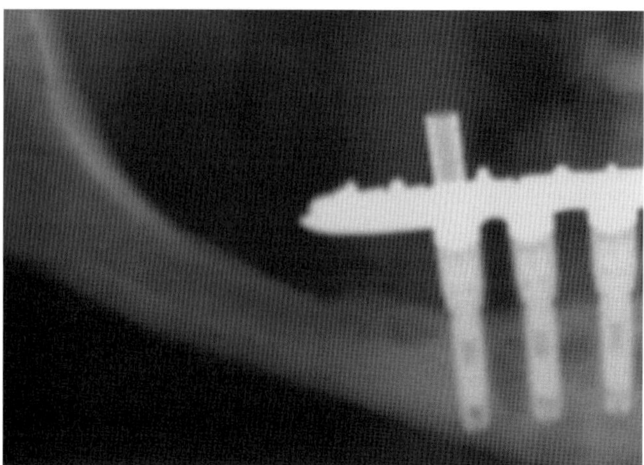

Figure 7.2. Close-up view of the right posterior segment in Figure 7.1. Note that the amount of bone resorption in the posterior mandibular segment and the proximity of the inferior alveolar canal to the crest of the alveolar ridge precluded placement of implants posterior to the mental foramen.

for the mandibular implants were 99.5% and 99.7%, respectively. The most common complications in the preceding 80-year-old group were soft tissue inflammation (mucositis) and cheek/lip biting. Veneer fractures of the denture teeth from the prostheses were the most common complaint of the younger-than-80 group. Engfors and others concluded that results of implant treatment in patients over 80 years of age were not significantly different from those of younger patients. However, there were more post-insertion complications and adjustment visits in the 80+-year-old group of patients.

With the development of osseointegration and the limited amount of motion inherent between an osseointegrated implant and the surrounding bone, accurate, passively fitting implant frameworks have been one of the goals in implant treatment (Brånemark and others 1977). An osseosintegrated implant has micro motion within the bone of approximately 10 μm; a natural tooth may move up to 100 μm (Assif and others 1996). This lack of flexibility between the bone/implant interface means that any forces induced into the system via an ill-fitting framework will almost certainly remain in the system and may result in biomechanical issues such as screw loosening and/or screw fracture.

Multiple authors have examined impressions and master cast accuracy in implant treatment (Carr 1991; Hsu and others 1993; Herbst and others 2000). Kari and others (2004) performed a laboratory study to determine the degree of passive fit in cement and screw-retained frameworks. They concluded that an absolute passive fit of implant superstructures is not possible using conventional clinical and laboratory procedures. They proposed that reference strain values from implant-retained prostheses that have functioned without apparent complications could help define a "biologically acceptable fit."

Titanium frameworks have been used as alternatives to gold castings for implant frameworks for more than 15 years. (Ortorp and Jemt 2004). Titanium is less expensive than noble alloys, is well tolerated in biologic environments, and has been shown to develop mucosal attachments, whereas gold alloys do not (Abrahamsson and others 1998). Computer numeric controlled (CNC) milling procedures with titanium alloys may allow better control of distortions inherent within the waxing/casting/finishing processes associated with conventional casting technology. Ortorp and Jemt (2004) reported on the results of a prospective clinical study with 129 edentulous patients who were treated with 67 CNC frameworks and 62 frameworks made with gold alloys and conventional casting techniques. Clinical and radiographic data were obtained over a five-year period.

They reported that problems were low in both groups (34% of the CNC group and 26% of the control group reported no problems during the study). The CSRs were 94.9% and 98.3% for implants and titanium prostheses, respectively. The respective corresponding CSRs for the control group were 97.9% and 98.2%. Metal fractures were seen only in the control group (casting). Mean marginal bone loss was 0.5 mm in both groups. They concluded that CNC titanium frameworks were a viable alternative to gold alloy castings in edentulous jaws. However, the degree of fit between implant abutments and frameworks was not quantitatively measured.

The following clinical case report demonstrates the treatment of an edentulous patient with implants and fixed implant-retained prostheses in both jaws. The edentulous maxillae were treated with CAD/CAM abutments and cement-retained fixed partial dentures. The edentulous mandible was treated with implants and a screw-retained fixed prosthesis. The mandibular framework was made using CAD/CAM technology (CAM StructSURE™ Precision Milled Bar, Implant Innovations, Inc.®, Palm Beach Gardens, FL). The maxillary abutments/prostheses are not illustrated.

CLINICAL CASE PRESENTATION

Appointment 1. Initial examination (3/4 Hour)

A 43-year-old female patient presented to the author with a chief complaint: "My dentures don't fit and I want implants."

History of the Present Illness

This patient had had her teeth extracted approximately 12 months prior to this visit. They were replaced with immedi-

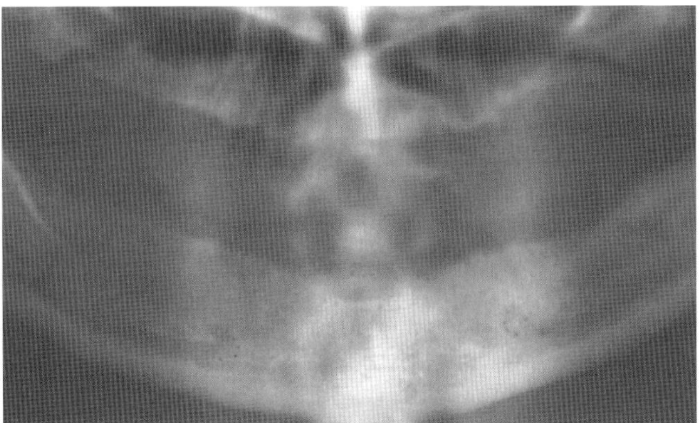

Figure 7.3. Panoramic radiograph 12 months post extraction of the natural teeth.

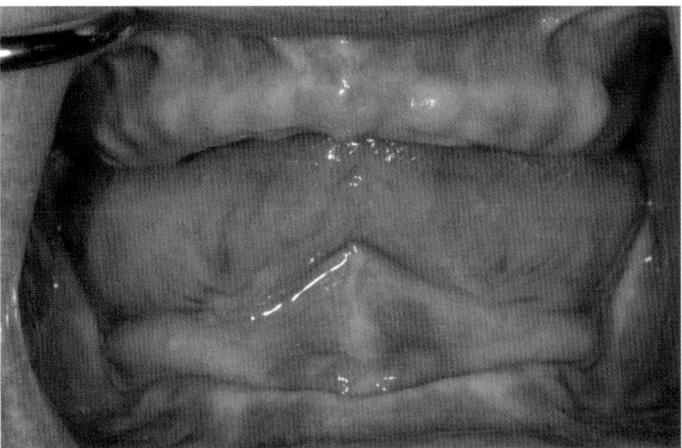

Figure 7.4. Intra-oral view of edentulous jaws.

ate dentures. The dentures were relined with tissue-conditioning material at appropriate time intervals and were processed with laboratory relines six months after the natural teeth were extracted. The patient reported that she liked the appearance of the dentures relative to lip support, incisal displays at rest, speaking and smiling, and phonetically. She felt that she could not eat with the dentures in place. She was not happy with her masticatory function.

Radiographic Examination

The initial panoramic radiograph demonstrated adequate bone volume for implant placement in the anterior segments of the jaws. There was inadequate bone volume in the posterior maxillae. There was no pathology present (Figure 7.3).

Physical Examination

The physical examination revealed moderate vertical and facial/lingual bone resorption, mild generalized mucositis, and adequate restorative volume for prosthetic replacement of the teeth (Figure 7.4). Neither jaw demonstrated significant anterior/posterior resorption (Figure 7.5).

Diagnosis

The following diagnoses were established at the end of the first visit:

1. Edentulous maxillae with mild resorption anteriorly, moderate/significant resorption posteriorly
2. Edentulous mandible with mild resorption
3. Well-fitting dentures with appropriate vertical dimension of occlusion, aesthetics, and lip support
4. Mild mucositis secondary to tobacco abuse
5. Mild xerostomia

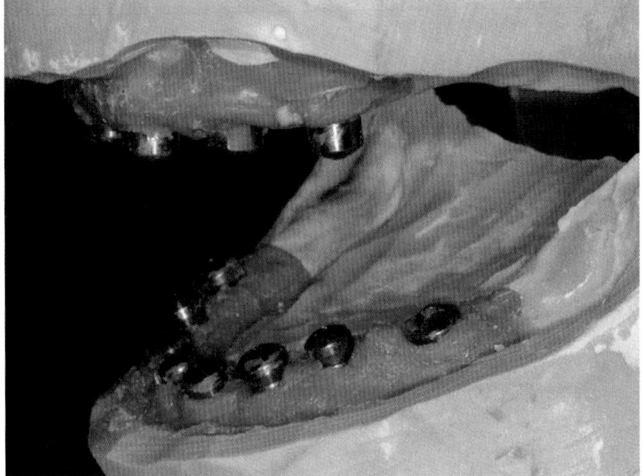

Figure 7.5. Laboratory articulator mounting of the master casts that demonstrated minimal anterior/posterior resorption of both edentulous jaws.

6. Inability to manage complete dentures
7. Class II (Moderately Compromised) Classification System for Edentulous Patients, American College of Prosthodontists (McGarry and others 2002)

Appointment 2. Consultation Restorative Dentist/Patient (1/2 Hour)

A definitive consultation appointment was scheduled as the patient left the office from the first visit. The time between the first and second appointments allowed for development of the treatment options for this particular patient.

Treatment Options

The first treatment option included an oral surgical consultation in order to assess the viability of multiple implant placements in both jaws that would support fixed implant-retained prostheses (Table 7.1). It was assumed that if bone grafting was needed, it could be accomplished to support the requisite number of implants in both jaws. New dentures were not required because the preexisting dentures were clinically acceptable in terms of stability, lip support, centric jaw relationships, aesthetics, and phonetics.

A second treatment plan was developed that incorporated implants in the anterior mandible for an implant-retained overdenture. The edentulous maxillae would be treated with a complete denture, with the potential for implants in the future (Table 7.2). It was assumed that if bone grafting was needed, it could be accomplished to support the requisite number of implants in both jaws. New dentures were

TABLE 7.1. Treatment Plan #1. (Maxillary/Mandibular Bone Grafting/Fixed Implant Prostheses)

Diagnosis:

1. Edentulous maxillae with mild resorption anteriorly, moderate/significant resorption posteriorly
2. Edentulous mandible with mild resorption
3. Well-fitting dentures with appropriate vertical dimension of occlusion, aesthetics and lip support
4. Mild mucositis secondary to tobacco abuse
5. Mild xerostomia
6. Inability to manage complete dentures

Prosthetic Services	**ADA #**	**Fee**
Comprehensive oral evaluation	D0150	
Diagnostic casts	D0470	
Panoramic radiograph	D0330	
Surgical guides	D6190	

Referral to oral surgical office:

1. Evaluate and treat for placement of 6-8 OSSEOTITE® implants (4.1 mm diameter) in the maxillae for fixed implant-retained prosthesis. Implants should be placed directly behind the teeth in the surgical guide. Embrasure placement will compromise the prosthetic results.
2. Evaluate and treat for placement of 4–6 implants in the edentulous mandible for fixed implant-retained prosthesis. Implants may be placed according to the edentulous protocol; embrasure placement would be permissible.
3. Bone grafting as needed to obtain the above results.
4. Single-stage surgical protocol, if possible.
5. Healing abutments should have the following profiles:
   - **a.** Mandible: 4.1 mm restorative platforms, 5 mm emergence profiles.
   - **b.** Maxillae: 5 mm restorative platforms, 6 mm emergence profiles for the first molars, cuspids, and central incisors; 4.1 mm restorative platforms, 5 mm emergence profiles for premolars and lateral incisors. Occlusal surfaces should be 1 mm supra-gingival.
6. Post-operative instructions.
7. Schedule a denture tissue-conditioning appointment 10 days post implant surgery.
8. Discharge to prosthodontist for prosthetic care.

Fees and services will be determined by the oral surgeon.

	ADA #	**Fees**
Healing/osseointegration		
Tissue conditioning of preexisting dentures, per time	D5851	
	D5850	
Prosthodontic re-evaluation	D0140	
Diagnostic casts	D0470	
Maxillary Prosthesis		
Custom abutments (7)	D6057	
Fixed Partial Dentures	D6059, D6240	
Maxillary right		
Maxillary anterior		
Maxillary left		

TABLE 7.1. Treatment Plan #1. (Maxillary/Mandibular Bone Grafting/Fixed Implant Prostheses) (*continued*)

Mandibular Screw-Retained Hybrid Prosthesis (CAD/CAM framework)	D6078
Yearly recall appointment	D0120
Periapical radiographs	D0220

Benefits of Treatment Plan #1

With osseointegration of all of the implants, both prostheses will be fixed and not removable by the patient. The patient should enjoy improved function. The occlusion (bite) will be made optimal; facial aesthetics should be maintained, consistent with the patient's desires. The patient should enjoy a good, long-term prognosis. Long-term bone loss will be minimized in both jaws.

Limitations of Treatment Plan #1

Cost, complexity, and length of treatment (9–15 months, depending on bone grafting). Implants are generally successful in the edentulous jaws approximately 96–99% of the time. The implants have to be placed optimally for the above treatments to be accomplished. If the implants cannot be placed optimally, changes in the treatments (surgical and prosthetic), fees, and designs will be likely. Neither prosthesis will be removable by the patient. In certain situations, one or both prostheses may need to be removed at any of the follow-up visits. The patient needs to return to this office at least once per year for follow-up, which will include radiographs (x-rays) to assess osseointegration of the implants, fit and occlusion of the prostheses, health of the soft tissues, and the integrity of the implant/abutment connections. This treatment plan itemizes only the prosthetic phase of treatment.

Patient signature ______________________

Date ______________________

Witness ______________________

Date ______________________

ADA #'s, CDT 2005 Current Dental Terminology, Council on Dental Benefit Programs, American Dental Association, 211 East Chicago Avenue, Chicago, IL 60611

not required because the preexisting dentures were clinically acceptable in terms of stability, lip support, centric jaw relationships, aesthetics, and phonetics.

A third treatment option was presented that did not include any definitive prosthetic treatment (Table 7.3).

Appointment 3. Consultation Restorative Dentist/Surgeon (1 Hour)

Prosthesis Design

This appointment generally takes place before or after normal business hours and should precede the surgeon's examination appointment. It may occur at lunch, at either practitioner's office, or at another convenient location. This consultation is critical for the long-term functional and aesthetic success of implant treatment. It is essential that the restorative dentist explain to the surgeon the physical and radiographic findings, the diagnosis, and the treatment options that were explained to the patient, as well as the treatment option that the patient has tentatively selected. This particular treatment option was technically demanding and the consultation between restorative dentist and the surgeon required approximately one hour.

Type/Number/Size of Implants

In this case, the patient was edentulous in both jaws and had not adapted to either denture. Because this case would involve multiple, splinted implants, the author felt comfortable with using external hex implants in both jaws. Unfortunately, there was some miscommunication and the surgeon placed 4.1 mm diameter implants in all maxillary and mandibular implant sites, instead of placing 5 mm diameter implants in the maxillary central incisor, cuspid, and first molar sites. The surgeon determined the shape of the implant body and preselected tapered implants.

Abutment/Prosthesis Design

This case presentation concentrates on the mandibular prosthesis (CAD/CAM). The maxillary restorations are mentioned only briefly.

TABLE 7.2. Treatment Plan #2. (Two Implants Anterior Mandible, Mandibular Implant-Retained Overdenture, Maxillary Complete Denture)

Diagnosis:

1. Edentulous maxillae with mild resorption anteriorly, moderate/significant resorption posteriorly
2. Edentulous mandible with mild resorption
3. Well fitting dentures with appropriate vertical dimension of occlusion, aesthetics and lip support
4. Mild mucositis secondary to tobacco abuse
5. Mild xerostomia
6. Inability to manage complete dentures

Prosthetic Services	**ADA #**	**Fee**
Comprehensive oral evaluation	D0150	
Diagnostic casts	D0470	
Panoramic radiograph	D0330	
Surgical guide	D6190	

Referral to oral surgical office:

1. Evaluate and treat for placement of two OSSEOTITE® implants in the edentulous mandible for an implant-retained overdenture (resilient attachments). Implants should be placed per the locations identified in the surgical guide.
2. Bone grafting as needed to obtain the above results.
3. Single-stage surgical protocol, if possible
4. Healing abutments should have the following profiles:
   a. Mandible: 4.1 mm restorative platforms, 5 mm emergence profiles
5. Post-operative instructions.
6. Schedule a denture tissue-conditioning appointment 10 days post implant surgery.

Discharge to prosthodontist for prosthetic care.

Fees and services will be determined by the oral surgeon.

	ADA #	**Fees**
Healing/osseointegration		
Tissue conditioning of preexisting mandibular denture, per time	D5851	
Prosthodontic reevaluation	D0140	
Placement of LOCATOR® Abutments	D6199	
Laboratory processed reline of preexisting mandibular denture	D5751	
Yearly recall appointment	D0120	
Periapical radiographs	D0220	

Benefits of Treatment Plan #2

With osseointegration of the implants, the lower denture should have significantly more retention and stability, which should improve the patient's function. The denture occlusion (bite) will be improved; facial aesthetics should be maintained to be consistent with the patient's desires. The patient should enjoy a good, long-term prognosis. Bone loss will be minimized in the front part of the lower jaw.

Limitations of Treatment Plan #2

Cost, complexity and length of treatment (3–6 months). Implants are generally successful in the front part of the lower jaw approximately 96–99% of the time. The implants have to be placed optimally for the above treatments to be accomplished. If the implants cannot be placed optimally, changes in the treatments (surgical and prosthetic), fees, and designs will be likely. Both dentures will move, the upper denture more so than the lower denture. Bone loss will continue in the upper jaw without implants. If the denture/implant experience is unsatisfactory, additional

TABLE 7.2. Treatment Plan #2. (Two Implants Anterior Mandible, Mandibular Implant-Retained Overdenture, Maxillary Complete Denture) (*continued*)

implants may be placed in one or both jaws, at additional cost. The patient will be asked to take the dentures out during nighttime sleep. The patient needs to return to this office at least once per year for follow-up, which will include radiographs (x-rays) to assess osseointegration of the implants, fit and occlusion of the dentures, health of the soft tissues, and the integrity of the implant/abutment connections. This treatment plan itemizes only the prosthetic phase of treatment.

Patient signature ______________________
Date ______________________
Witness ______________________
Date ______________________

ADA #'s, CDT 2005 Current Dental Terminology, Council on Dental Benefit Programs, American Dental Association, 211 East Chicago Avenue, Chicago, IL 60611

TABLE 7.3. Treatment Plan #3. No Definitive Prosthetic Treatment

Diagnosis:

1. Edentulous maxillae with mild resorption anteriorly, moderate/significant resorption posteriorly
2. Edentulous mandible with mild resorption
3. Well-fitting dentures with appropriate vertical dimension of occlusion, aesthetics, and lip support
4. Mild mucositis secondary to tobacco abuse
5. Mild xerostomia
6. Inability to manage complete dentures

Prosthetic Services	**ADA #**	**Fee**
Comprehensive oral evaluation	D0150	
Diagnostic casts	D0470	
Panoramic radiograph	D0330	
Yearly recall	D0120	
Panoramic radiograph	D0220	

Benefits of Treatment Plan #3

The patient will undergo no additional treatments and no further expenses except what is noted above on a yearly basis.

Limitations of Treatment Plan #3

Both dentures will continue to move. The patient likely will continue to experience recurring soreness. Her ability to chew certain types of food will be limited. She will be asked to take both dentures out during nighttime sleep. Bone loss will continue in both jaws without implants. If the denture experience continues to deteriorate, implants may be considered in one or both jaws for improved retention and stability of the dentures. The patient needs to return to this office at least once per year for follow-up, which will include radiographs (x-rays), fit and occlusion of the dentures, and the health of the soft tissues. This treatment plan itemizes only the prosthetic phase of treatment.

Patient signature ______________________
Date ______________________
Witness ______________________
Date ______________________

ADA #'s, CDT 2005 Current Dental Terminology, Council on Dental Benefit Programs, American Dental Association, 211 East Chicago Avenue, Chicago, IL 60611

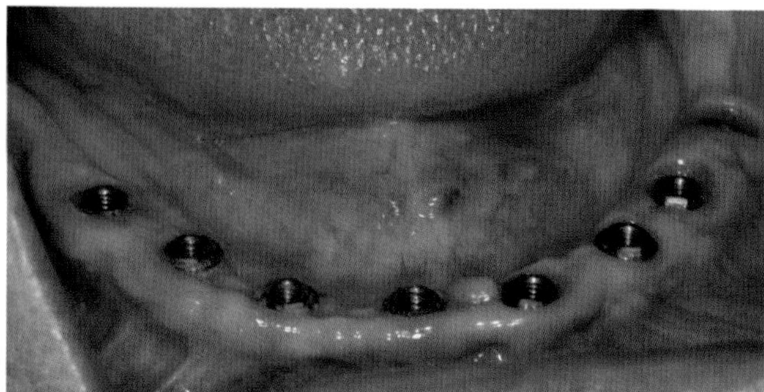

Figure 7.6. Clinical facial/occlusal view of mandibular implant restorative platforms.

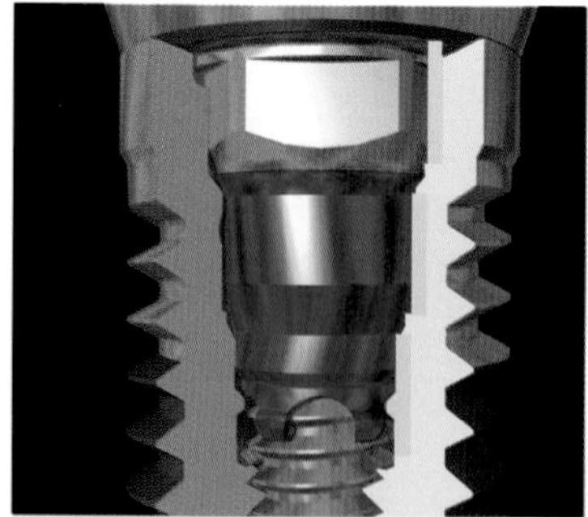

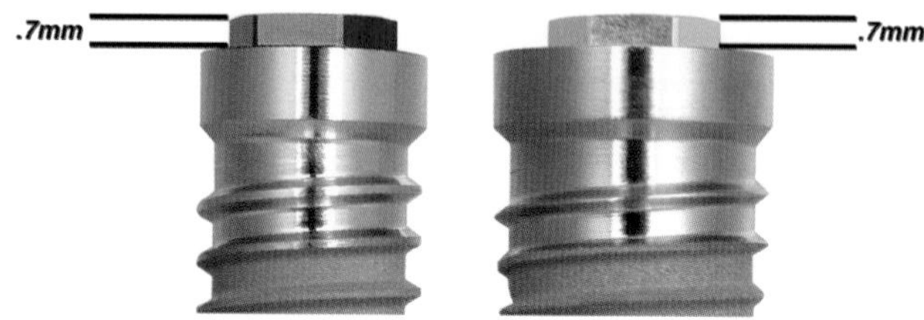

Figure 7.7. Cross sections of the OSSEOTITE® Certain® internal connection (top) and OSSEOTITE® external hex implant connections (bottom, 4.1 mm restorative platform left; 5 mm restorative platform right).

Because there was minimal anterior/posterior resorption, the edentulous maxillae were to be treated with CAD/CAM abutments and three fixed partial dentures. The tooth positions would be determined by the tooth positions within the preexisting maxillary denture. The fixed partial dentures would be independent from one another and cement-retained. Six to eight maxillary implants would be required for this type of prosthetic treatment.

The edentulous mandible would be treated with 5–8 implants for use with a screw-retained prosthesis. The metal framework was to be fabricated with CAD/CAM technology. The framework was to be fabricated directly onto the implant restorative platforms. Abutments, cylinders, and retaining screws would not be used (Figure 7.6).

Implant/Abutment Connection

The original design called for the ***3i®*** internal connection implant system (OSSEOTITE® Certain®) to be used for the maxillary restorations and the OSSEOTITE® implant system to be used for the mandibular prosthesis (Figure 7.7).

Surgical Protocol

The author requested that a single-stage protocol be used if possible because patients more easily tolerate it than the traditional two-stage protocols. Healing abutments would be placed in a manner consistent with the teeth being replaced in the maxillae; 5 mm healing abutments were to be used in the mandible. The occlusal surfaces of the healing abutments were to be slightly supra-gingival after the soft tissues had healed.

Surgical Guides

Surgical guides were fabricated by duplicating the preexisting maxillary and mandibular dentures (Figure 7.8). Holes in anticipation of optimal implant placement were placed bilaterally in the first molar, first premolar, and lateral incisor areas. This would provide for the largest anterior/posterior spread and would also minimize cantilevered extensions (McAlarney and Stavropoulos 1996).

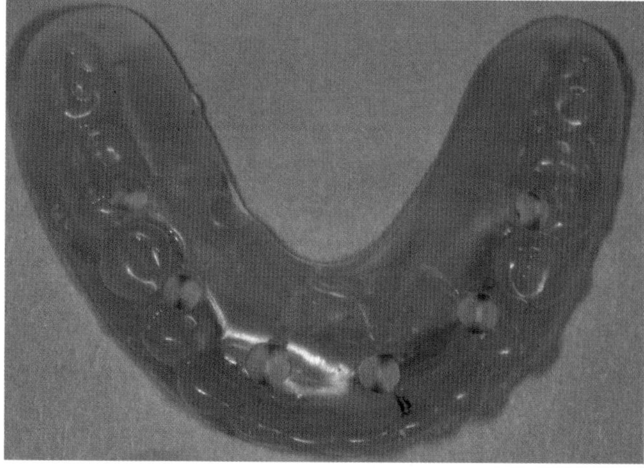

Figure 7.8. Mandibular surgical guide was made as a duplicate of the preexisting denture.

Anticipated Healing Time

The implant surgeon anticipated Type I and Type II bone in the mandibular implant sites. He also anticipated using a single-stage surgical protocol. Therefore, the prosthetic protocol could commence approximately 10 weeks post implant placement (Testori and others 2002).

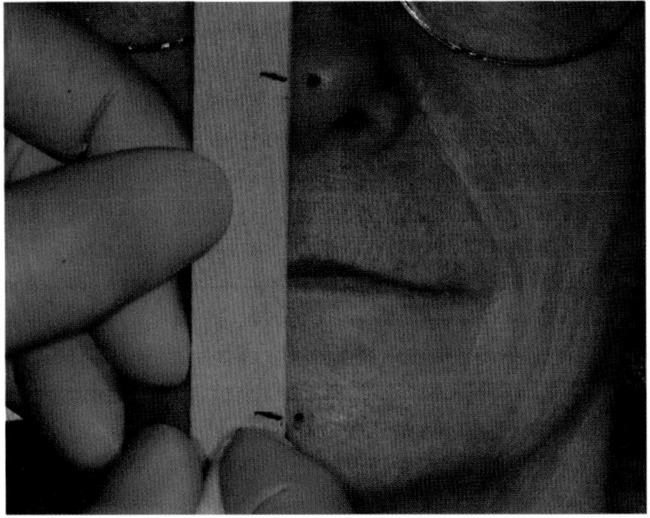

Figure 7.9. The pre-operative vertical dimension of occlusion was identified by placing marks on the patient's nose and chin. This distance was transferred to a tongue blade.

Appointment 4. Implant Placement (2 1/2 Hours)

The vertical dimension of occlusion was marked pre-operatively, with the patient seated upright, by placing a dot on her nose and another dot on her chin. Her head was unsupported and the marks were transferred to a tongue blade (Figure 7.9). This measurement would be used intra-operatively to provide the surgeon with a reference point relative to the amount of bone reduction (if needed) required that would not interfere with the requisite restorative volume needed for the implant restorative components and prosthesis.

This patient was treated with IV sedation and local anesthesia. A full thickness mucoperiosteal flap was reflected from the right second molar to the left second molar. The surgical guide was adjusted as needed to fit onto the edentulous mandible without increasing the vertical dimension of occlusion (Figure 7.10).

Eight straight wall implants were placed (OSSEOTITE®, ***3i®***, Palm Beach Gardens, FL). All of the implants had insertional torque values of at least 30 Ncm. The implants were considered to have achieved adequate primary stability and the single stage protocol was implemented. Healing abutments for 4.1 mm implant restorative platforms, 5 mm emergence profiles, and 2 or 4 mm collar heights were placed according to the heights of the peri-implant soft tissues (THA452, THA454) (Figure 7.11). These were hand tightened with a large hex driver (PHD02N).

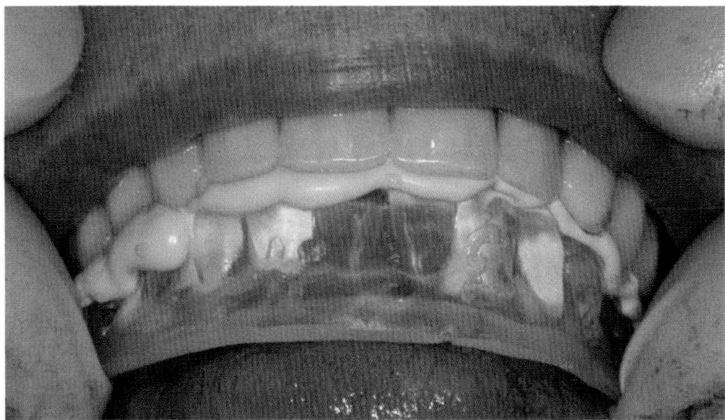

Figure 7.10. Mandibular surgical guide in place, in centric occlusion against the maxillary denture, after reflection of the soft tissues, prior to osteotomy preparation.

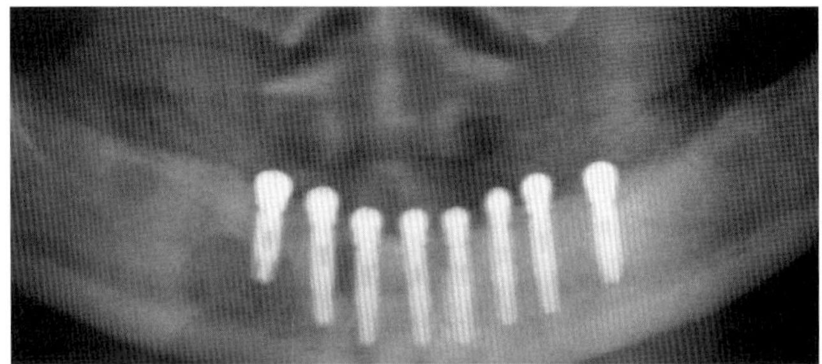

Figure 7.11. Panoramic radiograph immediately post implant placement. Healing abutments were placed at the time of surgery.

The patient was discharged by the surgical office with instructions not to wear the preexisting mandibular denture until the first restorative follow-up appointment in 10 days. She was instructed to maintain a soft diet and perform twice daily rinsing with 0.12% chlorhexidine.

Appointments 5–7. Prosthetic Follow-Up Appointments (3/4 Hour)

Ten Days

The patient reported to the author's office at the appointed time. She reported minimal discomfort and swelling immediately post operatively. She did require narcotic analgesics for the first two days and then was quite comfortable with nonsteroidal anti-inflammatory medications.

The surgical incision was healing nicely (Figure 7.12).

Tissue Conditioning

The preexisting mandibular denture was thoroughly relieved and polished. It was relined with tissue conditioning material (Visgo-gel, Dentsply Inc., York, PA) with the patient

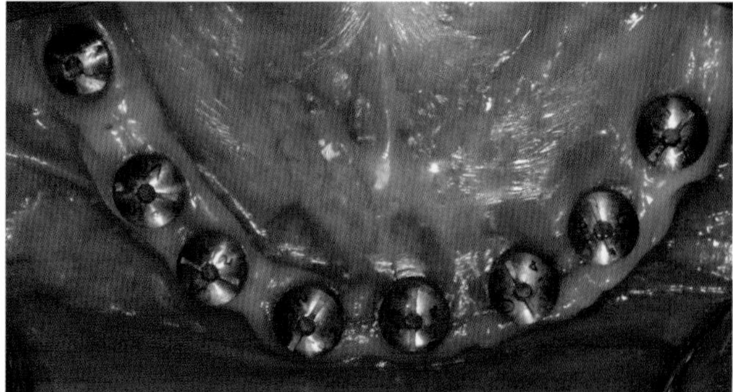

Figure 7.12. Occlusal view of the edentulous mandible with healing abutments in place 10 days post implant placement.

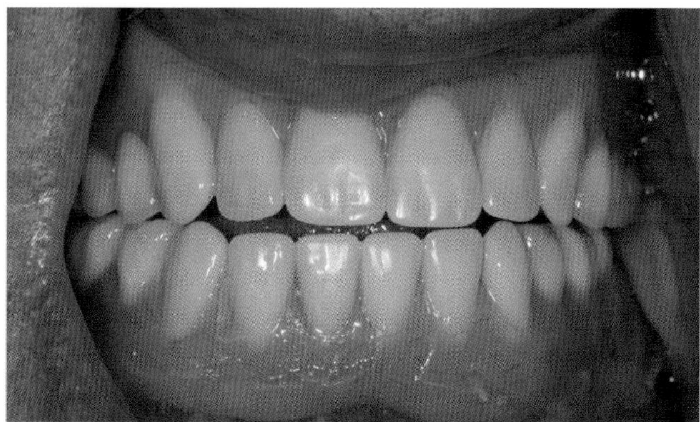

Figure 7.13. Anterior view of patient in centric occlusion as the tissue conditioning material set intra-orally for five minutes.

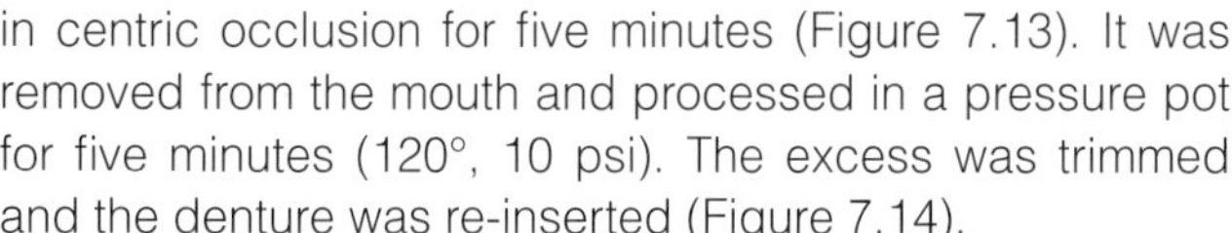

in centric occlusion for five minutes (Figure 7.13). It was removed from the mouth and processed in a pressure pot for five minutes (120°, 10 psi). The excess was trimmed and the denture was re-inserted (Figure 7.14).

The patient was instructed to continue with the soft diet, the chlorhexidine rinses, and oral hygiene in and around the healing abutments with a soft toothbrush and/or cotton swabs (Figure 7.15).

The patient's next scheduled visit was made for four weeks.

Four Weeks (1/2 Hour)

The patient continued to do well. She reported no particular problems relative to discomfort, oral hygiene, diet, and denture function. The healing abutments were highly polished and stable (Figure 7.16). The tissue-conditioning material was satisfactory. Dietary and oral hygiene instructions were reinforced and the patient was discharged to return again in four weeks.

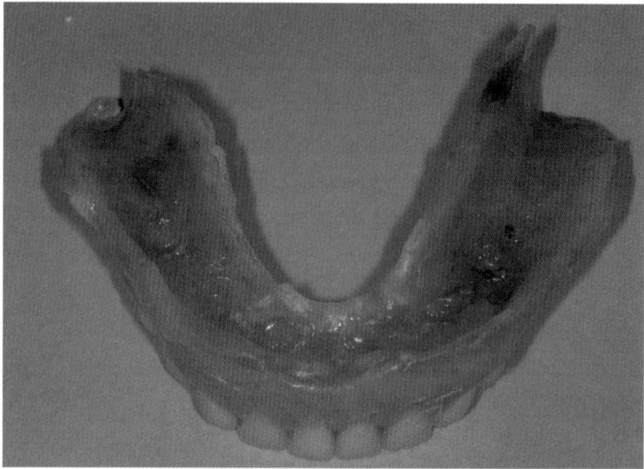

Figure 7.14. Intaglio surface of the mandibular denture after laboratory processing (five minutes, 120° water, 10 psi) of the tissue conditioning material.

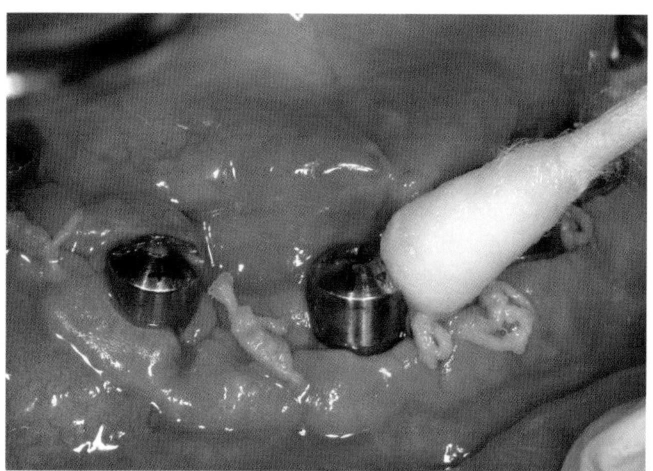

Figure 7.15. Post operative hygiene instructions include discussion and demonstrations of dipping a cotton swab into the chlorhexidine mouth rinse and applying slight pressure in and around the healing abutments to remove plaque and place the medication topically in and around the surgical sites. This photograph was taken 10 days after the implants were uncovered.

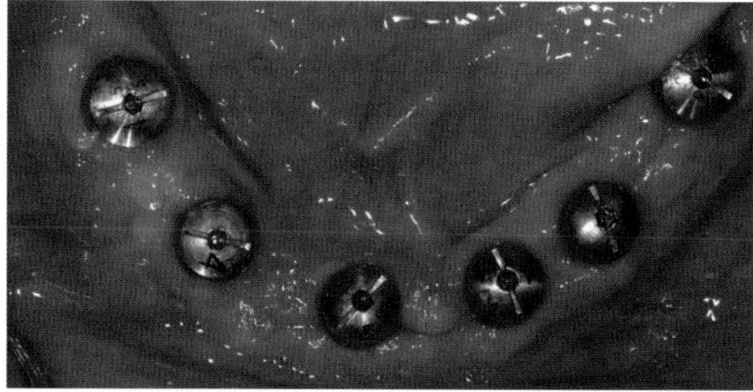

Figure 7.16. Occlusal view of mandibular healing abutments four weeks post implant placement.

Eight Weeks—Tissue Conditioning (¾ Hour)

The patient continued to do well and was anxious to proceed with the prosthetic portion of the treatment plan. She reported no particular problems relative to discomfort, oral hygiene, diet, and denture function. The healing abutments were highly polished and stable. The tissue-conditioning material was no longer satisfactory and was replaced in conventional fashion. The patient was discharged and scheduled to return in two weeks for reevaluation, preliminary impressions, diagnostic casts, and construction of a custom impression tray.

Appointment 8. Reevaluation (1/2 Hour)

The patient continued to do well and had no complaints.

Diagnostic Impressions and Diagnostic Casts

Alginate impressions were made of both edentulous jaws, as well as the preexisting immediate dentures in stock impression trays. The casts were poured in dental stone (Figure 7.17).

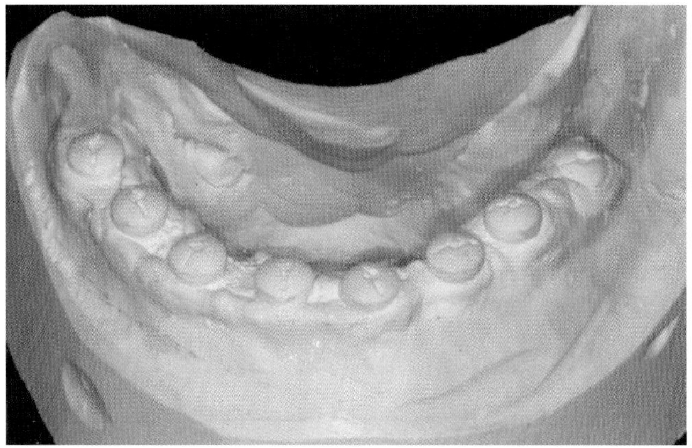

Figure 7.17. Mandibular diagnostic cast made from an alginate impression approximately 10 weeks post implant placement.

Tentative Abutment Selection

The casts identified the locations of the healing abutments, implants, and the locations of the gingival margins. Because all of the healing abutments were 4 mm in height and the occlusal and axial walls of the healing abutments were visible, the decision was made that the framework could be made directly to the implant restorative platforms. With peri-implant sulcular depths greater than 4 mm, implant level impressions are generally more difficult to make. The restorative implant coordinator was instructed to locate eight pick-up implant impression copings for 4.1 mm implant restorative platforms with 5 mm emergence profile diameters prior to the impression appointment (IIC12) (Figure 7.18).

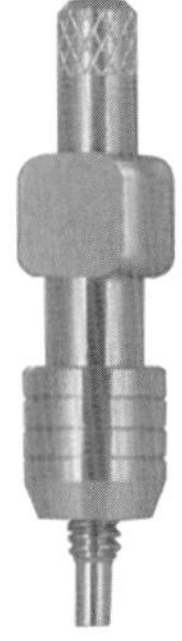

Figure 7.18. Pick-up implant impression coping for 4.1 mm external hex implant restorative platform, with 5 mm emergence profile diameter.

Custom Impression Tray

The author prefers the pick-up type implant level impression protocol. This protocol requires the use of open impression trays. One layer of baseplate wax was placed over the healing abutments on the diagnostic cast and a light cured resin was used to fabricate the tray. (Triad®, Dentsply International, York, PA) A handle was placed on the anterior segment in such a way that it supported the lower lip. After the material had polymerized, the tray was adjusted to provide adequate coverage of the hard and soft tissues lateral to the implants. Windows were placed in the occlusal aspect of the impression tray that would allow access to the pick-up implant impression copings (Figure 7.19).

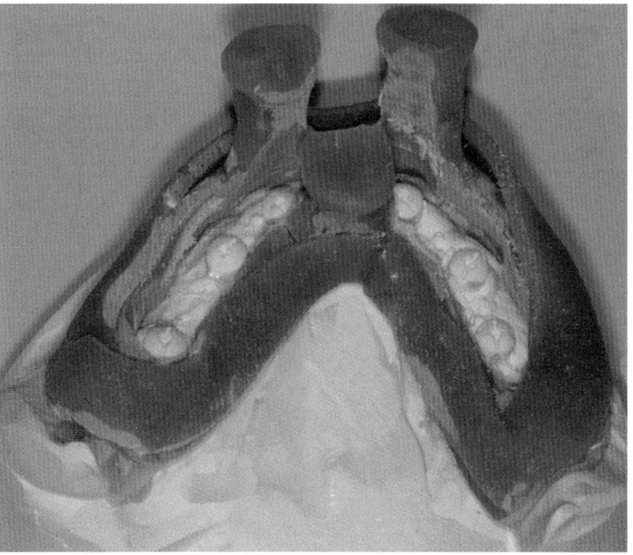

Figure 7.19. Occlusal view of custom open impression tray. The windows were designed to allow access to the pick-up implant impression copings.

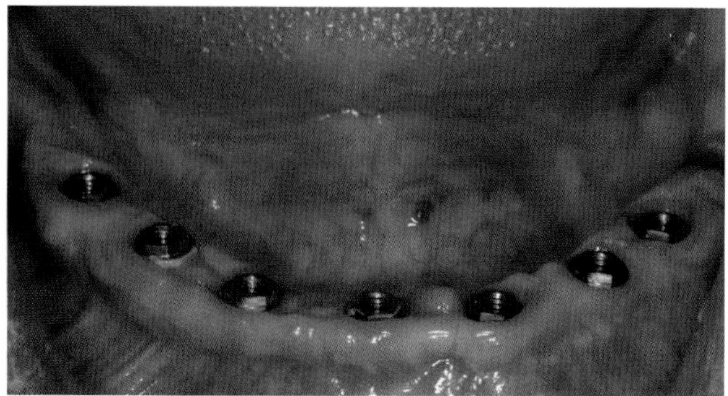

Figure 7.20. Implant restorative platforms after the healing abutments were removed. All of the restorative platforms were completely exposed.

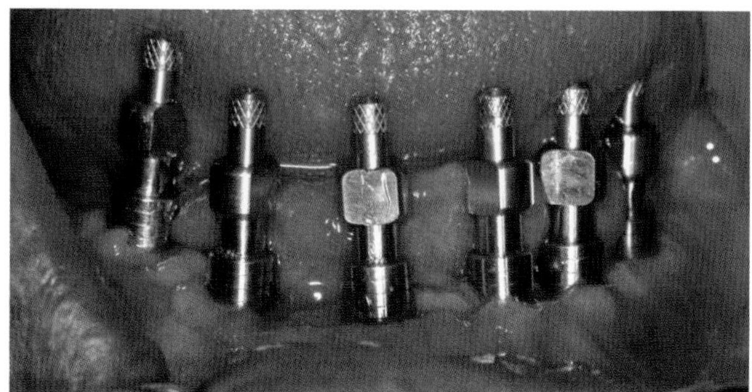

Figure 7.21. Pick-up implant impression copings in place on the mandibular implants.

Appointment 9. Implant Level Impression (One Hour)

The patient again reported no difficulties and was ready to proceed.

Clinical Procedures

The healing abutments were removed with the large hex posterior hex driver (PHD02). The soft tissues had healed consistent with the shape of the healing abutments (Figure 7.20).

The implant impression copings were placed onto the external hexes of the implants. The impression coping screws were hand tightened with the large hex posterior hex driver (PHD02) (Figure 7.21).

The custom impression tray was adjusted to fit without interference from any of the impression copings (Figure 7.22).

Adhesive, specific to the vinyl polysiloxane impression material (Splash!, Discus Dental, Culver City, CA) was applied to the intaglio surface of the impression tray and allowed to dry.

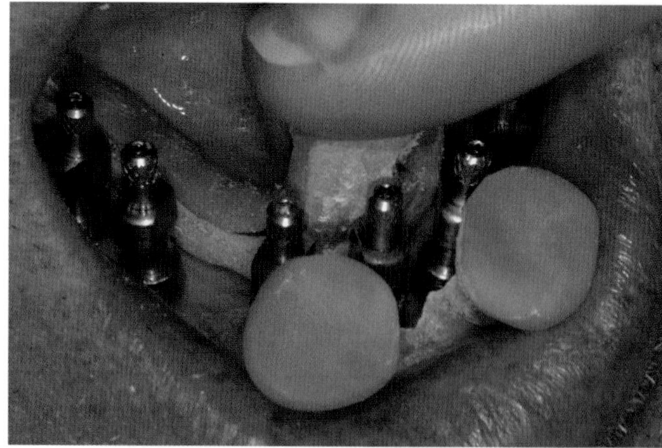

Figure 7.22. The custom impression tray was adjusted to fit around the impression copings.

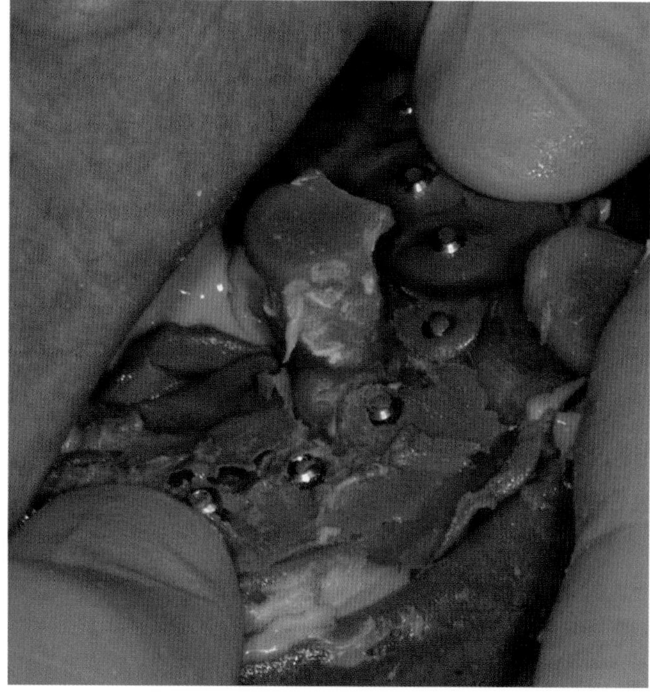

Figure 7.23. Intra-oral occlusal view of the mandibular impression tray in place. Note that the impression coping screws were visible within the windows of the impression tray.

One dental assistant mixed the putty portion of the impression material and loaded it into the impression tray. A second dental assistant retracted and suctioned intra-orally while the author injected the injection type vinyl polysiloxane impression material around the impression copings. The impression tray was then seated, excess impression material was removed from the windows in the tray, and all of the impression coping screws were exposed (Figure 7.23).

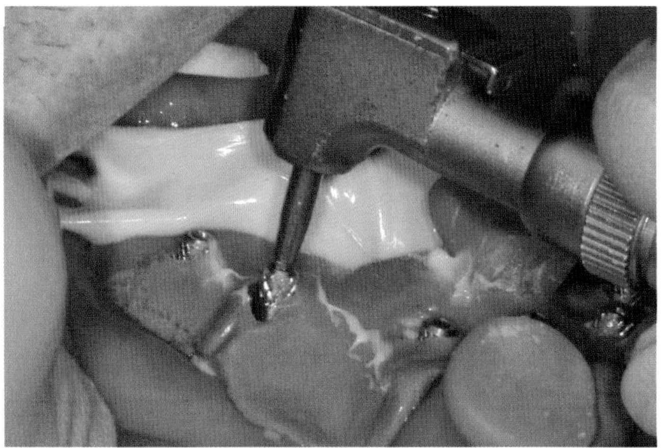

Figure 7.24. The Contra Angle Torque Driver (CATDB) with a large hex driver tip, long (RASH8N) was used to unscrew the impression coping screws.

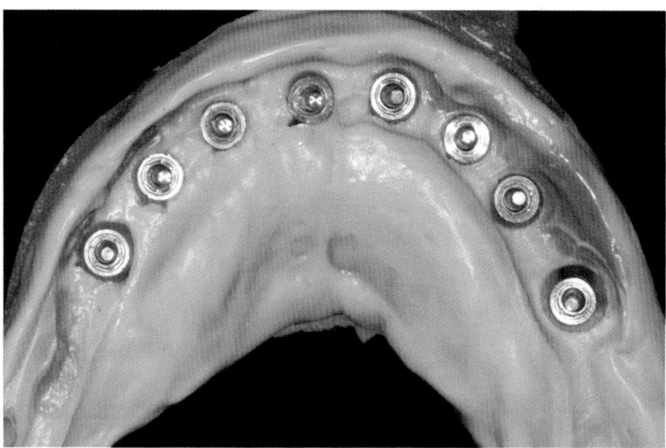

Figure 7.26. The intaglio surface of the mandibular implant impression. All of the impression copings were "picked up" within the impression.

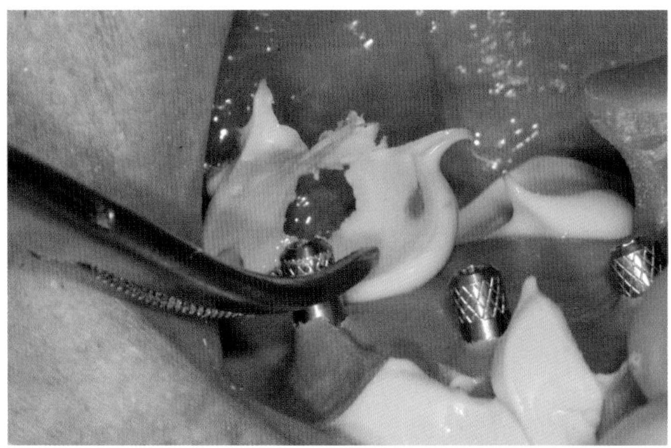

Figure 7.25. A hemostat was used to ensure that the impression coping screws were completely free of the implants before removing the impression tray.

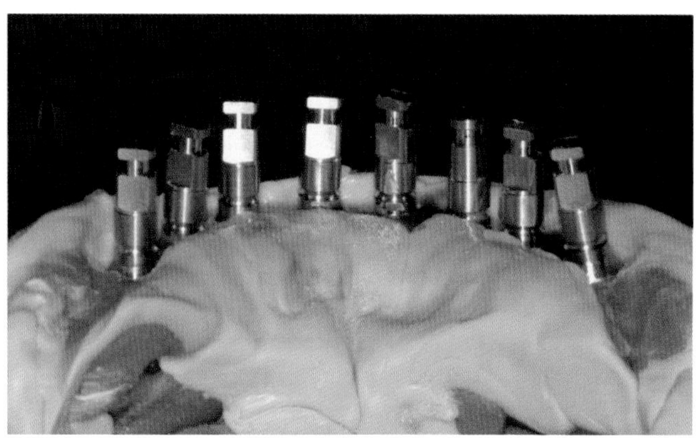

Figure 7.27. Implant lab analogs for 4.1 mm external hex implant restorative platforms in place within mandibular impression. It is critical to visualize metal-to-metal contact between implant analogs and implant impression copings.

The impression material was allowed to completely set and the impression coping screws were unscrewed with the Contra Angle Torque Driver (CATDB) and large hex driver tip, long (RASH8N) (Figure 7.24). A hemostat was used to ensure that the impression coping screws were completely free of the implants prior to removing the impression tray from the mouth (Figure 7.25).

The intaglio surface of the impression tray was evaluated for accuracy and that all of the impression copings were completely surrounded by impression material (Figure 7.26).

The healing abutments were placed back onto the implants and the patient was discharged to return in one week for fabrication of the verification index.

Laboratory Procedures/Laboratory Work Orders

Implant Analogs

Implant analogs are exact replicas of implant restorative platforms. In this case, eight implant analogs (ILA20) were required to fabricate the initial master cast (Figure 7.27).

TABLE 7.4. Laboratory Work Order for Fabrication of Mandibular Master Cast

Enclosed:

1. Mandibular final impression with eight implant impression copings, 4.1 mm external hex implants, 5 mm emergence profiles.
2. Place individual implant analogs (***3i***®, ILA20) onto each impression coping.
3. Visualize metal-to-metal contact between all analogs and implant impression copings.
4. Inject resilient soft material of your choice around each implant/abutment connection.
5. Mix die stone per the manufacturer's instructions relative to powder weight and liquid volume.
6. Pour master cast.

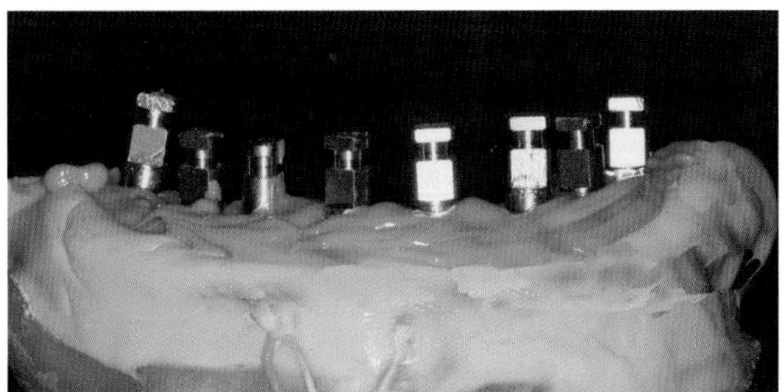

Figure 7.28. Resilient impression material was injected around the implant impression coping/implant analog connections.

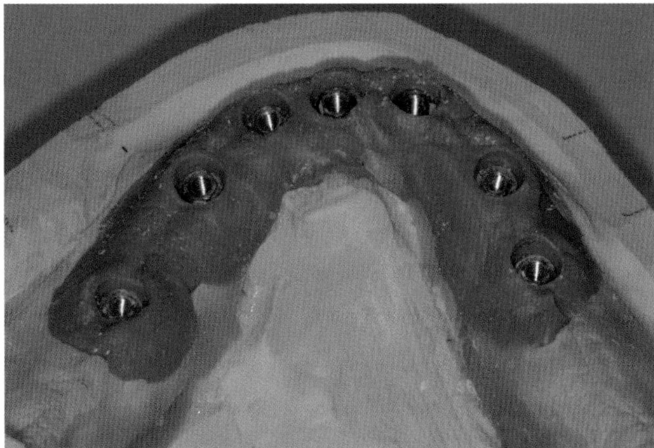

Figure 7.29. Mandibular master cast with resilient soft tissue that replicated the peri-implant soft tissue margins around each implant.

Master Cast Work Order

The work order for fabrication of the master cast is located in Table 7.4 (Figures 7.28 and 7.29).

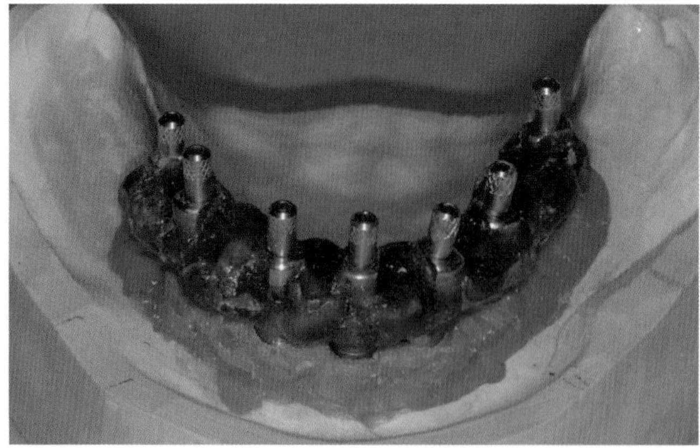

Figure 7.30. The impression copings were removed from the impression and placed back onto the implant analogs of the master cast. Autopolymerizing acrylic resin was mixed and placed around the impression copings and allowed to set overnight.

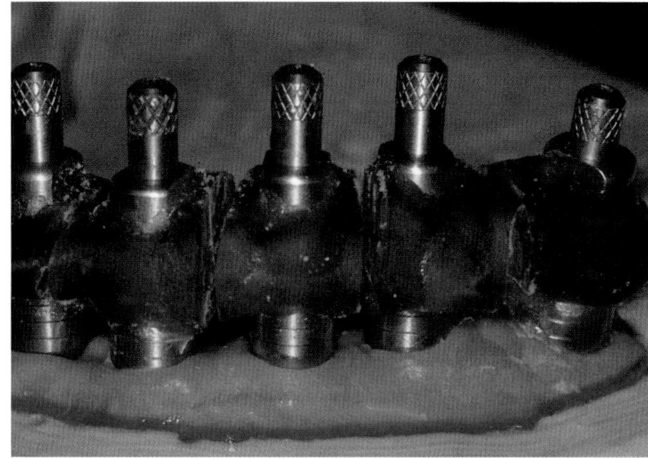

Figure 7.31. The verification index was sectioned in preparation for the clinical appointment.

Verification Index

The original protocol for mandibular screw retained implant prostheses included luting the impression copings together with an autopolymerizing acrylic resin at the time of the final impression (Zarb and Jansson 1985). Although this procedure has proven to be effective, it requires a significant amount of clinical time. The author prefers to fabricate a verification index on the initial master cast as described previously (Relate Acrylic Resin, Parkell BioMaterials Division, Farmingdale, NY). This index was allowed to polymerize overnight and then was sectioned in the laboratory (Figures 7.30 and 7.31). These segments were to be placed onto the implants intra-orally to fabricate the verification index.

TABLE 7.5. Laboratory Work Order for Fabrication of a Verification Index

1. After the master cast has been made, remove the impression copings from the impression.
2. Place the impression copings back onto the implant lab analogs in the master cast. Make sure that you visualize metal-to-metal contact between all of the impression copings and the implant analogs.
3. Mix Relate Acrylic Resin and place the resin around each of the impression copings, making sure to engage the undercuts of the impression copings.
4. Allow the resin to polymerize overnight.
5. Section the verification index into individual segments with a fine separating disc.
6. Return the master cast and verification index for try-in.

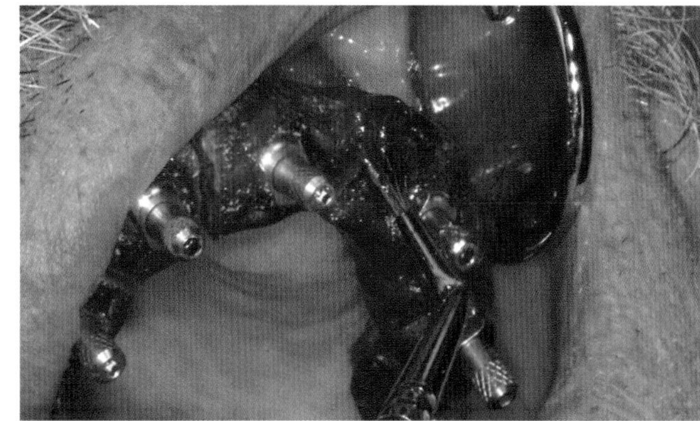

Figure 7.33. In this photo, additional acrylic resin was placed into the spaces between the segments for a maxillary prosthesis using a paintbrush.

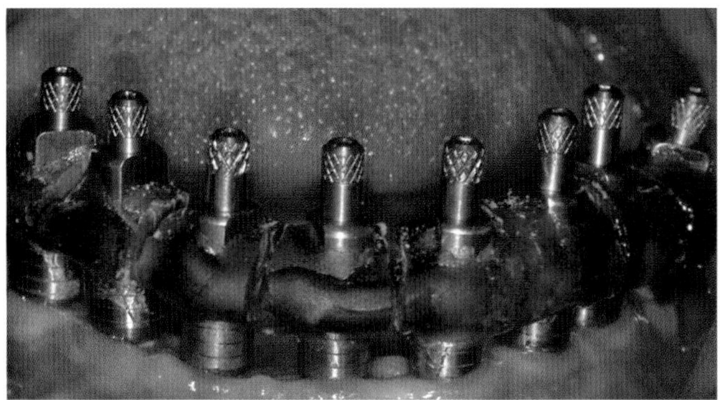

Figure 7.32. Intra-orally, the individual segments were placed onto their respective implants. There should be space visible between the segments.

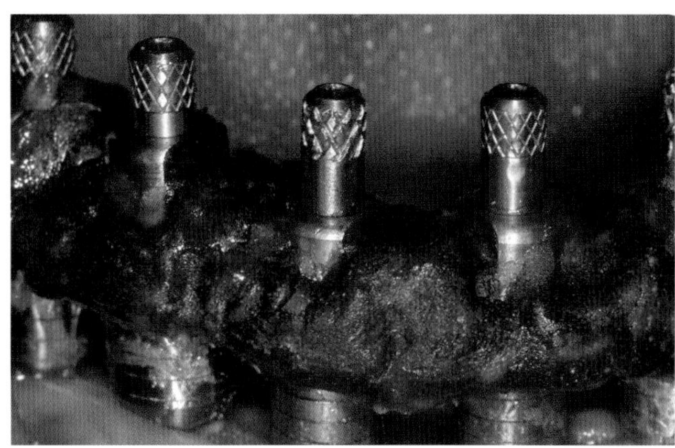

Figure 7.34. The resin was allowed to polymerize for 15 minutes.

Work Order

The work order for fabrication of the verification index has been described in Table 7.5.

Appointment 10. Verification Index/Definitive Impression (3/4 Hour)

The patient returned for the above procedures. She again reported no problems or concerns with the prosthetic phase of treatment.

Clinical Procedures

The healing abutments were removed from the mandibular implants. The individual segments were placed onto their respective implants (Figure 7.32).

The segments were luted together with the same acrylic resin. These additions were allowed to polymerize for 15 minutes (Figures 7.33 and 7.34).

The CAD/CAM protocol for CAM StructSURE™ Precision Milled Frameworks requires that the soft tissues on the master cast be replicated in a resilient material that can be removed and replaced back onto the master cast. The author prefers to make a new impression and fabricate a definitive master cast according to the above technique.

Laboratory Procedures/Laboratory Work Orders

Master Cast (Definitive)

A new master cast was fabricated using the same protocol as described previously. The laboratory work orders for fabrication of the definitive master cast are exactly the same as for development of the first master cast (Table 7.4).

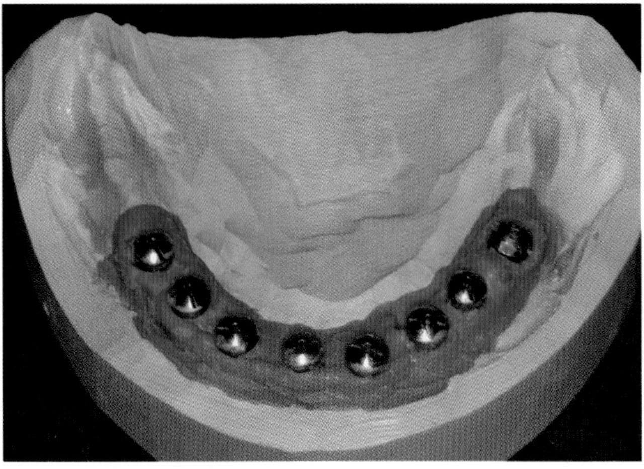

Figure 7.35. Healing abutments that were identical to those in the mouth were placed onto the implant analogs on the master cast.

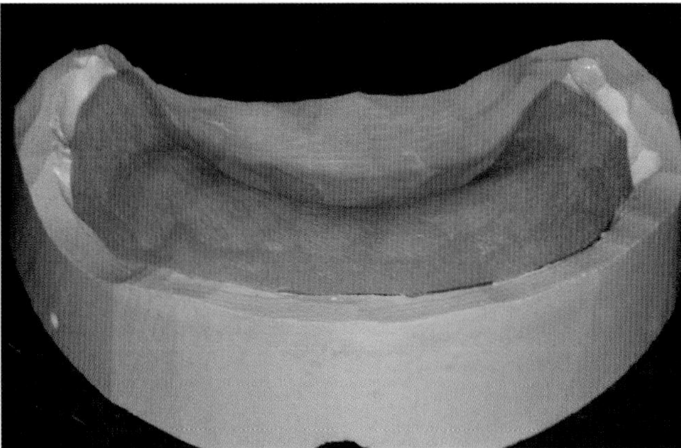

Figure 7.36. The mandibular record base in place on the master cast.

Maxillary Occlusion Rim/Mandibular Record Base

The next clinical appointment would include initial jaw relation records and tooth selection procedures. The author prefers to make the jaw relation records on the master cast with duplicate healing abutments in place. In this case, this was similar to an 8-unit mandibular overdenture. This was accomplished by noting the size of the clinical healing abutments in order to place similar healing abutments onto the master cast prior to fabrication of the mandibular record base (Figure 7.35).

The mandibular record base was made from a light cured resin material directly on the master cast and healing abutments (Figure 7.36). Record bases constructed in this fashion are extremely stable secondary to the presence of the healing abutments. This generally results in accurate jaw relation records and minimizes the need for remount procedures.

The laboratory work orders for fabrication of the mandibular record base are located in Table 7.6.

TABLE 7.6. Laboratory Work Order for Fabrication of Mandibular Record Base

1. On the enclosed master cast, place the following healing abutments:
   a. THA54
2. Make sure that the healing abutments are completely seated.
3. Fabricate the mandibular record base directly on top of the healing abutments and master cast per conventional removable prosthodontic principles for extension and retro molar pad coverage.
4. Polish the peripheral borders.
5. Return for the jaw relation records appointment

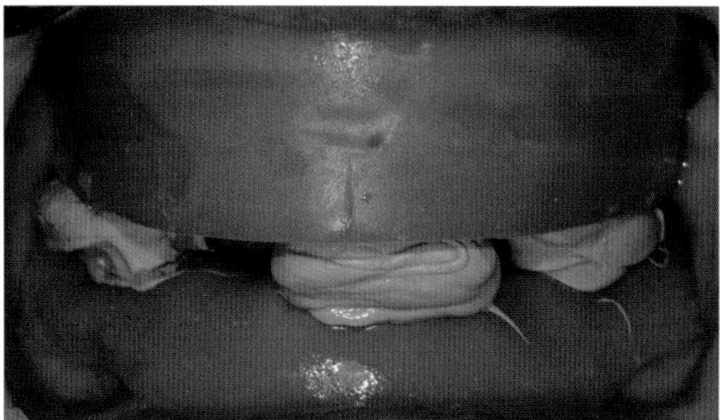

Figure 7.37. Initial jaw relation record with maxillary occlusion rim and mandibular record base, in centric relation at the predetermined vertical dimension of occlusion.

Appointment 11. Jaw Relation Records, Tooth Selection (1/2 Hour)

The patient was happy with the vertical dimension of occlusion, lip support, tooth arrangement, and incisal display of the existing dentures. Because the record bases were made on duplicate healing abutments on the master cast, clinically there was no reason to remove them.

Clinical Procedures

The patient was pleased with the overall aesthetic results of the preexisting dentures. This vertical dimension of occlusion and centric jaw relation record were duplicated using conventional removable prosthodontic techniques and materials (Pound 1970) (Figure 7.37).

Laboratory Procedures

Articulator Mounting

The casts were mounted on a semi-adjustable articulator (Table 7.7 and Figure 7.38).

TABLE 7.7. Laboratory Work Order for the Articulator Mounting of the Edentulous Casts and Initial Denture Set-Up

1. Mount the edentulous casts in the center of the articulator with the occlusal plane horizontal.
   a. The midline was marked on the maxillary occlusion rim.
2. Set the maxillary and mandibular denture teeth to be consistent with the occlusal plane established by the maxillary occlusion rim.
3. Return for wax try-in.

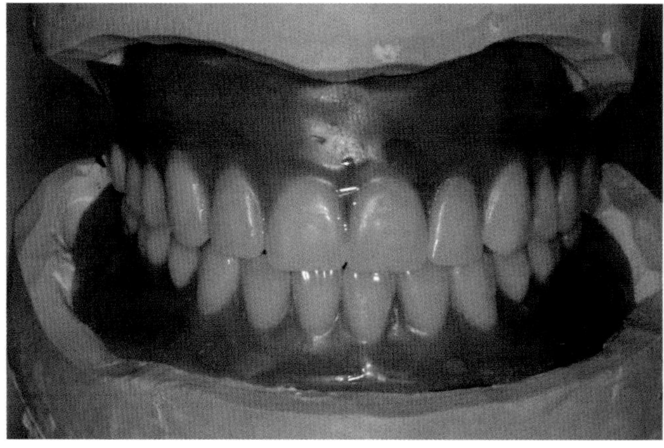

Figure 7.39. Denture teeth were set per the parameters established by the maxillary occlusion rim and mandibular record base.

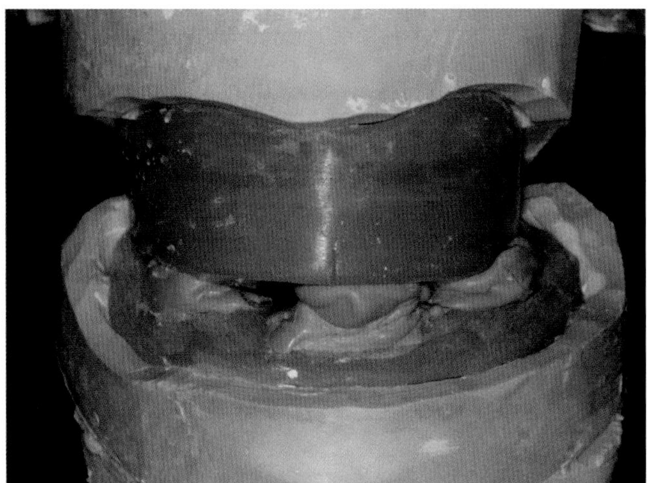

Figure 7.38. The master casts mounted on a semi-adjustable articulator.

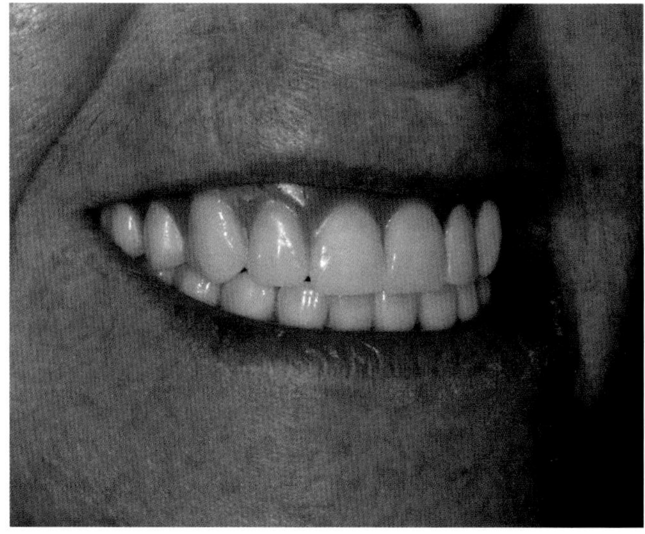

Figure 7.40. Clinical smile with wax dentures in place.

Initial Denture Set-Up

Denture teeth were set per the parameters of the maxillary occlusion rim relative to midline location, incisal edge position, and tooth arrangement (Figure 7.39).

Appointment 12. Wax Try-In (1/2 Hour)

The patient was comfortable and agreed to proceed with the wax try-in appointment. Because the record bases were made on duplicate healing abutments on the master cast, clinically there was no reason to remove them.

Verification of Jaw Relation Records

The wax dentures went to place. The jaw relation record was verified and the patient signed off on the vertical dimension of occlusion, lip support, incisal display during speaking/smiling, and tooth arrangement (Figure 7.40).

CAD/CAM Protocol

The CAD/CAM protocol for ***3i***®'s system is similar to the original protocol developed by Brånemark in the early 1980s (Adell and others 1981).

CAM StructSURE™ Precision Milled Bar

The protocol for fabrication of this type of prosthesis requires the following items for design and fabrication:

1. Wax denture
2. Verified master cast with resilient soft tissue
3. Verification index
4. Completed work order with a signature by the dentist that the master cast has been verified as accurate (Figure 7.41).

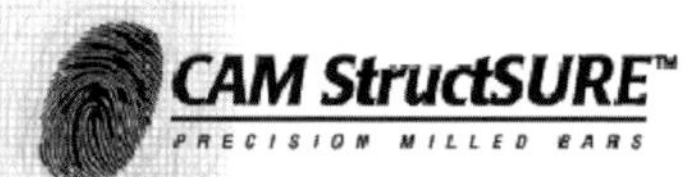

Work Order

* 1. Account Information

* Lab Name: ____________________

3i Account#: ____________________

* Contact: ____________________

* Phone: ____________________

Fax: ____________________

* Email: ____________________

* Patient ID: ____________________

* Ship To: ____________________

____

Bill To: ____________________

____

2. Preparing Your Case For Shipment

- __Only__ use new or undamaged implant analogs.
- Please __do not__ send the articulator.

Please include __only__ the following items:

❑ Verified/Accurate Soft-Tissue Cast
❑ Intraorally Verified Index, Disinfected (optional)
❑ Verified Wax Try-In, Disinfected
❑ Copy of the Completed Work Order
❑ Other Materials Included: ____________________

3. 3i Screw Ordering

❑ I would not like to order screws at this time.

__Certain® Abutment Screws__	__Qty.__
Gold-Tite™ Hexed Large Diameter (ILRGHG)	____
Titanium Hexed Large Diameter (ILRGHT)	____
__External Hex Abutment Screws__	
Gold-Tite Square (UNISG)	____
Gold-Tite Hexed (UNIHG)	____
Titanium Hexed (UNIHT)	____
Laboratory Square Try-in Screw -5 pack (UNITS)	____
__Retaining Screws__	
Gold-Tite, 2mm(H) (GSH20)	____
Gold-Tite, 3mm(H) (GSH30)	____
Gold-Tite, 7mm(H) (GSH70)	____
__Waxing Screws__	
Certain - Implant Level Waxing Screw, 16mm (IWSU30)	____
External Hex - Implant Level Waxing Screw, 15mm (WSU30)	____
Abutment Level Waxing Screw, 10mm (WSK10)	____
Abutment Level Waxing Screw, 15mm (WSK15)	____

4. 3i Polishing Protector Ordering

	__Qty.__
4.1mm (PPIA3)	____
5mm (WPP50)	____
6mm (WPP60)	____
Standard (PPSA3)	____
Conical (PPCA3)	____
IOL® (IOLPP)	____

5. Attachment Ordering

	__Qty.__
LOCATOR® Bar Attachment (LOAB)	____
LOCATOR Replacement Housing Kit (LORHK)	____
Hader Clip Gold (ORCG1)	____
Hader Clip Plastic (ORCY)	____

Job #: ____________________

Issued By: ____________________

* REQUIRED FIELD

6. Case Information

Tooth Position	Implant Brand**	Implant System	Implant Platform Diameter		Abutment Type
				or	
				or	
				or	
				or	
				or	
				or	
				or	
				or	

**See Compatibility Chart In CAM StructSURE Manual (ART868)

* 7. Structure Type

❑ Hader
❑ Dolder
❑ Primary ____ ° Taper
❑ Fixed Hybrid

8. Design Instructions

- See design matrix in CAM StructSURE Manual (ART868)
- Maximum implant divergence is 30°.
- Minimum distance between implants is 2mm.

❑ Design Bar according to the drawings below
❑ Position the bar within the confines of the verified wax try-in

* __Distal Extensions__
Patients Left ____mm
Patients Right ____mm

Bar Height ____mm (min. height 3mm)
Space Between Tissue and Bar ____mm (min. 1mm)

Tap areas for attachment:

❑ LOCATOR ❑ TSB Ball ❑ CEKA

● = Implant Position ■ = Clip Placement ▲ = Attachment

Maxillary **Mandibular**

9. Special Instructions

____

____

____

❑ Please see back or attached page.

*10. Certification

I certify that the analog positions on the cast and the wax try-in have been verified for accuracy and the stated information is correct. All items that have contacted the oral environment have been disinfected. This form authorizes *3i* to fabricate the CAM StructSURE Precision Milled Bar using and consistent with the information provided on this work order.

Technician Signature ____________________

Date ____________________

Implant Innovations, Inc.
4555 Riverside Drive
Palm Beach Gardens, FL 33410
800.443.8166

ART880
REV C 09/05

Figure 7.41. Blank work order for the CAM StructSURE Precision Milled Bar. This has to be completed by the dental laboratory technician before sending the case to *3i*®.

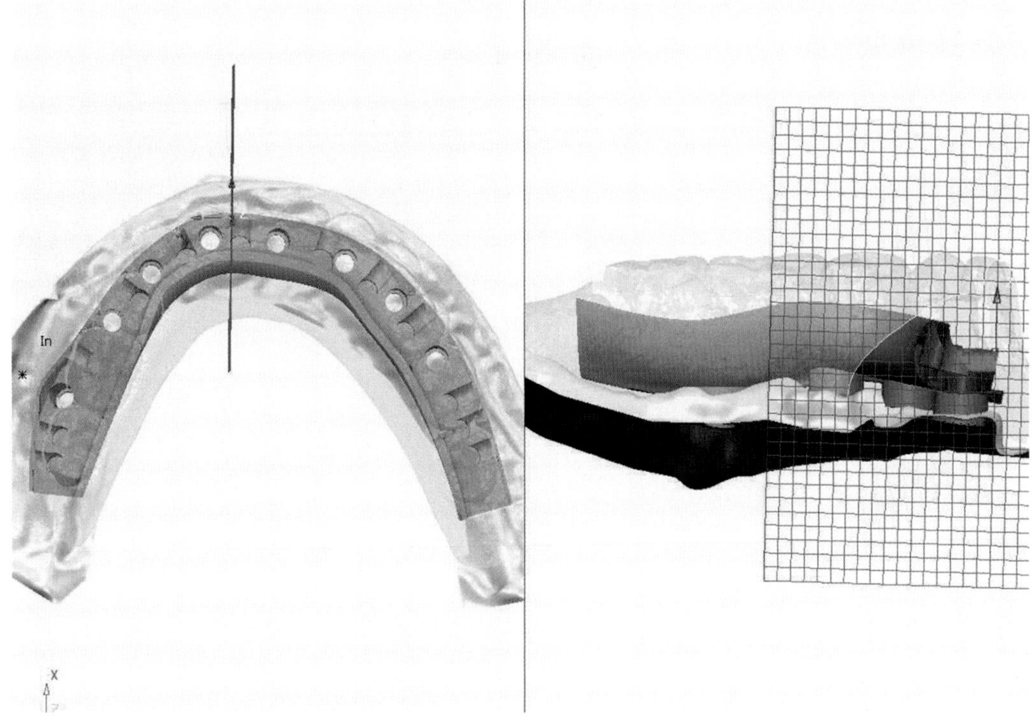

Figure 7.42. These are the virtual designs of the mandibular framework as developed by the CAD/CAM operator. They were emailed to the author's dental laboratory technician for review and modifications as needed.

All the items listed above were sent to the ARCHITECH PSR™ Center, Palm Beach Gardens, FL. Most restorative dentists will be working closely with a commercial dental laboratory and the laboratory will be involved in the CAD/CAM protocol relative to coordinating the prosthetic treatments.

Virtual Design of Framework

The master cast and wax denture were digitally scanned and the information was digitized. A dental laboratory technician designed the framework according to the work order and sent the tentative design to the author's dental laboratory technician for review and potential design changes (Figure 7.42).

Mill Framework

The framework was milled per the design illustrated in Figure 7.42. It was milled from a solid blank of titanium alloy (Figure 7.43). The framework was silicoated prior to the clinical try-in (Figure 7.44).

Laboratory Evaluation of Framework/Master Cast Fit (Square Try-In Screws)

The framework was evaluated for fit on the master cast with a one-screw test. One screw was placed into the screw access opening of the left posterior implant. A passive fit is

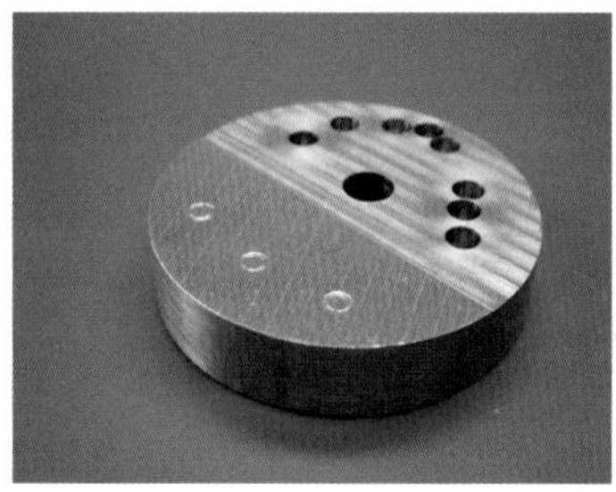

Figure 7.43. Solid blank of titanium alloy before milling the CAD/CAM mandibular framework.

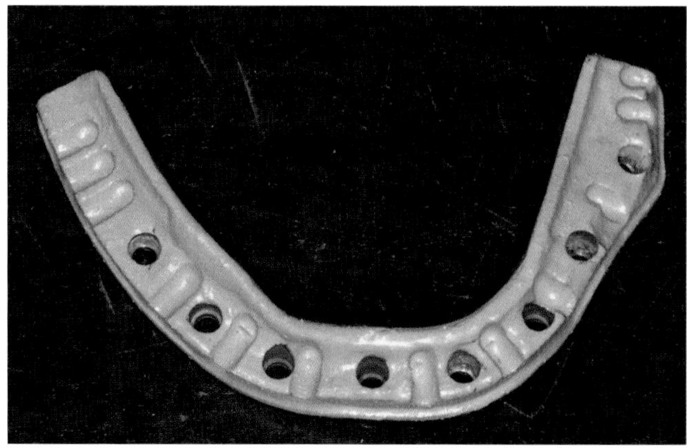

Figure 7.44. The CAD/CAM mandibular framework was milled and silicoated prior to the clinical try-in appointment.

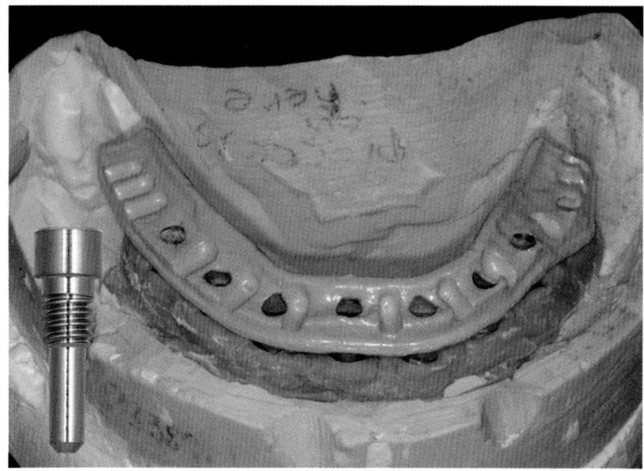

Figure 7.45. The CAD/CAM framework passed the 1-screw test on the master cast. The Square Try-In Screws (UNITS) should be used for all of the laboratory and clinical try in procedures (UNITS, inset).

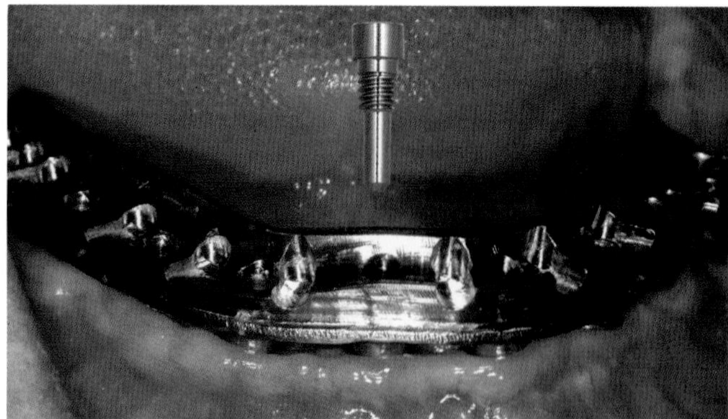

Figure 7.46. Facial view of CAD/CAM framework in place with one try-in screw (inset) in the left most distal implant. Note the fit between the framework and the implants.

indicated when no movement is observed on the contralateral most distal implant. The procedure was reversed and the framework was noted to fit the master cast accurately (Figure 7.45).

Appointment 13. Clinical Framework Try-In (3/4 Hour)

The patient presented for the clinical framework try-in appointment and remained asymptomatic.

Clinical One-Screw Test

The healing abutments were removed and all of the implant restorative platforms were visible (See Figure 7.20). The framework was tried in using Square Try-In Screws (UNITS). (Figures 7.46 and 7.47). One advantage of try-in screws is that the screws go quickly to place with two turns of the driver.

Radiographic One-Screw Test

Clinically, the framework was also noted to fit passively with one try-in screw in the middle implant and no screw in a posterior segment (Figures 7.48 and 7.49).

The framework was removed and the original healing abutments were placed back onto the implants. The patient was discharged and reappointed for the framework/wax try-in.

Laboratory Procedures

Silicoat Framework

Silicoating a framework provides a chemical bond and an opaque covering that masks the metallic color of the framework. The framework was returned to the commercial dental laboratory for silicoating (Figure 7.50).

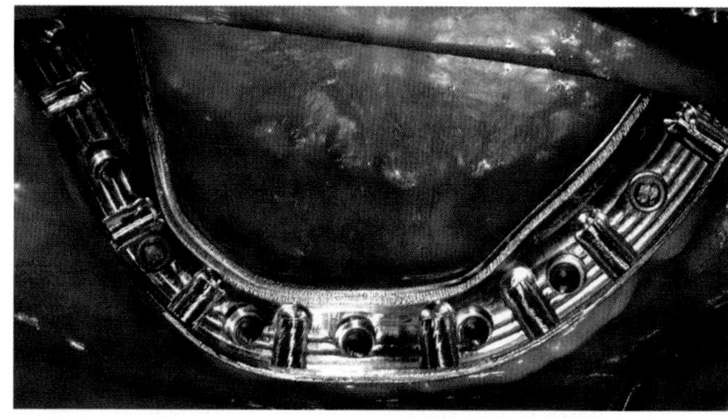

Figure 7.47. Occlusal view of CAD/CAM framework in place with one try in screw in the left most distal implant.

Denture Set-Up

Denture teeth were set per the parameters established by the mandibular record base (Figure 7.51).

Appointment 14. Wax Try-In with Framework (3/4 Hour)

The patient returned for this appointment with her significant other.

Verification of Jaw Relation Records, Approval of Aesthetics, Vertical Dimension, Centric Relation, Lip Support, Incisal Display, and Tooth Arrangement

The healing abutments were removed with the Posterior Hex Driver (large)(PHD02N) from the mandibular implants, and the wax denture/CAD/CAM framework went to place with the square try-in screws and Standard Square Driver, 24 mm (UNITS and PSDQD1N) (Figure 7.52). The patient

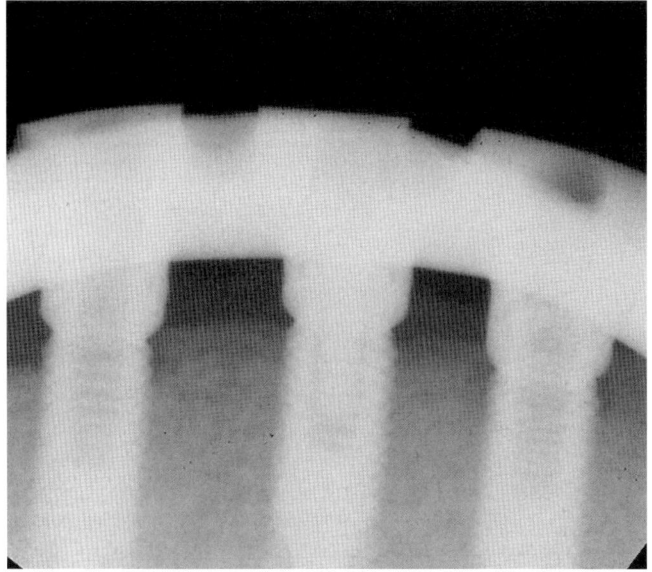

Figure 7.48. Radiograph of the middle implants with the framework retained by one try-in screw in the middle implant.

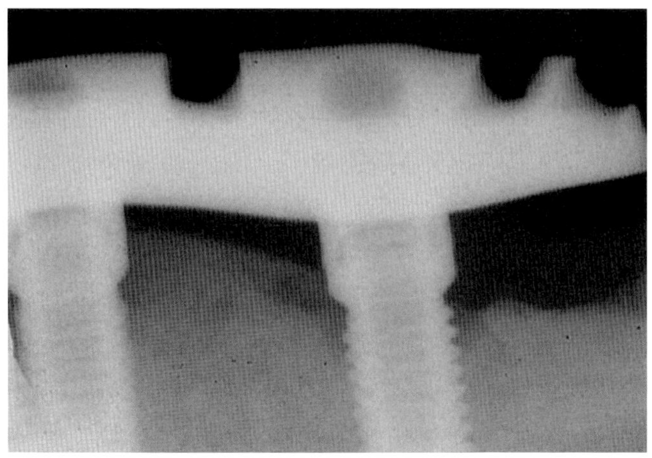

Figure 7.49. Radiograph of the left posterior segment that indicated a precise fit between the framework and the implant restorative platforms with one screw in the center implant as in Figure 7.48.

had a thorough chance to evaluate the tooth arrangement, vertical dimension of occlusion, and incisal display during speaking and smiling. She and her significant other approved of the wax denture tooth arrangement.

The wax denture/CAD/CAM framework was removed with the Standard Square Driver, 24 mm and the healing abutments were placed back onto the implants. The patient was discharged and reappointed for the clinical insertion appointment.

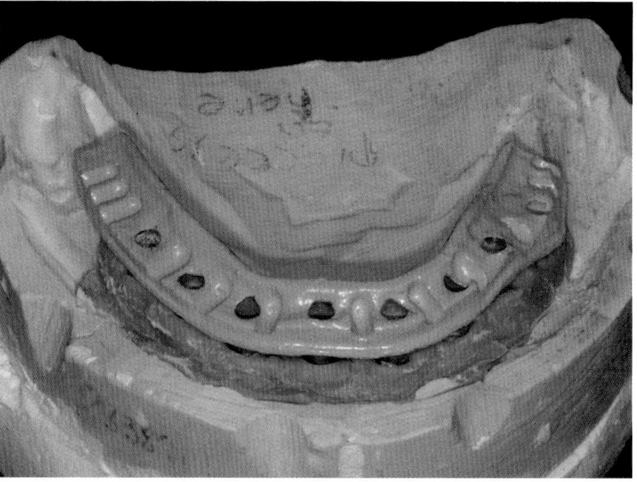

Figure 7.50. Laboratory view of silicoated CAD/CAM framework.

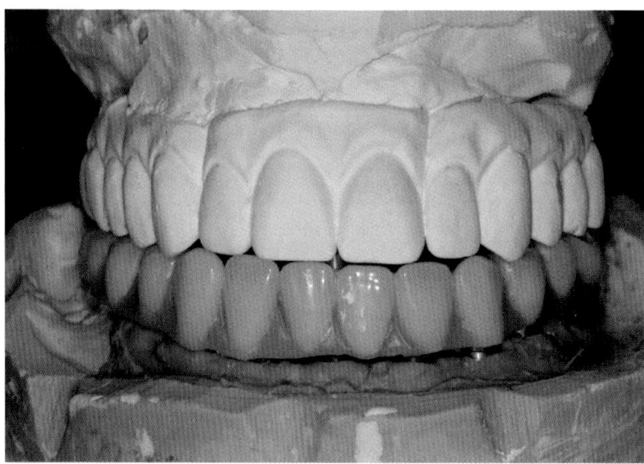

Figure 7.51. Laboratory view of mandibular framework with teeth set per the wax denture set up in Figure 7.39 prior to try-in.

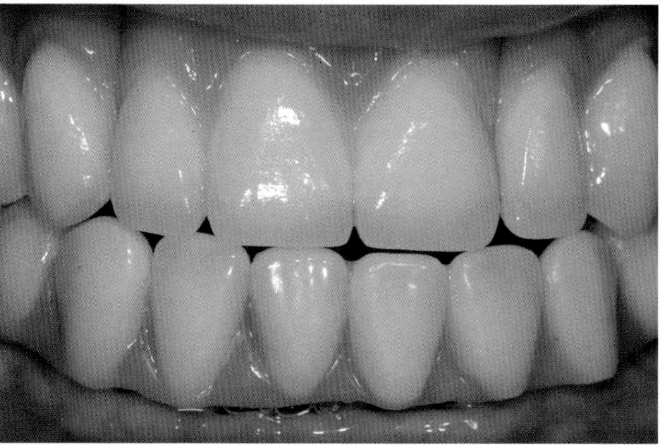

Figure 7.52. Clinical anterior view of the mandibular wax denture/CAD/CAM framework against the porcelain fused to metal maxillary restorations.

TABLE 7.8. Laboratory Work Orders for Processing the Mandibular CAD/CAM Prosthesis

The patient approved of the aesthetic arrangement of the denture set-up.

1. Re-establish optimal centric occlusal contacts in the posterior teeth. Set posterior teeth in tight centric occlusion.
2. Right and left working movements should be Group Function.
3. Leave mandibular anterior teeth where they are in the wax denture. (Patient specifically requested this tooth arrangement.)
4. Numbers s 8 and 9 should disclude in protrusive with posterior balancing contacts.
5. Wax the denture portion of the prosthesis to optimal gingival contours.
6. Process in acrylic resin.
7. Remount and adjust occlusion after processing.
8. Remove the prosthesis from the master cast.
9. Place polishing protectors to protect the machined interfaces.
10. Finish and polish.

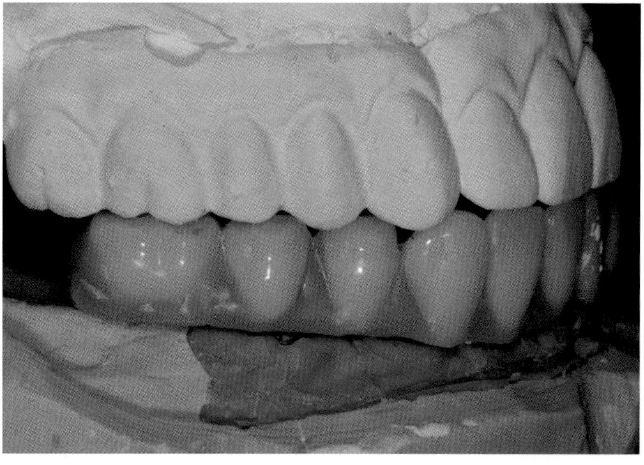

Figure 7.53. Right posterior laboratory view of mandibular wax denture/CAD/CAM prosthesis with teeth in maximum intercuspation.

Laboratory Procedures and Laboratory Work Orders

The laboratory work orders are located in Table 7.8 (Figures 7.53 through 7.57).

Appointment 15. Prosthesis Insertion (3/4 Hour)

Removal of Healing Abutments

The healing abutments were removed with the PHD02N (Standard Large Hex Driver, 24 mm). The soft tissues had healed consistent with the shape of the healing abutments,

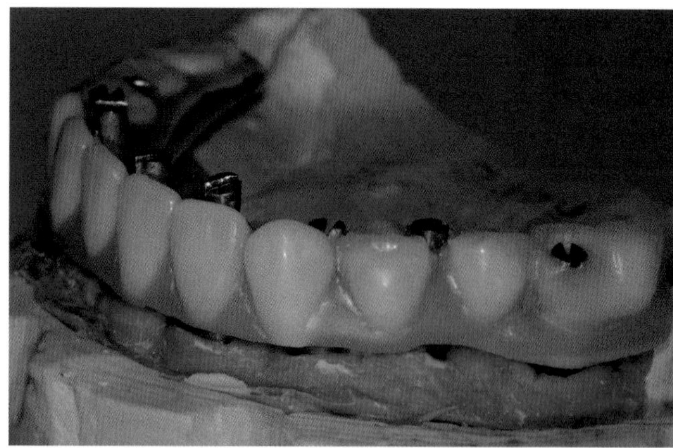

Figure 7.54. Left posterior laboratory view of mandibular wax denture/CAD/CAM prosthesis, waxed to full contour, prior to processing. Note that the screw access opening for the mandibular first molar was lateral to the buccal cusp.

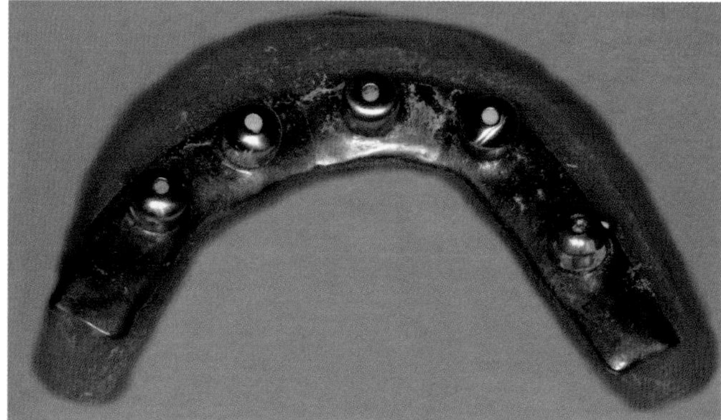

Figure 7.55. Polishing protectors in place on the machined surfaces of the mandibular prosthesis. These should be placed onto the framework after removal from the master cast, prior to polishing.

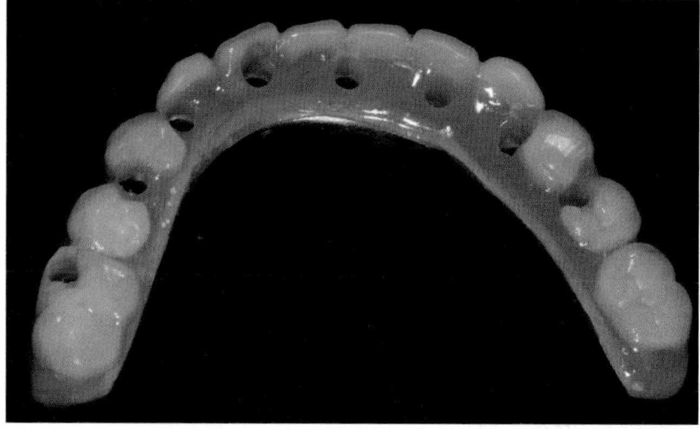

Figure 7.56. Laboratory occlusal view of the mandibular prosthesis after polishing.

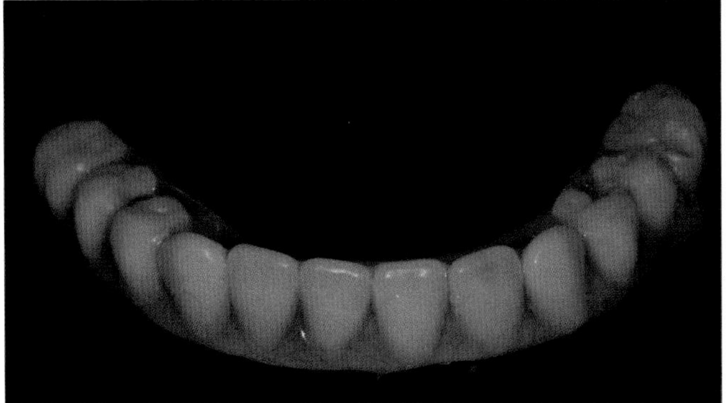

Figure 7.57. Laboratory facial view of the mandibular prosthesis after polishing.

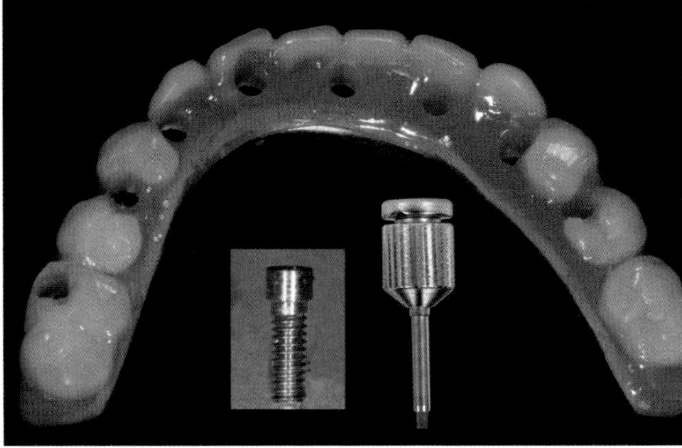

Figure 7.58. The definitive mandibular prosthesis went to place with the abutment screws (UNISG). The Standard Square Driver, 24 mm (PSQD1N) was used to hand tighten the screws (UNISG, left inset; PSQD1N, right inset).

and the patient reported no pain during this procedure (Figure 7.20). The implants were assumed to be osseointegrated.

Insertion of Mandibular Prosthesis

Abutment Screws

The prosthesis went to place with the definitive abutment screws (Gold-Tite™ Square Abutment Screws, UNISG). This abutment screw is made from a high-strength gold palladium alloy with a 0.76 μm 24-carat-gold coating. In laboratory studies, Gold-Tite™ abutment screws achieve a greater degree of preload torque compared to titanium, gold alloy, and coated titanium screws. Gold-Tite™ is a dry lubricant between mating threads that reduces friction between screws and implants and allows 62% more screw turn during tightening than non-Gold-Tite screws. This is significant in that the preload increases within the screw joint without increasing the force generated on the screw head. The Standard Square Driver (PSQD1N) was used to hand tighten the abutment screws (Figure 7.58).

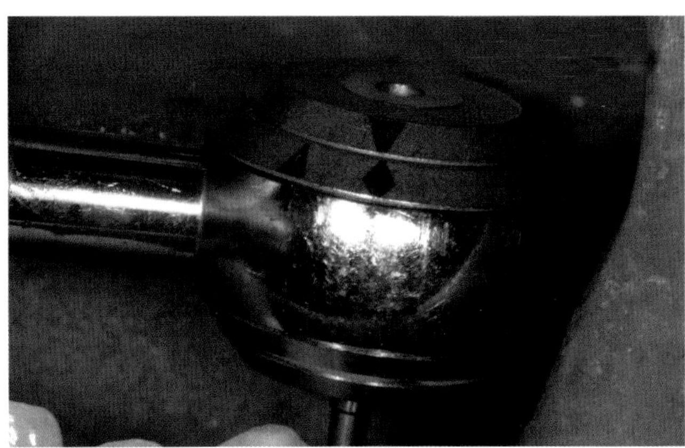

Figure 7.59. The head of a Restorative Torque Indicator. The triangle to diamond indicated that 35 Ncm of preload was generated to the abutment screw.

Torque

In the OSSEOTITE® Implant System (external hex implant/abutment connection), square abutment screws are the abutment screws of choice. These screws can be torqued to 32 to 35 Ncm. In this case, the screws were torqued to 35 Ncm with the Restorative Torque Driver and 32 Ncm torque controller (RTI230, CATC3, respectively) (Figure 7.59).

After the screws were torqued according to the above procedures, the screw access openings were partially blocked out with cotton and then restored with light cured composite resin (Figure 7.60).

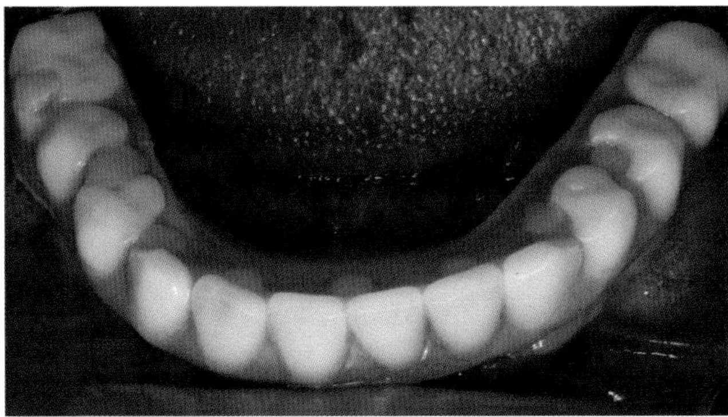

Figure 7.60. Occlusal view of mandibular implant-retained prosthesis. Light cured composite resin was used to seal the screw access openings.

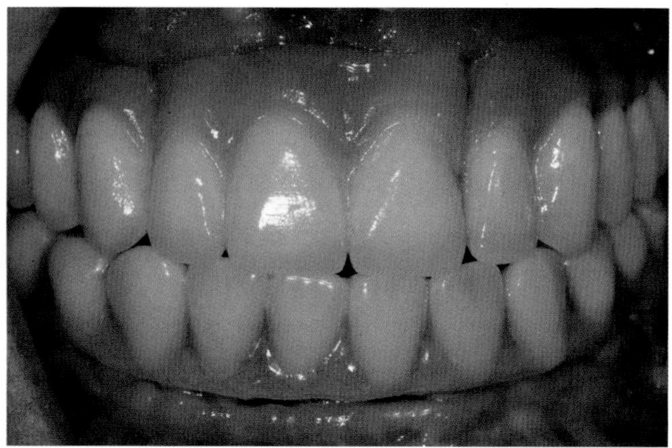

Figure 7.61. Anterior view of completed prostheses at the mandibular prosthesis insertion appointment.

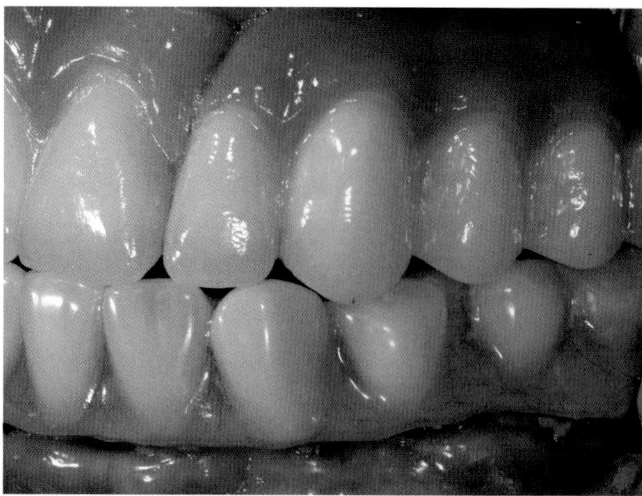

Figure 7.63. Left lateral view of completed prostheses at the mandibular prosthesis insertion appointment.

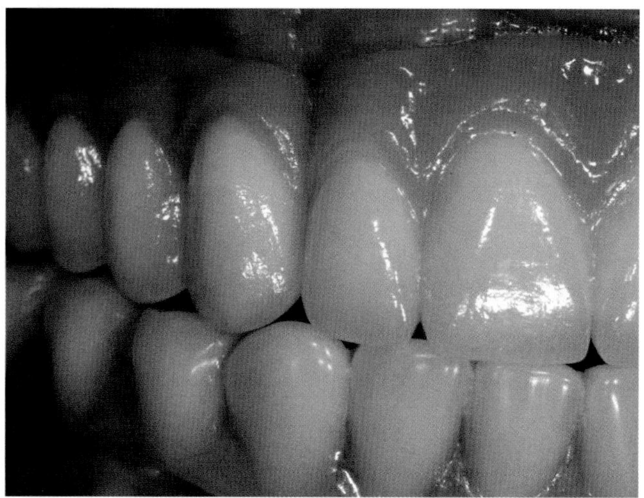

Figure 7.62. Right lateral view of completed prostheses at the mandibular prosthesis insertion appointment.

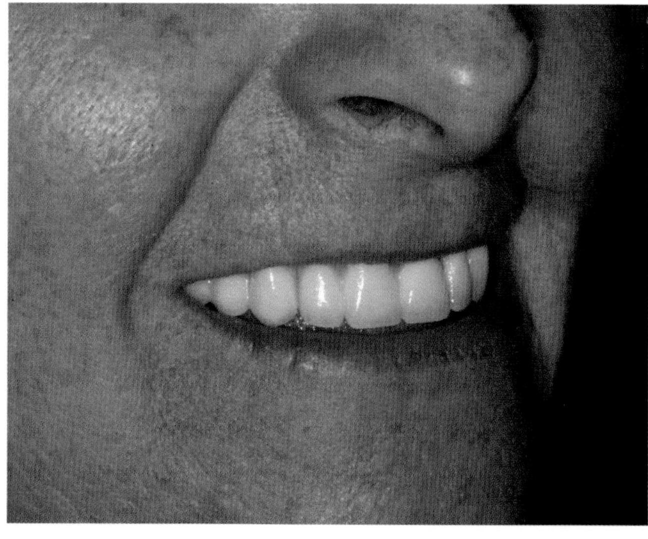

Figure 7.64. Extra-oral view of the patient's smile at the insertion appointment.

Final Prostheses

The patient was discharged with the completed prostheses in place (Figures 7.61, 7.62, 7.63, 7.64).

Oral Hygiene Instructions

The patient was introduced to several different methods for oral hygiene for both the maxillary fixed partial dentures and the mandibular implant prosthesis. The use of Superfloss® and manual and electric toothbrushes was demonstrated to the patient. The author has found that dispensing oral hygiene supplies at the insertion appointment to be the most effective means of increasing patient compliance (Figures 7.65, 7.66, 7.67 and 7.68).

Appointments 16 and 17. Prosthetic Follow-up Appointments: Two Weeks, Six Months (1/2 Hour)

This patient was seen approximately two weeks after the prostheses were inserted. She was extremely pleased with the aesthetic, phonetic, and functional results of the prosthetic treatment. She reported no difficulties with either prosthesis. Her oral hygiene was excellent. No treatment was required at either appointment.

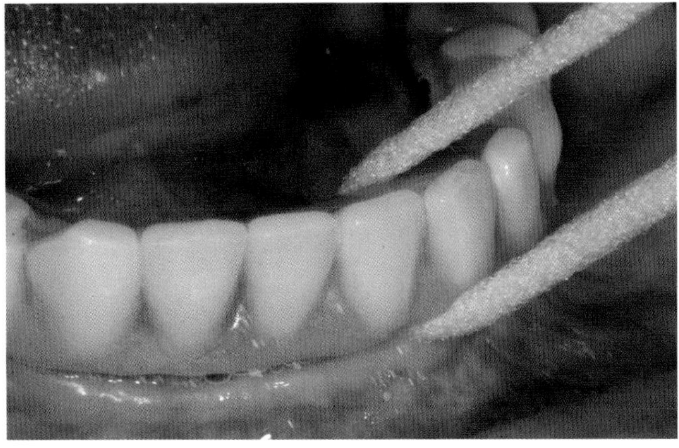

Figure 7.65. Superfloss® can be used for plaque removal around the implant/framework connections, as well as the intaglio surface of the implant-retained prosthesis.

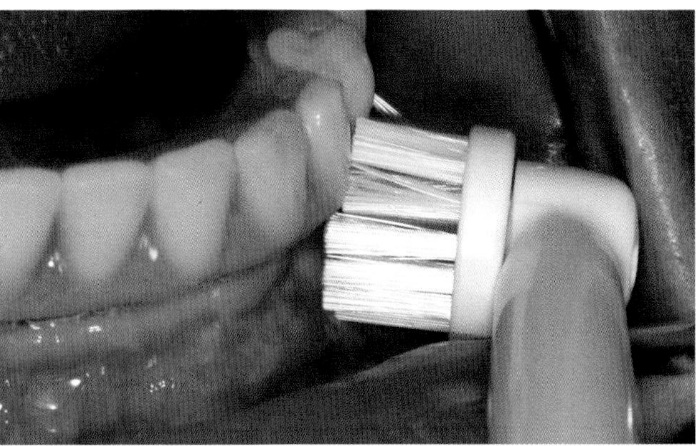

Figure 7.67. An electric toothbrush (Oral B® Professional Care 7000 Series, St. John, NB) also can be an effective tool for plaque removal around the implant/framework connections, especially for patients with limited manual dexterity.

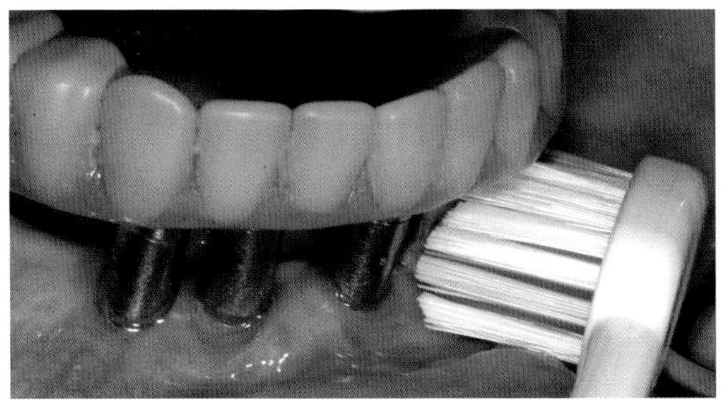

Figure 7.66. A manual toothbrush can be an effective instrument for plaque removal around the implant/framework connections. It may not be as effective on the intaglio or lingual surfaces of an implant-retained prosthesis.

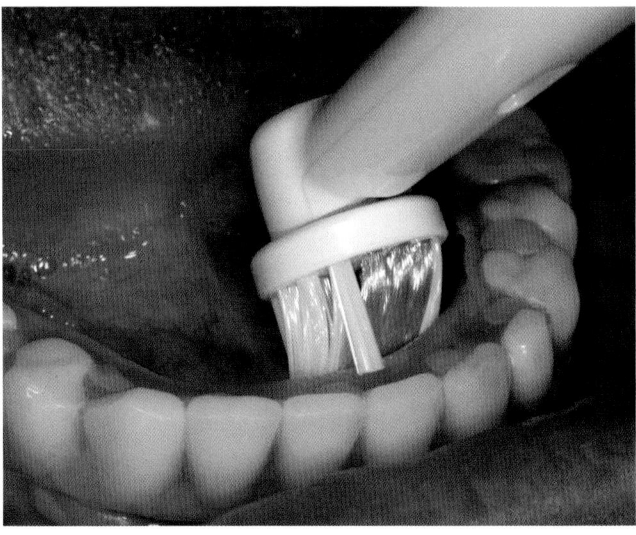

Figure 7.68. An electric toothbrush (Oral B® Professional Care 7000 Series, St. John, NB) can also be effective for plaque removal in and around the lingual surfaces of a screw-retained prosthesis.

Appointment 18. One-Year Recall

Again, the patient reported no problems with either prosthesis. She was still extremely pleased with the aesthetic, phonetic, and functional results of the prosthetic treatment.

Radiographs

In the absence of symptoms, a panoramic radiograph was ordered for the one-year recall appointment (Figure 7.69). If the patient had reported any symptoms related to pain, or discomfort in or around the implants, periapical radiographs would have been ordered and evaluated. In certain instances in which a patient presents with chronic, vague symptoms, clinicians may order periapical radiographs of individual implants. In this instance, there was less than 1 mm of crestal bone loss noted around the implants.

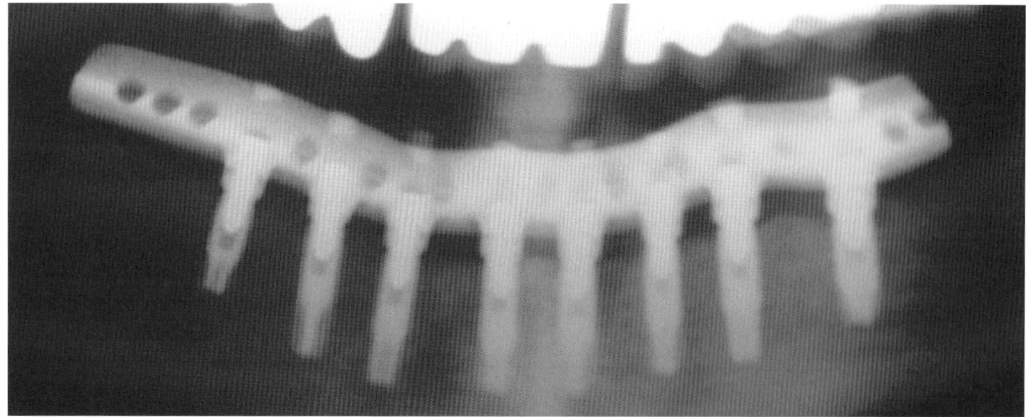

Figure 7.69. Panoramic radiograph at the one-year recall appointment. There was less than 1 mm of crestal bone loss around any of the implants. There was excellent bone/implant contact around all of the implants. There were no radiolucenies.

Clinical Examination

The prostheses were evaluated intra- and extra-orally. The vertical dimension of occlusion, as well as the Class I posterior occlusal relationships, were maintained. The maxillary fixed partial dentures were stable and the soft tissue contours were within normal limits. The mandibular implant-retained prosthesis was stable and without macroscopic movement. The patient's oral hygiene was excellent.

If a patient's oral hygiene is not satisfactory (Figure 7.70), calculus may be removed with the prosthesis in place. If the calculus is significant, the implant-retained prosthesis may need to be removed. In these instances, the author has found it more efficient to reappoint the patient for removal of the prosthesis, clinical polishing of the abutments, and laboratory finishing of the prosthesis (Figure 7.71).

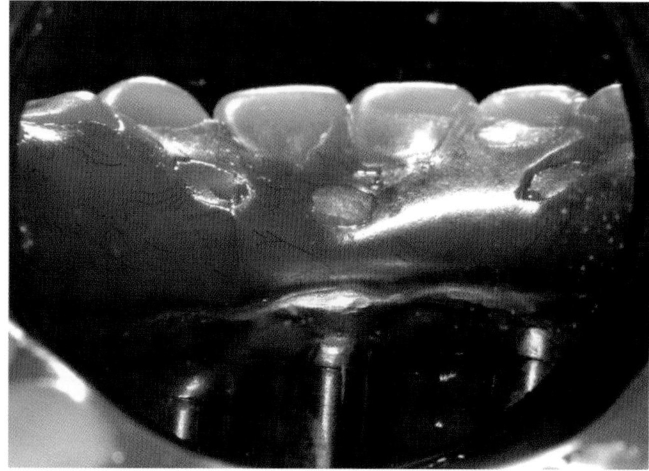

Figure 7.70. Moderate accumulations of supra-gingival plaque and calculus in and around a mandibular implant-retained prosthesis. These deposits were removed intra-orally with plastic scalers. The prosthesis did not need to be removed.

Future Recall Appointments

The author recalls this type of patient once yearly. Radiographs are taken every year for the first three years. In the absence of signs or symptoms of pathology, radiographs would be taken every two to three years thereafter.

Costs/Fees/Profitability

The following discussion (Table 7.9) relative to fees is reflective of 2006 in the Midwestern United States. The costs of the implant components are retail prices from Implant Innovations, Inc., Palm Beach Gardens, Florida.

Surgeon: Ajit Pillai, DMD, Gundersen Lutheran Medical Center, LaCrosse, Wisconsin

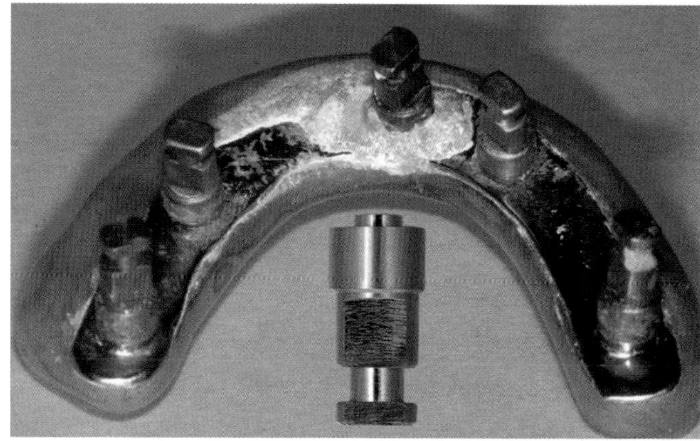

Figure 7.71. Laboratory view of an implant-retained prosthesis with heavy accumulations of plaque and calculus on the intaglio surface. In this case, abutment lab analogs (SLA20, inset) were used to protect the machined interfaces of the abutments inside the casting.

TABLE 7.9. Lab Fees, Component Costs, Overhead, Fees, and Restorative Profits

Fixed			
Chair Time	**Overhead**	**Laboratory Expenses**	
		Casts	$ 60
		Articulation	$ 50
		Record bases	$ 50
		Denture set up	$250
		Processing	$100
5.5 hours	**$350/hr = $1925**	**Sub Total**	**$510**
		Implant Components	
		CAM StructSURE Precision Milled Bar	$2100
		Polishing protectors	$90
		Lab screws	$150
		Abutment Screws	$330
		Sub Total	$2670
TOTALS	$1925		$3180
Professional Fee			**$7500**
Costs (fixed overhead and laboratory expenses)			**$5105**
Profit (fees less costs)			$2395
Profit per hour ($2395/5.5)			$ 435

Impression copings, lab screws, and polishing protectors may be used multiple times, therefore costs will be decreased for each succeeding case and profits will be increased. Analogs should not be re-used.

Dental Laboratory Technicians: Andrew Gingrasso, Gundersen Lutheran Medical Center, LaCrosse, Wisconsin; Thomas Peterson, MDT, CDT, NorthShore Dental Laboratory, Lynn, Massachusetts

BIBLIOGRAPHY

Abrahamsson, I, Berglundh, T, Glantz, P, Lindhe, J, 1998. The mucosal attachment at different abutments. An experimental study in dogs. *J Clin Periodontol* 25:721–727.

Adell, R, Lekholm, U, Rockler, B, Brånemark, P-I, 1981. A 15 year study of osseointegrated implants in the treatment of the edentulous jaw. *Int J Oral Surg* 10:387–416.

Albrektsson, T, Zarb, G, Worthington, P, Eriksson, A, 1986. The long-term efficacy of currently used dental implants: a review and proposed criteria of success. *Int J Oral Maxillofac Implants* 1:11–25.

Allen, P, McMillan, A, Walshaw, D, 1999. Patient expectations of oral implant-retained prostheses in a UK dental hospital. *Br Dent J* 186: 80–84.

Assif, D, Marshak, B, Schmidt, A, 1996. Accuracy of implant impression techniques. *Int J Oral Maxillofac Implants* 11:216–222.

Awad, M, Feine, J, 1998. Measuring patient satisfaction with mandibular prostheses. *Community Dent Oral Epidemiol* 26:400–405.

Awad, M, Llund, J, Duresne, E, Feine, J, 2003. Comparing the efficacy of mandibular implant-retained overdentures and conventional dentures among middle-aged edentulous patients: satisfaction and functional assessment. *Int J Prosthodont* 16:117–122.

Brånemark, P-I, Hansson, B, Adell, R, 1977. Osseointegrated implants in the treatment of the edentulous jaw. *Scand J Plast Reconstr Surg* 16:1–132.

Carlsson, G, Otterland, A, Wennstrom, A, 1967. Patient factors in appreciation of complete dentures. *J Prosthet Dent* 17:322–328.

Carr, A, 1991. Comparison of impression techniques for a five-implant mandibular model. *Int J Oral Maxillofac Implants* 6:448–455.

DeBoer, J, 1993. Edentulous implants: overdenture versus fixed. *J Prosthet Dent* 69:386–390.

Engfors, I, Ortorp, A, Jemt, T, 2004. Fixed implant supported prostheses in elderly patients: a 5-year retrospective study of 133 edentulous patients older than 79 years. *Clin Implant Dent Rel Res* 6:190–198.

Feine, J, Dufresne, E, Boudrias, P, Lund, J, 1998. Outcome assessment of implant-supported prostheses. *J Prosthet Dent* 79:575–579.

Herbst, D, Nel, J, Driessen, C, Becker, P, 2000. Evaluation of impression accuracy for osseointegrated implant-supported superstructures. *J Prosthet Dent* 83:555–561.

Hsu, C, Millstein, P, Stein, R, 1993. A comparative analysis of the accuracy of implant transfer techniques. *J Prosthet Dent* 69:588–593.

Kari, M, Winter, W, Taylor, T, 2004. In vitro study on passive fit in implant-supported 5-unit fixed partial dentures. *Int J Oral Maxillofac Implants* 19:30–37.

Lindquist, L, Rockler, B Carlsson G, 1988. Bone resorption around fixtures in edentulous patients treated with mandibular fixed tissue-integrated prosthesis. *J Prosthet Dent* 59:59–63.

Lindquist, L, Carlsson, G, Jemt, T, 1996. A prospective 15-year follow-up study of mandibular fixed prostheses supported by osseointegrated implants. Clinical results and marginal bone loss. *Clin Oral Implants Res* 7:329–336.

Melas, F, Marcenes, W, Wright P, 2001. Oral health impact on daily performance in patients with implant-stabilized overdentures and patients with conventional complete dentures. *Int J Oral Maxillofac Impl* 16:700–712.

McAlarney, M, Stavropoulous, D, 1996. Determination of cantilever length-anterior-posterior spread ratio assuming failure criteria to be the compromise of the prosthesis retaining screw-prosthesis joint. *Int J Oral Maxillofac Implants* 11:331–339.

McGarry, T, Nimmo, A, Skiba, J, 2002. Classification system for partial edentulism. *J Prosthodont* 11:181–193.

Morin, C, Lund, J, Sioufi, C, Feine, J, 1998. Patient satisfaction with dentures made by dentists and denturologists. *J Can Dent Assoc* 63:205–212.

Ortorp, A, Jemt, T, 2004. Clinical experiences of computer numeric control-milled titanium frameworks supported by implants in the edentulous jaw: a 5-year prospective study. *Clin Impl Dent Rel Res* 4:199–209.

Pound, E, 1970. Utilizing speech to simplify a personalized denture service. *J Prosthet Dent* 24:586–600.

Testori T, Del Fabbro M, Feldman S. 2002. A multicenter prospective evaluation of 2-months loaded Osseotite implants placed in the posterior jaws. 3-year follow-up results. *Clin Oral Implants Res* 13:154–161.

Wright, P, Glantz, P, Randow, K, Watson, R, 2002. The effects of fixed and removable implant-stabilized prostheses on posterior mandibular residual ridge resorption. *Clin Oral Impl Res* 13:169–174.

Zitzmann, N, Marinello, C, 2002. A review of clinical and technical considerations for fixed and removable implant prostheses in the edentulous mandible. *Int J Prosthodont* 15:65–72.

Zarb, George, and Jansson, Tomas. 1985. "Prosthodontic Procedures." In *Tissue-Integrated Prostheses: Osseointegration in Clinical Dentistry*, P-I Brånemark, George Zarb, and Tomas Albrektsson, eds. Chicago: Quintessence Publishing Co., Inc., p. 251–257.

Chapter 8: Treatment of the Edentulous Mandible with an Immediate Occlusal Loading® Protocol

LITERATURE REVIEW

Dentistry has moved through a number of evolutions over the last several decades. For many years, treatment of the edentulous mandible using conventional complete dentures has been the standard of care for dentistry, even though the term "standard of care" can have multiple definitions (Feine and others 2002; Fitzpatrick 2006). Conventional mandibular complete dentures still are frequently made for edentulous patients but often can be frustrating for clinicians and patients due to severe resorption and the resultant instability of the dentures.

The Pre-Osseointegration Era

The pre-osseointegration era was so defined by Philip Worthington (2005). He described this period as one in which pre-prosthetic surgical procedures were accomplished to facilitate prosthetic treatment in patients with significant anatomical compromises. The surgical procedures developed in this era were directed toward two goals:

1. The surgical removal of obstacles to prosthetic treatment
2. Procedures to increase the denture-bearing area

The most durable contribution made during this time was that of orthognathic and pre-prosthetic surgery that eliminated osseous asymmetries correcting problems prior to denture construction. Conventional prosthodontic treatment resulted in accurately fitting prostheses. However, there were numerous patients who still could not manage their dentures.

The Osseointegration Era

This era expanded knowledge of bone biology relative to osseous wound healing and its interactions with dental implants and their surfaces. Roughened surfaces and the requirement for minimal micromotion fostered a stable implant/bone connection and allowed the creation of fixed implant-retained prostheses. Albrektsson and others (1986) described the osseointegration era as halfway biotechnology.

Implantology struggled during this period of time with failures and successes. In 1982, at a conference organized in Toronto, Canada, by Dr. George Zarb, dental professionals realized that their interaction and understanding of bone biology was, in fact, progressing and many solid partnerships were being forged.

However, as quoted by Worthington (2005), the Scottish poet, Robert Burns (1971) reminded us it is not always easy to see ourselves as others see us and what perhaps was evolving was that the surgeons looking at themselves might see someone who was innovative, resourceful, and dexterous, whereas the prosthodontic colleague might see someone who was overconfident, unrealistic, and perhaps ineffective. On the other hand, the prosthodontist might look at himself and see a true artist with the hardest job of all—satisfying the patient. His surgical colleagues might see the prosthodontist as someone who was not only very demanding but also grudging in acknowledgement of the surgical contribution (Worthington 2005) (Figures 8.1 and 8.2).

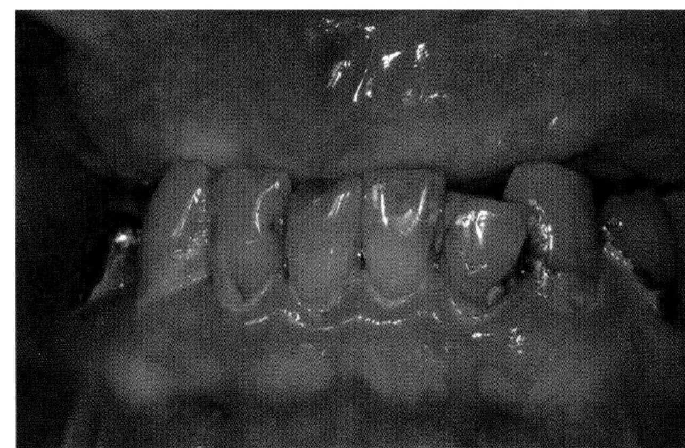

Figure 8.1. Pre-operative clinical anterior view of edentulous maxillae and partially edentulous mandible.

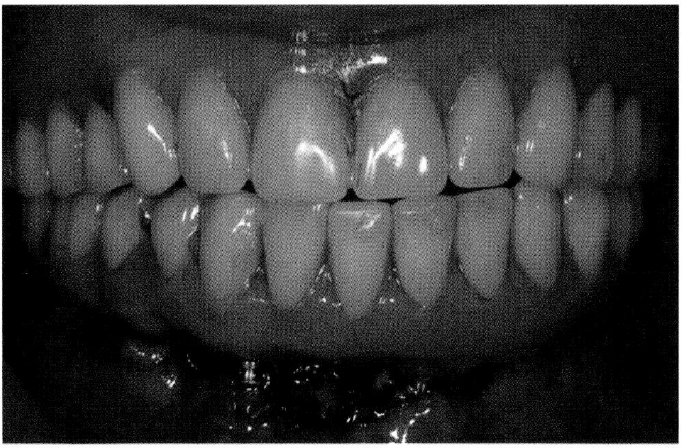

Figure 8.2. Immediate postoperative clinical anterior view of the patient in Figure 8.1.

Brånemark's protocol (Brånemark and others 1977) for dental implants included the following:

1. Machined commercially pure titanium implants
2. Two-stage surgical protocol with unloaded healing times of six months in edentulous maxillae and three to four months in edentulous mandibles
3. Atraumatic surgery
4. Sterile protocol
5. No intra-operative radiographs
6. Acrylic resin occlusal surfaces for screw-retained prostheses

This strict protocol led to high cumulative survival rates at up to 36 months post implant placement of 90.7% for implants with diameters less than 4 mm; 94.6% for implants with diameters of 4–5 mm; 66.7% for 7 mm-long implants and 96.4% for 16 mm-long implants (Winkler and others 2000).

Brånemark and others (1983) divided osseointegration into three phases: primary fixation; callus formation; and remodeling into mature, lamellar bone. Nonintegration of dental implants occurred when this sequence of events was disturbed (Brånemark 1985). The potential etiologies for nonintegration of dental implants included preparation trauma, infection, premature occlusal loading, and post occlusal overload. However, scientific evidence for premature occlusal loading has been disputed (Testori and others 2001; Testori and others 2002).

Immediate Occlusal Loading® in the Edentulous Mandible

Immediate Occlusal Loading® in the edentulous mandible has taken on several different names: DIEM™ (Implant Innovations, Inc., Palm Beach Gardens, FL) and Teeth in a Day™ (Prosthodontics Intermedica, Fort Washington, PA). Immediate Occlusal Loading® of multiple, splinted implants with a fixed, implant-retained prosthesis in the maxillae is evolving at the time of this publication but requires further investigation and long-term follow-up.

Immediate Occlusal Loading® (IOL®) in the edentulous mandible has been defined as implant placement with adequate primary stability and a fully functional occlusion at the time of implant placement (Schnitman and others 1997). This definition is specific regarding time and function of the implants (Figure 8.3).

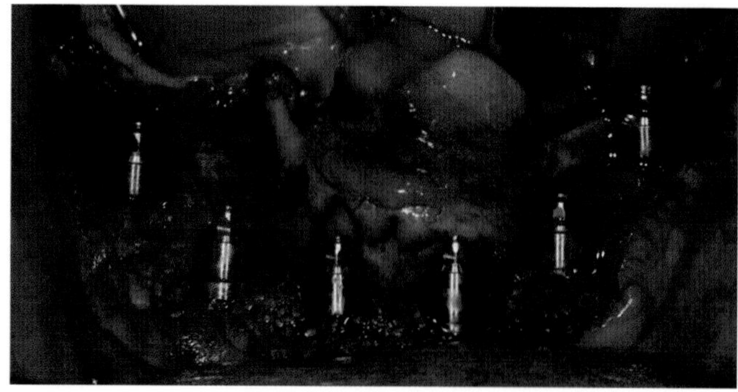

Figure 8.3. Patient with IOL® Abutments in place immediate post implant placement, prior to transfer to the author's office.

Immediate Occlusal Loading® has proven to be predictable when implants are placed with insertional torque values of at least 30 Ncm or greater (Testori and others 2001). This torque value is a quantitative measurement and correlates well with primary stability. Micromotion is the movement of an implant within an osteotomy. Tarnow (1997) quoted Brunski (1997) as stating that micromotion can be deleterious at the bone-implant interface, especially if the micromotion occurred soon after implantation. Brunski further stated that micromotion of more than 100 micrometers should be avoided because motion greater than this level would cause the wound to undergo fibrous repair rather than the desired osseous regeneration. Movement in the range of 50–100 micrometers is tolerated by implants and allows osseointegration.

Cross arch stabilization is accomplished when implants are splinted from one side of the arch to the other. This bilateral arrangement provides biomechanical advantages when connected by a rigid prosthesis. Cross arch stabilization is also a function of the anterior-posterior spread (AP) of implants in a given arch (McAlarney and Stavropoulos 1996). AP spread is measured by drawing a horizontal line across the most anterior implants and a second horizontal line through the middle of the most posterior implants. In definitive implant-retained prosthesis with a metal framework, the development of a cantilever distal to the last implants may range from 1.5 times the distance to one-half of this distance (English 1992).

Early investigators of Immediate Occlusal Loading® of dental implants included Schnitman, Tarnow, and Testori. Schnitman (1997) reported a 10-year study of 63 3.75 mm diameter machined, commercially pure titanium implants placed in 10 patients followed for 10 years. The 10-year cumulative survival rate (CSR) of all implants was 93.4%. The immediate loaded implants had a CSR of 84.7%, and the nonloaded implants had a CSR of 100%. Tarnow (1997) completed a five-year study and reported on the immediate loading of threaded implants in edentulous arches. Six of the patients had edentulous mandibles; four had edentulous maxillae. Fifty-nine implants were immediately loaded; 38 were nonloaded and healed without occlusal function. Fifty-seven of the 59 immediate loaded implants integrated, and 37 of the 38 submerged nonloaded implants integrated. Tarnow's conclusion was that immediate loading of multiple implants rigidly splinted, with cross-arch stabilization, can be a viable treatment option for edentulous patients.

Testori and others (2001) evaluated the healing of OSSEOTITE® implants with a submerged, traditional unloaded protocol and an immediate loading protocol in a single patient. It was a case report that quantified bone/implant contact surface area for two immediately loaded and one nonloaded implant eight weeks post implant placement. The case report described the treatment for one patient with 11 implants: five were allowed to heal with the traditional protocol and six were immediately loaded. Eight weeks post implant placement and immediate occlusal loading, three implants were removed and analyzed for bone implant contact. The two immediately loaded implants had significantly greater bone/implant contact (68%) than the nonloaded implants (34%). Immediate Occlusal Loading® of implants did not impede osseointegration and bone remodeling on the OSSEOTITE® surface.

Testori and others (2003) followed this clinical report with a study in which six patients received definitive prosthesis in occlusal function within 36 hours of implant placement surgery. All of the implants were clinically successful. They concluded that the treatment of edentulous mandibles with this Immediate Occlusal Loading® protocol supported by OSSEOTITE® implants seemed to be a viable option to the traditional nonloading healing protocol. High implant clinical survival rates and minimal bone loss were obtained with the immediate loading protocol immediately or up to a 36-hour period post implant placement. Drago and Lazzara (2005) reported similar findings with Immediate Occlusal Loading® of edentulous mandibles 12 months post implant placement. The CSR for the implants was 96.8%; the CSR for the prostheses was 100%.

DIEM™ Protocol

These investigators' efforts opened the door in 2003 for the transition into the DIEM™ protocol (Implant Innovations Inc., Palm Beach Gardens, FL). The protocol involves placement of at least four implants into an edentulous mandible, with insertional torque values of at least 30 Ncm and restoring the implants with a screw-retained prosthesis on the same day. Implant restorative components have been developed to facilitate fabrication of this type of prosthesis. It provides patients with a fixed, screw-retained implant prosthesis with a fully functional occlusion on the day of implant placement. The protocol can be adapted to dentulous patients who have had their teeth extracted on the day of implant placement, as well as edentulous patients who can leave the office with fixed, screw-retained implant prostheses on the same day.

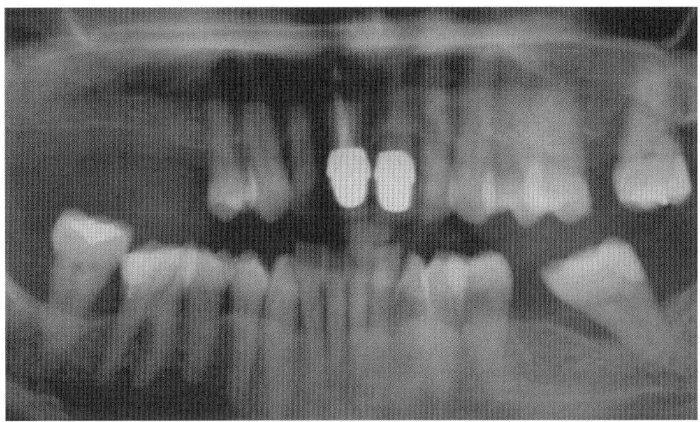

Figure 8.4. Pre-operative panoramic radiograph that demonstrated moderate to advanced bone loss throughout the dentition.

This type of dentistry clearly requires a team concept for restorative dentists, implant surgeons, and laboratory technicians. This protocol is restoratively driven but surgically determined in that all of the criteria for Immediate Occlusal Loading® have to be satisfied prior to the loading of the implants on the day of placement. If one or more of the criteria are not satisfied, implants may be placed and not loaded or grafting may be required prior to implant placement at a later date. Restorative dentists have the role of coordinating treatment logistics. Extensive pre-operative treatment planning is necessary to determine such details as to whether the patient will be treated at the surgical and restorative offices on the same day or whether the procedures will be extended to occur over a 36-hour period.

CLINICAL CASE PRESENTATION

Appointment 1. Initial Examination (Surgical Office; One Hour)

This patient was self-referred. The receptionist at the front desk sent this patient a personal letter welcoming her to the practice prior to the initial examination appointment. This letter introduced the entire staff to the patient and also discussed the philosophy of the practice. After the patient arrived at the office, the receptionists introduced themselves in person and again welcomed the patient to the practice.

The surgical implant coordinator re-explained what would be accomplished at this visit, noting that the initial visit would last approximately 60 minutes and that this visit was one of potentially two diagnostic visits in the treatment process. The patient was also asked to bring a family member or individual to accompany the patient at any future appointments.

Radiographs

Radiographs were taken at this time (Figure 8.4).

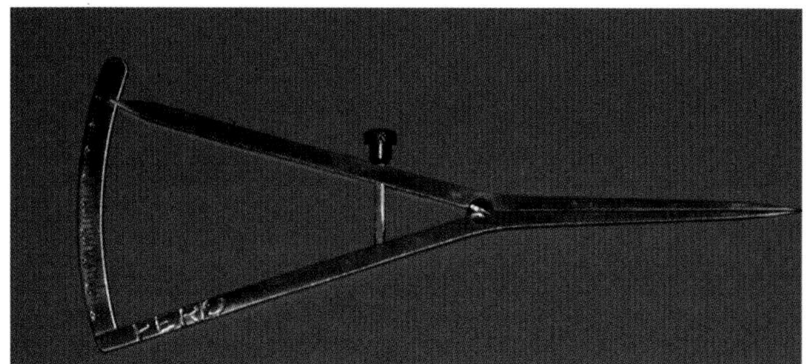

Figure 8.5. Castroviejo caliper used to measure the amount of interocclusal distance available for osteotomy and implant placement.

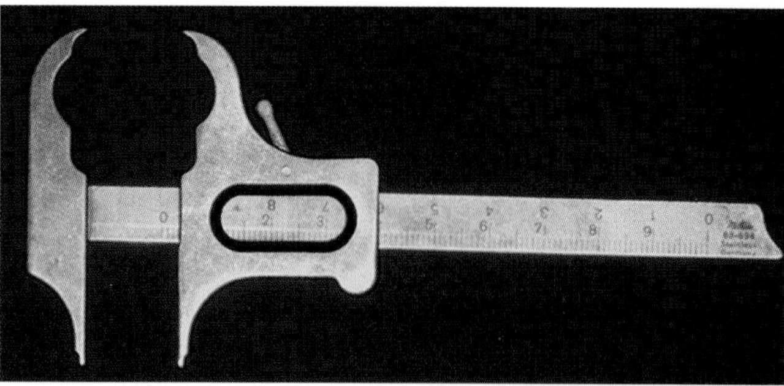

Figure 8.6. Boley gauge used to measure the width of the alveolus pre-operatively.

Chief Complaint

A 56-year-old female presented for care. The patient's chief complaint was: "My teeth hurt and I want them removed. I also want to consider dental implants for my treatment." The medical and dental histories with all medications were recorded.

Physical Examination

Extra- and intra-oral physical examinations were completed including periodontal pocket measurements and tooth mobility. Measurement of the patient's ability to open at potential implant sites was recorded with a long Castroviejo caliper (Ace Surgical Supply Co., Inc., Brockton, MA) (Figure 8.5). The bone and tissue thickness were recorded with Boley gauge calipers (Boley Gauge, Ace Surgical Co., Brockton, MA) at the same sites (Figure 8.6).

Diagnosis

1. Type III and Type IV chronic periodontitis, with lack of attached gingiva for teeth 20 and 29 (Figure 8.7)
2. Partially edentulous maxillae and mandible (Figure 8.8)
3. Dental caries
4. Class II malocclusion
5. Adequate bone volume for implant placement in the mandible
6. Moderate anxiety toward dental treatment

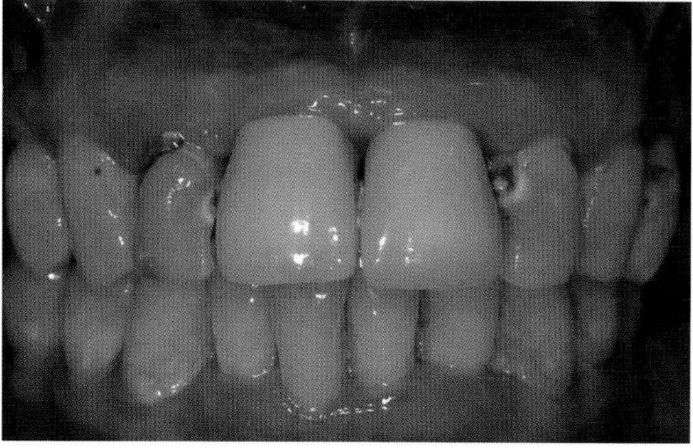

Figure 8.7. Pre-operative anterior clinical image that demonstrated advanced periodontal disease.

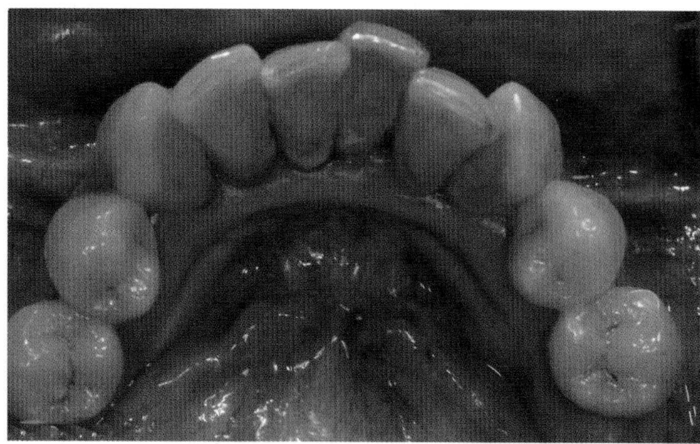

Figure 8.8. Pre-operative mandibular occlusal image that demonstrated a satisfactory anterior/posterior spread of the natural teeth.

Prognosis

The deterioration of the dentition at such an early age was projected to continue, and the patient agreed that the dentition would require a significant effort to restore. Multiple treatment plans were discussed including periodontal surgery, endodontics, crowns, fixed partial and removable partial dentures, complete dentures, overdentures, and dental implants with and without the Immediate Occlusal Loading® protocol (IOL®). The patient's lack of commitment to maintain reasonable oral hygiene, the cost to replace the missing teeth and restore the remaining teeth, and the potential for recurrent caries and periodontal disease, was beyond her means and desires. Maintenance of the natural dentition could require additional costly treatment in the future, and the prognosis considering her care and retention of the restored dentition was extremely poor.

The prognosis for extractions, alveolectomy, implant placement, and Immediate Occlusal Loading® for a mandibular denture and a complete maxillary denture was favorable, and she accepted it as her treatment option. The costs over the long term were figured to be less than the treatment option that included maintenance of her natural dentition. The IOL® denture should provide better function, aesthetics, and phonetics on a long-term basis. The interest and commitment to proceed expressed by the patient resulted in completion of the radiographic examinations, which included a computerized tomogram of the mandible and individual periapical and bitewing radiographs (Figures 8.9, 8.10, 8.11).

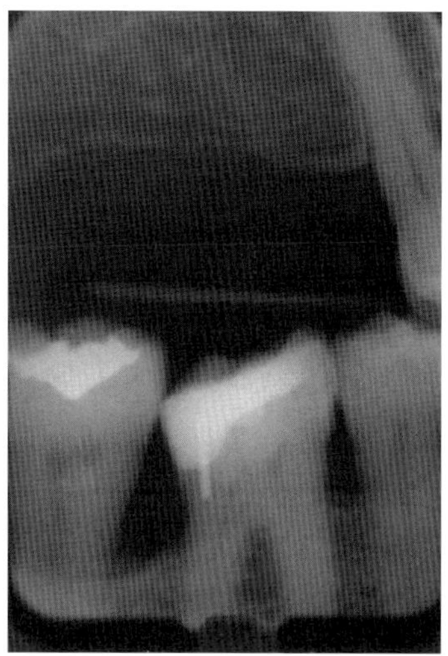

Figure 8.9. Right bitewing radiograph of the posterior right segment.

Appointment 2. Examination/Consultation Restorative Dentist/Patient (One Hour)

The patient was referred by the periodontist to the author for examination, diagnosis, and treatment planning relative to extraction of the remaining mandibular teeth, placement of dental implants, and Immediate Occlusal Loading®.

Examination

Because the patient had already been examined by the periodontist, additional radiographs were not necessary. The physical examination was unremarkable. The findings were consistent with the findings of the periodontal examination.

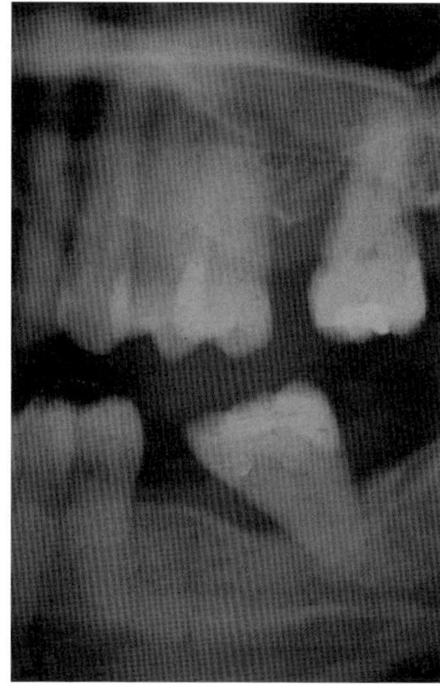

Figure 8.10. Left bitewing radiograph of the posterior left segment.

Diagnosis

1. Type III and Type IV chronic periodontitis, with lack of attached gingiva for teeth 20 and 29
2. Partially edentulous maxillae and mandible
3. Dental caries
4. Class II malocclusion
5. Adequate bone volume for implant placement in the mandible
6. Adequate restorative volume for implant restoration with a fixed implant-retained mandibular prosthesis
7. Moderate anxiety toward dental treatment

Treatment Options

The first treatment option described the extraction of the maxillary teeth and replacement with an immediate denture. It then included the extraction, alveolectomy, and placement of four to six implants in the edentulous mandible by the periodontist. The patient would be transferred to the prosthodontic office for placement of a screw-retained prosthesis (Table 8.1). The second treatment option described the extraction of the remaining teeth and replacement with immediate complete dentures. If the

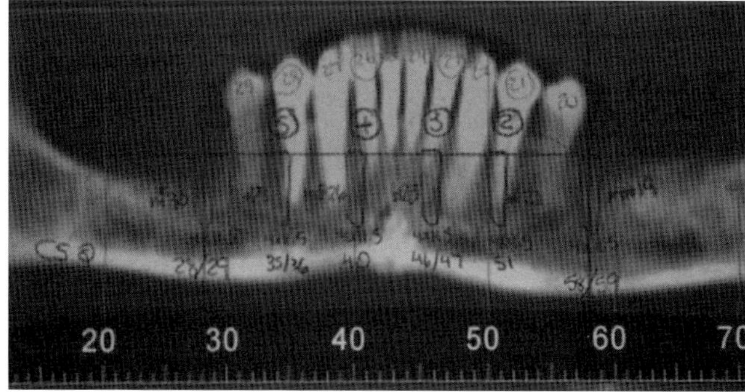

Figure 8.11. Panoramic CT image with diagnostic work up relative to proposed implant sites and implant sizes.

TABLE 8.1. Treatment Plan #1 (Maxillary Immediate Denture; Mandibular Extractions, Implant Placement and Immediate Occlusal Loading® of a Screw-Retained Prosthesis)

Diagnosis: Type III and Type IV chronic periodontitis

Restorative Services	**ADA #**	**Fee**
Comprehensive oral evaluation	D0150	
Diagnostic casts	D0470	
Panoramic radiograph	D0330	
Maxillary immediate complete denture	D5130	
Referral to periodontal office:		
1. Extract the maxillary teeth and insert maxillary immediate denture		
2. Discharge to prosthodontist for denture follow-up care		
3. Tissue conditioning of immediate maxillary complete denture	D5850	
Fees and services will be determined by the periodontist.		
Restorative reevaluation	D0140	
Fabrication of IOL® denture	D9999	

Referral to periodontal office:

1. Extract all mandibular teeth, perform alveolectomy to provide adequate restorative volume for the IOL® denture
2. Place 4–6 OSSEOTITE® implants from first molar to first molar, with an adequate A/P spread
3. Implants should achieve insertional torque values of at least 30 Ncm to be included in the DIEM denture
4. Place IOL® Abutments so that the collar heights are slightly above the gingival margin
5. Discharge to prosthodontist for fabrication of the IOL® denture

Follow-up prosthetic care	D9999	
Year recall	D0120	
Panoramic radiograph	D0330	

Benefits of Treatment Plan #1

Periodontal disease of all teeth will be taken care of via extraction of all teeth. The upper teeth will be replaced with a complete denture; the lower teeth will be replaced with a screw-retained implant prosthesis that will not be removable by the patient. Patient should enjoy improved function with a good long-term prognosis. Patient should also have improved aesthetics.

Limitations of Treatment Plan #1

Cost, complexity, and length of treatment (2–3 months). The upper denture will move. Bone loss will continue beneath the upper denture. Implants are generally successful in the lower jaw about 96–98% of the time. The implants have to obtain a high enough insertional torque value so as to achieve primary stability. At least four highly stable implants are required for the immediate loading protocol to be successful. If fewer than four implants achieve a high enough insertional torque value, the patient will leave with a conventional denture. A definitive screw-retained prosthesis will be constructed approximately 2–3 months after implant placement. The implants have to be placed optimally for the above treatment to be accomplished. If the implants are not placed optimally, changes in the treatments, designs, and fees will be likely. The patient will be asked to take the upper denture out during nighttime sleep. The patient will be expected to return for scheduled post-insertion office visits that may include radiographs, clinical examinations, and potential removal of the fixed prosthesis in the lower jaw.

Patient signature ______________________________

Date ______________________________

Witness ______________________________

Date ______________________________

ADA #'s, CDT 2005 Current Dental Terminology, Council on Dental Benefit Programs, American Dental Association, 211 East Chicago Avenue, Chicago, IL 60611

denture experience was unsatisfactory, implants could be considered at a later date for increased retention and stability of one or both dentures (Meijer and others 1996; Awad and others 2003) (Table 8.2). The third treatment option deferred prosthetic treatment at this time (Table 8.3).

Benefits and limitations of each treatment option were described in detail on the written treatment plans. The prosthodontic fees, or ranges of fees for each procedure, were also listed on each treatment plan. The patient was given copies of the treatment plans, and after some consideration, the patient agreed to proceed with the first treatment plan including implant placement and insertion

TABLE 8.2. Treatment Plan #2 (Maxillary Immediate Denture; Mandibular Immediate Denture)

Diagnosis: Type III and Type IV chronic periodontitis

Restorative Services	**ADA #**	**Fee**
Comprehensive oral evaluation	D0150	
Diagnostic casts	D0470	
Panoramic radiograph	D0330	
Maxillary immediate complete denture	D5130	
Mandibular immediate complete denture	D5140	
Referral to periodontal office:		
1. Extract all of the maxillary and mandibular teeth and insert maxillary and mandibular immediate dentures		
2. Discharge to prosthodontist for denture follow-up care		
3. Tissue conditioning of immediate maxillary complete denture	D5850	
4. Tissue conditioning of immediate mandibular complete denture	D5851	
Fees and services will be determined by the periodontist.		
Prosthetic reevaluation	D0140	
If denture experience has been successful		
Laboratory processed reline maxillary immediate denture	D5750	
Laboratory processed reline mandibular immediate denture	D5751	
If denture experience has been unsuccessful		
Consideration for implants in one or both jaws		
Fees and services to be determined		

Benefits of Treatment Plan #2

Periodontal disease of all teeth will be taken care of via extraction of all teeth. The upper and lower teeth will be replaced with immediate complete dentures. Patient should have improved function with a fair long-term prognosis. Patient should also have improved aesthetics.

Limitations of Treatment Plan #2

Cost, complexity, and length of treatment (4–6 months). Both dentures will move. The patient will be asked to take both dentures out during nighttime sleep. Bone loss will continue beneath both dentures. The patient will be expected to return for scheduled post-insertion office visits that may include radiographs and clinical examinations. Both dentures will have to relined at appropriate times to compensate for resorption of the jawbones and resulting ill fit of one or both dentures.

Patient signature ______________________________

Date ______________________________

Witness ______________________________

Date ______________________________

ADA #'s, CDT 2005 Current Dental Terminology, Council on Dental Benefit Programs, American Dental Association, 211 East Chicago Avenue, Chicago, IL 60611

TABLE 8.3. No Definitive Treatment

Diagnosis: Type III and Type IV chronic periodontitis		
Restorative Services	**ADA #**	**Fee**
Comprehensive oral evaluation	D0150	
Diagnostic casts	D0470	
Panoramic radiograph	D0330	
Prosthetic reevaluation	D0140	

Benefits of Treatment Plan #3

Patient will retain all remaining natural teeth.

Limitations of Treatment Plant #3

Patient's dentition will be at risk for loss secondary to periodontal disease. Patient will be at risk for dental infections and toothaches. Bone loss secondary to periodontal disease will continue and may compromise the bone volume if implants are to be placed.

Patient signature ______________________

Date ______________________

Witness ______________________

Date ______________________

ADA #'s, CDT 2005 Current Dental Terminology, Council on Dental Benefit Programs, American Dental Association, 211 East Chicago Avenue, Chicago, IL 60611

of a fixed implant-retained prosthesis on the same day. She was referred to the first author for the surgical diagnostic work-up.

Appointment 3. Consultation Restorative Dentist/Surgeon (1/2 Hour)

Number/Size of Implants

The surgeon discussed the height and width of the mandibular arch in anticipation of implant placement. The surgeon preferred the OSSEOTITE NT® implant system. The tentative size was decided to include 4.1 mm restorative platforms with 11.5 mm lengths. Optimal A/P spread includes placing implants distal to the mental foramen, which generally means the mesial occlusal fossae of the mandibular first molars. However, this procedure requires a CT scan so that the location of the inferior alveolar canals can be identified. Implants placed distal to the mental foramen sometimes require adequate bone reduction to allow adequate space for the implant abutments, temporary cylinders, and denture. This reduction must remain above the inferior alveolar canal and within the vertical dimension of occlusion (VDO) originally measured by the restorative dentist. Implants are generally placed a minimum of 8 mm on center.

Implant surgical volumes need to be approximately 6 mm in width to accommodate 4 mm diameter implants. Alveolar ridge width generally increases as the height of the residual ridge is reduced with the alveolectomy. Mandibular bone is generally harder than maxillary bone, which results in increased likelihood for primary stability in excess of 30 Ncm of insertional torque. Computerized tomo-

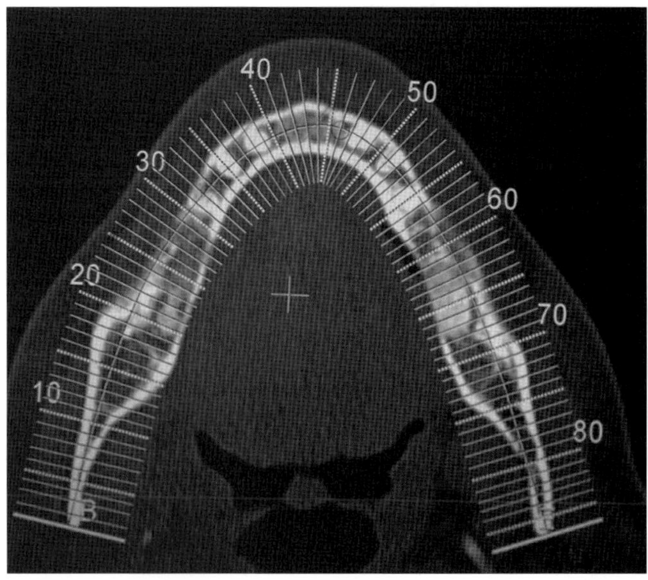

Figure 8.12. Mandibular occlusal CT scan with individual markings 1 mm apart that identified and allowed accurate transfer of information from the CT scan to the mouth.

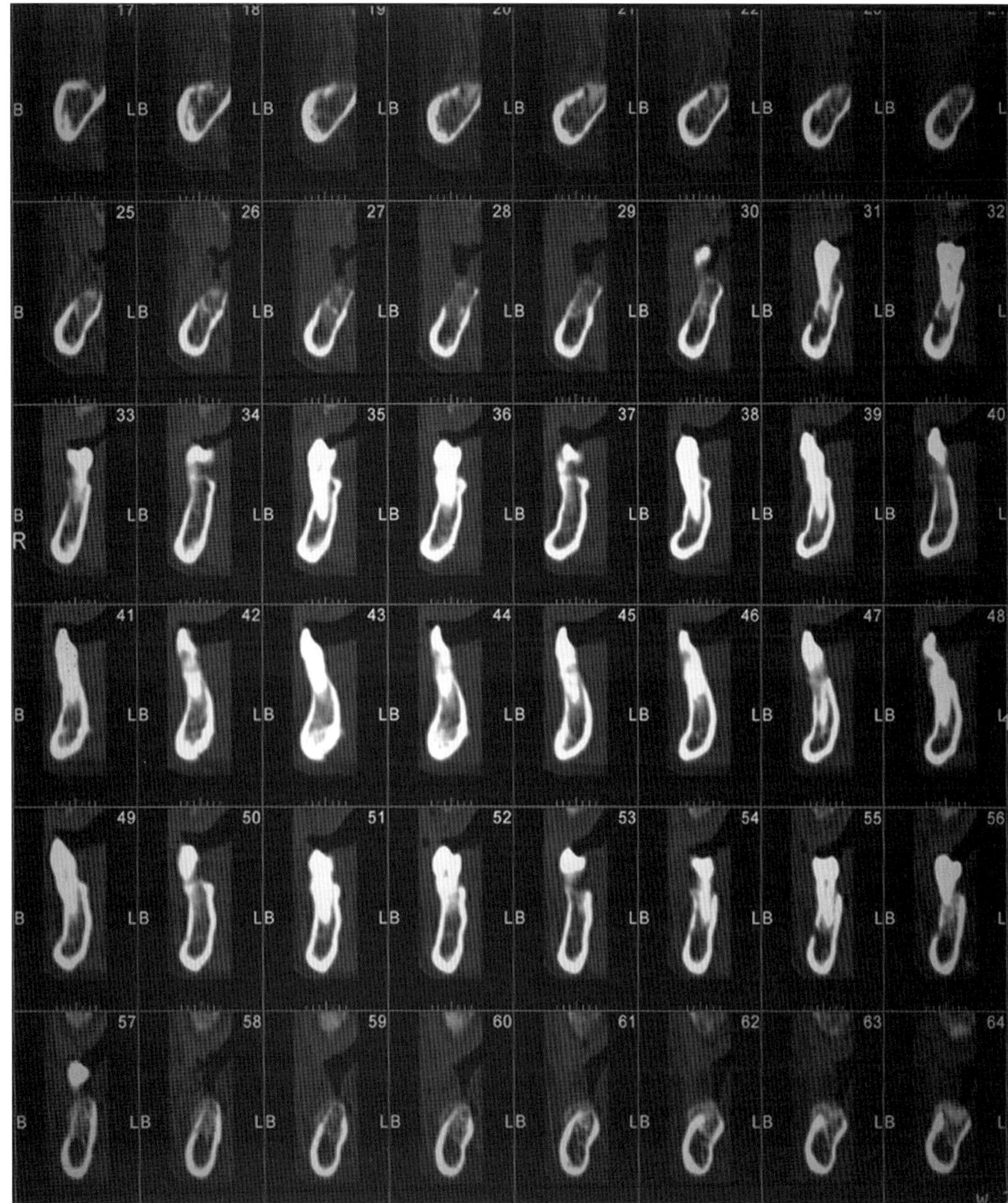

Figure 8.13. Cross sectional oblique CT images. The numbers of each view correspond to the numbers in the occlusal CT scan in Figure 8.12.

grams (CT cross section obliques) (Figures 8.12 and 8.13) are extremely helpful for determining the buccal/lingual width pre-operatively. If there is inadequate width, the IOL® protocol may not be possible. Bone grafting may be required prior to implant placement. Bone grafting delays the treatment time. However, the IOL® protocol may still be accomplished after the bone graft has healed.

The treatment option identified for this patient consisted of an immediate maxillary denture, followed by healing and adaptation prior to the maxillary complete denture before performing the IOL® protocol in the mandible. This treatment plan was thought to have a better prognosis than treating both jaws at one visit. Six implants (4 × 11.5 mm) were decided as the ideal number for the mandibular treatment.

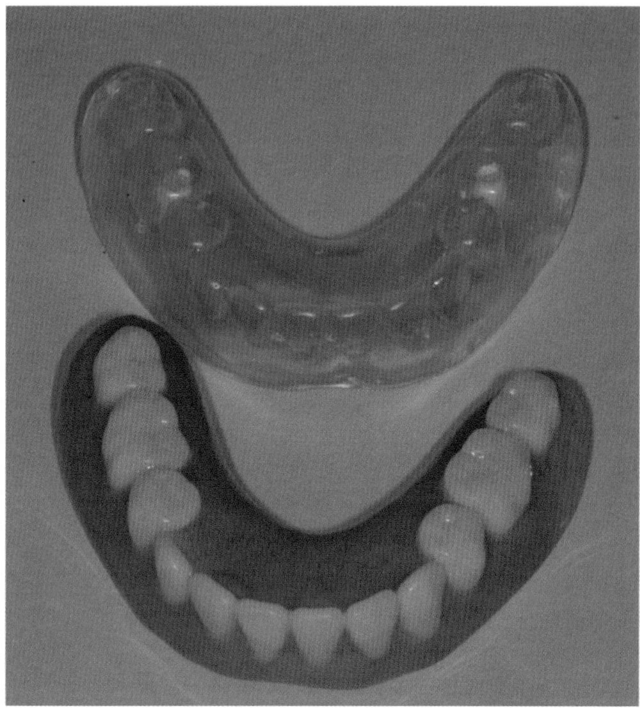

Figure 8.14. The surgical guide (top) was fabricated as a duplicate of the mandibular DIEM™ denture (bottom).

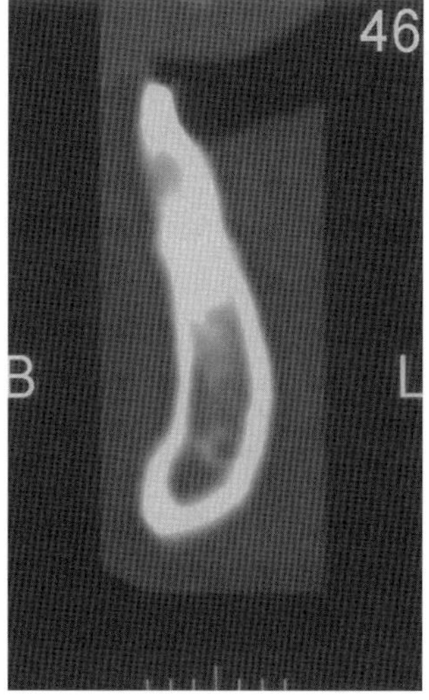

Figure 8.15. Lateral oblique CT scan of proposed implant location.

The surgical guide was fabricated as a duplicate of the mandibular prosthesis (Figure 8.14). Using the CT cross section obliques, six implant locations were identified, as well as the required reduction of mandible after extraction of the natural teeth, to permit adequate bulk for the mandibular IOL® denture without impinging on the predetermined Vertical Dimension of Occlusion (Figures 8.15, 8.16, 8.17, 8.18, 8.19, 8.20).

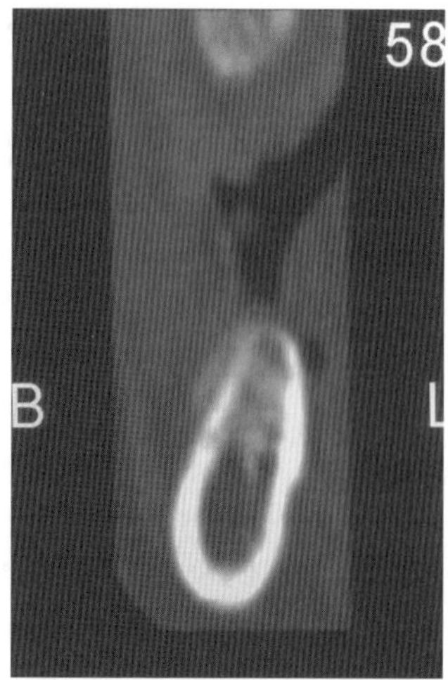

Figure 8.16. Lateral oblique CT scan of proposed implant location.

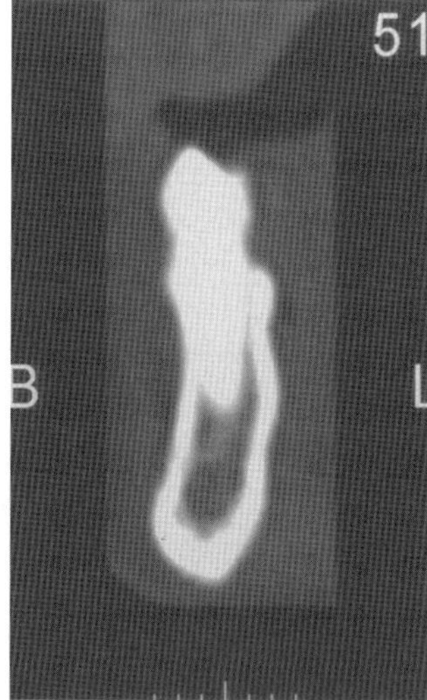

Figure 8.17. Lateral oblique CT scan of proposed implant location.

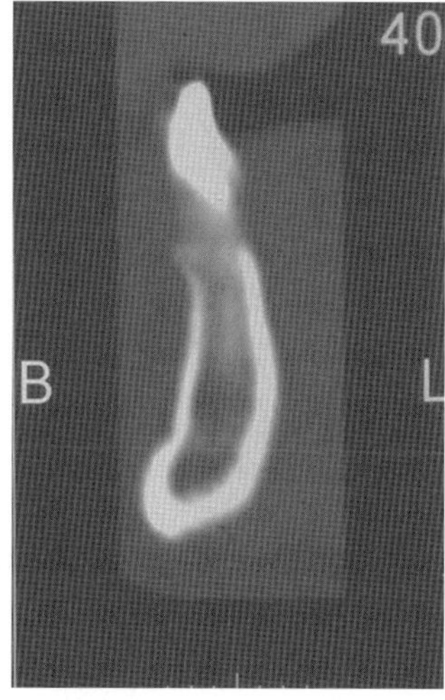

Figure 8.18. Lateral oblique CT scan of proposed implant location.

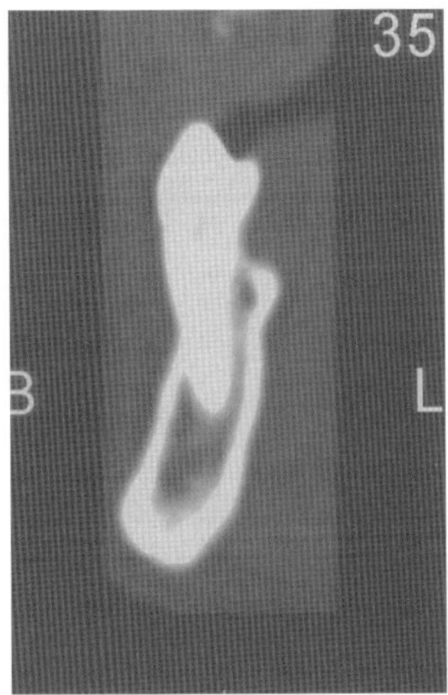

Figure 8.19. Lateral oblique CT scan of proposed implant location.

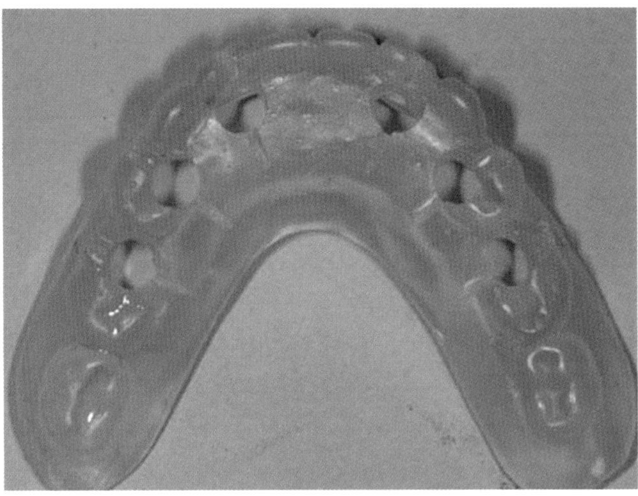

Figure 8.21. Occlusal view of mandibular surgical guide with holes corresponding to the proposed implant sites prepared as part of the preoperative surgical work-up.

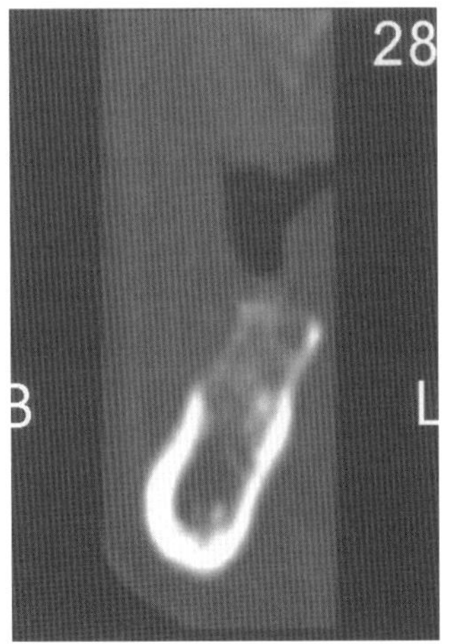

Figure 8.20. Lateral oblique CT scan of proposed implant location.

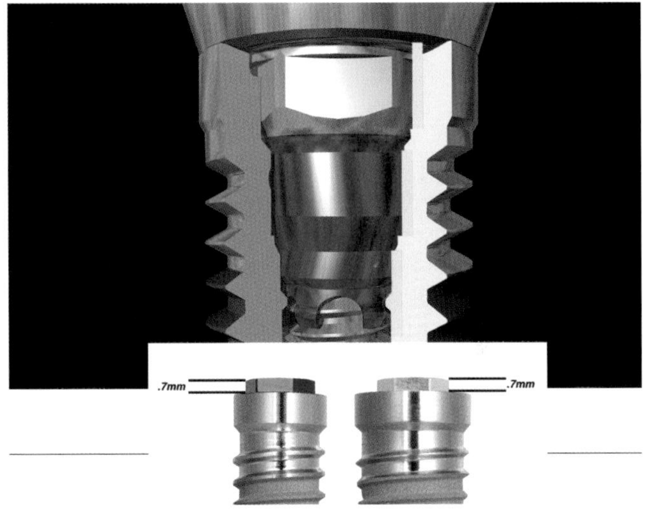

Figure 8.22. Diagrammatic representation of internal connection (top) and external hex (bottom) implant/abutment connections.

Prosthesis Design

A screw-retained prosthesis was agreed upon to be the treatment of choice. This required optimal implant placement within the occlusal surfaces of the posterior teeth and lingual to the facial surfaces of the anterior teeth (Figure 8.21).

Implant/Abutment Connection

3i®'s implant systems are available with both internal and external implant/abutment connections (Figure 8.22). In full arch edentulous situations, both connections have worked well. In this case, the surgeon placed OSSEOTITE NT® implants (external hex implant/abutment connections).

Surgical Work-Up and Protocol

The periodontist determined the long axis and inclination of the teeth in the locations selected for implant placement by using the CT scans: sagittal, panoramic, and cross section oblique views. The implant locations were identified and the amount of bone reduction for each alveolectomy was determined. The surgical guide as received from the prosthodontist was opened at the sites identified from the CT scan. The center of each potential implant site was marked with a burr on the buccal and lingual flanges of the surgical guide.

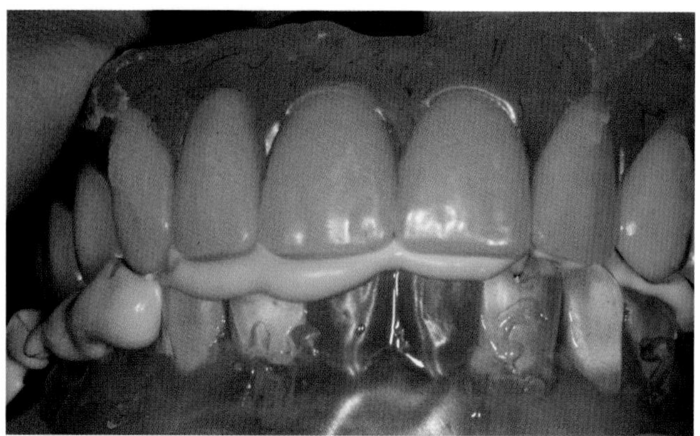

Figure 8.23. Pre-operative laboratory inter-occlusal record between the maxillary denture and surgical guide.

Selection of implants on the large full plate of lateral oblique views was identified from 1–6, number 1 on the left being the largest number cross section oblique (CSO) and number 6 on the right being the smallest numbered CSO.

The tentative surgical protocol involved the use of directional guide pins placed in a sequence that allowed the handpiece unobstructed movement. In this instance the surgeon planned on placing the first implant in the anterior left quadrant in the location of tooth #23 (CSO 46). The second implant was placed in the mesial fossa of the mandibular left first molar (CSO 58). Its angulation related to the orientation of the first anterior left directional guide pin. The remaining placements were planned as follows: the third implant, tooth #21 (CSO 51); the fourth implant, tooth #27 (CSO 40); the fifth implant, tooth #28 (CSO 35); the sixth implant in the mesial fossa of the mandibular right molar (CSO 28).

A laboratory centric occlusion registration (Figure 8.23) was made to orient the maxillary and mandibular dentures and surgical guide. This step would facilitate correctly orienting the denture and guide during the surgical appointment. The surgical guide was reduced along the flanges and the retromolar pad areas.

Appointment 4. Surgical Reevaluation (1/2 Hour)

The patient returned for a reevaluation with the implant surgeon. The radiographic studies were interpreted for her. The benefits and limitations of the surgical treatment were discussed, as were some of the prosthetic benefits and limitations. The type of sedation was also discussed. All of the questions asked by patient and her spouse were answered. The surgical appointment was scheduled for 120 minutes and pre-operative photographs were taken. The prescription medications were discussed and given to her, along with a detailed schedule for ingestion. For example, the patient was instructed to take the antibiotic early in the morning prior to the surgical appointment. The surgical consent forms were signed and witnessed by one dental assistant at the end of the reevaluation appointment.

The patient was discharged to the prosthodontist for the prosthetic phase of treatment including extraction of the maxillary teeth and insertion of the maxillary immediate denture. This portion of the treatment is not discussed.

Appointment 5. Definitive Impressions and Jaw Relation Record (1/2 Hour)

The patient presented for this appointment without complaints and was quite pleased with the maxillary immediate denture.

Because the DIEM® denture would be retained by the implants, there was no need to make a traditional border molded impression. Alginate impressions were made of the partially edentulous mandible and of the maxillary immediate denture.

A jaw relation record was made at the existing vertical dimension of occlusion with a poly vinylsiloxane bite registration material. Because the patient was already pleased with the aesthetic results associated with the maxillary complete denture, this appointment was relatively quick and did not involve the conventional prosthodontic steps associated with construction of complete dentures (Pound 1970; Landa 1952).

Diagnostic Casts

The impressions were poured in dental stone (Figures 8.24 and 8.25).

There was an adequate number of posterior teeth, so a mandibular record base was not required for the articulator mounting. The maxillary denture was already deemed acceptable, so the centric jaw relation record was made at the existing vertical dimension of occlusion. However, a maxillary record base and occlusion rim was fabricated for the initial jaw relation records appointment for construction of the maxillary immediate denture.

Articulator Mounting

The articulator mounting was actually done in conjunction with the maxillary immediate denture (Figure 8.26). The teeth were removed from the diagnostic casts in preparation for the maxillary immediate complete denture and the mandibular DIEM denture. Tooth and alveolar ridge reduction on the mandibular cast was minimized (Figure 8.27). This allowed the inner volume of the mandibular denture to be greater than a conventional immediate denture (Figure

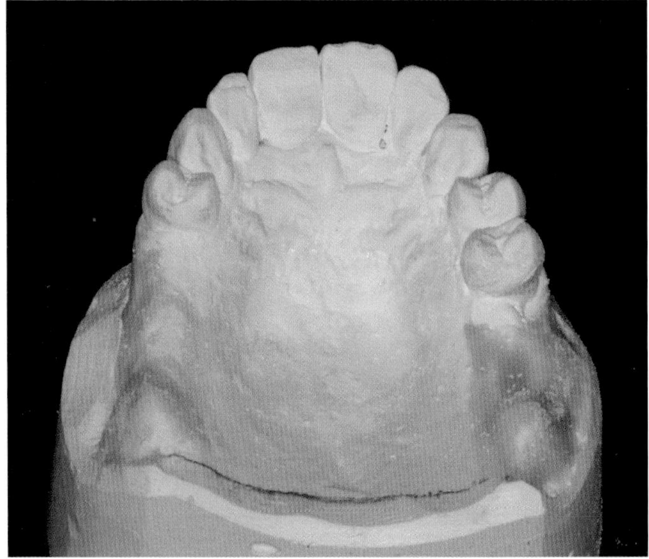

Figure 8.24. Maxillary diagnostic cast.

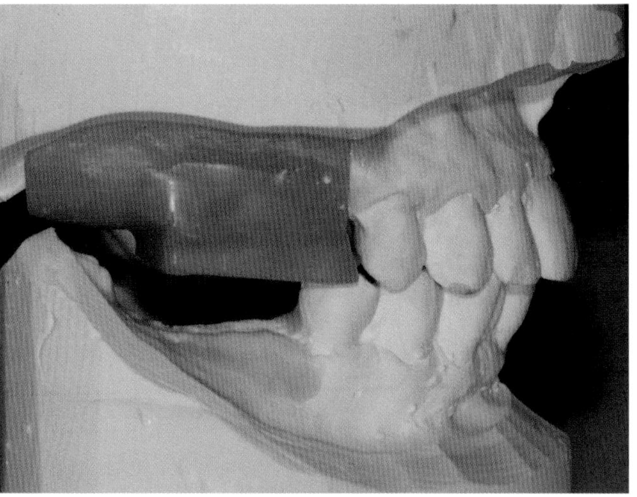

Figure 8.26. Laboratory articulator mounting at the preexisting vertical dimension of occlusion.

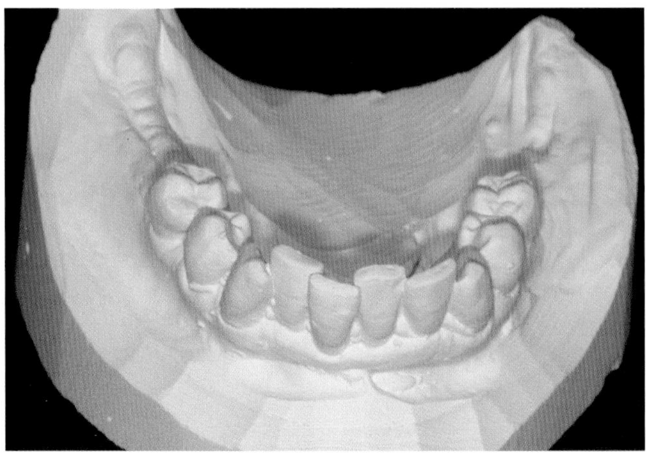

Figure 8.25. Mandibular diagnostic cast that was used to fabricate the DIEM™ denture.

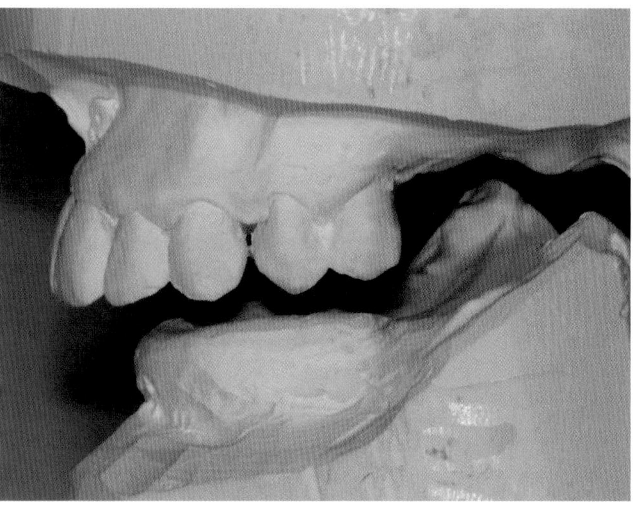

Figure 8.27. Laboratory lateral view after the mandibular teeth were extracted from the mandibular diagnostic cast.

8.28). The result was a larger volume within the intaglio surface, which would mean less adjustment at the insertion appointment.

Appointment 6. Wax Try-In (1/2 Hour)

The wax try-in was accomplished in conjunction with the maxillary immediate denture series of appointments (Figure 8.29).

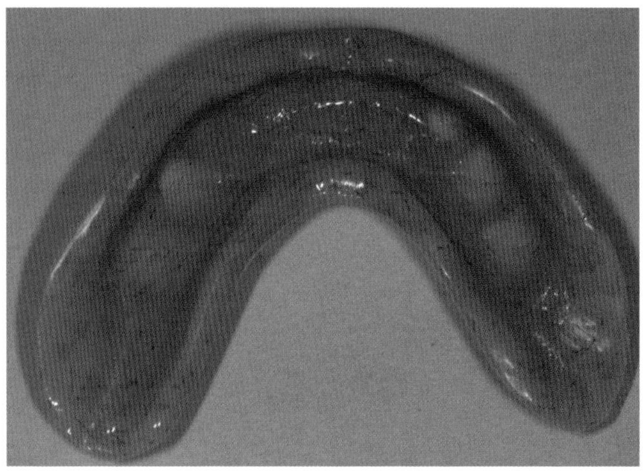

Figure 8.28. Intaglio surface of the DIEM™ denture. The volume was significantly bigger than a traditional immediate denture.

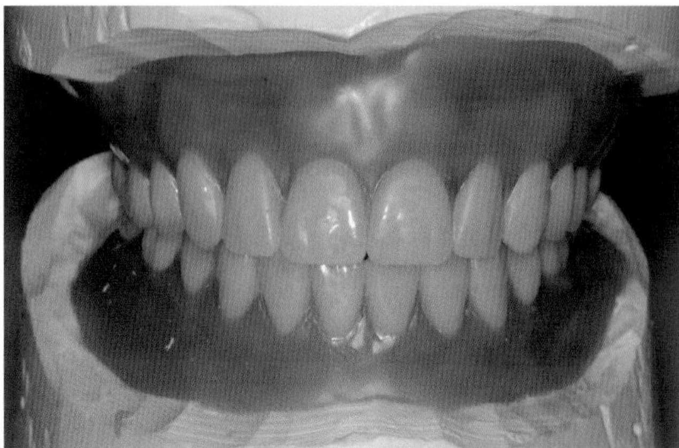

Figure 8.29. Waxed dentures prior to processing.

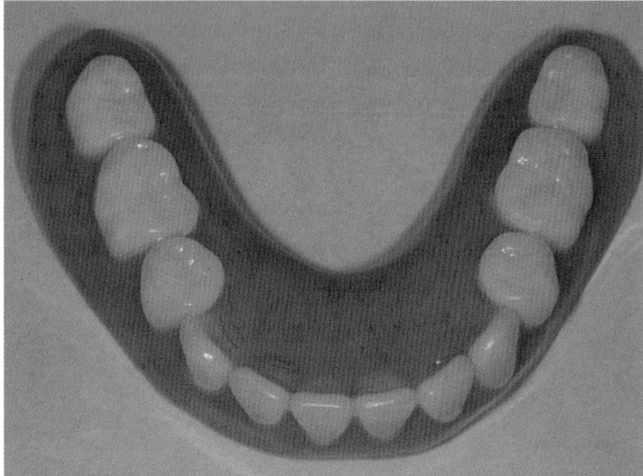

Figure 8.30. The processed mandibular DIEM™ denture.

Laboratory Procedures/Work Orders for Processing Dentures

The dentures were waxed, processed, and finished in conventional fashion. The maxillary denture was inserted first, as previously noted. The DIEM denture was completed at the same time (Figure 8.30). The DIEM denture was contoured significantly differently as compared to a conventional immediate denture. The flanges were significantly shorter and the retromolar pads were not covered. The DIEM denture was duplicated in clear acrylic resin for use as a surgical guide (Figure 8.31).

The work orders for the DIEM denture and surgical guide are located in Table 8.4.

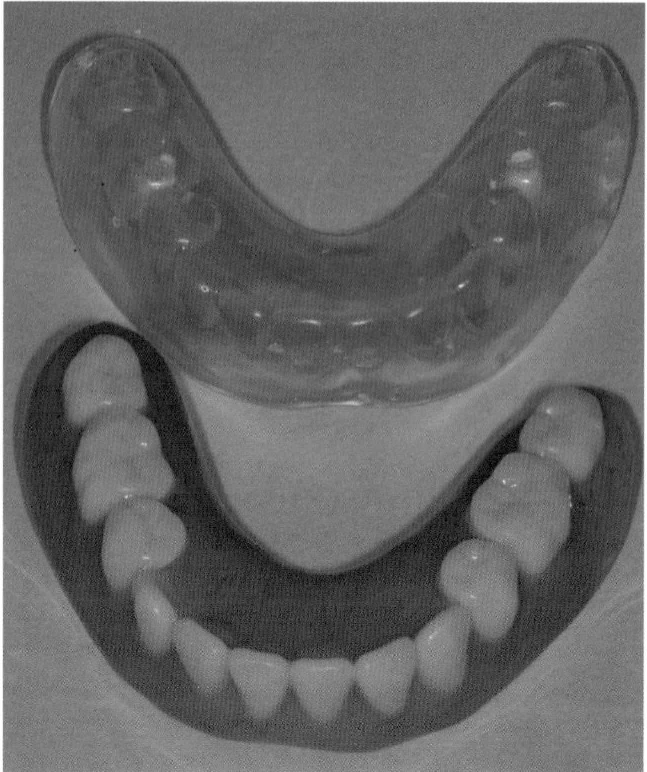

Figure 8.31. The processed surgical guide was made in clear acrylic resin (top); DIEM™ denture (bottom).

TABLE 8.4. Work Orders for Fabrication of DIEM Denture

Enclosed:

1. Articulator mounting of maxillary diagnostic cast of a complete denture
2. Mandibular waxed denture
3. Set teeth in tight Class I centric occlusion
4. Balancing contacts are not required
5. Wax final contours
6. Process in heat-cured acrylic resin
7. Remount and correct for occlusal processing error
8. Finish and polish
9. Duplicate in clear acrylic resin for use as a surgical guide
10. Finish and polish the surgical guide
11. Return to the periodontal office

Appointment 7. Implant/Prosthesis Placement

Surgical Protocol (2 1/2 Hours)

The pre-operative consent form was signed and witnessed. It was confirmed by the surgical implant coordinator that the pre-operative antibiotics were taken and the patient was ready to proceed.

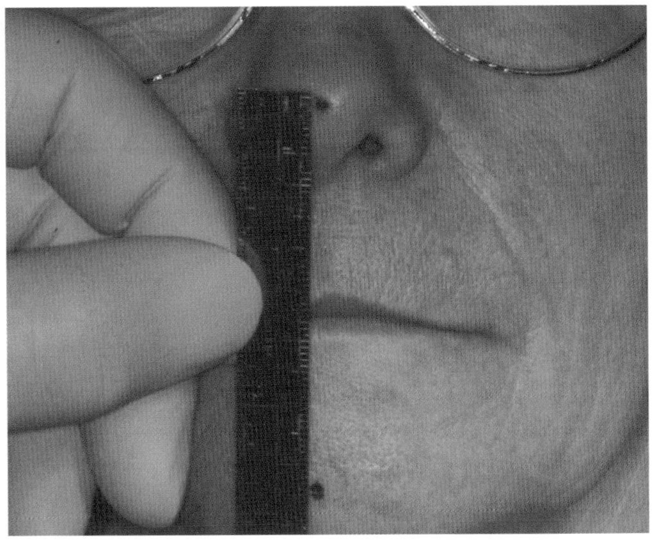

Figure 8.32. With the patient seated upright and her head unsupported, dots were placed on the patient's nose and chin. This measurement was recorded.

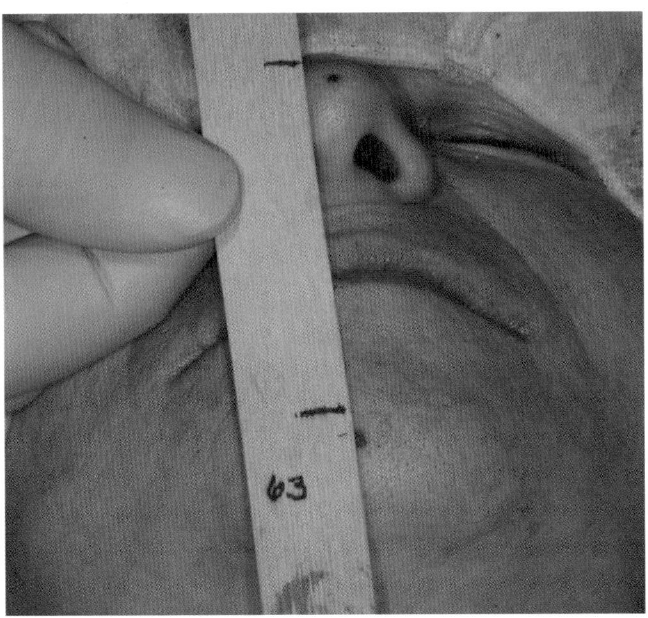

Figure 8.33. This photograph identified the increase in the vertical dimension of occlusion as measured with a reclined patient.

The patient was gowned and moved into the surgical suite. While she was seated upright, with her head unsupported, the vertical dimension of occlusion (VDO) (Figures 8.32 and 8.33) was identified by placing marks on the nose and chin. These marks were transferred to a tongue blade and measured. Typical measurements generally range between 60 and 70 mm.

Monitoring equipment was placed on the patient for blood pressure, EKG, and oxygen saturation. The intravenous

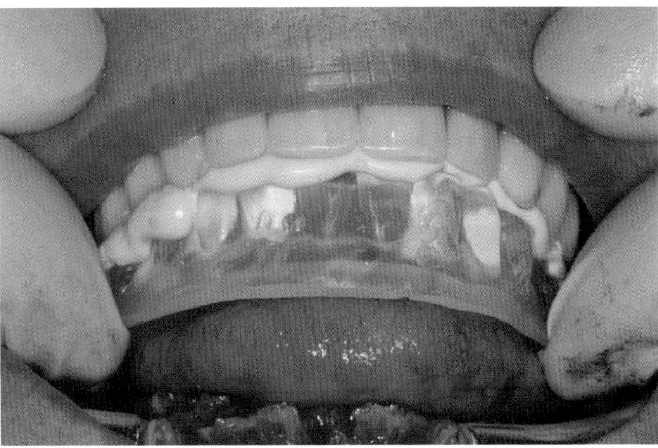

Figure 8.34. Intra-oral image with surgical guide/inter-occlusal record/maxillary denture in place. The inter-occlusal record facilitated accurate repositioning of the surgical guide against the maxillary denture.

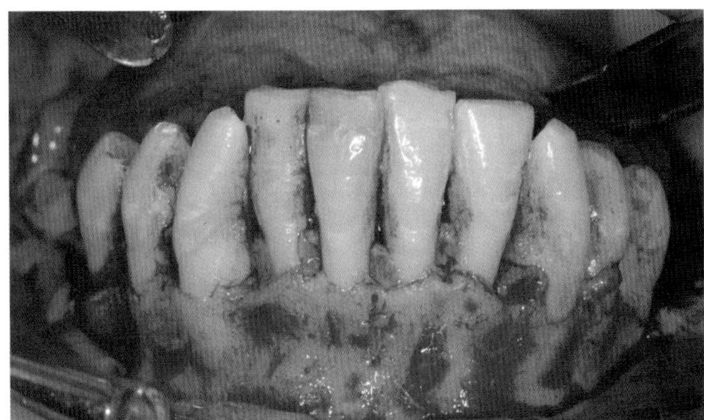

Figure 8.35. A full thickness mucoperiosteal flap was reflected prior to extraction of the remaining mandibular teeth.

line was placed and sedation was started with Diazepam (Diazepam Injection, USP, Hospira, Inc., Lake Forest, IL). Local anesthesia was administered via bilateral inferior alveolar nerve blocks along with papillary and sulcular infiltration with 2% Xylocaine (Lidocaine) with 1:100,000 and 1:50,000 epinephrine. The pre-operative inter-occlusal record that was made in the laboratory using the maxillary denture and the DIEM denture was tried in (refer to Figure 8.23). This registration was made as a full arch record and has proven to be useful in aiding implant surgeons with accurate positioning of the surgical guides and DIEM dentures during surgery (Figure 8.34).

The remaining mandibular teeth were removed (Figure 8.35). The appropriate amount of alveolar bone reduction was determined from the radiographic studies and is critical for successful treatment. The initial amount of alveolar

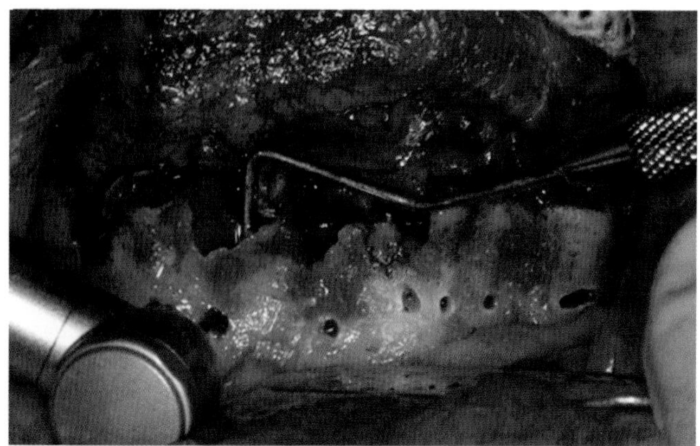

Figure 8.36. The tentative level of the alveolectomy was identified with a #2 round bur.

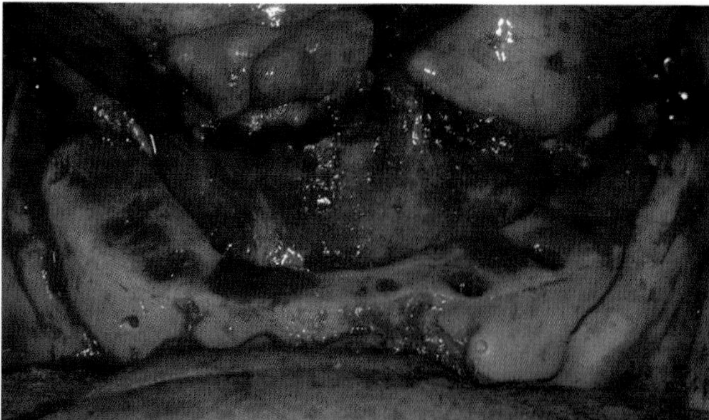

Figure 8.38. The edentulous mandible immediately post alveolectomy, prior to preparation of the osteotomies.

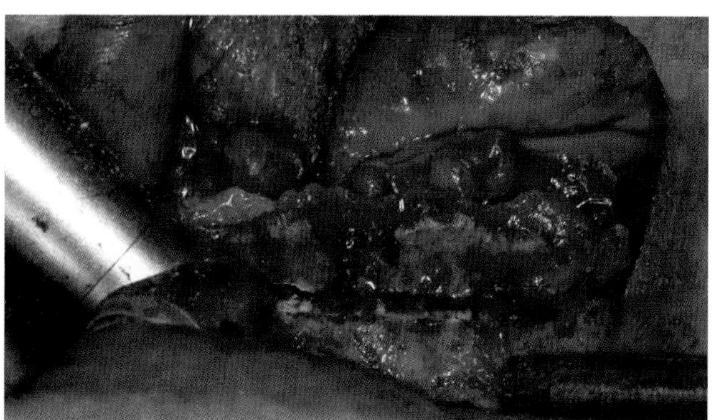

Figure 8.37. The perforations were connected with a coarse diamond bur.

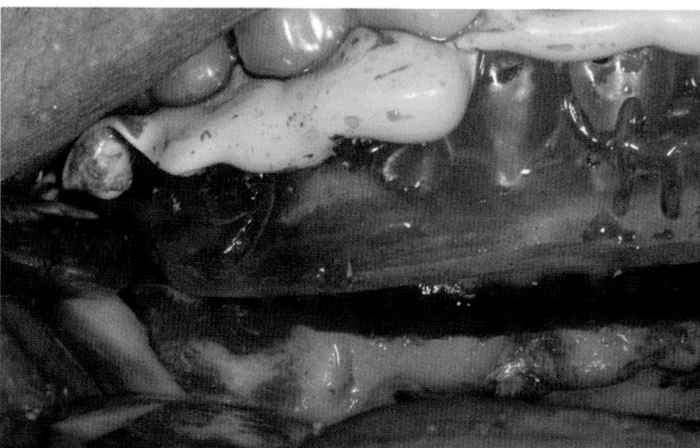

Figure 8.39. The surgical guide in place with the inter-occlusal record against the maxillary denture at the predetermined vertical dimension of occlusion. Adjustments were made in both the alveolus and the surgical guide in order to accurately seat the surgical guide at the pre-operative VDO.

reduction was marked on the labial aspect of the alveolus using a #2 round bur (Figure 8.36). This mark was pushed through the alveolus to penetrate the lingual plate. Connecting the perforations with a cutting bur completed the alveolectomy (Figure 8.37).

The occlusal aspect of the alveolus was flattened with a slight lingual inclination from the distal-most implant site on the right to the distal-most implant site on the left (Figure 8.38). The surgical guide was positioned and the VDO was evaluated for accuracy by guiding the patient into centric occlusion with the inter-occlusal record. Adjustments were made in both the surgical guide and the mandibular alveolar ridge. The flanges of the surgical guide were reduced. These adjustments permitted the surgical guide to be accurately positioned into the surgical site without increasing the VDO. Accurate positioning of the surgical guide facilitated accurate implant placement. The windows corresponding to the planned implant locations within the surgical guide were enlarged or connected by removing the interdental septum.

After the alveolectomy was completed, the inter-occlusal record (Blu Mousse®, Parkell Bio-Materials Division, Farmingdale, NY) was positioned on the maxillary denture and the surgical guide was inserted into the bite registration (Figure 8.39). This was inserted into the mouth and the patient closed into the intaglio surface of the surgical guide. Vertical marks were cut on the acrylic resin labial flange of the surgical guide and were extended on to the labial bone. These lines aided in accurately positioning the surgical guide in its correct position relative to the alveolectomy and planned osteotomy sites.

A round bur was used in the planned implant locations with the surgical guide in place. Twist drills were next used to sufficient depths to accept the guide pins (Figure 8.40). A panoramic radiograph was taken that identified the two-dimensional positions of the osteotomies and guide pins relative to the mental foramen and inferior alveolar nerves (Fig-

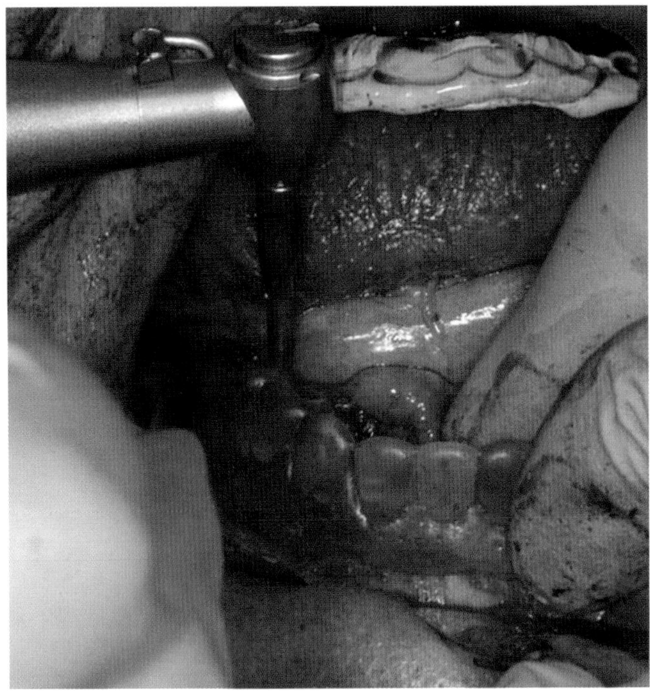

Figure 8.40. Twist drills were used to prepare the osteotomies to sufficient depths for placement of the directional guide pins.

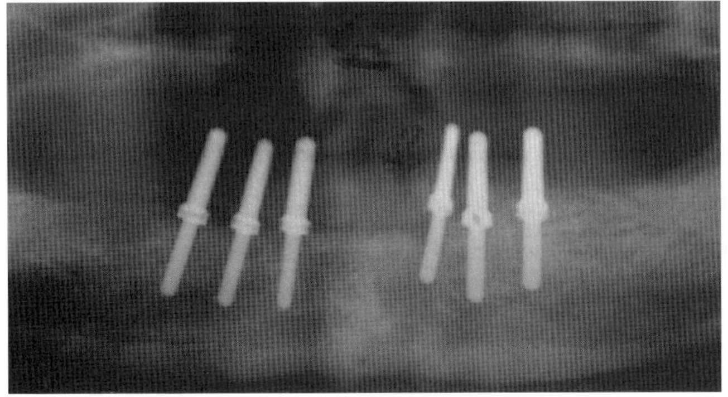

Figure 8.41. Intra-operative panoramic radiograph with directional guide pins in place.

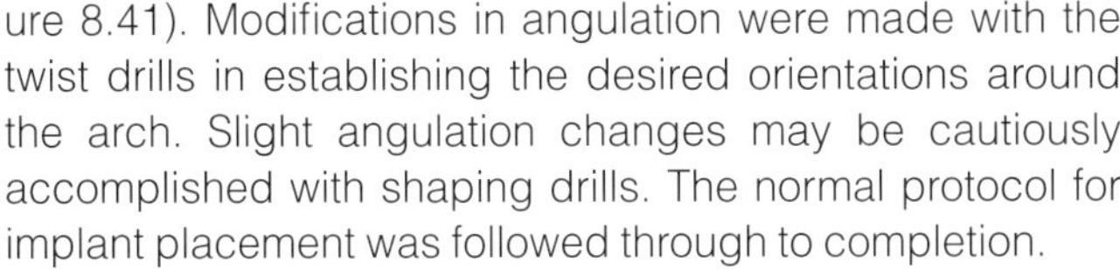

ure 8.41). Modifications in angulation were made with the twist drills in establishing the desired orientations around the arch. Slight angulation changes may be cautiously accomplished with shaping drills. The normal protocol for implant placement was followed through to completion.

The osteotomies were completed and six implants were placed. All of the implants obtained insertional torque values of at least 30 Ncm. This value is recommended as the minimal threshold for primary stability. If 30 Ncm is not obtained for a given implant, it should not be used to retain the DIEM denture. At least four implants are recommended for a successful DIEM protocol.

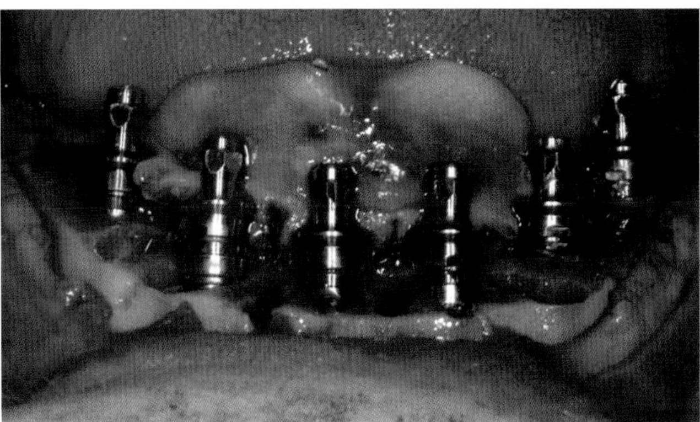

Figure 8.42. Clinical appearance of six mandibular implants with fixture mounts in place.

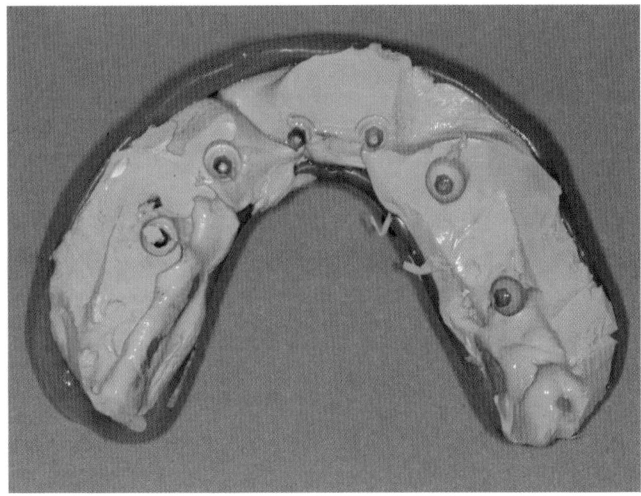

Figure 8.43. Intaglio surface of the DIEM™ denture after an impression was made of the implants and fixture mounts prior to abutment placement.

While the fixture mounts were still on the implants (Figure 8.42), an impression (Blu Mousse®, Parkell Bio-Materials Division, Farmingdale, NY) was made using the DIEM denture as the impression tray (Figure 8.43). The preexisting inter-occlusal record was in place on the occlusal surface of the maxillary denture and the patient was guided into centric occlusion. This impression was transferred to the prosthodontist's laboratory technician to facilitate preparation of the DIEM denture. The prosthodontic laboratory technician created holes within the DIEM denture base

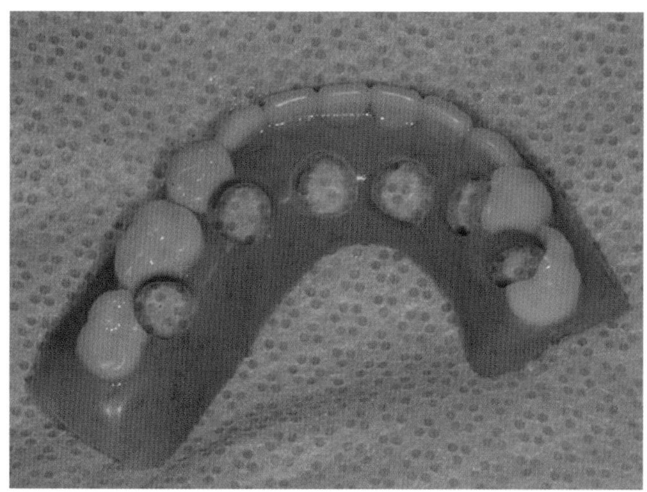

Figure 8.44. Holes were prepared completely through the denture base corresponding to the locations of the fixture mounts within the impression.

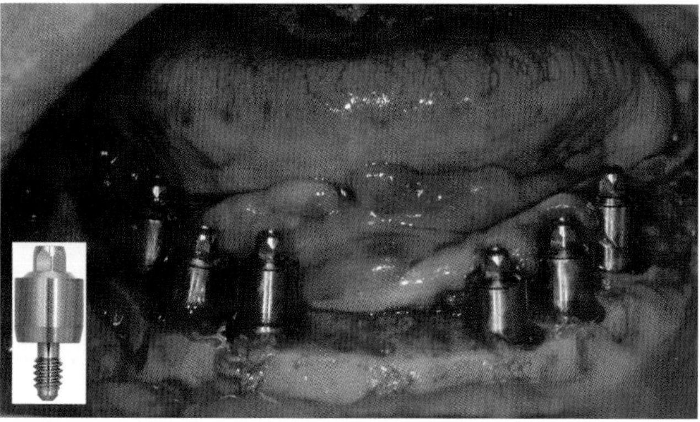

Figure 8.45. IOL® Abutments in place prior to flap closure (IOL® Abutment, inset).

consistent with the impressions of the fixture mounts (Figure 8.44).

In previous protocols, this impression was made and the holes were placed after the patient had been transferred from the surgical office to the prosthodontist's office. This procedure usually required approximately 20 minutes to complete. With this newer protocol, the DIEM™ denture was being prepared at the same time as the surgeon was closing the wound. This modification has decreased operating times by 30 minutes.

IOL® Abutments (IOL30, IOL40) were placed onto the implants and the tissue was sutured around them (Figure 8.45). The abutments were torqued to 20 Ncm with a torque driver. IOL® Abutments were selected so that the collars were at or above the gingival margins of the tissue after suturing. The patient was transferred to the prosthodontist's office for completion of the prosthetic phase of treatment. If the completion of the prosthesis will not be accomplished on the same day as the surgery, the surgeon prior to discharge would place IOL® Healing caps.

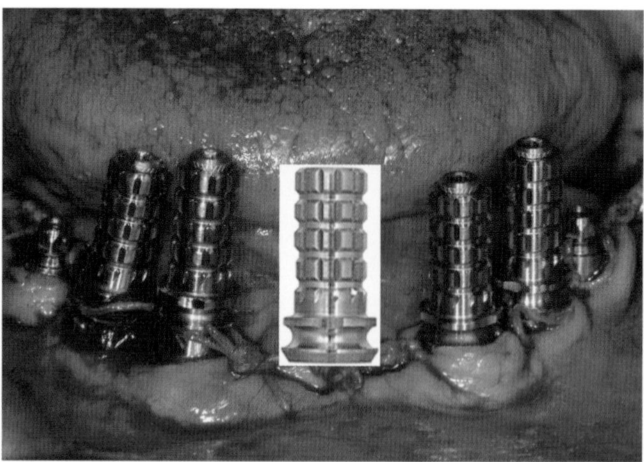

Figure 8.46. IOL® Temporary Cylinders in place on the anterior four implants (IOL® Temporary Cylinder, inset).

Prosthetic Protocol (2 1/2 Hours)

The patient was seated in the prosthodontic operatory. IOL® Temporary Cylinders (IOLTC) were placed onto the IOL® Abutments with laboratory screws (WSK15) (Figure 8.46). The initial adjustments were made so that the DIEM denture fit around the cylinders without regard to occlusal interferences.

After these adjustments were made, estimates were made relative to the heights of each IOL® Temporary Cylinder. The temporary cylinders were removed from the abutments and were sectioned with a separating disc in the laboratory. The lab screws also had to be reduced in height. Slots were prepared into the occlusal aspects of the screws as the large hexes were removed with the preparations. Adjustments were made until the DIEM denture went to place without violating the pre-operative VDO. In this case, only the posterior IOL® Temporary Cylinders had to be adjusted (Figure 8.47).

A rubber dam (Hygenic Non-Latex Flexi-Dam, Coltene/Whaledent Inc., Mahwah, NJ) was cut to fit around the IOL® Temporary Cylinders (Figure 8.48). The rubber dam served to separate the surgical field from the prosthetic field. Autopolymerizing acrylic resin was mixed per the manufacturer's instructions. A dental assistant loaded the intaglio surface of the DIEM denture, while the author injected resin around the IOL® Temporary Cylinders intra-orally. The denture was seated and the patient was guided into centric relation via the preexisting inter-

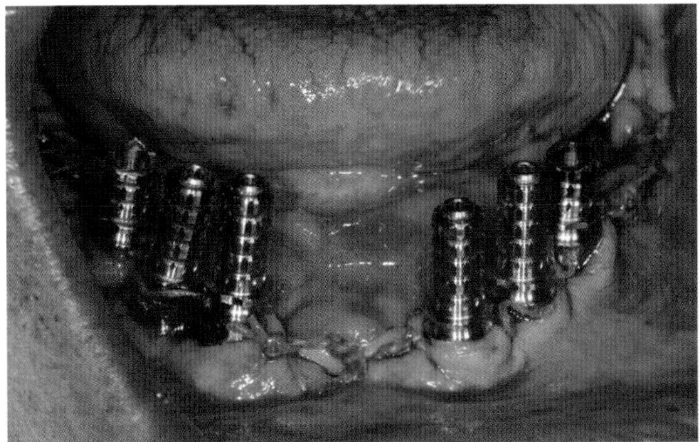

Figure 8.47. The posterior IOL® Temporary Cylinders on both sides had to be adjusted to provide adequate inter-occlusal clearance.

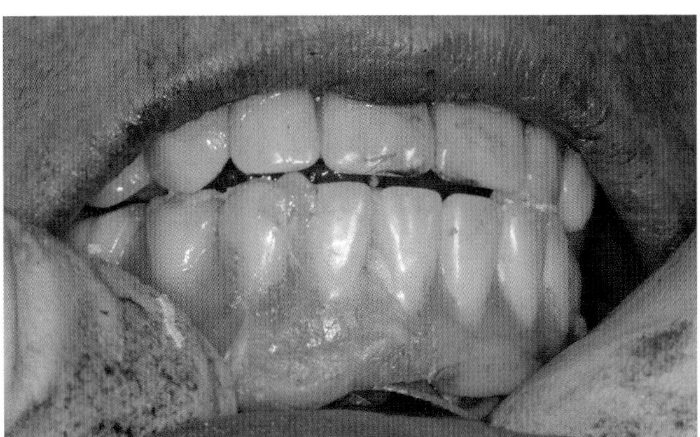

Figure 8.49. The patient was guided into centric occlusion after autopolymerizing acrylic resin was injected around the IOL® Temporary Cylinders and the intaglio surface of the DIEM™ denture was filled with the same resin.

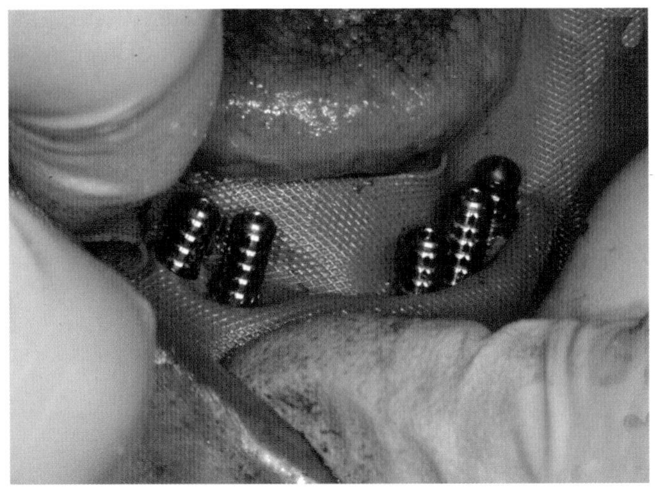

Figure 8.48. Rubber dam in place around the IOL® Temporary Cylinders.

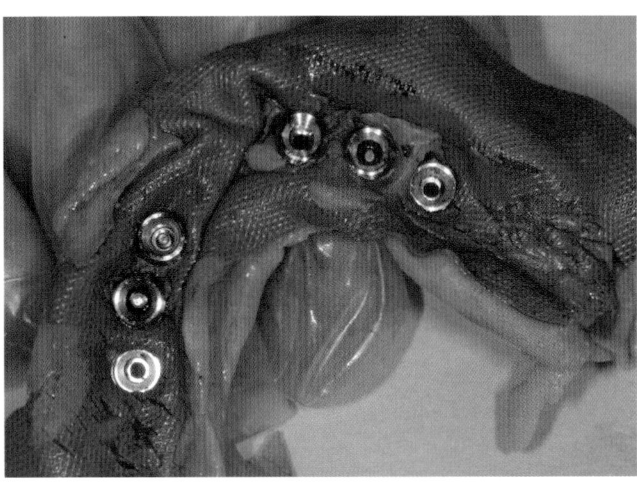

Figure 8.50. The rubber dam was retained around the IOL® Temporary Cylinders.

occlusal record, at the predetermined VDO (Figure 8.49). Water irrigation was used, along with high vacuum suction to minimize the amount of heat generated as the resin polymerized.

After the resin completed its set, the screws that retained the DIEM denture to the IOL® Abutments were removed. With removal of the DIEM denture, the rubber dam remained attached to the intaglio surface of the prosthesis (Figure 8.50). The rubber dam was removed from the denture and IOL® Abutment analogs were placed onto the apical portions of the IOL® Temporary Cylinders within the denture (Figure 8.51).

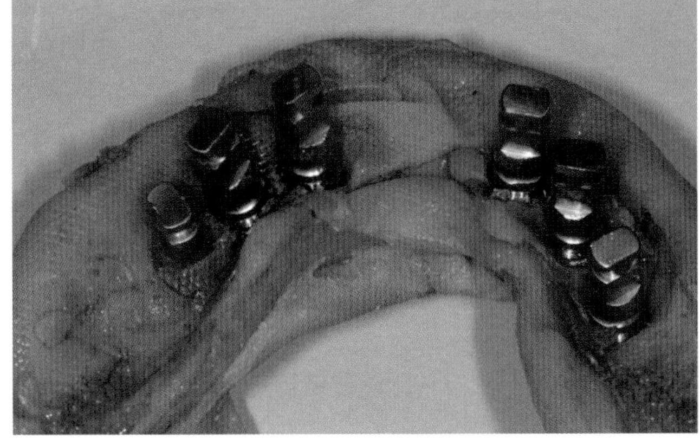

Figure 8.51. IOL® Abutment lab analogs were placed onto the apical surfaces of the IOL® Temporary Cylinders prior to filling any voids with acrylic resin.

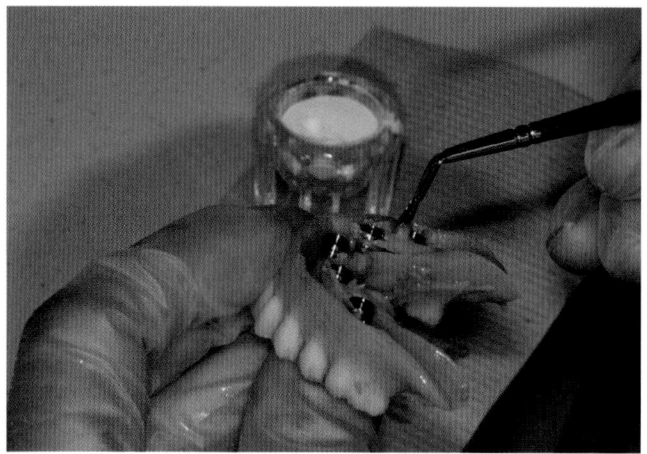

Figure 8.52. Acrylic resin was added to fill any voids that existed around the IOL® components.

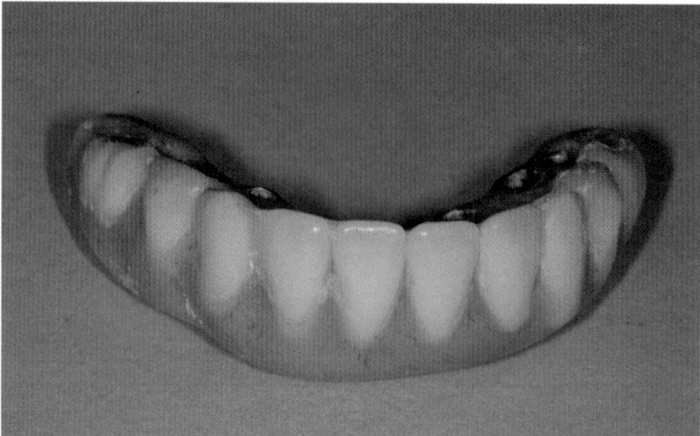

Figure 8.53. Laboratory anterior view of completed DIEM™ denture.

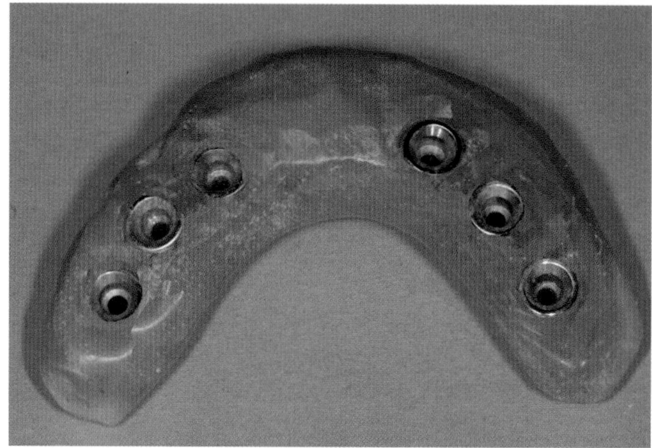

Figure 8.54. Laboratory view of the completed intaglio surface of the DIEM™ denture.

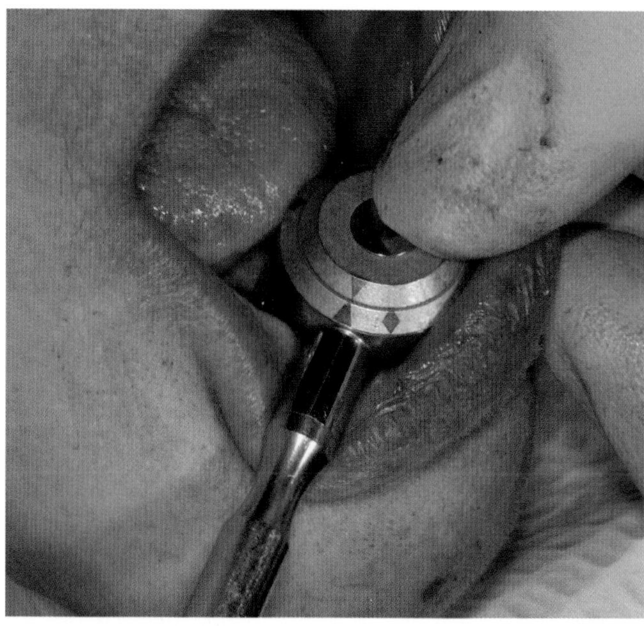

Figure 8.55. The IOL® Abutments were torqued to 20 Ncm with the Restorative Torque Indicator-triangle to triangle.

Additional resin was used to fill voids around the implant restorative components on the occlusal and intaglio surfaces of the DIEM denture (Figure 8.52). The denture was placed into a pressure pot (120° water, 15 psi) for 10 minutes. The DIEM denture was finished and polished per conventional prosthodontic techniques (Figures 8.53 and 8.54).

The IOL® Abutments were torqued to 20 Ncm with the Restorative Torque Indicator (RTI2035) (Figure 8.55). The DIEM denture was placed onto the IOL® Abutments with laboratory screws and the occlusion was adjusted to provide even occlusal contacts throughout the prosthesis. The DIEM denture was placed onto the IOL® Abutments definitively with Gold-Tite™ Hexed Screws (GSH30) that were torqued to 10 Ncm with the Restorative Torque Driver. Cotton was placed into the screw access openings (Figure 8.56) and the openings were restored with light cured composite resin (Figure 8.57). The patient was discharged with a fully functional occlusion approximately five hours after multiple extractions, alveolectomy and implant placement (Figures 8.58, 8.59, 8.60, 8.61).

Postoperative Instructions

Postoperative instructions were given to the patient in both written and verbal formats (Table 8.5). The patient was discharged in excellent condition.

Appointment 8. Prosthetic Follow-Up Appointments (1/2 Hour)

24-Hour Follow-Up Appointment (1/2 Hour)

The patient returned for this appointment and reported that she was extremely pleased with the results of yesterday's

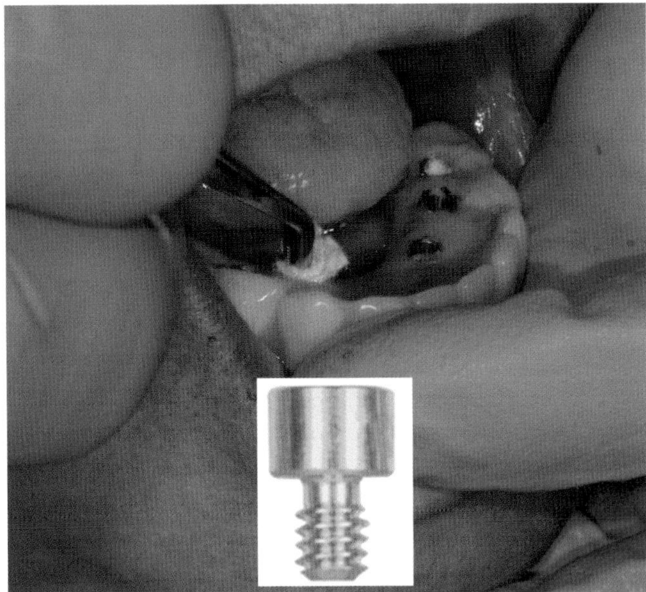

Figure 8.56. Cotton was placed into each screw access opening as fillers prior to restoring with composite resin (Hexed Gold-Tite™ screw [GSH30], inset).

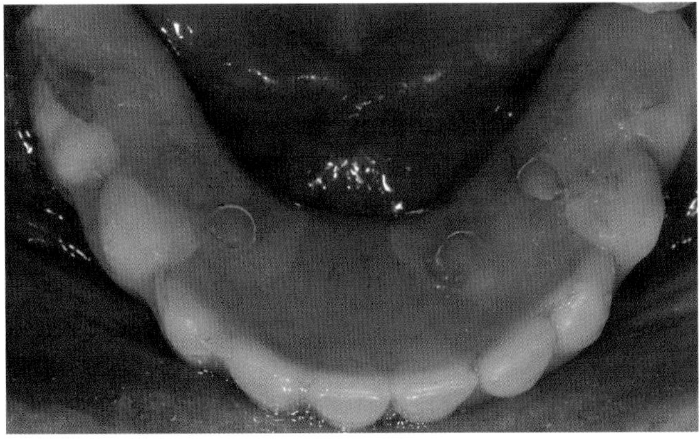

Figure 8.57. Clinical occlusal view of the completed DIEM™ denture with composite resin restorations in place.

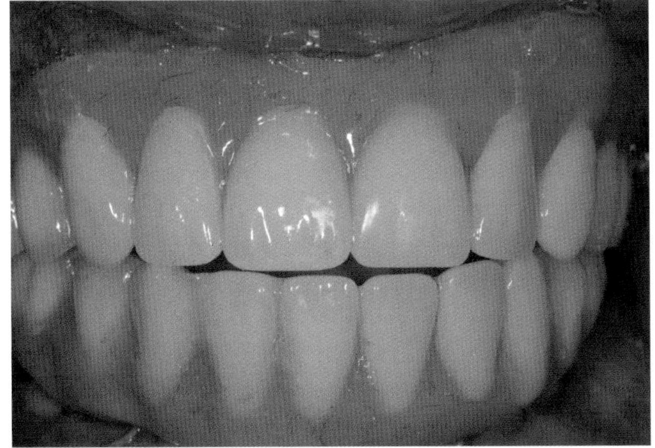

Figure 8.58. Anterior clinical view of patient in centric occlusion just prior to discharge.

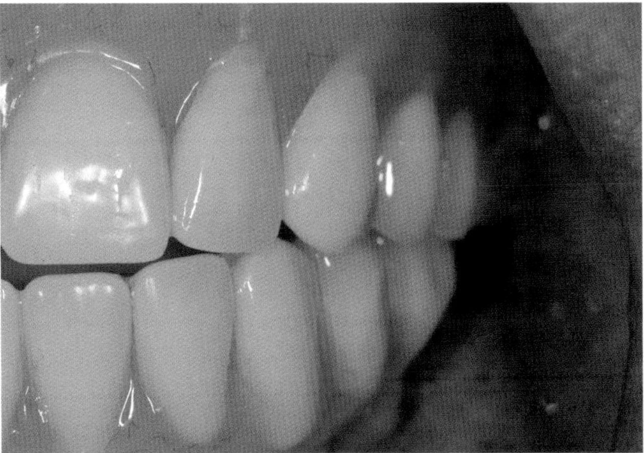

Figure 8.59. Left anterior clinical view of patient in centric occlusion just prior to discharge.

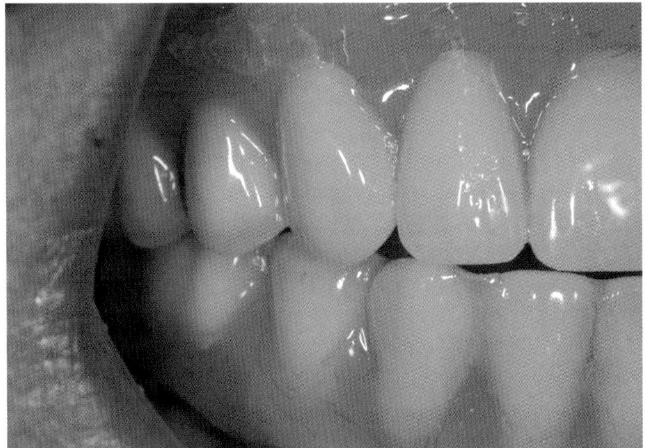

Figure 8.60. Right anterior clinical view of patient in centric occlusion just prior to discharge.

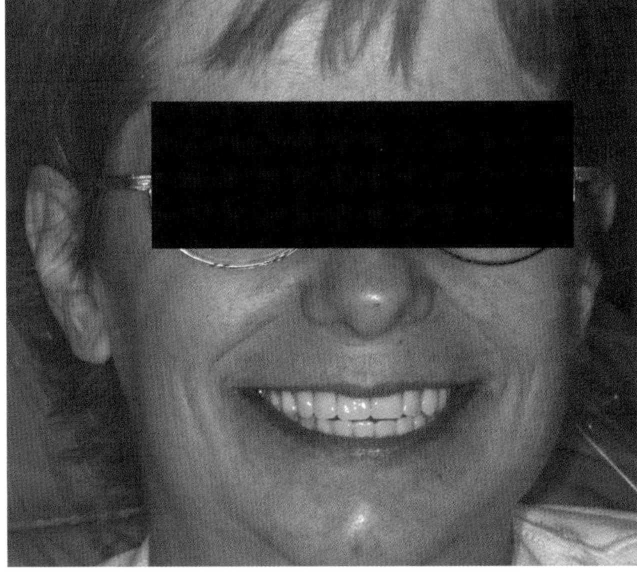

Figure 8.61. Clinical extra-oral facial view of the patient at the time of discharge.

TABLE 8.5. Post Operative Instructions

1. Place ice compresses to the right and left sides of your lower jaw: 20 minutes on, 20 minutes off for the next 12 hours.
2. Maintain a liquid diet with dietary supplements such as Instant Breakfast, Ensure, and so on.
3. Take the antibiotics as prescribed.
4. Take the pain pills as prescribed.
5. Do not worry about your oral hygiene at this time.
6. Take your upper denture out for nighttime sleep.
7. Sleep with one extra pillow.
8. Do not suck on straws.
9. Return for the first postoperative visit tomorrow.
10. Get a good night's sleep.

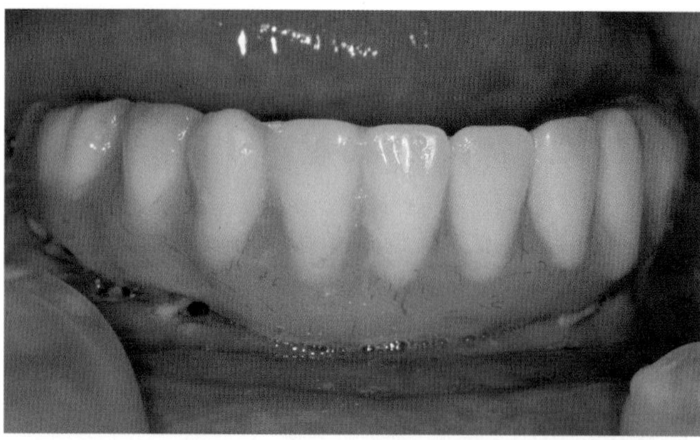

Figure 8.63. Clinical facial intra-oral view of the mandibular DIEM™ denture one week postoperative.

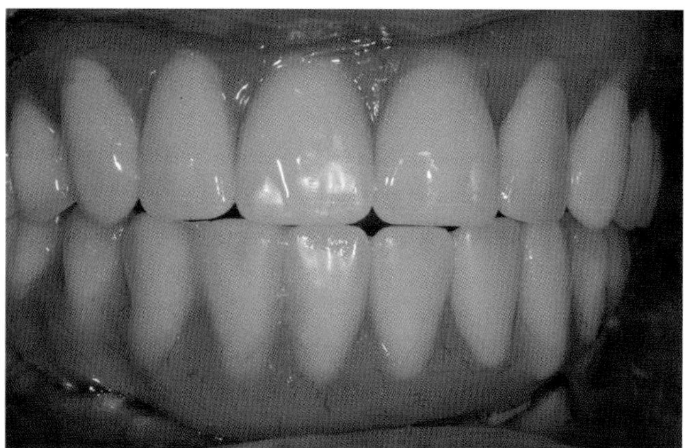

Figure 8.62. Clinical facial intra-oral view of the patient one day postoperative.

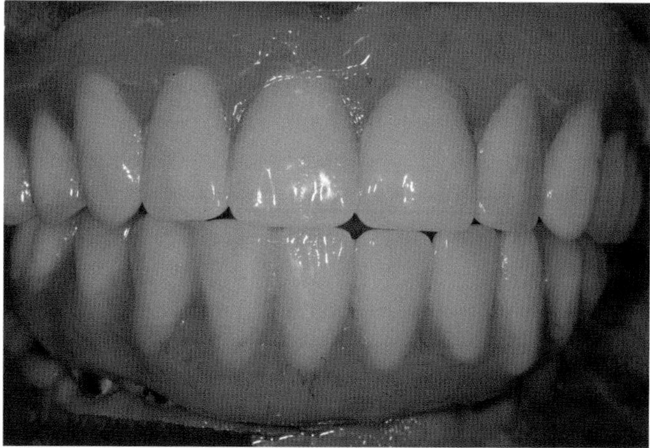

Figure 8.64. Clinical facial intra-oral view of the mandibular DIEM™ denture four weeks postoperative.

treatment. She had minimal discomfort and swelling. She was pleased with the aesthetic results of treatment as well (Figure 8.62).

Oral hygiene was demonstrated to the patient with a soft toothbrush. The toothbrush was to be placed at the junction of the DIEM denture, IOL® Abutments, and mandibular peri-implant soft tissues. The brush was to be moved back and forth, with minimal pressure. At this point in time, the brush was used to remove macroscopic debris. Chlorhexidine (0.12%) was to be placed onto the toothbrush to place the mouthwash in and around the surgical sites. This was to be accomplished two times per day until the next scheduled visit in one week.

The patient was advised to continue taking the antibiotics until all of the pills were taken.

She was urged to continue with the soft diet as prescribed immediately post operative.

One-Week Follow-Up Appointment (1/2 Hour)

The patient presented for this appointment and continued to do well. She reported a complete absence of pain and was no longer taking any analgesics. Her mouth felt comfortable. She was very pleased with the results of treatment (Figure 8.63).

Four-Week Follow-Up Appointment (1/2 Hour)

The patient continued to do well. She was still eating a soft diet. She noticed more space inferior to the intaglio surface of the DIEM denture (Figure 8.64).

Superfloss® (Oral B Laboratories, Iowa City, IA) was introduced to the patient at this appointment and she was advised that she could discontinue the use of 0.12% chlorhexidine.

The patient was discharged after being scheduled to return in four weeks for continued follow up.

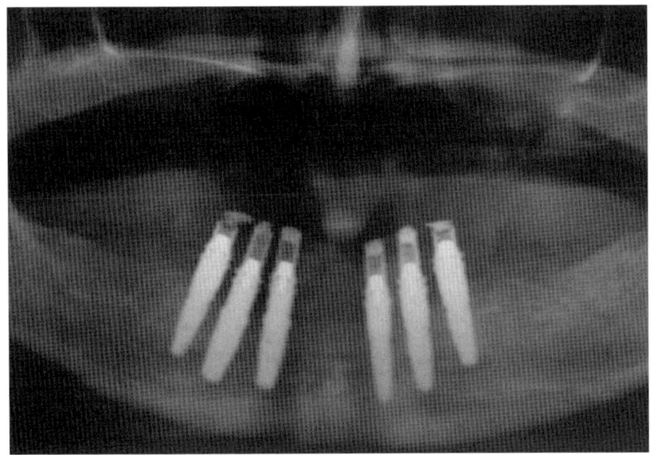

Figure 8.65. Panoramic radiograph one year post insertion of the DIEM(TM) denture.

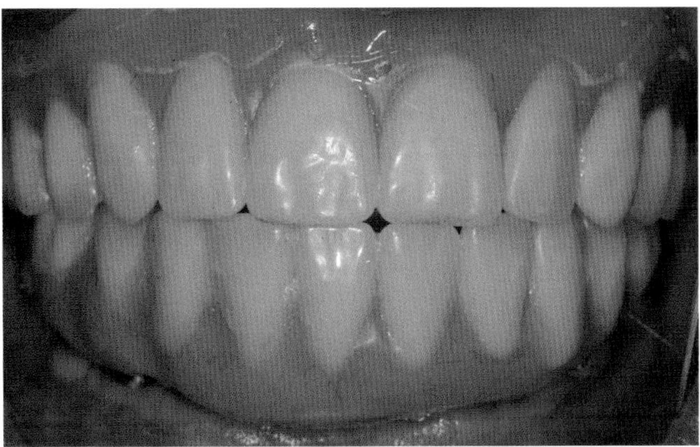

Figure 8.66. Clinical anterior intra-oral view of patient one year post insertion of the DIEM(TM) denture.

Eight-Week Follow-Up Appointment (1/2 Hour)

The patient continued to do extremely well. She was very pleased with the aesthetic, phonetic, and functional results of treatment. She reported no difficulties with any oral hygiene procedures.

The physical examination was within normal limits. The occlusion was stable with bilateral posterior contacts. The intra-oral soft tissues were normal and her plaque removal was excellent.

She was advised to return to a normal diet and complete function without any restrictions.

Appointment 9. One-Year Recall (3/4 Hour)

The patient returned approximately one-year post extraction, alveolectomy, implant placement, and insertion of the DIEM denture. She was extremely pleased with the aesthetic, phonetic, and functional portions of the treatment. She had absolutely no complaints relative to diet or oral hygiene.

Radiographs

Prior to this visit, a panoramic radiograph was taken (Figure 8.65). It demonstrated minimal occlusal bone loss and excellent macroscopic bone/implant contact. There were no radiolucencies.

Clinical

The clinical examination consisted of evaluating the occlusion, soft tissue contours, and oral hygiene (Figures 8.66, 8.67, 8.68). All of these were within normal limits.

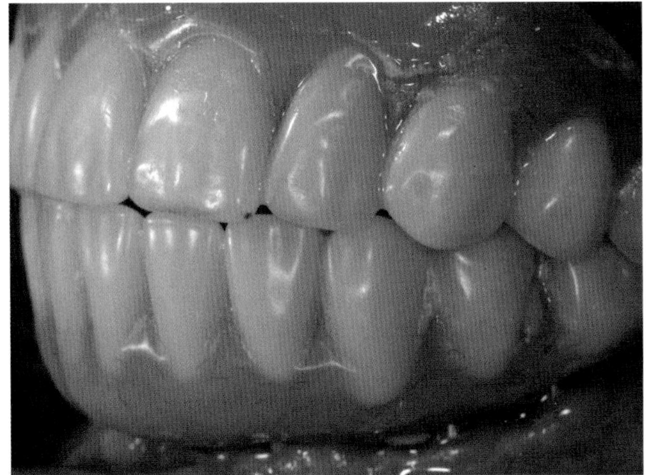

Figure 8.67. Clinical left lateral intra-oral view of patient one year post insertion of the DIEM(TM) denture.

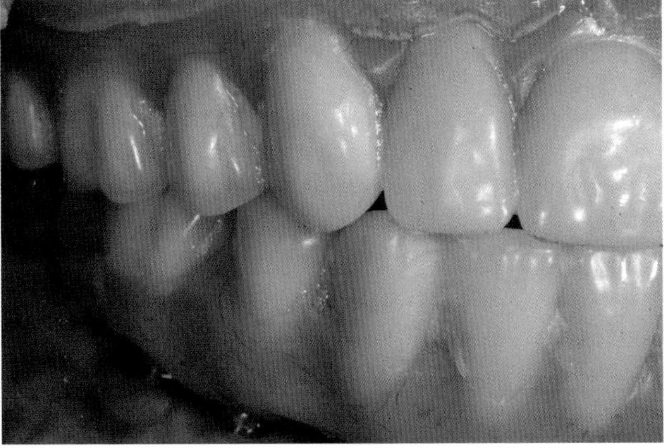

Figure 8.68. Clinical right lateral intra-oral view of patient one year post insertion of the DIEM(TM) denture.

TABLE 8.6. Lab Fees, Component Costs, Overhead, Fees, and Restorative Profits

Fixed				
Chair Time	**Overhead**	**Laboratory Expenses**		
		Casts	$ 60	
		Articulation	$ 50	
		Record bases	$ 50	
		Denture set up	$250	
		Processing	$100	
4 hours	**$350/hr = $1400**	**Sub Total**	**$510**	
		Implant Components		
		IOL® Temp cylinders	$210	
		IOL® Analogs	$111	
		Polishing protectors	$ 90	
		Lab screws	$150	
		Abutment Screws	$330	
		Sub Total	**$891**	
TOTALS	**$1400**		**$1401**	
Professional Fee				**$4000**
Costs (fixed overhead and laboratory expenses)				**$2801**
Profit (fees less costs)				**$1191**
Profit per hour ($1191/4 hr)				**$ 300**

Impression copings and lab screws may be used multiple times, therefore costs will be decreased for each succeeding case and profits will be increased. Analogs should not be re-used.

In the absence of any clinical problems, the author did not remove the DIEM denture. However, if there had been any abnormalities, the DIEM denture could have been removed by removing the composite resin screw access opening restorations, locating the retaining screws, and unscrewing them from the IOL® Abutments. The IOL® Abutments would then have been evaluated for tightness and mobility. The IOL® Abutment screws would have been retorqued to 20 Ncm with a torque instrument. Depending on the clinical conditions, radiographs would have been taken and evaluated (Figure 8.69).

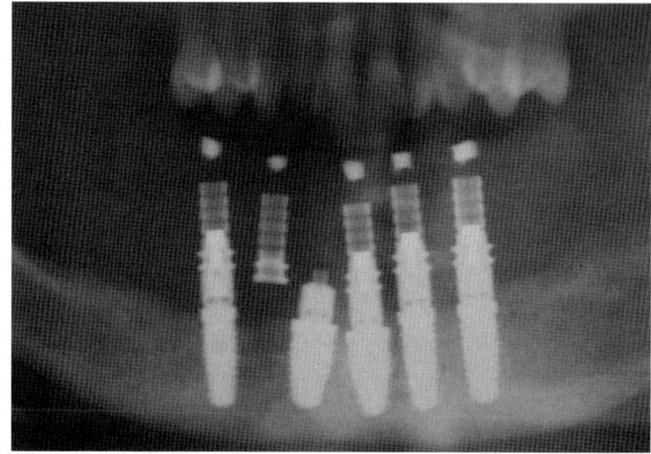

Figure 8.69. Panoramic radiograph of a patient who lost one implant approximately eight weeks post implant placement. The unused implant did not achieve an insertional torque value of 20 Ncm and therefore was not used per the DIEM™ protocol.

Definitive Prosthesis (CAD/CAM Framework)

The DIEM™ Protocol calls for fabrication of a definitive prosthesis with a CAD/CAM framework as discussed in Chapter 7 (Lazzara and others 2003).

Costs/Fees/Profitability

The following discussion (Table 8.6) relative to fees is reflective of 2006 in the Midwestern United States. The costs of the implant components are retail prices from Implant Innovations, Inc., Palm Beach Gardens, Florida.

Surgeon: C Garry O'Connor, DDS, MS, Gundersen Lutheran Medical Center, LaCrosse, Wisconsin

Dental laboratory technician: Andrew Gingrasso, Gundersen Lutheran Medical Center, LaCrosse, Wisconsin

BIBLIOGRAPHY

Albrektsson, T, Zarb, GA, Worthington, P, Ericksson, AR, 1986. The long-term efficacy of currently used dental implants; a review and proposed criteria of success. *Int J Oral Maxillofac Implants* 1:11–25.

Awad, M, Lund, J, Dufresne, E, Feine, J, 2003. Comparing the efficacy of mandibular implant-retained overdentures and conventional dentures among middle-aged edentulous patients: satisfaction and functional assessment. *Int J Prosthodont* 16:390–396.

Brånemark, P-I, 1983. Osseointegration and its experimental background. *J Prosthet Dent* 50:399–410.

Brånemark, P-I, 1983. "Introduction to osseointegration." In: *Tissue Integrated Prostheses.* Brånemark, P-I, Zarb, GA, Albrektsson, T, eds. Chicago: Quintessence Publishing Co., Inc., p. 11–76.

Brånemark, P-I, Hansson, B, Adell, R, 1977. Osseointegrated implants in the treatment of the edentulous jaw. Experience from a 10-year period. *Scan J Plast Reconstr Surg* 16(suppl):1–132.

Brunski, JB, 1997. Avoid pitfalls of overloading and micromotion of intraosseous implants [interview]. *Dental Implantol Update* 4:77–81.

Burns, Robert, 1971. "To a louse, on seeing one on a lady's bonnet at church." In: Burns R. *Complete Poems and Songs,* James Kinsley, ed. Oxford U.K.: Oxford University Press, p. 156.

Drago, CJ, Lazzara, RJ, 2006. Immediate loading of implants with a fixed prosthesis in the edentulous mandible. *J Prosthodont,* 15:187–194.

English, C, 1992. The critical A-P spread. *Implant Soc* 3:14–15.

Feine, J, Carlsson, G, Awad, M, Chehade, A, Duncan, W, Gizani, S, 2002. The McGill consensus statement on overdentures. *Int J Prosthodont* 15:413–414.

Fitzpatrick, B, 2006. Standard of care for the edentulous mandible: a systematic review. *J Prosthet Dent* 95:71–78.

Landa, J, 1952. Free-way space and its significance in the rehabilitation of the masticatory apparatus. *J Prosthet Dent* 2:756.

Lazzara, RJ, Testori, T, Meltzer, A, Misch, C., Porter, S, Del Castillo, R, Goéne, R, 2003. Immediate Occlusal Loading® (IOL®) of dental implants: Predictable results through DIEM™ Guidelines. Implant Innovations, Inc., Palm Beach Gardens, FL.

McAlarney, M, Stavropoulos, D, 1996. Determination of cantilever length-anterior-posterior spread ratio assuming failure criteria to be the compromise of the prosthesis retaining screw-prosthesis joint. *Int J Oral Maxillofac Implants* 11:331–339.

Meijer, H, Raghoebar, G, van't Hof, M, 2003. Comparison of implant-retained mandibular overdentures and conventional complete dentures: a 10-year prospective study of clinical aspects and patient satisfaction. *Int J Oral Maxillofac Implants* 18:879–885.

Schnitman, P, Wohrle, P, Rubenstein, J, DaSilva, J, Wang, N, 1997. 10-year results for Brånemark implants immediately loaded with fixed prosthesis at implant placement. *Int J Oral Maxillofac Implants* 12:495–503.

Tarnow, D. Emtiaz, S, Classi, A, 1997. Immediate loading of threaded implants at stage I surgery in edentulous arches: ten consecutive case reports with 1- to 5-year data. *Int J Oral Maxillofac Implants* 12:319–324.

Testori, T, Szmukler-Moncler, S, Francetti, L, Del Fabbro, M, Scarano, A, Piattelli, A, Weinstein, RL, 2001. Immediate loading of Osseotite implants: A case report and histologic analysis after 4 months of occlusal loading. *Int J Perio Restor Dent* 21:451–459.

Testori, T, Del Fabbro, M, Feldman, S, Vincenzi, G, Sullivan, D, Rossi, R, Jr, Anitua, E, Bianchi, F, Francetti, L, Weinstein, R, 2002. A multicenter prospective evaluation of 2-months loaded Osseotite implants placed in the posterior jaws: 3-year follow-up results. *Clin Oral Implants Res* 13:154–161.

Testori, T, Bianchi, F, Del Fabbro, M, Szmukler-Moncler, S, Francetti, L, Weinstein, RL, 2003. Immediate non-occlusal loading vs. early loading in partially edentulous patients. *Pract Proced Aesthet Dent* 15:787–794.

Winkler, S, Moore, H, Ochi, S, 2000. Implant survival to 36 months as related to length and diameter. *Ann Periodontol* 5:22–31.

Worthington, P, 2005. The changing relations between the allied disciplines. *J Calif Dent Assoc* 71:330–333.

Chapter 9: Immediate Non-Occlusal Loading Provisional Restoration; Definitive Restoration Maxillary Central Incisor

LITERATURE REVIEW

Since the advent of Brånemark's concept of osseointegration, the two-stage surgical approach has been the accepted protocol for endosseous implants (Brånemark and others 1977). Other researchers questioned the validity of this protocol by introducing the concept of a single stage surgical protocol but using the original unloaded healing times of 3–6 months (Buser and others 1988). More current reports suggest that implants designed for two-stage surgical protocols can osseointegrate in predictable fashion, with high Cumulative Survival Rates (CSRs), with single-stage surgical protocols (Becker and others 1997; Garber and others 2001; Cooper and others 2001).

Immediate Occlusal Loading® of multiple, splinted implants has already been discussed in Chapter 8 and is not repeated here. The reader is reminded that Immediate Occlusal Loading®, with high CSRs, has been recognized as a protocol involving multiple, splinted mandibular implants that have been placed and restored within three days of the surgical procedures (Schnitman and others 1997; Testori and others, 2003).

Treatment in the aesthetic zones of partially edentulous patients presents clinicians with numerous challenges including, but not limited to: the presence or absence of gingival papillae; gingival symmetry; location of implant restorative platforms; emergence profiles of the implant restorations; and clinical restorations that replicate the remaining natural teeth (Saadoun and Sebbag 2004).

Alterations in both the hard and soft tissues in extraction sites and the adjacent natural teeth may result in edentulous sites that are not appropriate for implant placement without additional surgical procedures (Figure 9.1). With older protocols, a healing time of 9–12 months was recommended after extraction prior to implant placement (Adell and others 1981). Other researchers have advocated immediate or delayed immediate implant placement (Schulte and Heimke 1976; Tarnow and Fletcher 1993; Cooper and others 2001). Aesthetic success in the aesthetic zone depends on harmony and anatomical contours of the hard and soft tissues (Wohrle 1998).

Wohrle reported on the success of 14 consecutive cases in which he extracted nonrestorable teeth, placed tapered implants with various surfaces, and restored them with provisional restorations on the same day (Wohrle 1998). It should be noted that none of the restorations had any occlusal contacts and patients were instructed to avoid using the implants and restorations for periods up to six months postoperatively. All of the implants achieved insertional torque values of at least 45 Ncm. This was a quantitative measurement of implant primary stability. Two of the implants were followed for 31–36 months; two for 25–30 months; five for 19–24 months; 12 for 13–18 months; 14 for 7–12 months; and 14 for 0–6 months. None of the implants was lost, and change in the levels of the soft tissues surrounding the restorations was greater than 1 mm in just two patients. Soft tissue loss never exceeded 1.5 mm for any restoration, and Wohrle considered that the harmony and continuity of the hard and soft tissues were predictably achieved in all cases (Figures 9.2 and 9.3).

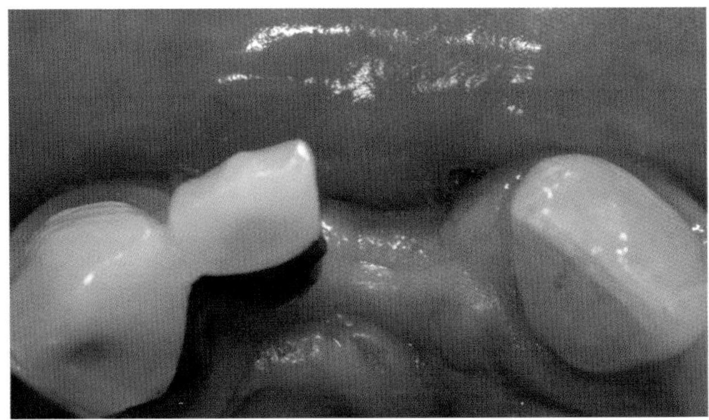

Figure 9.1. Occlusal view of a partially edentulous anterior maxillary ridge 14 months post extraction. Note the collapse of the ridge in the area of the missing right central incisor.

Hui and others (2001) reported on the results of a clinical study that provided immediate, non-occlusal loading restorations in the anterior maxillary aesthetic zone for 24 patients. Thirteen of the 24 patients had immediate implant placement after tooth extraction. Primary implant stability was defined as insertional torque values of at least 40 Ncm, and none of the restorations had occlusal contacts in centric or eccentric positions. The follow-up periods ranged from one to 15 months, and all of the implants were reported to be stable. The aesthetic results were considered to be satisfactory by all patients.

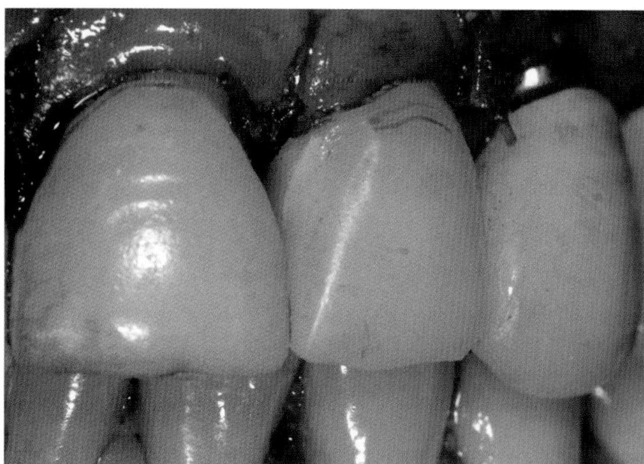

Figure 9.2. Intra-oral view of a provisional restoration (INOL) without occlusal contacts that restored an implant that replaced a maxillary left lateral incisor on the day of surgery.

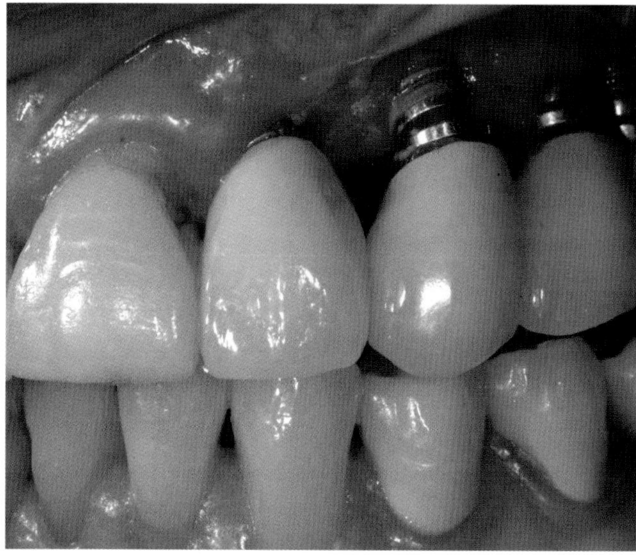

Figure 9.3. Definitive restoration 12 months post insertion of the implant in Figure 9.2.

Kan and others (2003) performed a study similar to those noted above with 35 patients. Thirty-five threaded hydoxyapatite-coated implants were placed and restored with non-occlusal load provisional restorations immediately post implant placement. The implants were placed with primary stability, but the authors did not define this term quantitatively. Kan reported that, at 12 months, all of the implants were osseointegrated with mean midfacial gingival level and mesial/distal papillae level changes from pretreatment to 12 months post treatment of -0.55 ± 0.53 mm, -0.53 ± 0.39 mm, and -0.39 ± 0.40 mm, respectively. Kan reported that all of the patients were pleased with the aesthetic results. Kan concluded that favorable

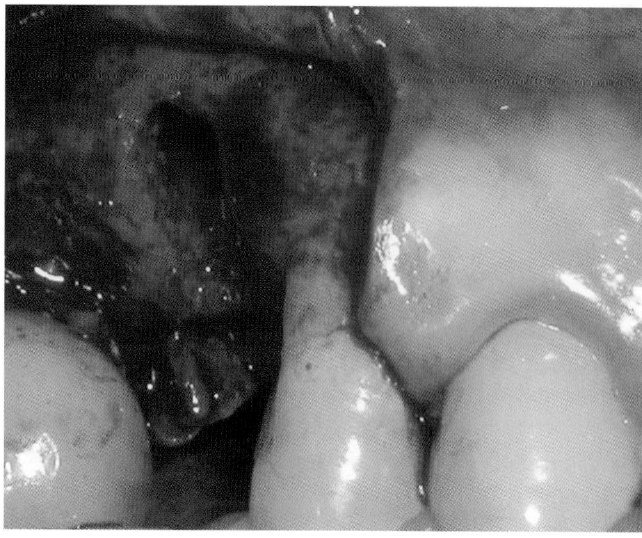

Figure 9.4. Intra-oral view of a large fenestration within the alveolus after extraction of the maxillary right second premolar. This patient was not a candidate for immediate implant placement because of the defect and the need for bone grafting prior to implant placement.

CSRs, peri-implant tissue responses and aesthetic outcomes could be achieved predictably with this protocol.

Other authors have also demonstrated predictable, high CSRs with minor variations of the immediate non-occlusal protocols (INOL) identified above (Saadoun and Sebbag 2004; Drago and Lazzara 2004). Successful treatment appears to be dependent on implant primary stability (insertional torque values of at least 35 Ncm at implant placement); the absence of infection or fenestrations of the alveolus (Figure 9.4); and provisional restorations that are out of occlusion in all mandibular movements.

However, there are also several studies that restored immediate, single-tooth, unsplinted provisional restorations with occlusal contacts at the time of implant placement (Ericsson and others 2000; Chaushu and others 2001). Ericsson reported that two of the 12 implants that were restored with this protocol failed within five months of implant placement. Chaushu reported that the one-year CSR for the immediately loaded single-unit implants, placed into fresh extraction sites, was 82.4%. For those implants that were placed into healed edentulous sites, the CSR was 100%. Chaushu and others concluded that an Immediate Occlusal Loading® protocol for single-unit implants may have higher-than-acceptable failure rates and that this protocol, if used, should be used only in healed extraction sites.

Immediate Non Occlusal Loading (INOL) is a protocol that is generally restorative driven, in that a fixed restoration is to be placed at the time of implant surgery. With this proto-

TABLE 9.1. Immediate Non-Occlusal Loading (INOL) Protocol for Single, Unsplinted Provisional Implant Restorations

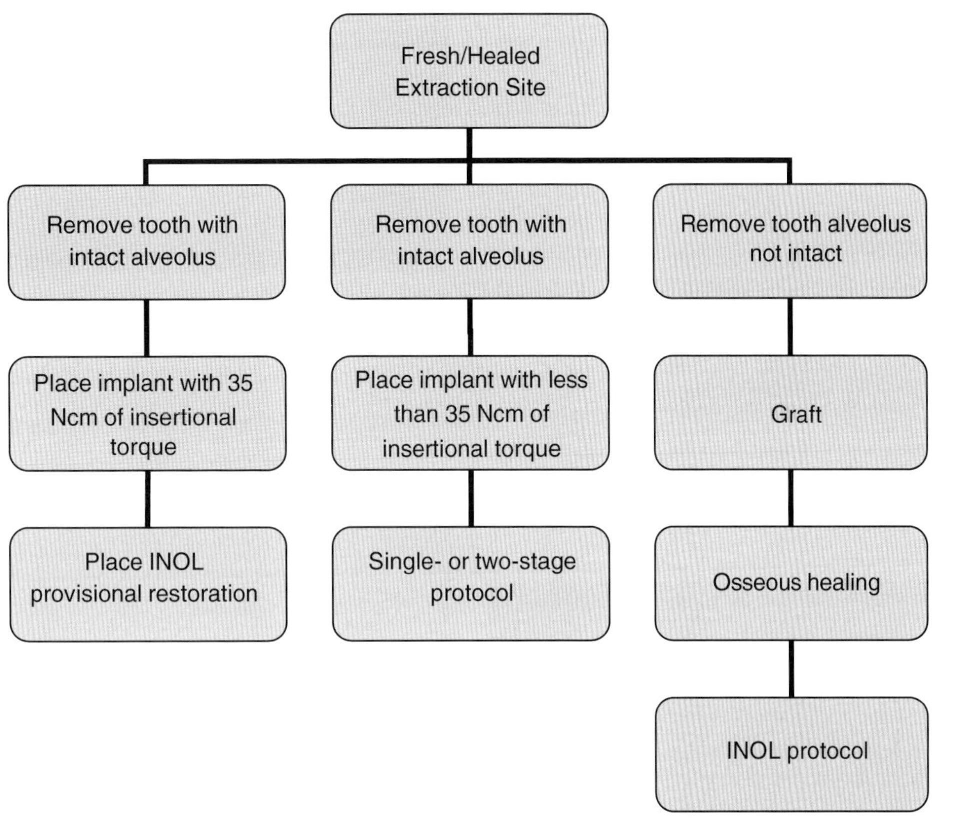

col, patients will not have to wear any sort of removable prosthesis. The implant surgeon and restorative dentist have to be prepared for multiple contingencies related to the proposed surgery: quality and quantity of bone; implant primary stability (35 Ncm); and location of the gingival margins. If any of the above criteria are not satisfied in a given situation, an implant may or may not be placed; a provisional implant restoration may or may not be placed (Table 9.1). This protocol may be said to be restorative driven but surgically determined.

CLINICAL CASE PRESENTATION

Appointment 1. Initial Clinical Visit (3/4 Hour)

A 19-year-old female patient presented to the author with a chief complaint of: "Evaluation of my missing upper-left front tooth."

History of the Present Illness

The dental history relative to tooth #9 included trauma to the anterior maxillae approximately five years previously. As reported by an oral surgeon, the incisal edge of the maxillary left central incisor was approximately 3 mm shorter than the right central incisor (Figure 9.5). Ankylosis

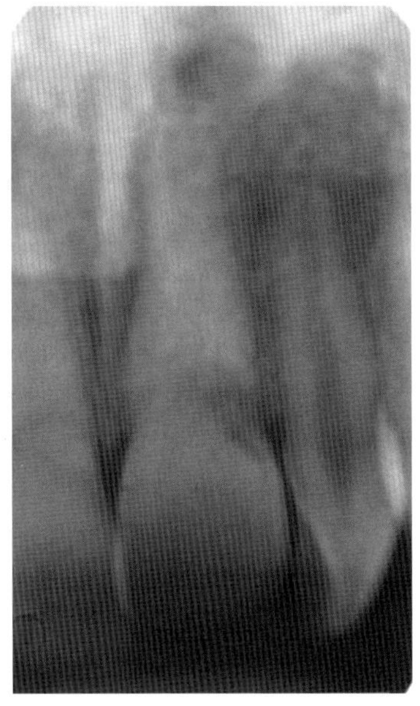

Figure 9.5. Radiograph at the time of the initial presentation that demonstrated ankylosis of the maxillary left central incisor.

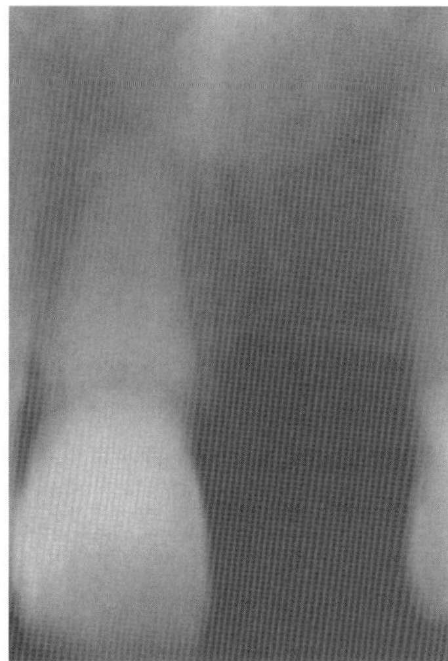

Figure 9.6. Radiograph approximately nine months post extraction of the maxillary left central incisor. There appeared to be adequate bone volume for implant placement.

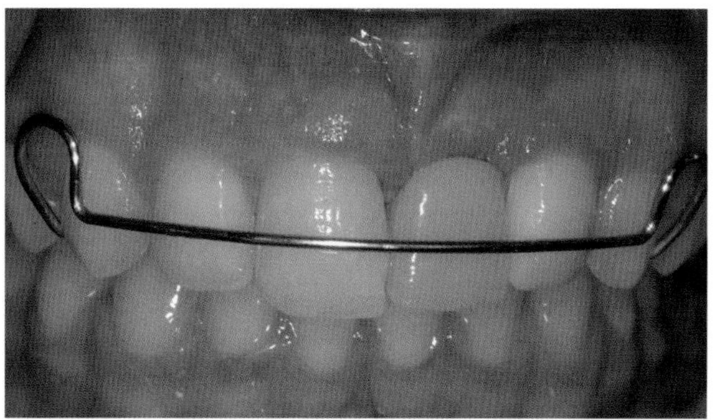

Figure 9.7. Pre-operative clinical view of the patient as she presented to the author, with the removable partial denture in place.

was the diagnosis, and the tooth was treatment planned for extraction and replacement with a removable partial denture. The tooth was extracted uneventfully and the oral surgeon placed the immediate partial denture. The extraction site was allowed to heal for nine months (Figure 9.6).

The patient presented to the author's office approximately 12 months post extraction (Figures 9.7 and 9.8).

Radiographs

Pre-operative radiographs consisted of single periapical and panoramic radiographs. Based on the clinical examination and anatomic location, the implant surgeon decided that a CT scan was not necessary.

Physical Examination

This patient presented with an otherwise intact dentition and mild gingivitis and was caries free (Figure 9.9).

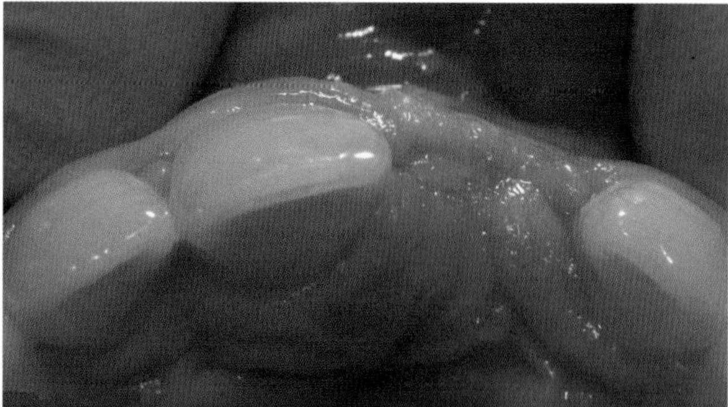

Figure 9.8. Pre-operative occlusal view of the anterior maxillary partially edentulous ridge. There appeared to be adequate buccal/lingual width for implant placement for the missing left central incisor.

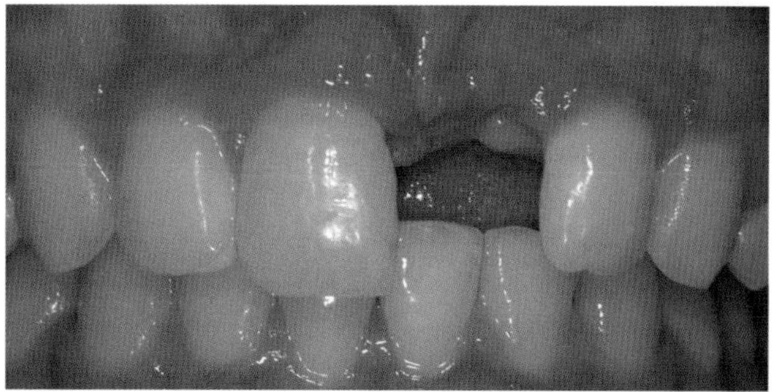

Figure 9.9. Pre-operative labial view of the anterior maxillary segment that demonstrated adequate restorative volume for an implant restoration for tooth #9.

Diagnostic Casts

Diagnostic casts were fabricated from alginate impressions. A denture tooth was used to identify the optimal location for the implant-retained crown (Figures 9.10 and 9.11).

Surgical Guide

The surgical guide was required to identify the optimal location of the planned implant restoration. The surgeon needed to know the three-dimensional position of the planned implant restoration in order to place the implant in its correct location. The surgical guide was made by duplicating the diagnostic cast with the denture tooth in place, pouring that impression in dental stone, and then making a vacuum-formed matrix (125 mm Biocryl Material, Great Lakes Orthodontics, Tonawanda, NY) (Figure 9.12). The author has found it prudent to make the surgical guide on a duplicate cast because the cast is generally damaged during fabrication of the surgical guide.

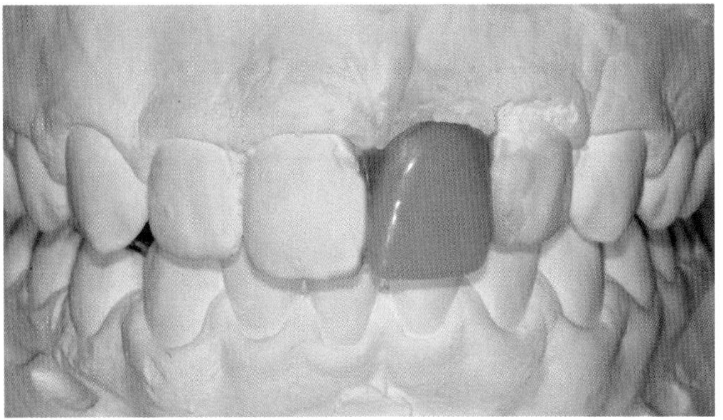

Figure 9.10. Labial view of the maxillary diagnostic cast with denture tooth in place before making the surgical guide.

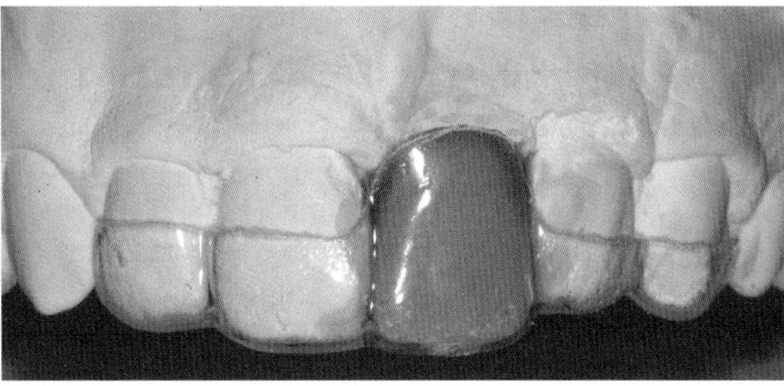

Figure 9.12. Surgical guide in place on the diagnostic cast. The guide was modified specifically to include the optimal location of the gingival margin for the implant restoration. The surgeon needed this landmark to place the implant in its proper vertical position.

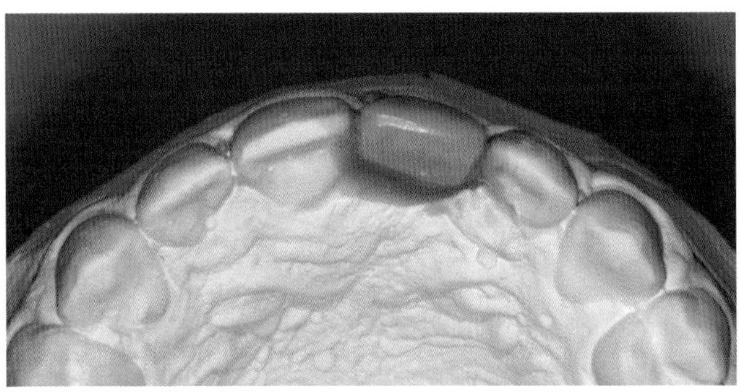

Figure 9.11. Laboratory occlusal view of the diagnostic cast with denture tooth in place before making the surgical guide.

Diagnoses

The following diagnoses were developed:

1. Partially edentulous maxilla secondary to trauma
2. Adequate bone volume for implant placement (Tooth #9)
3. Adequate restorative volume for implant restoration (Tooth #9)
4. Chronic mild gingivitis (Type I)

Prognosis

Based on the patient's age, residual alveolar ridge, occlusion, and overall general health, the author felt that the prognosis for this patient's treatment was excellent.

Appointment 2. Consultation Restorative Dentist/Patient (1/2 Hour)

Treatment Options

The patient returned for the definitive consultation appointment during which three treatment plans were presented. The first treatment option described placement of a 5 mm diameter implant with primary stability (at least 35 Ncm insertional torque), placement of an interim abutment and provisional crown without occlusal contacts, and osseointegration and fabrication of the definitive implant-retained crown (Table 9.2). The second treatment option described the replacement of the maxillary left central incisor with a 3-unit fixed partial denture (Table 9.3). The third treatment option deferred prosthetic treatment at this time (Table 9.4).

Benefits and limitations of each treatment option were described in detail on the written treatment plans. The prosthodontic fees, or ranges of fees for each procedure, were also listed on each treatment plan. The patient was given copies of the treatment plans. The patient agreed to proceed with the first treatment plan, including implant placement, and was referred to an oral surgeon for the surgical diagnostic work-up.

Appointment 3. Consultation Restorative Dentist/Surgeon (1/2 Hour)

This appointment generally takes place before or after normal business hours and should precede the surgeon's examination appointment. It may occur at lunch, at either practitioner's office, or at another convenient location. This consultation is critical for the long-term functional and aesthetic success of implant treatment. It is essential that the restorative dentist explain to the surgeon the physical and radiographic findings, the diagnosis, and the treatment options that were explained to the patient. This particular case presentation was technically demanding, and the consultation between restorative dentist and the oral surgeon was completed within 30 minutes.

Number/Size of Implant

In this case, the patient was missing a single tooth and appeared to have adequate space for both the surgical and prosthetic phases of implant treatment. The author

TABLE 9.2. Treatment Plan #1 (Implant Restoration)

Diagnosis: Partially edentulous maxilla secondary to trauma		
Restorative Services	**ADA #**	**Fee**
Comprehensive oral evaluation	D0150	
Diagnostic casts	D0470	
Panoramic radiograph	D0330	
Diagnostic wax pattern (#9)	D9999	
Surgical guide	D5988	

Referral to oral surgical office:

1. Evaluate and treat for replacement of the missing maxillary left central incisor with an Immediate Non Occlusal Loading Protocol (INOL).
2. Place a 5 mm diameter, internal connection implant with a single-stage protocol, if possible.
3. The implant should have primary stability as defined by insertional torque value of at least 35 Ncm. If the implant does not achieve this insertional torque value, place a healing abutment with the following dimensions: 5 mm restorative platform, 6 mm emergence profile, 2–4 mm collar height (IWTH562, IWTH563 or IWTH564).
4. An interim abutment (GingiHue® Post 5 mm restorative platform, 6 mm emergence profile, 4 mm collar height, IWPP564G) should be placed at the time of surgery. The abutment screw (IUNIHG) should be hand tightened.
5. Discharge the patient back to the author for fabrication of the INOL provisional restoration.
6. Postoperative instructions.

Restorative reevaluation	D0140	
Pre-machined interim implant abutment and INOL provisional restoration	D6056	
Osseointegration		
Custom implant abutment	D6057	
Abutment supported porcelain fused to metal crown (noble metal)	D6061	
Yearly recall appointment	D0120	
Periapical radiograph	D0220	

Benefits of Treatment Plan #1

The missing tooth in the front part of the upper jaw will be replaced with an implant restoration that will not be removable by the patient. Occlusion (bite) will be optimized. Patient should enjoy improved function with good aesthetics on a long-term basis. Some of the services may be eligible for payment under your medical insurance policy because the permanent tooth was lost secondary to an accident. The teeth adjacent to the missing tooth will not have to be prepared for crowns (caps).

Limitations of Treatment Plan #1

Cost, complexity, and length of treatment (4–12 months). Implants are generally successful in the front part of the upper jaw approximately 96–98% of the time. For this protocol to be successful, the patient must agree to COMPLETELY avoid placing food anywhere near or on the temporary crown for at least two months after the implant has been placed. Chewing on the temporary crown before the implant has bonded into the bone WILL jeopardize healing and may result in loss of the implant. If you admit to chewing on the implant, additional fees will be charged to you for redoing the treatment. Additional treatment, including bone grafting, may be necessary. The implant has to be placed optimally and be tight enough at the time of placement for the above treatments to be accomplished. If the implant cannot be placed optimally or it is not tight enough in the bone, changes in the treatments (surgical and prosthetic), fees, and designs will be likely. After the treatment has been completed, the patient needs to return to this office at least once per year (may be in conjunction with planned recall appointments) for follow-up, which will

TABLE 9.2. Treatment Plan #1 (Implant Restoration) (*continued*)

include radiographs (x-rays) to assess osseointegration of the implant, status of the occlusion, health of the soft tissues, and the integrity of the implant/abutment connection. This treatment plan itemizes only the prosthetic phase of treatment.

Patient signature ______________________
Date ______________________
Witness ______________________
Date ______________________

ADA #'s, CDT 2005 Current Dental Terminology, Council on Dental Benefit Programs, American Dental Association, 211 East Chicago Avenue, Chicago, IL 60611

suggested that a 5 mm diameter implant with an internal connection be placed because this size implant most closely approximated the size of the missing tooth. The surgeon would determine the shape of the implant body at the time of implant placement. In this case, the oral surgeon preselected a tapered implant (OSSEOTITE® Certain® IOSS515) (Figure 9.13).

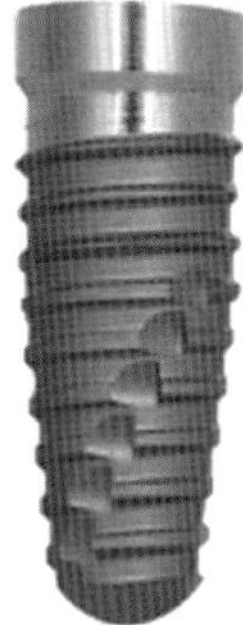

Figure 9.13. Profile view of OSSEOTITE® Certain® natural taper implant (IOSS515) used in this case.

Implant/Abutment Connection

The ***3i®*** internal connection implant was designed with a 4 mm long implant/abutment connection (refer to Chapter 5, Figure 5.15). The reader is referred to Chapter 5 for a review of the biomechanics of this connection.

Surgical Protocol

The surgical protocol for Immediate Non-Occlusal Loading requires a single stage surgical approach. The alveolus must be intact, and an insertional torque value of 35 Ncm is the critical threshold for successful treatment. The surgeon also must be sensitive to the standard parameters of implant placement.

Interim Abutment

There are several available abutments to select from for use with the INOL protocol: the Provide™ Abutment; the GingiHue® Post; the ZiReal™ Post; the STA® Abutment; and temporary cylinders and TG Posts. There are advantages and disadvantages associated with the above abutments. At the time this was written, the author found that GingiHue® Posts were the abutments of choice due to their versatility, numerous sizes (collar heights and emergence profile diameters), relative ease of preparation, and relative expense (Figure 9.14).

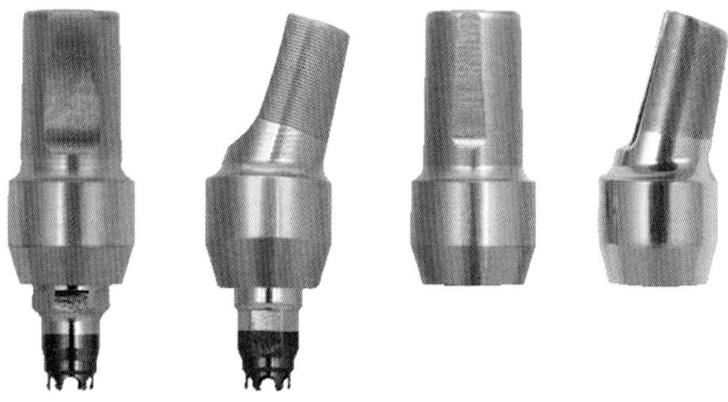

Figure 9.14. Laboratory product images of four GingiHue® Posts: internal connection straight and 15° Pre-Angled; external connection straight and 15° Pre-Angled, left to right.

In this instance the author provided the oral surgeon with a GingiHue® Post for a 5 mm diameter OSSEOTITE® Certain® implant with a 6 mm emergence profile and 4 mm collar height (IWPP564G) and a hexed try-in screw for the internal connection (IUNITS).

Implant Restorative Wish List

The above concepts have proven to be excellent starting points for discussions between the author and implant surgeons. A form was developed that incorporated all of the concepts noted above and is called the Implant Restorative Wish List (Table 9.5). It is now completed for each patient and sent to the implant surgeon prior to patient treatment.

TABLE 9.3. Treatment Plan #2 (Fixed Bridge)

Diagnosis: Partially edentulous maxilla secondary to trauma		
Restorative Services	**ADA #**	**Fee**
Comprehensive oral evaluation	D0150	
Diagnostic casts	D0470	
Panoramic radiograph	D0330	
Diagnostic wax pattern (#9)	D9999	
Tooth #8 (upper-right front tooth)		
Porcelain Fused to Metal Retainer	D6752	
Tooth #9 (missing front tooth)		
Porcelain Fused to Metal Pontic	D6242	
Tooth #10 (upper-left lateral incisor)		
Porcelain Fused to Metal Retainer	D6752	
Yearly recall appointment	D0120	
Periapical radiograph	D0220	

Benefits of Treatment Plan #2

The missing tooth in the upper jaw will be replaced with a fixed prosthesis that will not be removable by the patient. Occlusion (bite) will be optimized. Patient should enjoy improved function with good aesthetics on a long-term basis.

Limitations of Treatment Plan #2

Cost, complexity, and length of treatment (1–2 months). The teeth on either side of the missing tooth will have to be prepared (ground down) for crowns, even though neither one of them warrants such treatment. Local anesthesia will have to be used during the preparation appointment. The pulps (nerves) in one or both teeth may become irritated during the preparation procedures. The worst-case scenario would be that one or both of the teeth may warrant endodontic therapy (root canal treatment) during or after completion of the prosthesis. It may be slightly more difficult for you to accomplish satisfactory levels of oral hygiene in and around the prosthesis. One or both of the abutment teeth may be more likely to experience decay and/or periodontal (gum) disease. The patient needs to return to this office after treatment has been completed at least once per year (may be in conjunction with planned recall appointments) for follow-up, which will include radiographs (x-rays) to assess the integrity of the fit between the crowns and the abutment teeth, status of the occlusion, and health of the soft tissues. Fixed bridges generally have life expectancies of 5–12 years.

Patient signature ____________________________

Date ____________________________

Witness ____________________________

Date ____________________________

ADA #'s, CDT 2005 Current Dental Terminology, Council on Dental Benefit Programs, American Dental Association, 211 East Chicago Avenue, Chicago, IL 60611.

TABLE 9.4. Treatment Plan #3 (No Definitive Treatment)

Diagnosis: Partially edentulous maxilla secondary to trauma

Restorative Services	ADA #	Fee
Yearly recall appointment	D0120	
Bitewing radiographs	D0274	

Benefits of Treatment Plan #3

No invasive procedures will be performed in conjunction with the missing tooth in the front part of the upper jaw.

Limitations of Treatment Plan #3

The upper-front section of the mouth may be unstable and the adjacent teeth may be subject to drifting into the space of the missing tooth. Long-term function may be compromised by nonreplacement of the upper-front incisor. If the teeth in this section drift and then the patient decides to proceed with prosthetic treatment, orthodontics may be needed to put the teeth back into optimal positions prior to proceeding with definitive treatment.

Patient signature ________________________

Date ________________________

Witness ________________________

Date ________________________

ADA #'s, CDT 2005 Current Dental Terminology, Council on Dental Benefit Programs, American Dental Association, 211 East Chicago Avenue, Chicago, IL 60611.

TABLE 9.5. Implant Restorative Wish List

Tooth # 9 (Maxillary left central incisor)	
Type of Implant	OSSEOTITE® Certain®
Implant Restorative Platform	5.0 mm
Surgical Protocol	Single-stage/INOL
Implant/Abutment Connection	Internal (Certain)
Interim Abutment	GingiHue® Post: 5 mm × 6 mm × 4 mm
Occlusal Loading Protocol	Immediate Non-Occlusal Loading
Definitive restoration	3–6 months post implant placement

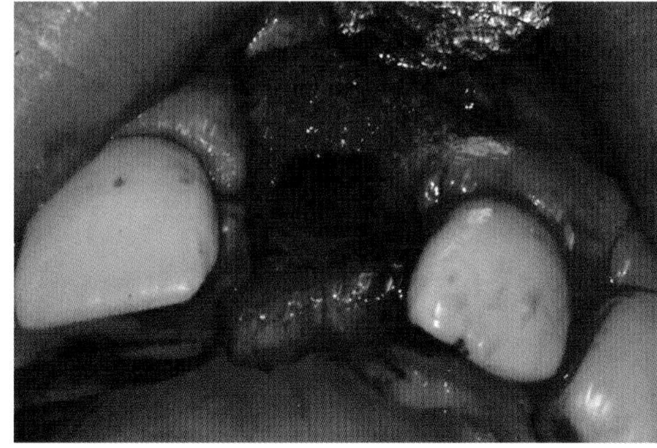

Figure 9.15. Occlusal view of the completed osteotomy for the natural taper implant used in this case.

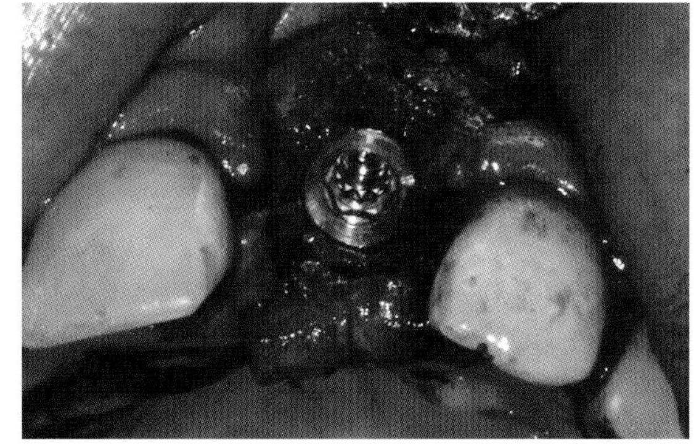

Figure 9.16. Occlusal view of the OSSEOTITE® Certain® implant in place.

Appointment 4. Implant and Interim Abutment Placement (Surgical Office—One Hour)

Implant Placement and Insertional Torque

The patient was premedicated with the appropriate antibiotic, and local anesthesia was administered. The osteotomy was prepared without incident. The surgeon was able to place a 5 × 15 mm implant with 40 Ncm insertional torque as registered on the drilling unit (Figures 9.15 and 9.16).

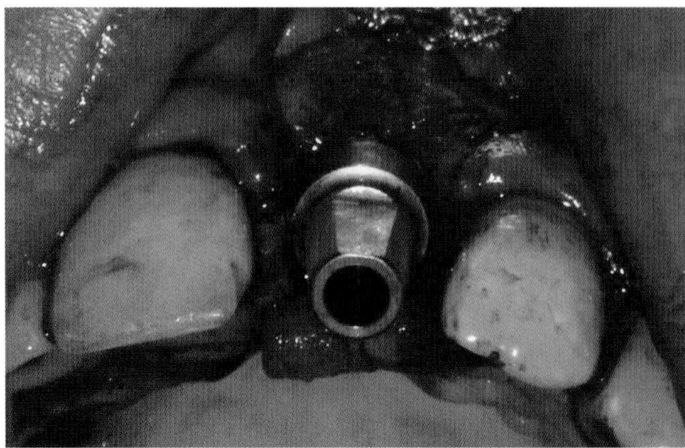

Figure 9.17. Occlusal view of the interim abutment in place prior to flap closure.

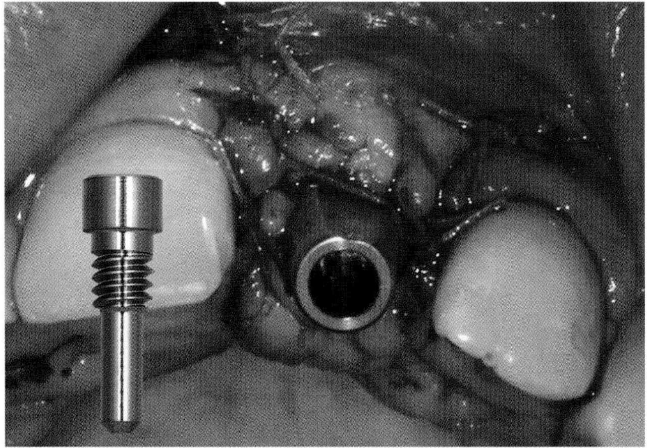

Figure 9.18. Occlusal view of the interim abutment in place after the flap was closed. The try-in screw (inset) that was provided by the author was hand tightened by the surgeon prior to discharge.

Interim Abutment Placement

The surgeon, prior to closure, placed the interim abutment and try-in screw that were provided by the author (Figure 9.17). It is essential for the surgeon to make sure that the interim abutment completely seats onto the implant restorative platform. If it does not, the surgeon would have to profile the surrounding bone in order to insure complete seating of the abutment.

The surgical wound was closed and the patient was discharged to the author for fabrication of the INOL provisional restoration (Figure 9.18).

Appointment 5. Restorative Appointment INOL Provisional Restoration—Same Day (3/4 Hour)

The patient was seated in the author's operatory. She still had satisfactory anesthesia.

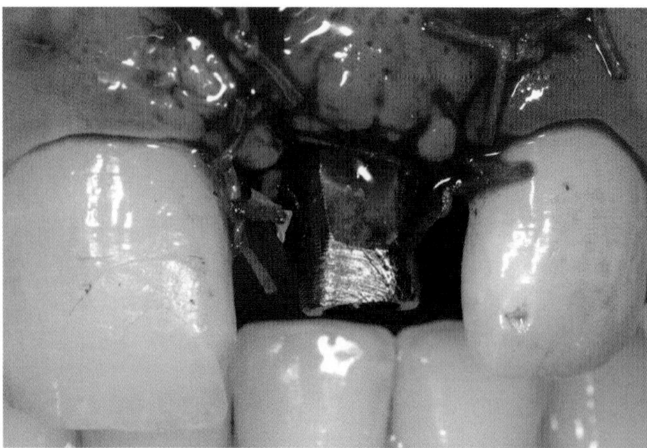

Figure 9.19. The interim abutment in place after the preparation was completed.

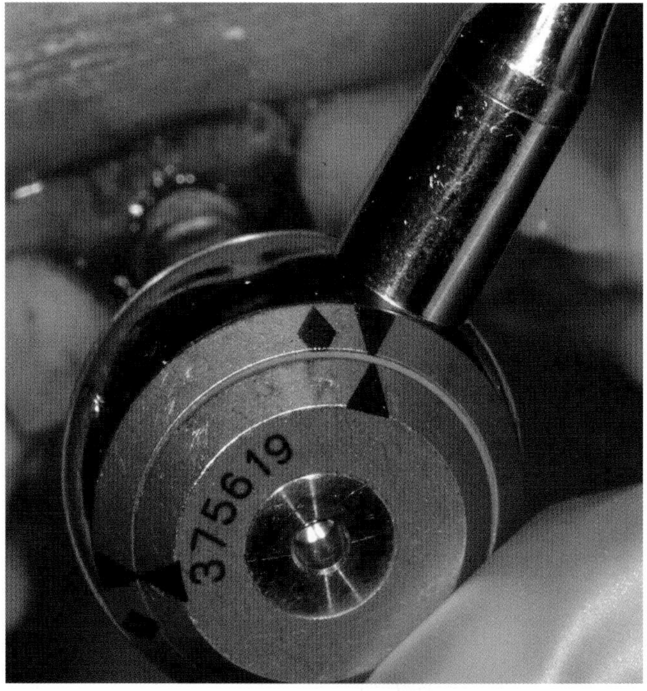

Figure 9.20. Occlusal view of the Restorative Torque Indicator (RTI2035) that demonstrated 20 Ncm of torque (triangle to triangle).

Abutment Preparation

The restorative procedures commenced with reducing the lingual/occlusal surfaces of the interim abutment to provide at least 2 mm of inter-occlusal clearance between the mandibular anterior teeth and the interim abutment (Figure 9.19). The bulk of the reduction was performed extra-orally so as to not generate heat or disrupt the fit between the implant and the osteotomy. The margins of the interim abutment were prepared so that they were approximately 1 mm sub-gingival.

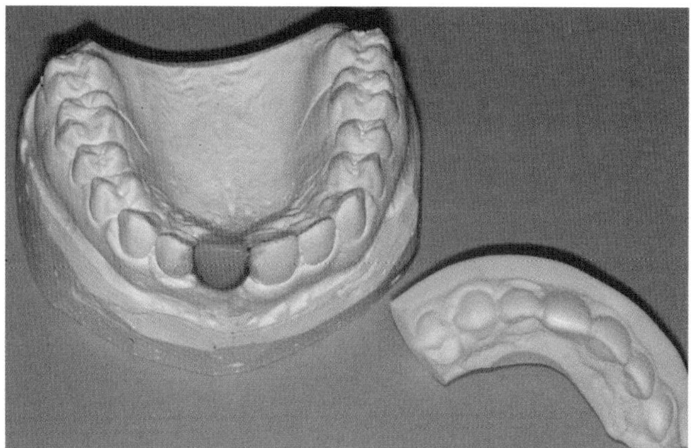

Figure 9.21. The silicone mold was made from the diagnostic cast to make the INOL provisional crown.

Immediate Non-Occlusal Loading Provisional Crown (INOL-No Centric/Eccentric Contacts)

After the preparation was completed, the try-in screw was removed and the definitive abutment screw (IUNIHG) was inserted and torqued to 20 Ncm with the Restorative Torque Indicator (RTI2035) and the Large Hex Driver Tip-Short (RASH3N) (Figure 9.20). The screw access opening was blocked out with cotton prior to fabrication of the INOL provisional restoration.

The INOL provisional restoration was made by using a mold from the denture tooth set in the original diagnostic cast (Figure 9.21). It was made using conventional fixed prosthodontic protocols and materials (Luxatemp®, DMG, Hamburg, Germany). The provisional crown was contoured for optimal emergence profiles. No occlusal contacts were permitted. It was cemented with temporary cement (IRM®, Dentsply Caulk, Milford, DE) (Figures 9.22 and 9.23).

Dietary and Oral Hygiene Instructions

Dietary restrictions were discussed for both the immediate postoperative period and long term as osseointegration occurred. The patient was instructed to use this implant and restoration for speaking and smiling only. There was to be absolutely no chewing on or near the provisional restoration and implant.

Oral hygiene was discussed and demonstrated to the patient with a typodont. A soft toothbrush (GUM® 468 Super Tip, Subcompact Soft, Sunstar Americas, Inc., Chicago, IL) was dispensed that was to clean macroscopic debris from around the surgical site and adjacent teeth. Chlorhexidine 0.12% was also dispensed and the patient was instructed to dip a cotton swab into the chlorhexidine and then massage it in and around the INOL provisional crown (Figure 9.24).

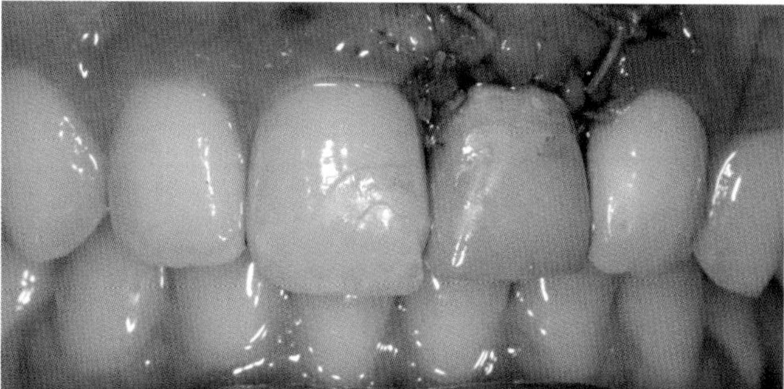

Figure 9.22. Facial view of the INOL provisional restoration in place prior to discharge on the day of implant placement. Centric or eccentric occlusal contacts were not permitted on this restoration.

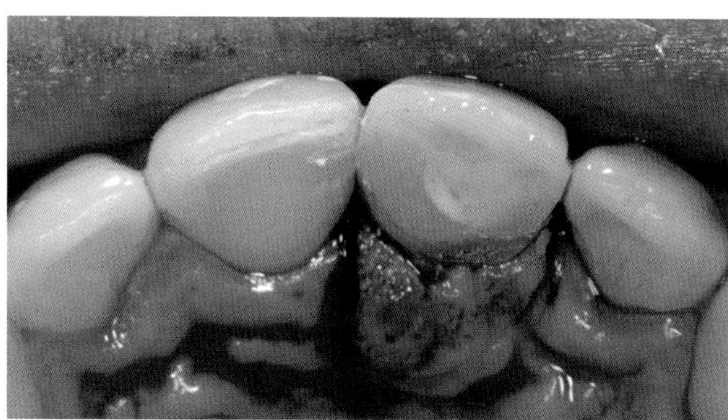

Figure 9.23. Occlusal view of the INOL provisional restoration in place prior to discharge.

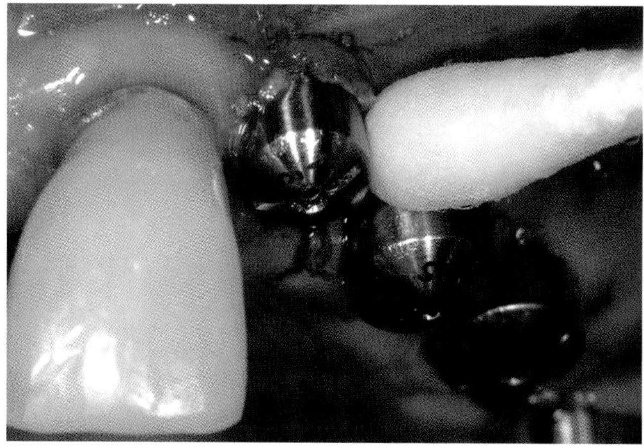

Figure 9.24. Clinical demonstration of cotton swab wetted with chlorhexidine used in and around healing abutments in a partially edentulous patient.

Appointment 6. Reevaluation Appointment—24 Hours (1/2 Hour)

History

The patient returned on the next day and reported absolutely no problems. Her pain was controlled with acetaminophen. She had minimal swelling and reported no change relative to phonetics. Overall, she was pleasantly surprised with the results of treatment.

Clinical Examination

There was minimal swelling. Her occlusion remained stable and there were no occlusal contacts on the INOL provisional restoration. There was no gingival recession noted at this appointment. The implant and provisional restoration were macroscopically stable and the soft tissues were healing consistent with the time frame.

Oral hygiene and dietary instructions were reinforced. The patient was discharged to return in two weeks or prn (as needed).

Appointment 7. Reevaluation Appointment—10 Days (1/2 Hour)

History

The patient reported no problems in the interim since the last appointment. She no longer needed any type of analgesic medications and had finished her antibiotic as prescribed. She remained pleased with the aesthetic and phonetic results.

Clinical Examination

The patient's occlusion remained stable and the INOL provisional restoration remained out of occlusion. The soft tissues were healing consistently with the time frame with minimal swelling. The implant and INOL provisional restoration remained macroscopically stable (Figure 9.25).

Oral hygiene and dietary instructions were reinforced. The patient was discharged to return in two weeks or prn.

Appointment 8. Reevaluation Appointment—10 Weeks (1/2 Hour)

History

The patient continued to do extremely well and reported no complaints. She reported no difficulties with oral hygiene and continued to avoid the INOL restoration with eating. She remained pleased with the results of treatment.

Clinical Examination

At this point, gingival recession was noted around the INOL provisional restoration (Figure 9.26). This soft tissue shrinkage was consistent with the time frame from the implant surgery. Fixed keratinized tissues were noted around the INOL provisional restoration. There was also reasonable gingival symmetry. The interdental papilla between the INOL provisional restoration and the maxillary cuspid was still lacking. The occlusion remained stable with the INOL provisional restoration out of contact in centric and eccentric occlusal positions.

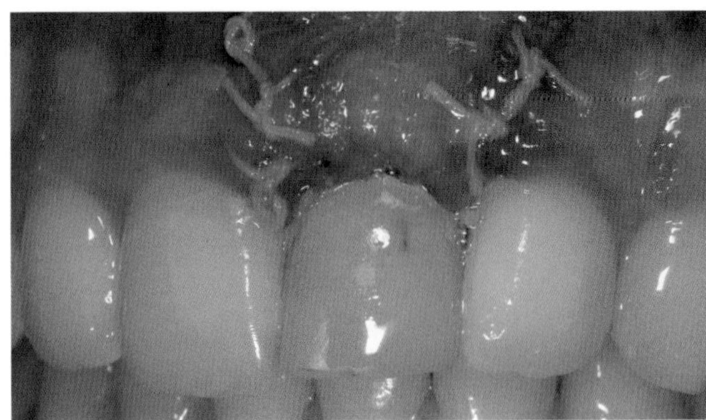

Figure 9.25. Clinical facial view of INOL provisional restoration 10 days post implant placement.

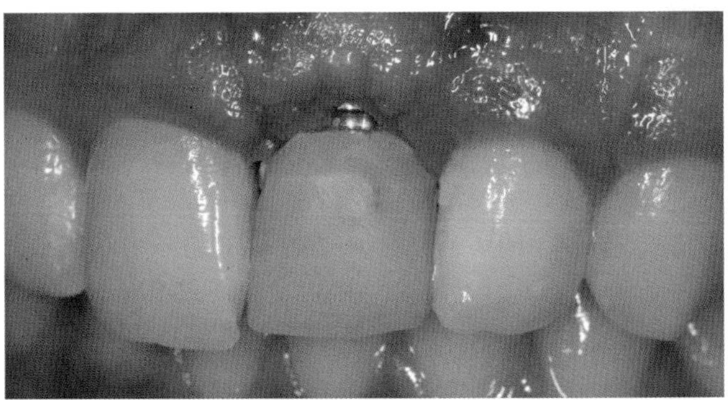

Figure 9.26. Clinical facial view of INOL provisional restoration 10 weeks post implant placement. Note the amount of gingival recession that has occurred when compared to the photograph in Figure 9.25.

At this point, the implant surgery was deemed to be successful. Another reevaluation appointment was scheduled in approximately six more weeks. At this appointment, definitive decisions would be made relative to osseointegration of the implant and gingival symmetry.

Appointment 9. Reevaluation—12 weeks (1/2 Hour)

History

The patient again reported no adverse signs or symptoms associated with the implant or the INOL provisional restoration. She was also pleased with the overall aesthetic results and did not want any additional surgery to "fine tune the gum tissues."

Clinical Examination

The patient's occlusion remained stable and the INOL provisional restoration remained without occlusal contacts. The soft tissues had healed and the gingival margins around the INOL provisional restoration appeared to be

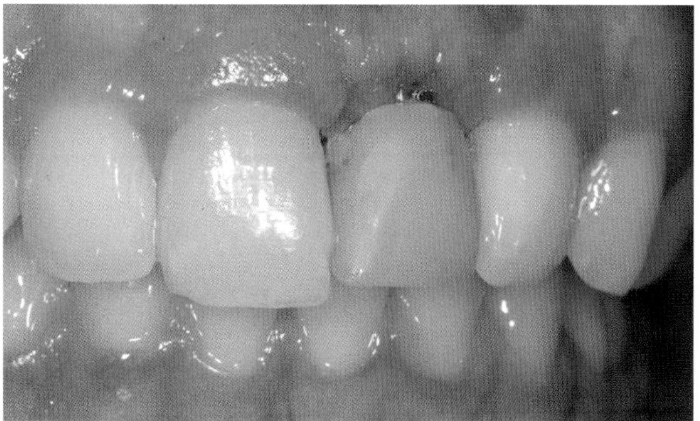

Figure 9.27. Clinical facial view of INOL provisional restoration 12 weeks post implant placement.

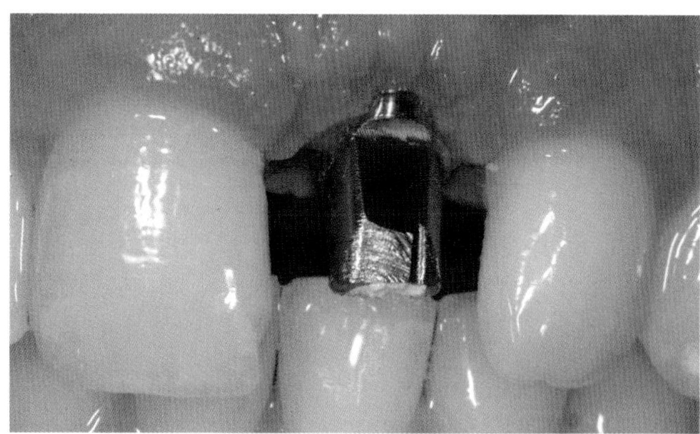

Figure 9.29. Interim abutment after removal of the INOL provisional crown. Note the amount of gingival recession that occurred with healing.

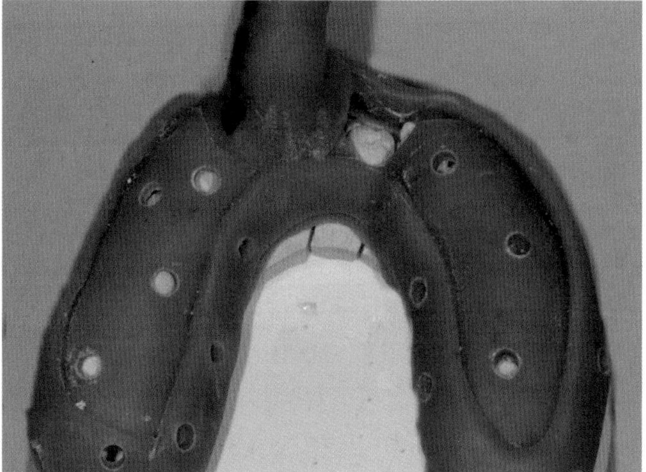

Figure 9.28. Occlusal laboratory view of custom open tray used in the pick-up implant impression protocol.

free of inflammation. The interdental papillae were still deficient (Figure 9.27).

The implant was determined to be osseointegrated. The clinical signs associated with osseointegration were the following: lack of mobility, tenderness, soft-tissue swelling, drainage, pain, and widened peri-implant space (radiograph).

Diagnostic Impressions/Casts (Optional)

In this case, diagnostic impressions were not required because the original diagnostic casts had been saved. New diagnostic casts can be made at this point, which would identify the locations of the implant and provisional restoration.

Custom Impression Tray (Pick-Up Technique)

The author prefers to use pick-up implant impression copings for implant impressions. This technique requires an open face impression tray (Figure 9.28). The laboratory work order for a custom open face impression tray is noted in Table 9.6.

TABLE 9.6. Laboratory Work Order for Custom Open Face Impression Tray

Patient name ______________________

Laboratory ______________________

Date ______________________

Enclosed:

1. Maxillary diagnostic cast

Please fabricate a custom open face acrylic resin impression tray (U-shaped).

1. Place one layer of baseplate wax over the maxillary teeth.
2. Adapt visible light cured acrylic resin material over the baseplate wax.
3. Light cure.
4. Prepare a window approximately 10 × 10 mm over the maxillary left central incisor.
5. Place multiple holes throughout the tray with a number 8 round bur.
6. Finish the borders.
7. Return.

Appointment 10. Implant Impression (3/4 Hour)

INOL Provisional Restoration and Interim Abutment

The INOL provisional restoration was removed and the interim abutment was completely visualized (Figure 9.29). The soft tissues had receded approximately 3 mm from the immediate post-implant insertion visit as determined from the amount the abutment facial margin was supra-gingival.

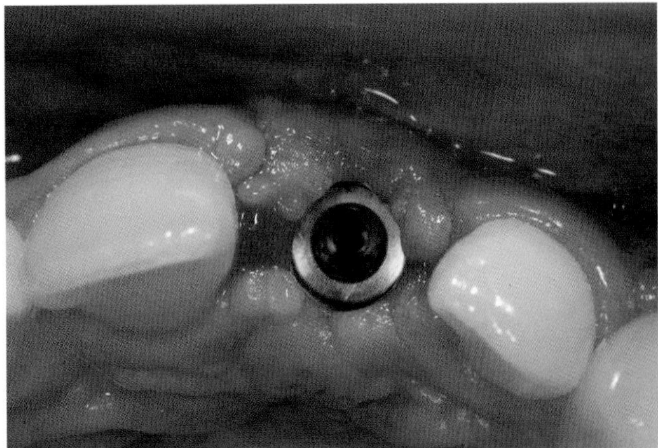

Figure 9.30. Implant restorative platform after removal of the interim abutment. The entire implant restorative platform must be visible in order to make an accurate implant level impression.

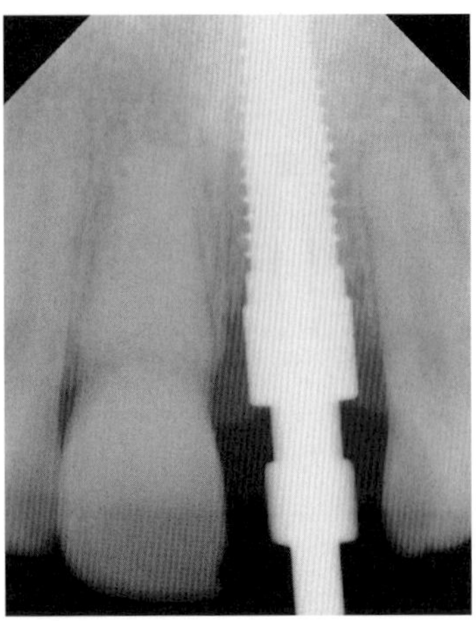

Figure 9.32. Radiograph that demonstrated an accurate fit between the implant impression coping and the implant.

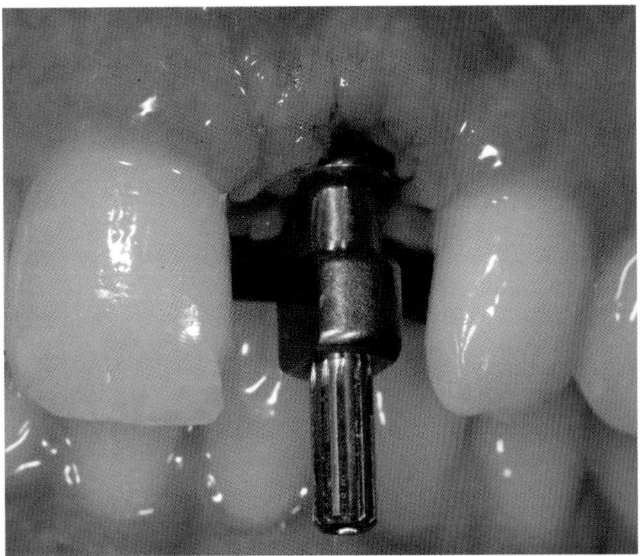

Figure 9.31. Implant impression coping (IWIP56) in place prior to the final impression.

A driver (PHD03N) was used to remove the hexed abutment screw from the interim abutment. The implant restorative platform was completely exposed and easy to visualize (Figure 9.30).

Implant Level Impression

An implant impression coping (IWIP56) consistent with the implant/abutment connection, emergence profile of the interim abutment, and implant restorative platform was placed onto the implant (Figure 9.31). A radiograph was taken to verify that the impression coping was accurately seated onto the implant restorative platform (Figure 9.32).

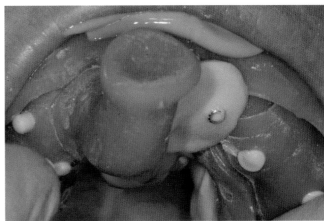

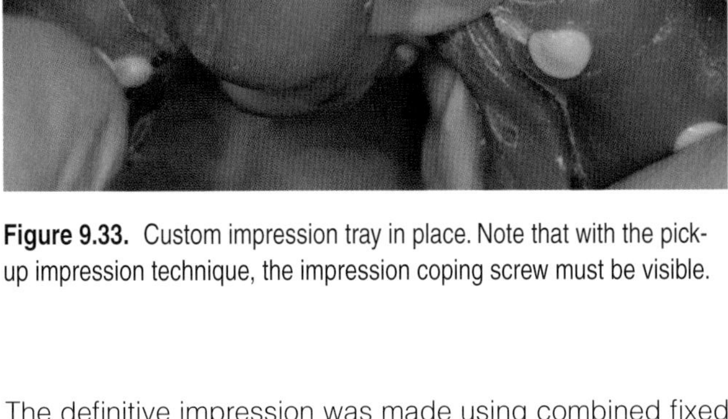

Figure 9.33. Custom impression tray in place. Note that with the pick-up impression technique, the impression coping screw must be visible.

The definitive impression was made using combined fixed prosthodontic and implant techniques by injecting light body polyvinyl siloxane impression material around the impression coping and loading the impression tray with a putty polyvinyl siloxane impression material (Exafast™, NDS, GC America, Alsip, IL) (Figure 9.33). With the pick-up impression technique, it is critical that the impression coping screw top remain visible during the impression procedure.

After the impression material polymerized, the excess material was removed from the hex of the implant impression coping screw with an explorer. The Standard Large Hex Driver, 24 mm (PHD03N) was used to loosen the screw (Figure 9.34). In order to ensure that the impression coping screw was completely free of the implant, a hemo-

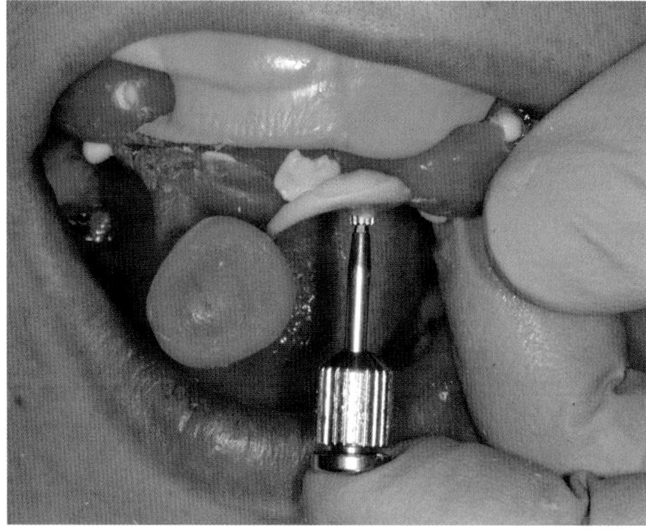

Figure 9.34. Posterior Large Hex Driver, 24 mm (PHDO3N) in place before removing the implant impression coping screw.

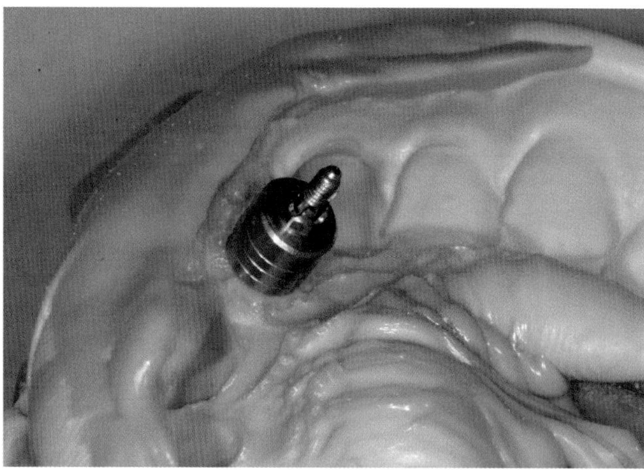

Figure 9.36. Intaglio surface of the definitive impression with the implant impression coping securely in place.

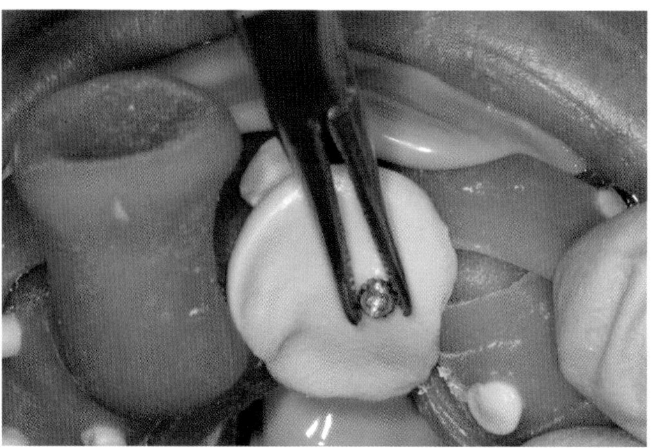

Figure 9.35. Hemostat in place that demonstrated that the impression coping screw was completely free of the implant and that the impression could safely be removed.

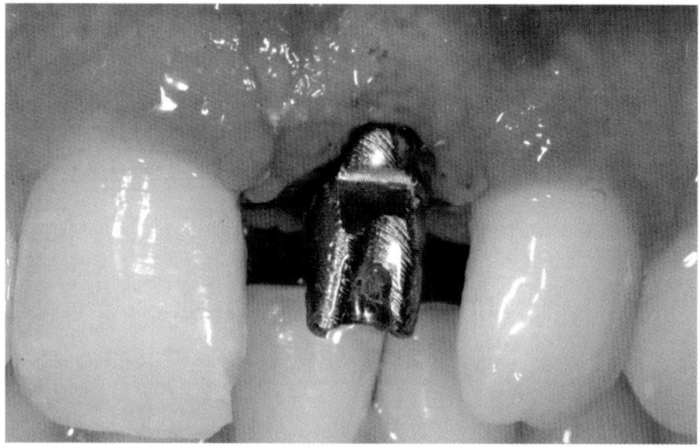

Figure 9.37. The interim abutment was placed back into the implant with the original abutment screw. The abutment screw was torqued to 20 Ncm and the abutment was re-prepared intra-orally with new facial subgingival margins.

stat was used to slightly pull the impression coping screw vertically (Figure 9.35). If the screw is not completely free of the implant, the impression tray must not be removed from the mouth because the impression coping will remain in the implant and the impression will not be accurate.

The impression tray was removed from the mouth and the pick-up implant impression coping remained inside the impression (Figure 9.36).

Interim Abutment Re-Preparation

The interim abutment was put back onto the implant with the Gold-Tite™ Hexed Abutment Screw and torqued to 20 Ncm with the Restorative Torque Indicator (RTI2035) and the Large Hex Driver Tip, Short (RASH3N). The abutment was re-prepared using coarse diamond burs so that the facial margin was slightly sub-gingival (Figure 9.37).

Provisional Crown with Occlusal Contacts

Cotton was used to block out the screw access opening and a new provisional crown was fabricated using conventional fixed prosthodontic materials and techniques (Figure 9.38). Because this implant was considered to be osseointegrated, this provisional crown was made with occlusal contacts in centric occlusion and shared disclusion in a protrusive position with the incisal edge of the maxillary right central incisor.

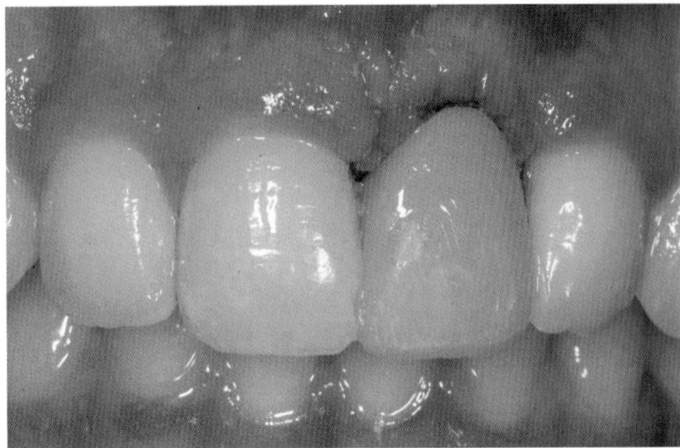

Figure 9.38. New provisional restoration in place. This restoration had occlusal contacts.

Laboratory Procedures for the Master Cast

The author's laboratory technician fabricated the master cast. However, a commercial dental laboratory may also fabricate the master cast (Table 9.7).

Implant Analogs

Implant analogs replicate implants that have been placed intra-orally. After the implant analogs have been placed appropriately within impressions and attached to the implant impression copings accurately, they will replicate the orientation of implants in the master cast. In this case, a 5 mm OSSEOTITE® Certain® implant lab analog was selected (IILAW5). The OSSEOTITE® Certain® Implant System features color-coding that facilitates accurate matching of implant restorative components for dental assistants, laboratory technicians, and restorative dentists. The components for 5 mm diameter implants are color-coded gold. The 5 mm OSSEOTITE® Certain® implant analog was placed into the apical surface of the implant impression coping that was inside the impression (Figure 9.39). Metal-to-metal contact must be visualized around the entire periphery of the impression coping/implant analog interface.

The soft tissues that surround implants should be replicated in a resilient material instead of die stone. This technique allows laboratory technicians to customize the sub-gingival emergence profiles of implant restorations consistently with the emergence profiles that were generated by clinicians via the emergence profiles of healing or interim abutments. In this case, a resilient material manufactured specifically for this purpose was used (Gingival Mask HP, Henry Schein®, Melville, NY). This material comes in a delivery system similar to impression materials and was injected around the impression coping/implant lab analog junction (Figure 9.40). It was allowed to set for approximately 10 minutes.

TABLE 9.7. Laboratory Work Order for Construction of Maxillary Master Cast (Implant Analog)

Patient name ________________

Laboratory ________________

Date ________________

Enclosed:

1. Mandibular diagnostic cast.
2. Definitive maxillary implant impression.
   a. 5 mm OSSEOTITE® Certain® implant
   b. 6 mm pick-up implant impression coping in impression

Please fabricate a maxilary master cast.

1. Place 5 mm OSSEOTITE® Certain® analog (IILAW5-gold color) onto the apical portion of the impression coping.
   a. Make sure there is metal-to-metal contact all around the impression coping/analog junction.
2. Place and fabricate the soft-tissue portion of the cast with a suitable material per the manufacturer's instructions.
3. Pour the cast with Type IV dental stone per the manufacturer's instructions.
4. Pin the cast as in conventional fixed prosthodontics.
5. Mount both casts on a simple hinge articulator.
6. Return to me for abutment selection.

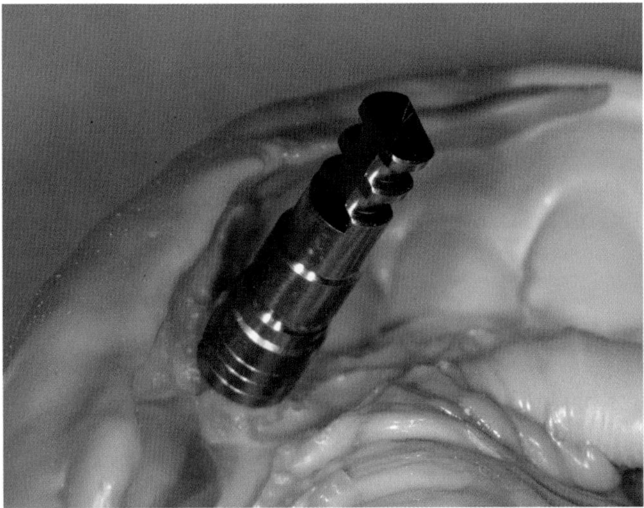

Figure 9.39. OSSEOTITE® Certain® 5 mm implant lab analog connected to the apical surface of the implant impression coping inside the impression.

Master Cast

The impression was poured in Type IV die stone. It was pinned in conventional fashion and mounted on a simple hinge articulator for abutment selection (Figures 9.41, 9.42).

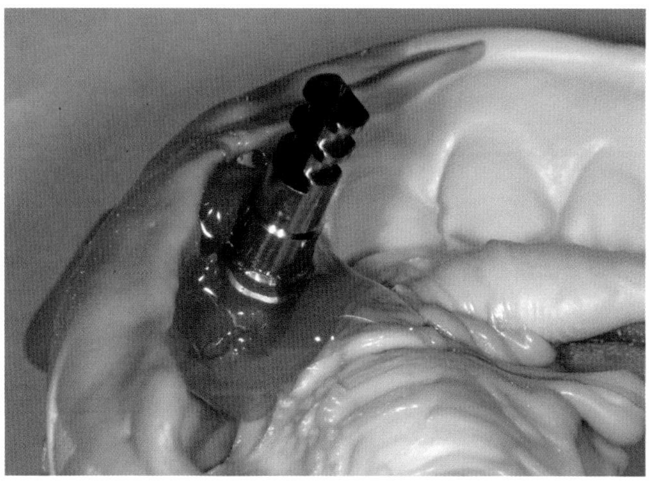

Figure 9.40. A resilient soft material was injected around the impression coping/implant lab analog junction to replicate the intra-oral peri-implant soft tissues.

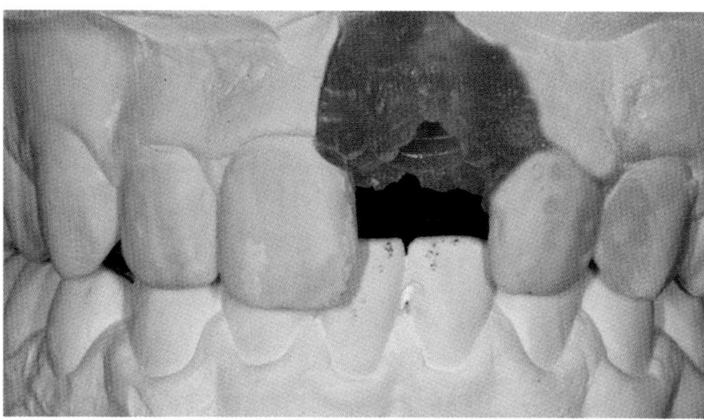

Figure 9.42. The master cast mounted on a simple hinge articulator prior to abutment selection.

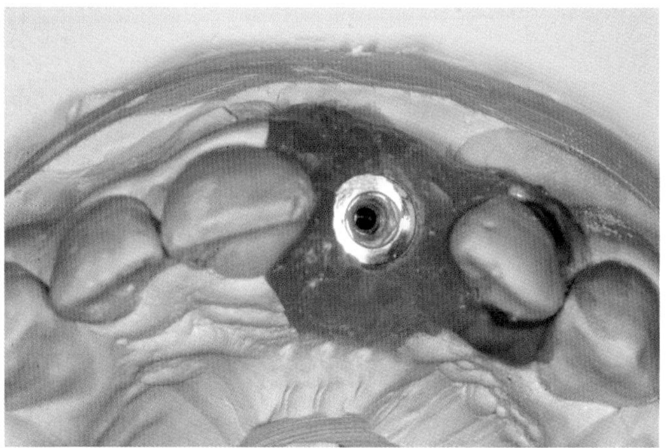

Figure 9.41. Laboratory occlusal view of the 5 mm diameter implant lab analog in the master cast.

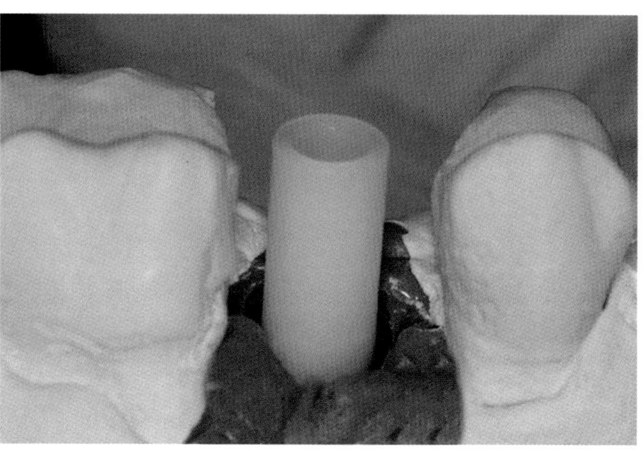

Figure 9.43. UCLA Abutment (IWGA51C) as received from the manufacturer in place on a master cast. The nylon portion of the abutment can be adjusted by carving and/or adding wax to develop the contours required for an aesthetic, functional implant-retained restoration.

Abutment Selection

There are six key factors in determining the most appropriate abutment for use in a given situation:

1. Implant/abutment connection
2. Implant restorative platform (diameter)
3. Emergence profile of the healing or interim abutment
4. Depth of the peri-implant soft tissues
5. Implant angulation
6. Inter-occlusal clearance

In this case, the inter-occlusal clearance from the implant restorative platform to the incisal edges of the mandibular incisors was greater than 12 mm. This fact precluded the use of stock abutments (GingiHue® Posts or ZiReal™ Posts). Screw-retained crowns are generally easier to remove in the event that the aesthetic veneer of an implant-retained crown fractures or an abutment screw becomes loose. However, screw-retained crowns may sacrifice occlusion and aesthetics, depending on the location of the screw access opening within the crown restoration (Hebel and Gajjar 1997).

The abutment selection process was therefore limited to custom abutments: UCLA Abutments or definitive Encode™ Abutments. UCLA Abutments were the original custom abutments (Figure 9.43). Stock abutments would not be appropriate in this case because the inter-occlusal clearance exceeded 10 mm. The most precise fitting UCLA Abutments are made with machined interfaces and a castable

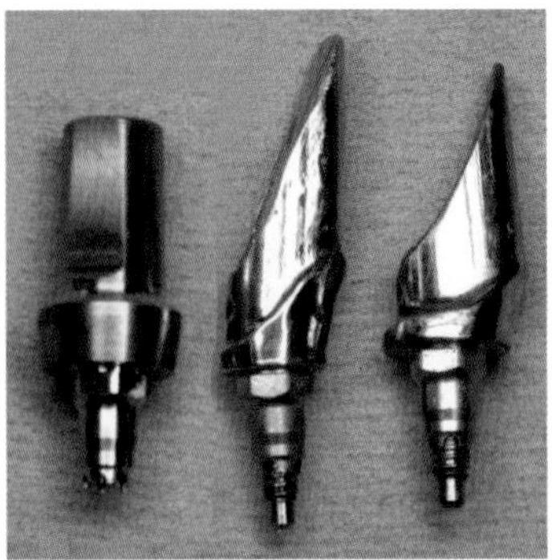

Figure 9.44. A pre-machined, stock abutment as received from the manufacturer (left); and two custom UCLA Abutments (right). Note the dramatic differences in the levels of the interproximal margins created in the custom abutments. These different levels could not have been prepared into the stock abutment on the left.

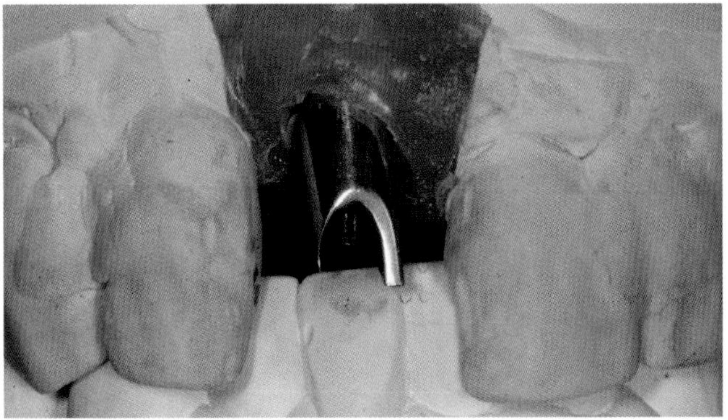

Figure 9.45. This is an example of a Final Encode™ Abutment with a gold titanium nitride coating for a maxillary right central incisor on a master cast.

nylon pattern (IGUCA1C) (Hurson 1996). The machined interface provides a precise implant/abutment connection, whereas the nylon castable pattern allows dental laboratory technicians to customize the contours of the custom abutment for individual clinical conditions (Figure 9.44).

Final Encode™ Abutments are made with CAD/CAM technology, as described in Chapter 6. The two major advantages with using this type of an abutment include precise CAD/CAM machining and a gold titanium nitride coating that can be applied to the abutment after it has been machined (Figure 9.45).

Protocol for Fabrication of Final Encode™ Abutment

The protocol for fabrication of a Final Encode Abutment includes a master cast of the Encode Healing Abutment, articulator mounting (Stratos® 100 articulator), and completion of the Encode Work Order. The cast with the Encode Healing Abutment must be poured in an appropriate die stone (GC FUJIROCK® EP, GC Europe, Leuven, Belgium). The cast can be made from an intra-oral impression of the Encode Healing Abutment in place on an implant or it can be made from a laboratory impression of an Encode Healing Abutment in place on an implant analog in the analog-containing master cast. In this case, the author made an implant level impression clinically and his technician attached an implant analog to the implant impression coping and poured the analog containing master cast.

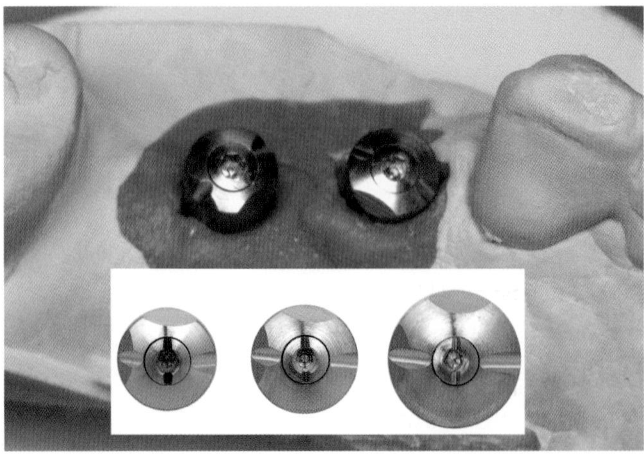

Figure 9.46. Two Encode Healing Abutments (IEHA454) in place on a master cast (top). The Encode Healing Abutments were selected consistent with the sizes of the teeth being replaced (maxillary first and second premolars). The codes on the occlusal surfaces of the Encode Healing Abutments must be supra-gingival in order for the optical scanner to recognize them. Occlusal surfaces of Encode Healing Abutments with 5, 6, and 7.5 mm emergence profile diameters (lower inset).

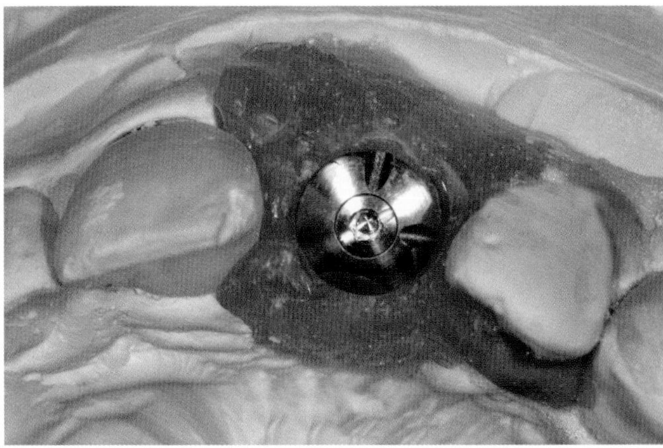

Figure 9.47. Laboratory occlusal view of the Encode Healing Abutment (IEHA564) in place on the master cast that was used in this case.

Laboratory Fabrication of Encode Master Cast

The foundation of this system is the codes that have been machined into Encode Healing Abutments (Figure 9.46). The codes have to be reproduced in die stone because

TABLE 9.8. Laboratory Work Order for Construction of Maxillary Master Cast (Encode Healing Abutment)

Patient name ______________________

Laboratory ______________________

Date ______________________

Enclosed:

1. Maxillary master cast with implant lab analog for 5 mm OSSEOTITE® Certain® implant.
2. Encode Healing Abutment (IEHA564-2 pieces):
   a. 5 mm restorative platform
   b. 6 mm emergence profile
   c. 4 mm collar height

Please fabricate a maxilary master cast.

1. Place Encode Healing Abutment into position on the above master cast. Make sure the healing abutment is completely seated onto the implant analog.
2. The codes of the healing abutment must be supragingival.
3. Make an impression of the cast with a vinyl polysiloxane impression material.
4. Pour this impression in GC FUJIROCK® EP per the manufacturer's instructions.
5. Mount the maxillary Encode cast and the mandibular cast on a Stratos 100 articulator (Ivoclar Vivadent) with magnetic mounting plates.
6. Complete the Final Encode Healing Abutment work order.
7. Ship the casts and the work order to the ARCHITECH PSR™ Center, Palm Beach Gardens, FL.

The Final Encode Abutment will be returned to you for fabrication of the crown.

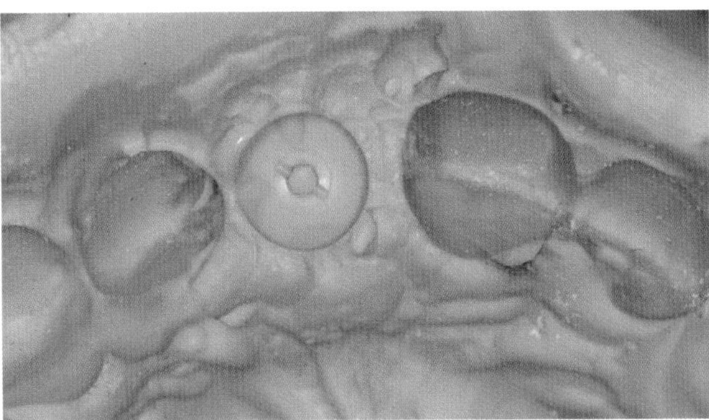

Figure 9.48. Intaglio surface of the vinyl polysiloxane impression of the Encode Healing Abutment in Figure 9.47.

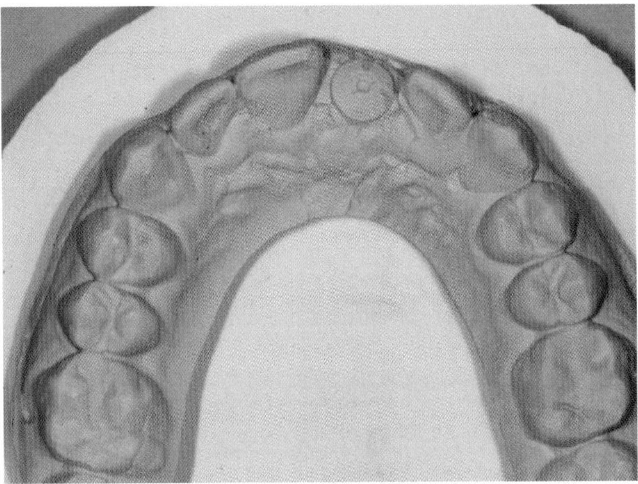

Figure 9.49. Laboratory occlusal view of the master cast with the Encode Healing Abutment in die stone. This cast was scanned as part of the protocol for fabrication of the Final Encode Abutment.

the scanner is not able to read the codes from the metallic healing abutments. These codes are optically scanned by a digital scanner and identify the implant/abutment connection, location of the implant hex, the location of the soft tissue margins, and the emergence profile of the healing abutment. Encode Healing Abutments can be used intraorally and in the laboratory. The following sequence illustrates the use of Encode Healing Abutments in the dental laboratory (Table 9.8).

An Encode Healing Abutment (IEHA564) was selected that was consistent with the size of the interim abutment (Figure 9.47). It was essential that all of the codes were supragingival because the optical scanner cannot read subgingival margins.

An impression was made of the master cast with the Encode Healing Abutment in place (Figure 9.48). This impression was poured in a low-chroma, low-value die stone (GC FUJIROCK® EP, GC Europe, Leuven, Belgium) (Figure 9.49).

This cast was mounted on a Stratos® 100 articulator (Ivoclar Vivadent, Amherst, NY). The author's dental laboratory technician completed the laboratory work order specific for Final Encode Abutments (Table 9.9). In this case, the author asked for sub-gingival labial and inter-proximal margins; the lingual margin was to be at the gingival crest. The design also included a circumferential shoulder preparation of 1.8 mm. The author also wanted a two-plane reduction on the labial surface of the abutment to allow for optimal thickness of porcelain and accurate reproduction of natural tooth contours, consistent with the contours of the contra lateral maxillary central incisor. The work order and the casts, not the articulator, were sent to the ARCHITECH PSR™ Center in Palm Beach Gardens, FL, for scanning and fabrication of the Final Encode Abutment.

TABLE 9.9. Laboratory Work Order for Construction of Final Encode Abutment

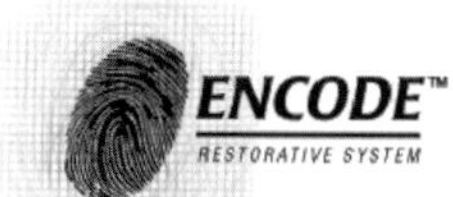

Work Order

* 1. Account Information

* Lab Name:________________

3i Account#:________________

* Contact:________________

* Phone:________________

Fax:________________

* Email:________________

* Patient ID:________________

* Ship To:________________

____

Bill To:________________

____

* 2. Preparing Your Case For Shipment

- *Use only **yellow** die stone for the Encode Casts.*
- *Verify that all of the codes on each healing abutment are completely visible on the cast.*
- *Section and pin the Encode Die Cast **(Please do not trim the Encode Die).***
- *Mount casts on Adesso Split Plates Articulator **only** (Stratos® or Baumann) and verify the vertical pin is set at zero and meets the occlusal table.*
- *Following mounting on the designated articulator please include the following in the shipment to **3i**:*
  - ❑ Pinned & Sectioned Encode Die Cast
  - ❑ Opposing Cast
  - ❑ Copy of the Completed Work Order
- *All un-articulated or mis-articulated casts will be returned to the lab*
- *Please **do not** send the articulator*

* 3. Case Information

Tooth Position	Connection Type		Gold Colored TiN** (Titanium Nitride) Yes or No
	Certain®	Ex-Hex	

** NOTE: TiN Coating will add two working days to the processing of your abutment. If a box is not checked the abutment will not be TiN coated.

* 4. Design Guidelines

Margin Style – Select One
❑ Shoulder
❑ Chamfer (Default)

Interocclusal Distance: _____mm

NOTE: Default on all margins = 1mm Subgingival

Buccal Margin Location
❑ Subgingival _____mm
❑ Flush with Gingiva

Lingual Margin Location
❑ Subgingival _____mm
❑ Flush with Gingiva
❑ Supragingival _____mm

* REQUIRED FIELD

5. Contour Guidelines

Please draw the approximate contour desired over the default images below. Note margin style. Please draw in tissue contour. (Minimum abutment height = 4mm and minimum collar height = .5mm)

Buccal Interproximal

Anterior

Posterior

6. Special Instructions

❑ Polish entire abutment (Default) ❑ Only polish the subgingival collar

____

____

____

❑ See back or attached page for additional instructions.

7. Screw Ordering

❑ I would not like to order screws at this time.

External Hex Abutment Screws	Qty.
Gold-Tite™ Square (UNISG)	____
Gold-Tite Hexed (UNIHG)	____
Titanium Hexed (UNIHT)	____
Laboratory Square Try-in Screw - 5 pack (UNITS)	____
Microminiplant™ Square Try-in Screw - 5 pack (MUNITS)	____

Certain Abutment Screws	Qty.
Gold-Tite Hexed (IUNIHG)	____
Titanium Hexed (IUNIHT)	____
Laboratory Hexed Try-in Screw - 5 pack (IUNITS)	____

* 8. Certification — must be signed

I certify that the stated information is correct and that the submitted materials are accurate. All items that have contacted the oral environment have been disinfected. This form authorizes *3i* to fabricate the patient specific abutment(s) using and consistent with the information provided on this work order.

Technician Signature ________________

Date ________________

Internal Use Only

Job #: ________________

Signature: ________________

3i Implant Innovations, Inc.
4555 Riverside Drive
Palm Beach Gardens, FL 33410
800.443.8166

ART881
REV E 10/05

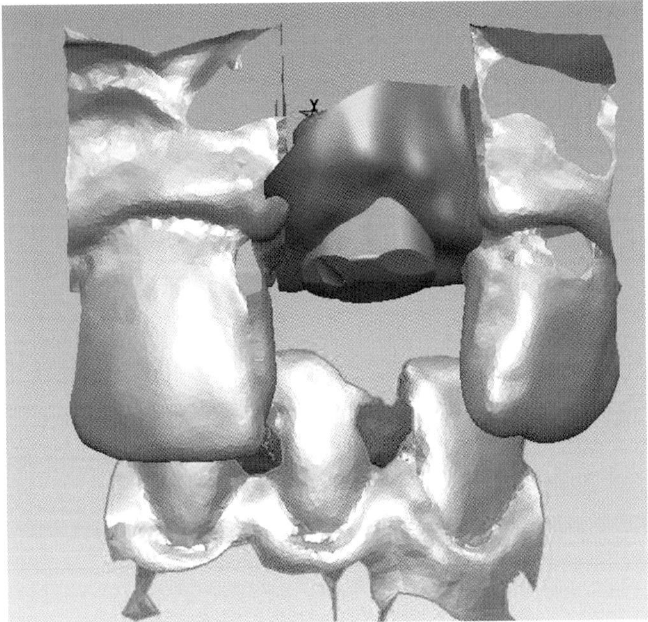

Figure 9.50. This image was the first image in the CAD design process. It was an image of the Encode Healing Abutment (die stone cast) in place.

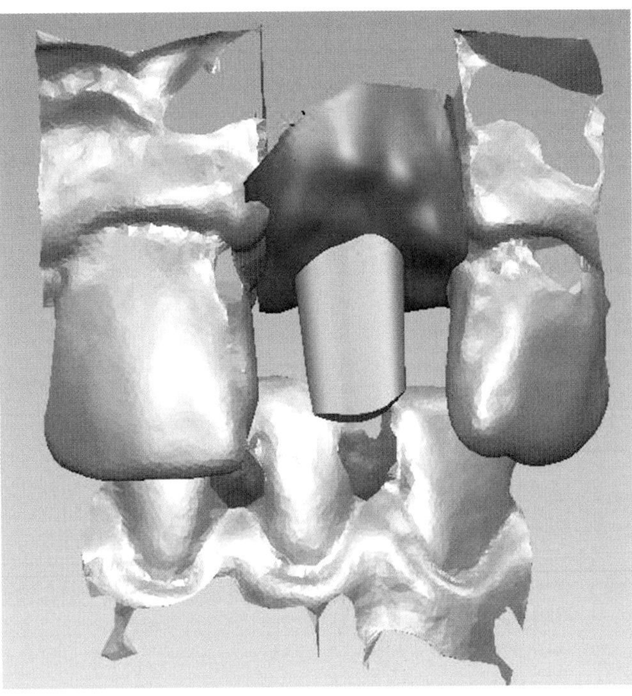

Figure 9.52. This image is similar to Figure 9.51 except that the soft tissue was not removed.

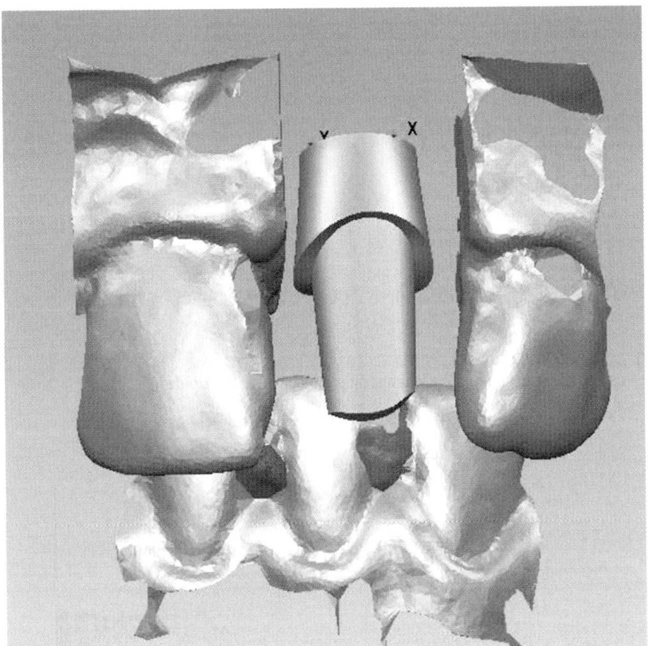

Figure 9.51. This was the image of the initial abutment preparation. The computer software program removed the soft tissue from around the abutment.

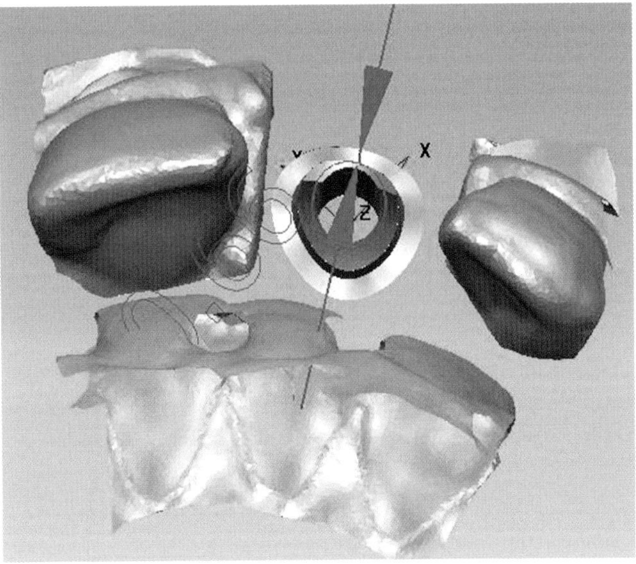

Figure 9.53. This is an occlusal view of the CAD design for the Final Encode Abutment. Note the circumferential shoulder.

After the above was received at the ARCHITECH™ PSR Center, the cast was scanned and the abutment was designed with a sophisticated computer software program (Figure 9.50). This design was emailed to the author for review and modification. The virtual design was then transferred to the computer-milling unit to fabricate the Final Encode™ Abutment (Figures 9.51, 9.52, 9.53).

TABLE 9.10. Laboratory Work Order for Construction of Porcelain Fused to Metal Crown on Final Encode Abutment

Patient name ________________

Laboratory ________________

Date ________________

1. Block out the screw access opening of the Final Encode Abutment with cotton.
2. Place two layers of die spacer on the abutment.
3. Wax the coping for implant #9 to full contour.
4. Cut back the wax pattern for use as a coping for a PFM crown.
5. Cast in 60% gold alloy (IPS d.SIGN 91, Ivoclar Vivadent).
6. Finish the casting.
7. Apply porcelain with contours that replicate those of the natural tooth #8.
8. Stain and glaze.
9. Return the crown and casts.

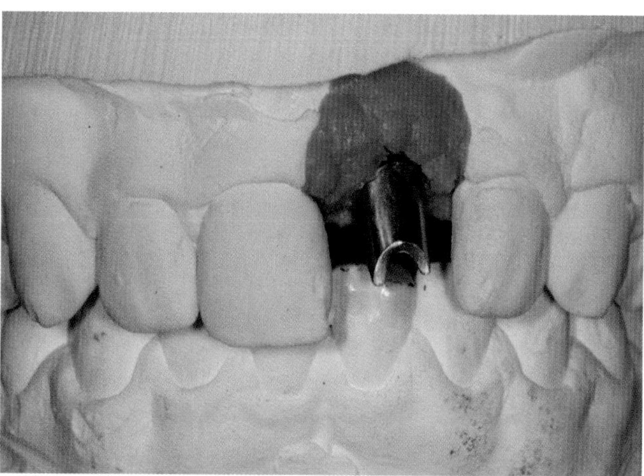

Figure 9.54. The Final Encode Abutment in place on the master cast with the implant analog. This image was taken at the commercial dental laboratory before waxing the coping for the porcelain fused to metal crown.

The Final Encode Abutment was completed and sent to the author's commercial dental laboratory for fabrication of the definitive crown per the original laboratory work order (Table 9.10) (Figures 9.54 through 9.59).

Laboratory Work Orders

See Tables 9.7 through 9.10, shown previously.

Appointment 11. Abutment and Crown Insertion (3/4 Hour)

This appointment occurred approximately four weeks after the definitive impression described above. The patient reported no symptoms or adverse occurrences and was pleased with the aesthetic, phonetic, and functional results of the provisional implant restoration.

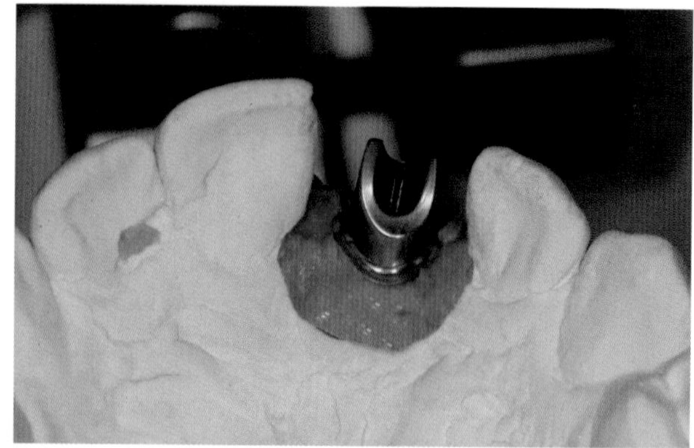

Figure 9.55. Lingual view of the Final Encode Abutment in place on the master cast. The author designed the lingual margin to be at the gingival crest.

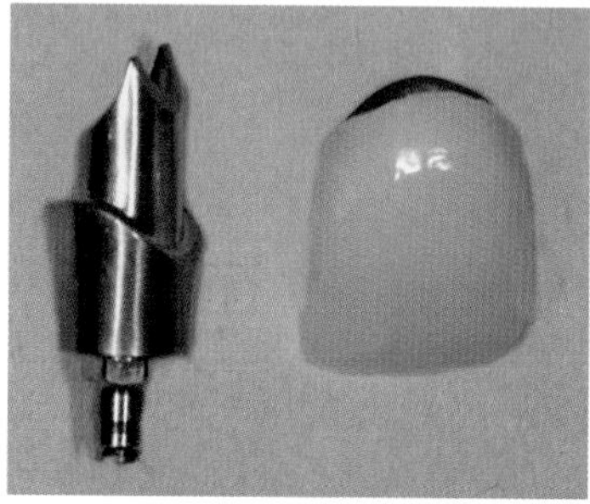

Figure 9.56. Laboratory view of the Final Encode Abutment and the definitive porcelain fused to metal crown.

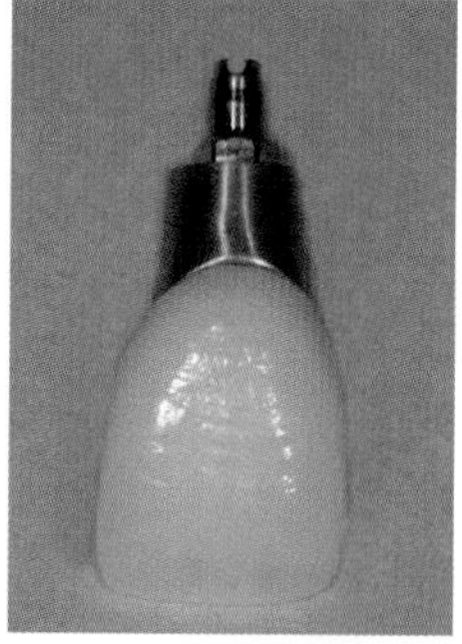

Figure 9.57. Laboratory view of the definitive crown on the Final Encode Abutment. Optimal emergence profiles were developed by the computer software program and milled into the abutment. The crown was cast and the porcelain applied in conventional fashion.

Interim Abutment and Provisional Crown Removal

The patient reported no problems with the provisional restoration or implant (Figure 9.60). The upcoming procedures were explained and she agreed to proceed.

The provisional crown was removed. The peri-implant soft tissues had healed and appeared to be stable (Figure

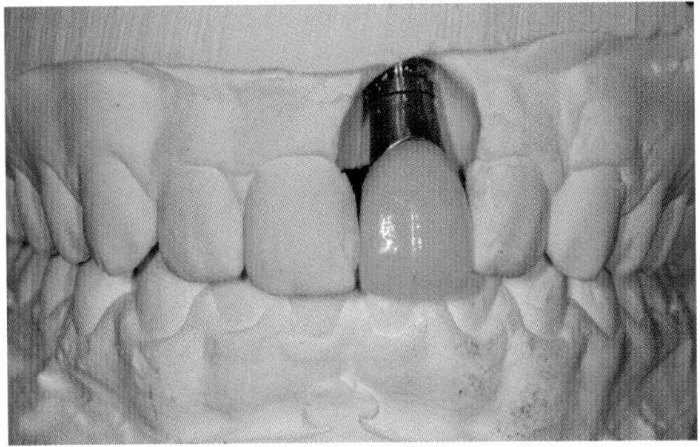

Figure 9.58. Facial view of the definitive crown in place on the abutment in the master cast. The soft tissue replica has been removed.

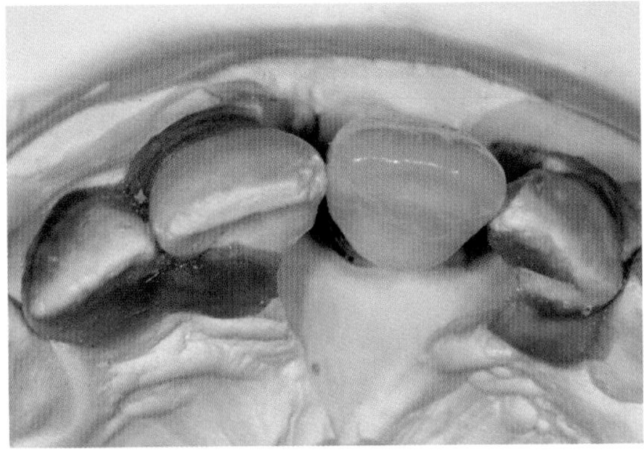

Figure 9.59. Occlusal view of the definitive crown in place on the abutment in the master cast.

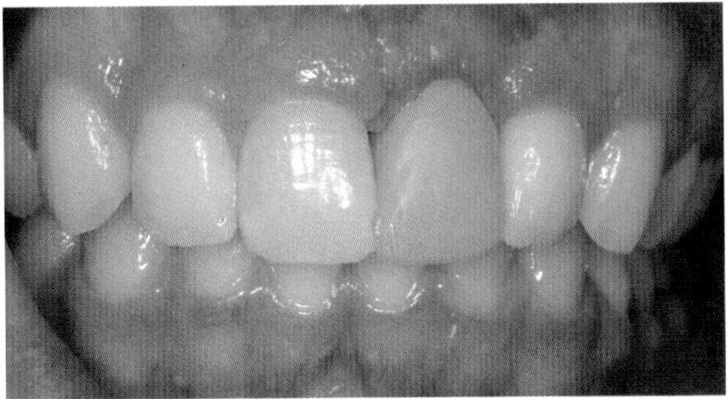

Figure 9.60. Clinical anterior view of the maxillary anterior segment with the provisional crown in place four weeks after the definitive implant level impression was made.

9.61). The interim abutment was removed and the implant restorative platform was completely exposed (Figure 9.62).

Definitive Abutment Placement

The Final Encode™ Abutment was placed by seating the abutment placement index onto the occlusal surfaces of the adjacent teeth (Figure 9.63). A hexed try-in screw (IUNIT) was used to retain the abutment to the implant (Figure 9.64). The abutment "clicked" into place by virtue of the Quick Seat™ Connection.

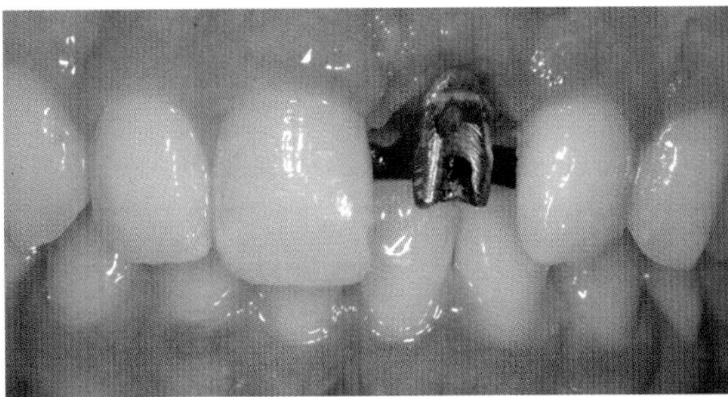

Figure 9.61. Clinical anterior view of the interim abutment after the provisional crown was removed. Note the stability of the gingival margin relative to the prepared facial margin of the interim abutment.

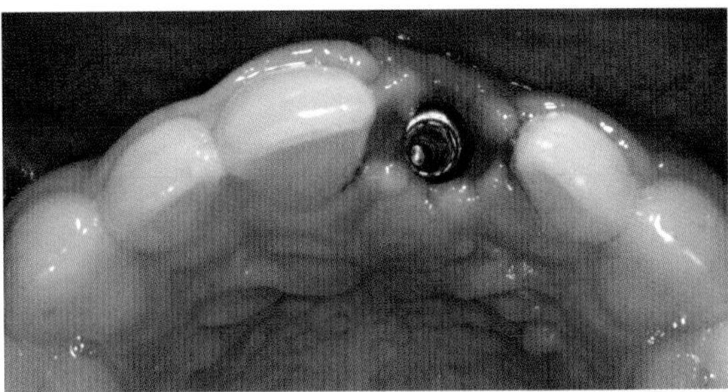

Figure 9.62. The implant restorative platform prior to insertion of the Final Encode Abutment.

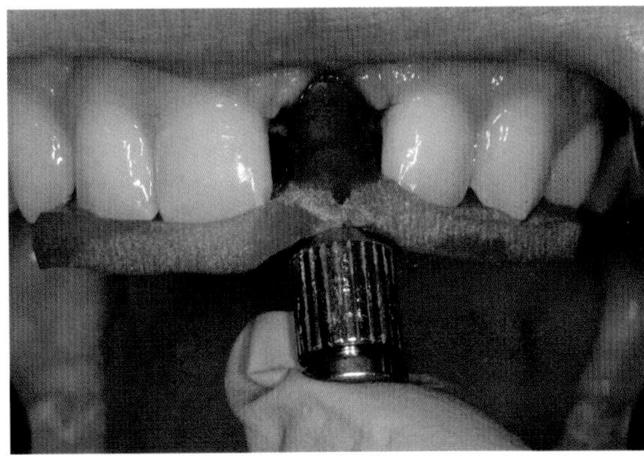

Figure 9.63. Clinical view of the abutment placement index seated onto the occlusal and incisal surfaces of the teeth adjacent to the implant site. The driver (PHD03N) is in place.

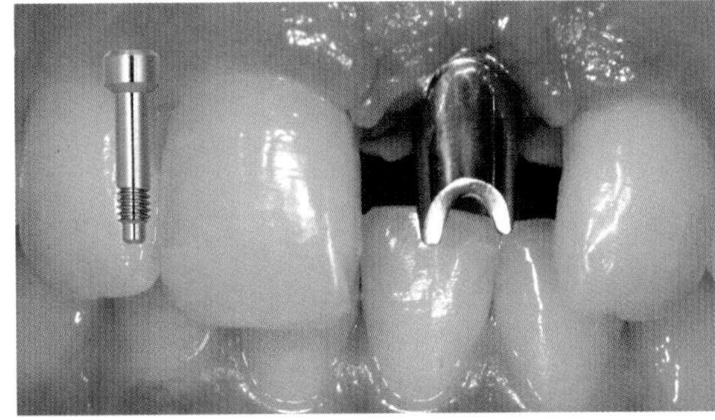

Figure 9.64. Clinical view of the definitive abutment in place. A hexed try-in screw (IUNIT) was used to attach the abutment to the implant (inset).

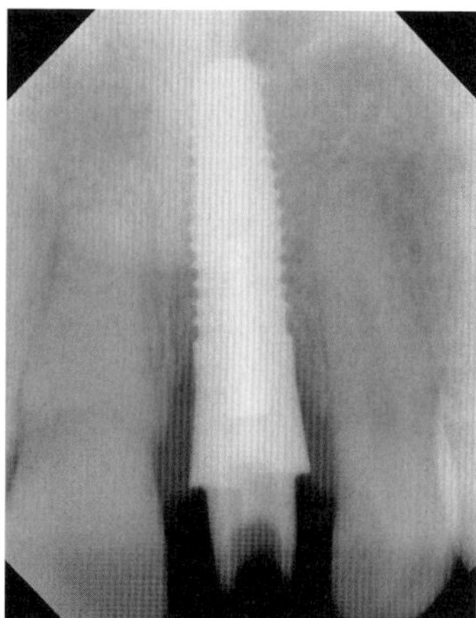

Figure 9.65. Radiograph that demonstrated that the abutment was accurately seated onto to the implant.

Radiographic Verification

A periapical radiograph (parallel technique) was taken after the abutment was seated to confirm that the abutment was seated completely into the internal connection of the OSSEOTITE® Certain® implant (Figure 9.65). Accurate seating of the abutment was virtually guaranteed with the use of the abutment placement index. If the abutment was not correctly seated into the implant, it would have to be removed and another attempt would be required to accurately seat the abutment. If the abutment could not be accurately seated, a new implant level impression would be indicated. The internal connection design featured in OSSEOTITE® Certain® implants has resulted in high levels of clinically successful implant/abutment connections (Drago 2006).

Torque

The hexed try-in screw was removed and replaced with a hexed Gold-Tite™ Abutment Screw (IUNIHG). This abutment screw was torqued to 20 Ncm with the Restorative Torque Driver and Large Hex driver tip (RTI2035, RASH3N) (Figure 9.66). There should be no pain or discomfort of any kind during this procedure. If the patient experiences any discomfort, careful examination is warranted. Discomfort that does not originate within the peri-implant soft tissues should be viewed critically by clinicians because the implant may not be osseointegrated.

Crown Try-In

The definitive crown was tried-in using conventional fixed prosthodontic protocols: physiologic interproximal contacts; accurate marginal adaptation between the abutment and crown; and optimal occlusal relationships. A radiograph was taken to verify accurate marginal adaptation between the abutment and crown (Figure 9.67).

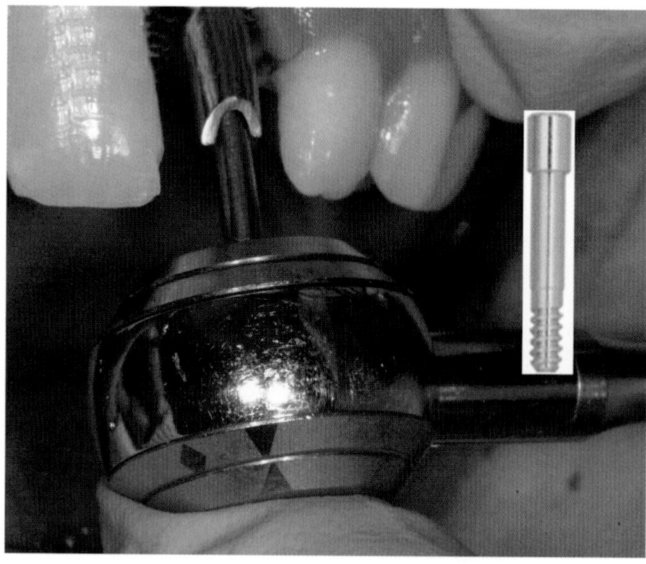

Figure 9.66. A hexed Gold-Tite™ Abutment Screw (IUNIHG) was used as the definitive abutment screw (inset). This screw was torqued to 20 Ncm with the Restorative Torque Indicator (RTI2035) and the large hex driver tip (RASH3N).

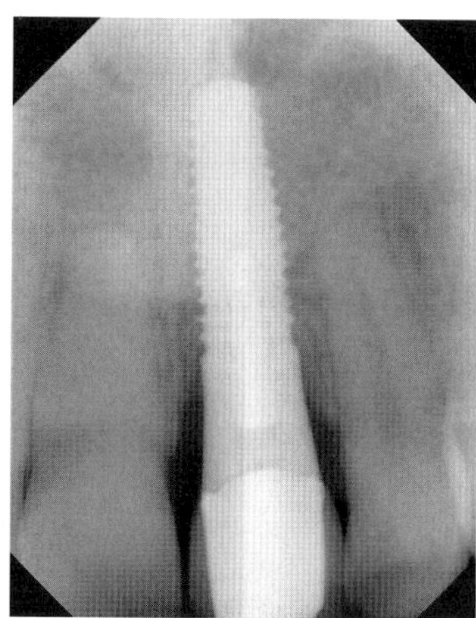

Figure 9.67. Radiograph demonstrated excellent marginal adaptation between the abutment and definitive crown.

Occlusion in the natural dentition has been extensively studied, but published articles are mainly empirical in nature, based on theories with little scientific basis for discussion (Taylor and others 2005). Most occlusion-related therapy may be deemed successful if it is assumed that results such as patient comfort, satisfaction, and restoration durability are acceptable outcomes. Relative to implant-supported restorations, authors have stated that nonaxial forces to dental implants should be avoided (Rangert and others 1989). Possible reasons to avoid nonaxial loading were that implants lack a periodontal ligament and potential high-stress concentrations instead of uniform compression along the implant/bone interface. Nonaxial loading may put the implant components at risk, specifically components fastened together with screws. Taylor and others (2005), in an extensive review of the literature, reported that evidence is lacking regarding the effect of nonaxial loading or overload on the integrity of the osseointegrated interface between bone and implants.

The author prefers to develop occlusal contacts on implant-retained crowns similar to the occlusal contacts on natural teeth: even centric occlusal contacts, no balancing interferences, and, in this case, protrusive disclusion that would be shared equally between the maxillary right and left central incisors (Figure 9.68).

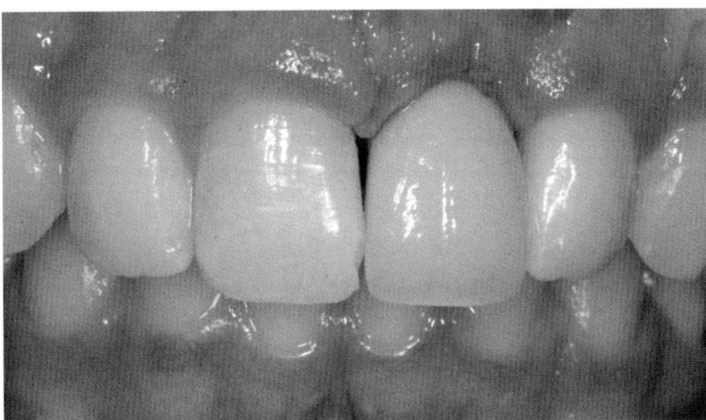

Figure 9.68. Anterior clinical view of the definitive porcelain fused to metal crown in place on the definitive abutment.

Cementation

Cement-retained crowns have several advantages when compared to screw-retained crowns. There are also several disadvantages, with the most prominent being the lack of easy, predictable retrievablility (Guichet and others 2000). Michalakis and others (2003) reviewed the dental literature relative to cement- and screw-retention for implant restorations and concluded that cement-retained crowns are better suited for implant restorations in terms of ease of fabrication, decreased cost, passivity of frameworks in multiple implant cases, occlusion, and aesthetics.

Maeyama and others (2005) studied the retentive strengths of metal copings cemented to prefabricated implant abutments (Easy Abutments, Nobel Biocare, Yorba Linda, CA) with different cements. Composite resin cement (Panavia F 2.0) and resin-reinforced glass inonomer cement (Fuji Luting) demonstrated the highest loads in Newtons for failure. Maeyama and others concluded that cements could be grouped into three distinct categories with increasing strength: zinc oxide eugenol-free temporary cement; zinc oxyphosphate and glass inonomer cements; and resin-reinforced glass inonomer and composite resin cements.

The crown was polished, air abraded with 50 μm aluminum oxide, and steam cleaned. The crown was cemented with reinforced glass ionomer luting cement (GC Fuji Plus, GC America Inc., Alsip, Il) mixed per the manufacturer's instructions. The cement was placed in and around the apical 2 mm of the crown and seated into place (Figure 9.69). The cement was allowed to set for 2.5 minutes and the excess was removed.

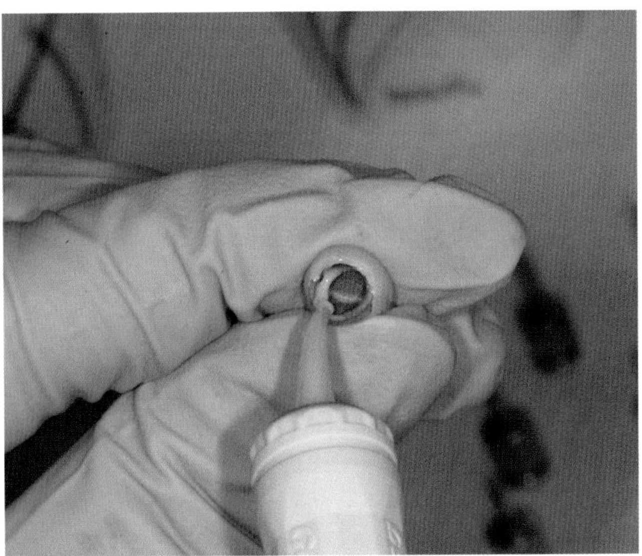

Figure 9.69. Definitive cement was placed in and around the apical 2 mm of the crown and seated onto the abutment.

Postoperative Instructions

The patient was told that there were virtually no dietary restrictions relative to the implant and implant-retained restoration. Brushing and flossing could be accomplished with techniques similar to that used on the natural teeth.

Appointment 12. Two-Week Follow-Up Appointment (1/4 Hour)

The patient returned two weeks post insertion of the abutment and crown and reported absolutely no symptoms. She was pleased with the aesthetic, functional, and phonetic results. She was also quite pleased in that the treatment was accomplished in such a short period of time and that she never had to go without a tooth.

Appointment 13. Six-Month Follow-Up Appointment (1/4 Hour)

History

This patient was lost to follow-up because she moved out of the area.

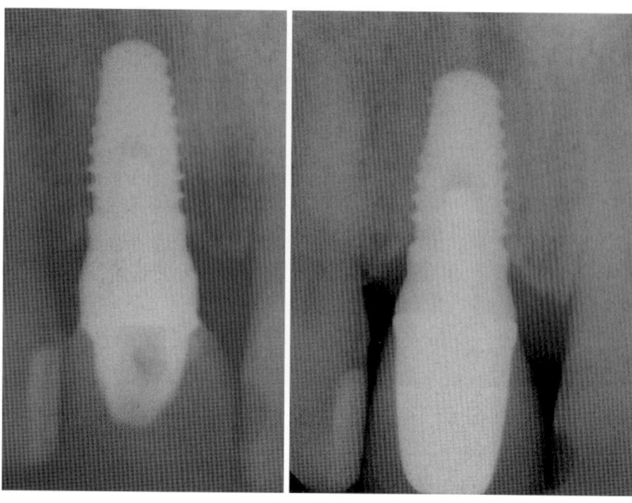

Figure 9.70. The periapical radiograph on the left was taken at the time the INOL provisional restoration was placed. The periapical radiograph on the right was taken at the one-year recall appointment.

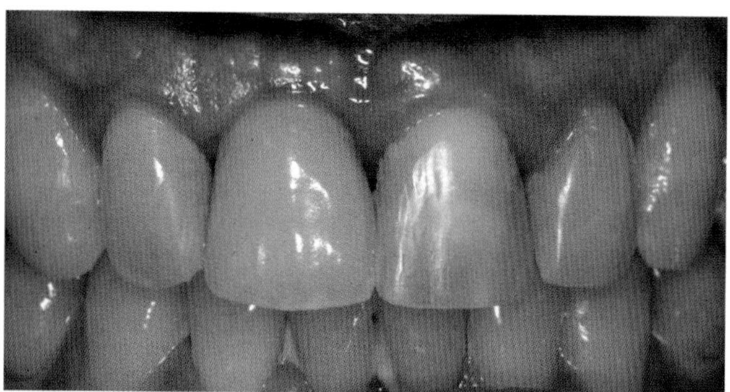

Figure 9.71. Anterior clinical view of an implant retained crown (maxillary right central incisor) made with the INOL protocol 12 months post implant placement.

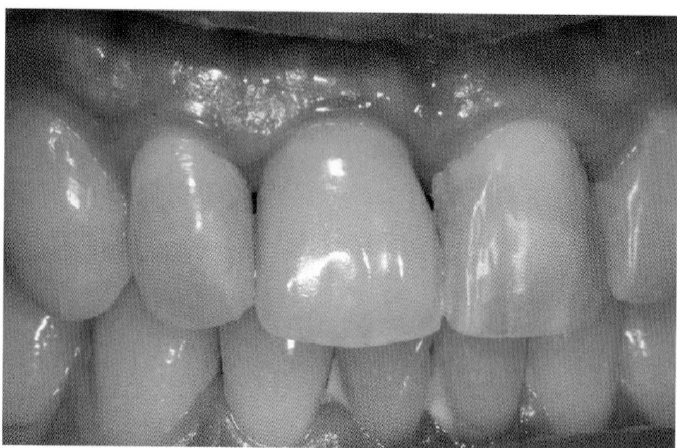

Figure 9.72. Right anterior clinical view of the implant-retained crown in Figure 9.71 one year post insertion.

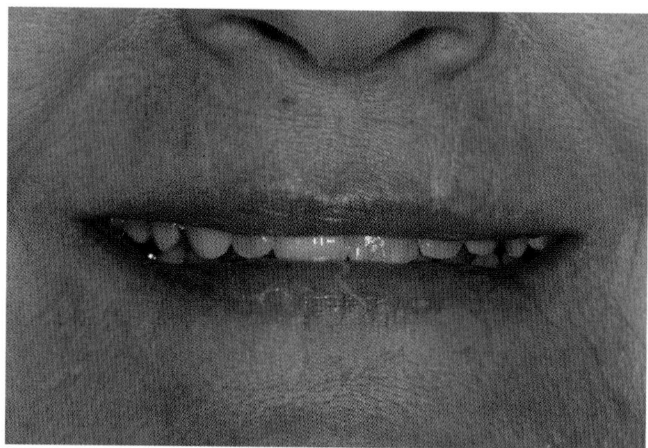

Figure 9.73. Clinical smile one-year post insertion of the implant-retained crown for the maxillary right central incisor. The lack of interdental papillae is not a clinical concern because the patient presented with a low lip line.

Clinical Examination

This patient was lost to follow-up because she moved out of the area. Clinical photographs were not available.

Appointment 14. One-Year Recall (1/2 Hour)

History

The patient described in this chapter was lost to follow-up. The patient who is illustrated for this appointment was a patient who was treated with the same INOL protocol that was illustrated in this chapter. This patient was very pleased with the results of treatment and had absolutely no complaints.

Radiograph

A periapical radiograph was taken at this appointment. It demonstrated less than 1 mm of crestal bone loss on either inter proximal surface when compared to the radiograph taken at the abutment and definitive crown insertion appointment (Figure 9.70). There were no peri-implant radiolucencies around the implant, and satisfactory bone/implant contact was visualized around the circumference of the implant. There were approximately 6 mm between the interproximal heights of bone and the interproximal contacts on both surfaces of the teeth adjacent to the implant-retained crown.

Clinical Examination

The occlusion was stable in both centric and eccentric movements. There was no fremitus. The gingival margins were stable around the implant restoration. The peri-implant and gingival tissues exhibited minimal inflammation. Gingival interdental papillae were not present on either interproximal surface of the implant-retained crown (Figures 9.71, 9.72). The interproximal heights of bone on

TABLE 9.11. Lab Fees, Component Costs, Overhead, Fees and Profits (INOL Protocol-Definitive Restoration)

Fixed				
Chair Time	**Overhead**	**Laboratory Expenses**		
		Casts	$ 60	
Impression		Articulation	$ 50	
3/4 hour	$350/hr = $213	Sub Total	$ 110	
		Implant Components		
		Final Encode Abutment	$250	
		Impression Coping	$ 45	
		Analog	$ 21	
		Lab screw	$ 25	
		Encode Cast	$ 50	
		Sub Total	**$ 391**	
Final Encode Abutment and Crown Insertion				
3/4 hour	$350/hr = $212			
TOTALS	**$525**		**$ 501**	
Professional Fee				**$1850**
Costs (fixed overhead and laboratory expenses)				**$1026**
Profit (fees less costs)				$ 824
Profit per hour ($ 824/1.75)				**$ 470**

Encode Healing Abutment, impression copings, and lab screws may be used multiple times, therefore costs will be decreased for each succeeding case and profits will be increased. Analogs should not be re-used.

either side of the implant-retained crown were approximately 6+ mm apical to the interproximal contact areas of the adjacent teeth. The clinical finding in this case (lack of interdental papillae) is consistent with Salama and others' (1998) research in which they found interdental papillae present in similar situations in less than 60% of cases.

The lack of interdental papillae did not present a clinical concern to either the patient or the author because the patient presented with a low lip line (Figure 9.73). The lack of interdental papillae would be a clinical concern if the patient presented with a high lip line that exposed the cervical one-third of the maxillary anterior teeth.

Due to the absence of any negative signs and/or symptoms, this implant was considered to be osseointegrated. The long-term prognosis for success with both the implant and implant restoration was considered to be excellent. The patient was discharged back to her family dentist for preventative and restorative care. She was scheduled to return to see the author in 12 months for an additional radiograph and clinical follow up.

Costs/Fees/Profitability

The following discussion relative to fees is reflective of 2006 in the Midwestern United States. The costs of the implant components are retail prices from Implant Innovations, Inc., Palm Beach Gardens, Florida (Table 9.11).

Surgeon: Michael Banasik, DDS, MS, Gundersen Lutheran Medical Center, LaCrosse, Wisconsin

Dental Laboratory Technicians: Thomas Peterson, CDT, MDT, NorthShore Dental Laboratory, Lynn, Massachusetts; Andrew Gingrasso, Gundersen Lutheran Medical Center, LaCrosse, Wisconsin

BIBLIOGRAPHY

Adell, R, Lekholm, U, Rockler, B, Brånemark, P-I, 1981. A 15-year study of osseointegrated implants in the treatment of the edentulous jaw. *Int J Oral Surg* 10:387–416.

Becker, W, Becker, B, Israelson, H, 1997. One-step surgical placement of Brånemark implants: a prospective multicenter clinical study. *Int J Oral Maxillofac Implants* 12:454–462.

Brånemark, P-I, Hansson, B, Adell, R, 1977. Osseointegrated implants in the treatment of the edentulous jaw. Experience from a 10-year period. *Scand J Plast Reconstr Surg* 11(Suppl 16):1–132.

Chaushu, G, Chaushu, S, Tzohar, A, Dayan, D, 2001. Immediate loading of single-tooth implants: immediate versus non-immediate implantation. A clinical report. *Int J Oral Maxillofac Implants* 16:267–272.

Cooper, L, Felton, D, Kugelberg, C, 2001. A multicenter 12-month evaluation of single-tooth implants restored 3 weeks after 1-stage surgery. *Int J Oral Maxillofac Implants* 16:182–192.

Drago, C, 2006. A clinical report on the 18-month cumulative survival rates of implants and implant prostheses with an internal connection implant system. *Compendium Cont Dent Ed* 27:266–271.

Ericsson, I, Nilson, H, Lindh, T, 2000. Immediate functional loading of Brånemark single-tooth implants. An 18 months' clinical pilot follow-up study. *Clin Oral Implants Res* 11:26–33.

Garber, D, Salama, H, Salama, M, 2001. Two-stage versus one stage—is there really a controversy? *J Periodontol* 72:417–421.

Guichet, D, Caputo, A, Choi, H, Sorensen, J, 2000. Passivity of fit and marginal opening in screw- or cement-retained implant fixed partial denture designs. *Int J Oral Maxillofac Implants* 15:239–246.

Hebel, K, Gajjar, R, 1997. Cement-retained versus screw-retained implant restorations: achieving optimal occlusion and esthetics in implant dentistry. *J Prosthet Dent* 77:28–35.

Hui, E, Chow, J, Li, D, Liu, J, Wat, P, Law, H, 2001. Immediate provisional for single-tooth implant replacement with Brånemark system: preliminary report. *Clin Implant Dent Rel Res* 3:79–86.

Hurson, S, 1996. Laboratory techniques to prevent screw loosening on dental implants. *J Dent Tech* 13:30–37.

Kan, J, Rungcharassaeng, K, Lozada, J, 2003. Immediate placement and provisionalization of maxillary anterior single implants: 1-year prospective study. *Int J Oral Maxillofac Implants* 18:31–39.

Maeyama, H, Sawase, T, Jimbo, R, Kamada, K, Suketa, N, Fukui, J, Atsuta, M, 2005. Retentive strength of metal copings on prefabricated abutments with five different cements. *Clin Implant Dent Rel Res* 7:229–234.

Michalakis, K, Hirayama, H, Garefis, P, 2003. Cement-retained implant restorations: a critical review. *Int J Oral Maxillofac Implants* 18:719–728.

Rangert, B, Jemt, T, Jorneus, L, 1989. Forces and moments on Brånemark implants. *Int J Oral Maxillofac Implants* 4:241–247.

Saadoun, A, Sebbag, P, 2004. Immediate implant placement and temporization: literature review and case studies. *Compendium* 25:277–294.

Salama, H, Salama, M, Garber, D, Adar, P, 1998. The interproximal height of bone: a guidepost to predictable aesthetic strategies and soft tissue contours in anterior tooth replacement. *Pract Perio Aesthet Dent* 10:1131–1141.

Schnitman, P, Wohrle, P, Rubenstein, J, DaSilva, J, Wang, N, 1997. Ten-year results for Brånemark implants immediately loaded with fixed prostheses implant placement. *Int J Oral Maxillofac Implants* 12:495–503.

Schulte, W, Heimke, G, 1976. The Tubingen immediate implant. *Quintessence* 27:17–23.

Tarnow, D, Fletcher, P, 1993. The 2–3 month post-extraction placement of root-form implants: a useful compromise. *Implants Clin Rev Dent* 2:1–8.

Taylor, T, Wiens, J, Carr, A, 2005. Evidence-based considerations for removable prosthodontic and dental implant occlusion: a literature review. *J Prosthet Dent* 94:555–560.

Testori, T, Del Fabbro, M, Szmukler-Moncler, S, Francetti, L, Weinstein, R, 2003. Immediate Occlusal Loading® of Osseotite implants in the completely edentulous mandible. *Int J Oral Maxillofac Implants* 18:544–551.

Wohrle, P, 1998. Single-tooth replacement in the aesthetic zone with immediate provisionalization: fourteen consecutive case reports. *Pract Perio Aesthet Dent* 10:1107–1114.

Chapter 10: Surgical Considerations in Implant Dentistry: Integration of Hard and Soft Tissues

INTRODUCTION

Without osseointegration and "soft tissue integration" between intra-oral tissues and implants, there are no restorative options. Today's surgeons and restorative doctors must work together to achieve the goals associated with fully integrated, functional, aesthetic, and hygienic prostheses. Surgeons must place implants in appropriate positions to allow for functional, aesthetic restorations. Implant materials and designs continue to evolve in efforts to increase the frequency of and decrease the time for integration. Equal emphasis should be placed on both osseointegration and on the so-called soft-tissue integration.

Osseointegration of dental implants involves a complex array of events relative to the healing and remodeling of bone and soft tissue. Osseointegration refers to an implant's direct bone contact providing anchorage that supports a prosthesis under occlusal forces. Per-Ingvar Brånemark at the University of Goteborg in Sweden developed the concept of osseointegration while studying microcirculation in bone repair. Brånemark and others (1977) defined osseointegration as "a direct structural and functional connection between ordered, living bone and the surface of a load carrying implant." During the 1950s, Brånemark discovered that there was a strong bond between titanium and bone. Over the next 25 years, Brånemark continued to modify and improve the technology and protocol associated with predictable, long-term osseointegration of dental implants. Brånemark presented the first two-staged threaded titanium root-form implant in North America in 1982. Since Brånemark's benchmark research was originally presented, there have been multiple modifications to the original protocol to enhance biocompatibility and retention for dental implants.

Several factors have been shown to influence implant osseointegration:

- Surgical technique including prevention of excessive heat during drilling
- Sterile technique
- Unloaded healing of dental implants (no micro-motion)
- Implant design, shape, length, surface topography (microsurface or macrosurface)
- Systemic health of patients

IMPLANT DESIGN

Commercially pure titanium has excellent biocompatibility and mechanical properties. However, strength issues with pure titanium led manufacturers to use a titanium alloy (Ti-6Al-4Va) to maximize dental implant strength. Today most practitioners prefer titanium alloy with varying compositions for dental implants. The surface oxide layer on commercially pure titanium and titanium alloy implants determines the biocompatibility of a particular implant. This oxide layer is the only portion of the implant in contact with host tissue (De Leonardi and others 1999).

Implant surface topography has been shown to enhance implant-to-bone contact. Adding titanium to implant surfaces through plasma-spray technology is one technique that modifies the surfaces of dental titanium alloy implants. Dental implants have also been modified by reduction techniques involving blasting and or acid etching implant surfaces. Cordioli reported five-week bone-to-implant contact values to be 72.4% for acid-etched surfaces, 56.8% for titanium plasma-sprayed surfaces, 54.8% for grit-blasted titanium surfaces, and 48.6% for machine surface implants (Cordioli and others 2000). Virtually all major implant manufacturers use some form of roughened surface texture for their endosseous dental implants.

HARD TISSUE INTEGRATION

Following a minimally traumatic drilling and surgical protocols for the placement of endosseous implants, bone and soft tissue healing must progress for osseointegration to occur. The biologic activity required to achieve osseointegration includes the following three phases: osteophyllic, osteoconductive, and osteoadaptive (Marx and others 1996). These three phases have also been called inflammatory, proliferative, and maturation phases.

Tissue trauma begins with the incision and continues through to the osteotomy and implant placement; the initial obvious result is immediate hemorrhaging. Multiple cells and pathways for inflammation and healing begin with the surgical insult to bone with preparation of the osteotomies. In cancellous bone, there is a surprisingly small implant-to-bone contact area. The remaining implant surface is in contact with extra cellular fluid and cells. A blood clot is formed at the interface between the implant and bone. The clot contains numerous cytokines and cells that regulate

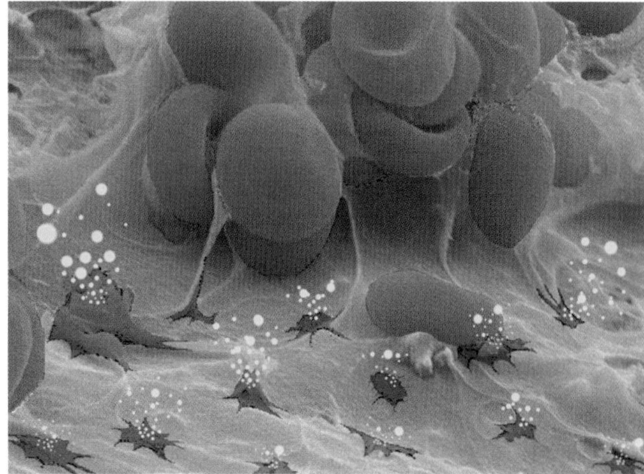

Figure 10.1. Enhanced scanning electron micrograph of an OSSEOTITE® implant that demonstrated platelet activation.

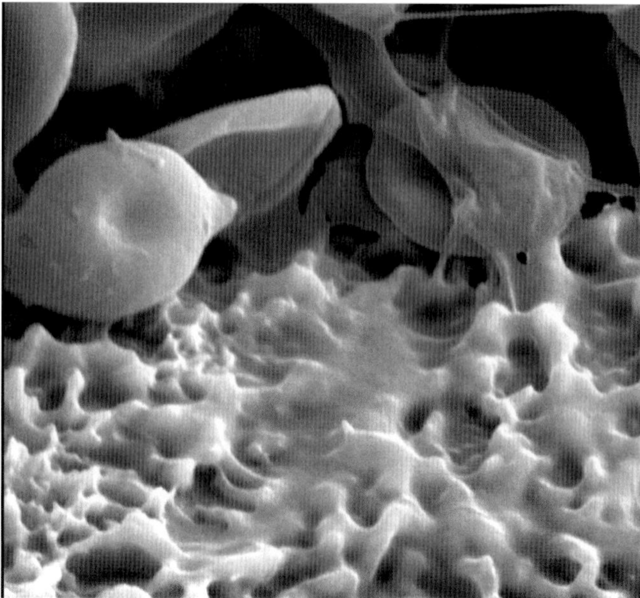

Figure 10.2. Scanning electron micrograph of the acid-etched surface of an OSEOTITIE® implant that shows red blood cells and platelet interactions. Courtesy of JE Davies and JY Park, University of Toronto.

bone metabolism. The clot provides a reservoir of growth factors and cytokines and serves as a scaffold for cell migration. Increased platelet adhesion has been shown to occur quicker on a micro-textured implant surface than on a smooth implant surface (Park and Davies 2001) (Figures 10.1 and 10.2). Several studies have concluded that rough surface implants have a significantly higher percentage of bone-to-implant contact and faster, stronger osseointegration when compared to machined surface titanium implants (Trisi and others 1999; De Leonardi and others 1999; De Leonardi and others 1997).

Platelet contacts with the micro and macro topography of implant surfaces causes secretion from intracellular granules and aides in healing injured tissue (Shetty and Bertolami 1992). After clot formation, an influx of inflammatory cells, responding to foreign antigens and the surgical insult, migrate to the surgical site. Also known as the inflammatory phase, these cells support vascular growth. The formation of new blood vessels (angiogenesis) is a vital step in wound healing. The vascular ingrowth begins about three days after implant placement and continues for three weeks (Zoldos and Kent 1995). In order to maintain cellular activity during bone repair and formation, angiogenesis must be active. Healing, during the osteophyllic phase, results in a mature vascular network during its approximately one-month duration. Osteocytes are activated and the osteophyllic phase transitions into the osteoconductive phase.

Bone formation is marked by osteoblast polarization and protein production. A collagenous matrix at the bone/implant interface matures and mineralizes. The initial formation of bone-type structure is referred to as the footplate or woven bone. The laying down of osteoid around the implant surface takes place over the next three months. This process is known as the osteoconductive phase. A "bone callus" covers the surface area of the implant. This cell-rich unorganized bone is referred to as woven bone. Woven bone formation predominates during this time period.

Bone deposition is thought to arise from two different mechanisms: distance osteogenesis and contact osteogenesis (Davies 2003). These two distinct processes involve the formation of bone "de novo" (Davies 2003). Distance osteogenesis is a gradual reparative process (Hoshaw and others 1994). It is thought to start from the edge of the osteotomy and proceed toward but not onto the implant surface. Contact osteogenesis occurs at the surface of the implant (Figure 10.3). Direct migration of osteogenic cells occurs through the clot matrix to the implant surface (Figure 10.4). Bone deposition onto the implant surface continues until it reaches a steady state at about four months (Zoldos and Kent 1995). Distance and contact osteogenesis work concurrently to obtain osseointegration. When these processes overlap, a favorable result is more likely to be achieved by optimization of contact osteogenesis.

The final phase in the osseointegration process is the osteoadaptive phase. This phase involves the remodeling of woven bone within a vascularized, connective tissue matrix at the implant/bone interface. Occlusal loading of dental endosseous implants stimulates the maturation of woven bone to lamellar bone. This change is in direct response to forces transmitted from the implant to the surrounding bone. Woven bone is gradually replaced by

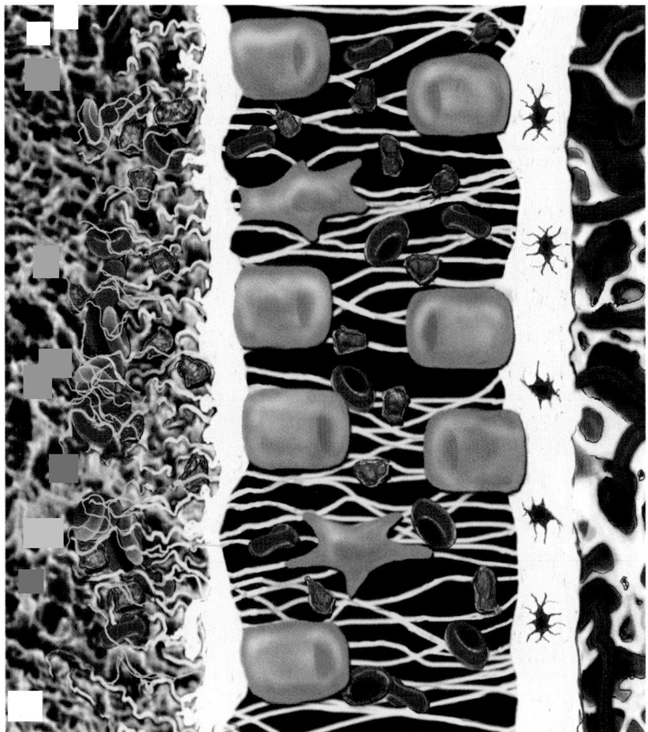

Figure 10.3. Schematic rendition of contact osteogenesis that demonstrates the direct migration of cells through the clot matrix to the implant surface. Courtesy of ***3i®***, Implant Innovations, Inc., Palm Beach Gardens, FL.

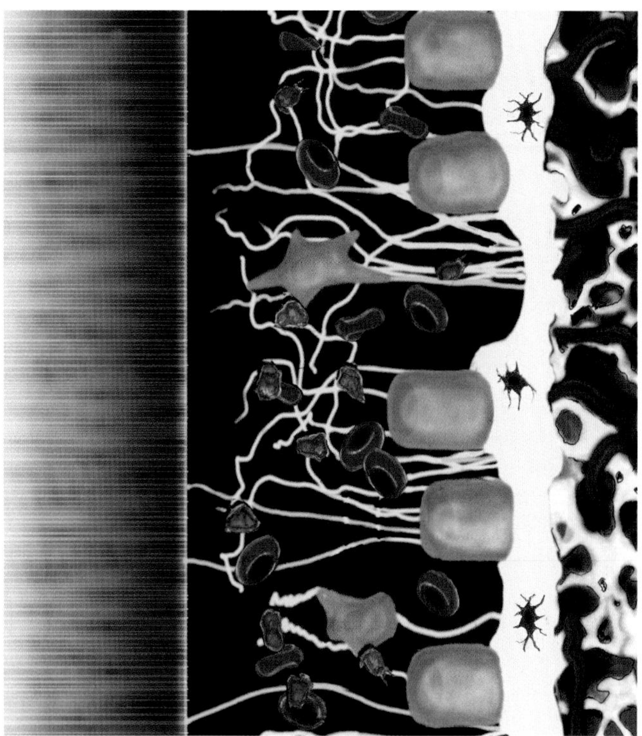

Figure 10.4. Schematic rendition of distance osteogenesis that demonstrates bone healing inward from the walls of the osteotomy toward the implant surface, but not onto the surface. Courtesy of ***3i®***, Implant Innovations, Inc., Palm Beach Gardens, FL.

lamellar bone (Berglundh and others 2003). The newly formed lamellar bone provides the necessary rigid fixation for the implant to function under occlusal loading. After four months, there does not appear to be a significant amount of increased bone/implant contact; however, the footplate thickens in response to loading (Garg 2004). How much of the implant surface is truly osseointegrated? Some authors have implied that 100% of the implant surface is rarely, if ever, achieved. Albrektsson suggested that successful clinical outcomes might be achieved with implant surface osseointegration of 60% (Albrektsson and others 1993).

SOFT TISSUE INTEGRATION

Soft tissue integration is now being used to describe the biologic process that occurs during the maturation of the peri-implant "soft tissue" connective tissue and epithelium (Figure 10.5). There is no question as to the importance of the relationship between natural teeth and the surrounding periodontium. Soft tissues that encompass implants must form seals around the emerging implants similarly to the relationships that exist in natural teeth.

Soft tissue integration has been defined as the biologic processes that occur during the formation and maturation

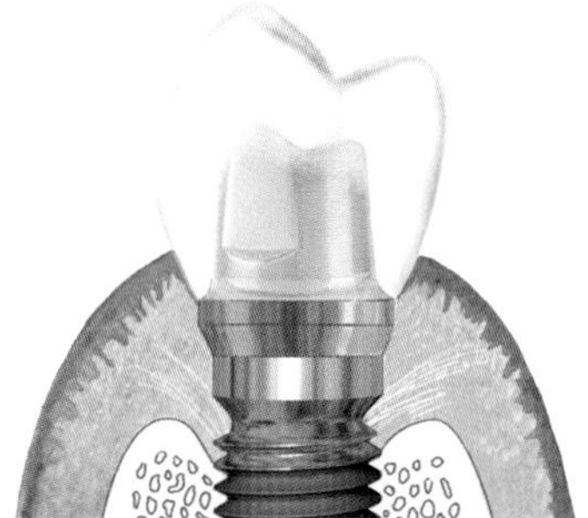

Figure 10.5. Cross sectional diagram of an implant-retained crown that was cemented onto a GingiHue® Post that demonstrates healthy junctional epithelium around the sub-gingival portions of the implant retained crown. Courtesy of ***3i®***, Implant Innovations, Inc., Palm Beach Gardens, FL.

between the transmucosal portion of the implant and soft tissue. The maintenance of soft tissue health is as important as osseointegration is for the long-term survival of an implant-supported prosthesis. Surgeons and restorative doctors must be versant in the management of the peri-implant soft tissue.

Sclar (2003) has referred to internal and external factors that affect the health of the peri-implant soft tissue. Internal factors include: age of the patient; general health; periodontal status of remaining dentition; host resistance; systemic disease; and periodontal phenotype. External factor differences include: tobacco uses; use of medication; oral hygiene; implant design and surface characteristics; and location of the implant.

The soft tissue histomorphology has some similarities and differences as it applies to natural teeth and titanium implants. It is the important similarities that make implant dentistry even possible. The periodontal histology and peri-implant histology of the junctional and sulcular epithelium are similar. Junctional epithelium attaches to the endosseous implant and is critical in providing a protective barrier around the implant. Sulcular epithelium provides cellular immunological protection.

Important differences between them render implants susceptible to failure. Dental implants lack periodontal ligament attachments, cementum, and well-vascularized connective tissues. Despite the lack of periodontal ligament or gingival sulcus, the epithelium has been shown to have a tight adaptation at the collar of implants when minimal plaque or inflammation is present (Schroeder and others 1981). The peri-implant connective tissue contains more collagen but fewer fibroblasts and a lack of vascular structures (Moon and others 1999). To overcome these challenges, the surgical placement and the final restoration must be in compliance with reliable and predictable principles of implantology.

The literature for implant placement within attached, keratinized soft tissues versus alveolar mucosa is without consensus. Fewer complications, healthier soft tissue, and better patient satisfaction have been reported with implants and restorations encompassed by attached (fixed) soft tissue (Schroeder and others 1981; Bauman and others 1993; Silverstein and others 1994; Silverstein and Lefkove 1994). Some authors have suggested that attached, keratinized soft tissues may have no long-term advantages over alveolar mucosa (Zarb and Schmill 1990; Wennstrom and others 1994). There is a consensus that many factors influence the health of the peri-implant hard and soft tissue and the ultimate success of osseointegrated implants. Based on the effectiveness of oral hygiene, resistance to recession, aesthetics, and predictability of the peri-implant soft tissue, this author concludes that a margin of attached soft tissue in contact with an emerging implant is critical for long-term hard and soft tissue integration.

TRADITIONAL/EARLY LOADING PROTOCOLS FOR DENTAL IMPLANTS

There has been significant discussion as to the time required for osseointegration to occur. Osseointegration is a time-dependent process (Johansson and Albrektsson 1987). The original protocol set forth by Brånemark, six months for maxillary implants and four to six months for mandibular implants, has been and continues to be challenged by modern researchers and clinicians (Adell and others 1981). Lazzara and others studied loading OSSEOTITE® implants two months after insertion. All of the implants were placed with a single-stage surgical protocol. The Cumulative Survival Rate (CSR) was 98.5% up to 12.6 months post loading. Testori and others (2001) also researched OSSEOTITE® implants per the protocol described by Lazzara (1998) above. The implants were placed in both jaws and were also loaded two months post implant placement. Their follow-up time period was three years. The results demonstrated CSRs of 97.7% for mandibular implants and 98.4% for maxillary implants. All of the implants that were studied in the above two studies were straight-wall commercially pure titanium implants. As implant science continues to "push the envelope" with protocols involving different implant loading protocols, it is likely that these timelines will continue to evolve.

QUANTITATIVE MEASUREMENTS OF IMPLANT SUCCESS

Several devices have been used to quantify primary stability and long-term osseointegration of dental implants. The usefulness and accuracy of these devices is still being determined. OSSTELL® (Integration Diagnostics, Inc., Savedalin, Sweden) has been approved by the United States Food and Drug Administration for such measurements. It uses resonance frequency to assess implant stability. Periotest® (Siemens AG, Bensheim, Germany) has also been used to measure the damping effect of the supporting tissues to a standardized force as an indicator of implant mobility/immobility.

A torque wrench test has also been used to quantitatively assess clinical osseointegration of dental implants. If a preload corresponding to a torque of 10 to 20 Ncm is applied to an implant and the implant remains stable, without discomfort, the implant can be considered to be osseointegrated (Martin and others 2000).

Although not scientifically supported, percussing implants and evaluating the sounds that are emitted from the implants may also test clinical osseointegration of dental implants. The implant is percussed with a blunt instrument and the sound evaluated by the clinician. There is a crisp sound when this occurs with osseointegrated implants and a duller sound when this occurs with non-integrated implants. A "ringing or pinging" sound is considered favorable for osseointegration, whereas a "dull and flat" sound may suggest fibrous tissue involvement. This test is simple and quick but may not be reliable for some implants in determining clinical osseointegration. Nevertheless, it is the author's opinion that percussion of dental implants tends to be the method of choice for most clinicians.

Smith and Zarb (1989) published criteria relative to assessing clinical osseointegration of dental implants:

1. Individual, nonsplinted implants that demonstrate no clinical mobility.
2. The absence of peri-implant radiolucencies on radiographs.
3. Mean vertical bone loss that averages less than 0.2 mm annually after the first year of occlusal loading.
4. The absence of pain, discomfort, or infection in or around implants.
5. An implant design that does not preclude placement of a crown or prosthesis with acceptable aesthetics.

IMPLANT FAILURE

Implant failure is a major concern and disappointment for patients, surgeons, and restorative dentists. The terms "ailing" and "failing" implants have been used as qualitative terms in assessing varying degrees of implant health. It has been proposed that an "ailing" implant is one that has radiographic evidence of bone loss and probing depths greater than 5 mm but remains clinically stable. A "failing" implant shows bleeding or purulence upon probing and increasing levels of bone loss with serial radiographs (Martin and others 2000). A non-osseointegrated implant will demonstrate clinical mobility, dullness to percussion, and peri-implant radiolucency. Non-osseointegrated implants must be removed.

Why, despite many years of improved materials, do some implants fail to become osseointegrated? Patient selection continues to relate to clinical success. A patient's past medical and dental histories are key places to start. Debate exists as to the absolute contraindications for implant placement. Recently, bisphosphonates have been found to lead to bisphosphonate-induced osteonecrosis of the jaws. This family of drugs has been identified as an absolute contraindication for dental implants (Marx and others 2005). Many more relative contraindications exist, including but not limited to smoking, uncontrolled diabetes, immunocompromised patients, bleeding disorders, poor systemic health with multiple co-morbidities, active periodontitis, high-dose radiation to the jaws, and anatomy not amenable to favorable placement.

The most important factors for implant success as published by Block and others were "surgery without compromise in technique, placing implants into sound bone, avoiding thin bone or implant dehiscence at the time of implant placement, avoiding premature implant exposure during the healing period, establishing a balanced restoration, and insuring appropriate follow-up hygiene care" (Block and Kent 1990). Implant mobility in a previously stable implant should be considered the ultimate sign of clinical non-integration. After an existing implant becomes unstable, the implant should be removed. A clinically mobile implant has not been observed to become re-osseointegrated (Garg 2004; Adell 1992). Successful treatment of nonmobile dental implants with radiolucencies is still controversial and unpredictable. The majority of implant failures are believed to occur in the first 12 months following implant placement.

MAINTENANCE

Dental implants have become an integral part of treatment planning for edentulous and partially edentulous patients. Significant emphasis has been placed on obtaining integration and achieving functional aesthetic restorations. But is the treatment really done? After an implant has become integrated, does it always remain integrated? Implants and their surrounding hard and soft tissues are susceptible to component failure, screw loosening, peri-implant mucositis, and peri-implantitis. Any or all of the previous factors may lead to loss of implants. Peri-implant mucositis refers to inflammation around implants that is considered to be reversible. Bone loss would not be part of the clinical appearance of peri-implant mucositis. Peri-implantitis involves bone loss and may occur in as many as 10% of osseointegrated implants (Mombelli and Lang 2000).

As alluded to earlier in this chapter, there are fundamental differences when comparing the soft and hard tissues surrounding natural teeth versus dental implants. The pathogenicity of oral bacteria seems to be particularly diminished in edentulous patients with or without dental implants. The composition of oral plaques around natural teeth and titanium implants are similar, and the initial microbiological colonizations follow similar patterns (Leonhardt and others 1993; Zitmann and others 2001) (Figure 10.6). Peri-implant inflammation may progress from the peri-implant mucosa

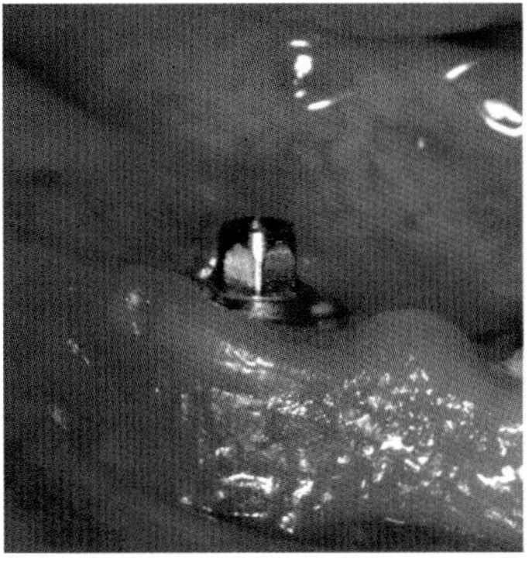

Figure 10.6. Peri-implant soft tissue inflammation around a nonintegrated implant. This implant was clinically mobile and was subsequently removed.

into the supporting bone, causing peri-implantitis. Therefore the long-term integrity of dental implants is influenced and maintained by, among other things, meticulous oral hygiene.

Anatomically contoured implant restorations play an important role in maintaining osseointegration. Physiologic implant restorative emergence profiles, consistent with the emergence profiles of natural teeth, provide patients with the opportunities to perform oral hygiene procedures with maximum efficiency and minimal difficulty.

Occlusal harmony distributes occlusal forces to those anatomic and restored structures that are best able to handle them. Overloading implants with excessive occlusal forces may be detrimental to the long-term success of the implants. Controversy remains as to the potential loss of an osseointegrated implant with occlusal overloading of the final restoration. A literature review published in 1998 by Esposito and others concluded that occlusal overload led to loss of integration and failure of dental implants. Subsequent studies in animal models have raised questions by demonstrating continued osseointegration in the presence of occlusal overload (Gotfedsen and others 2002). Nevertheless, intuitive thinking leads surgeons and restorative dentists to design occlusal schemes for dental implants without hyperocclusion.

Periodic periapical radiographs are needed for adequate follow-up (Figure 10.7). The most diagnostic films allow for the complete visualization of the implant threads. When these threads are clearly seen, an accurate radiograph has been taken that is 90 degrees to the long axis of the implant and the film has been placed parallel to the implant. Marginal bone loss or "saucerization" that may be progressive can be a sign of implant failure (Esposito and others 1998). One follow-up radiographic protocol for asymptomatic patients includes radiographs on a two- to three-year frequency (Grondahl 2003). Radiographs should be taken more frequently with clinical evidence of peri-implantitis (Mombelli and Lang 2000).

One European workshop on implantology defined clinical success as the absence of implant mobility and less than 1.5 mm marginal bone loss during the first year of function and less than 0.2 mm annually thereafter (Albrektsson and others 1994).

Probing in and around asymptomatic dental implants remains controversial. Etter and others have shown that light probing can be performed without permanent damage to the transmucosal attachment surrounding an implant (Etter and others 2002).

Professional polishing of supra- and sub-gingival implant components with plastic or carbon fiber curettes may also enhance patients' oral health. Conventional steel instrumentation or ultrasonic instruments should be avoided because these may cause damage to the implant surface (Matarasso and others 1996). Traditional adult prophylaxis including rubber cups and polishing paste is acceptable.

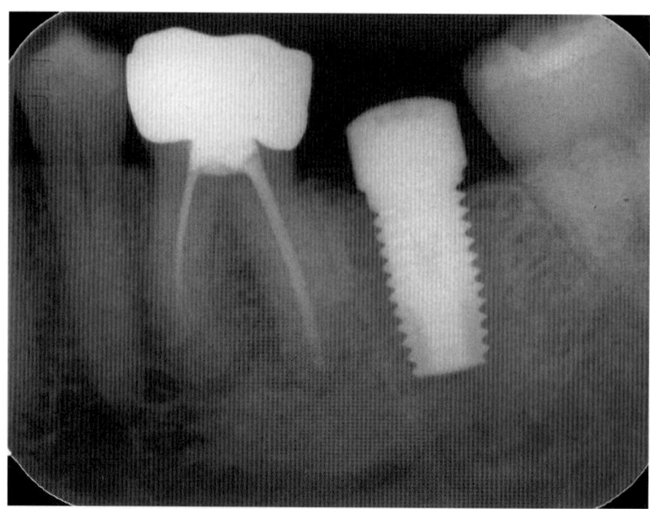

Figure 10.7. Radiographic example of a nonintegrated dental implant. Note the widened peri-implant space around the entire periphery of the implant.

CONCLUSIONS

The concept of teamwork in implant dentistry is required to produce satisfied patients and pleased doctors. Surgeons must find a balance among aesthetics, alveolar bone levels, and peri-implant soft tissue considerations at the time of implant placement. Restorative doctors must deal with the three-dimensional positioning of implants, proximity to adjacent teeth or implants, periodontal phenotype, emergence profiles, ideal crown-to-implant ratios, and more. Patient selection and thorough treatment planning is necessary for the development of a successful implant practice for both implant surgeons and restorative doctors. The concepts of hard and soft tissue integration are not completely understood. We do know that these codependent processes are intimately involved with clinical successes and failures. Appropriate surgical and restorative techniques are also vital in achieving high CSRs. Implant failure is multifactorial; however, the reversal of peri-implant mucositis, and prevention of peri-implantitis, can minimize implant failure.

BIBLIOGRAPHY

Adell, R, Lekholm, U, Brånemark, P-I, 1985. "*Surgical procedures.*" In: *Tissue integrated prostheses: osseointegration in clinical dentistry.* P-I Brånemark, GA Zarb, T Albrektsson, eds. Chicago (IL): Quintessence Publishing Co., Inc., p. 211–32.

Adell, R, Lekholm, U, Rockler, B, Brånemark, P-I, 1981. A 15-year study of osseointegrated implants in the treatment of the edentulous jaw. *Int J Oral Surg* 10:417–422.

Albrektsson, T, 1993. On long-term maintenance of the osseointegrated response. *Aust Prosthet J* 7:15–24.

Albrektsson, Tomas, and Isidor, Fleming, 1994. "Consensus report of session IV." In *Proceedings of the First European Workshop on Periodontology*. Niklaus P. Lang and Thorkild Karing, eds. London: Quintessence Publishing Co., Inc., p. 365–369.

Bauman, GR, Rapley, JW, Hallmon, WW, Mills, M, 1993. The peri-implant sulcus. *Int J Oral Maxillofac Implants* 8:273–280.

Berglundh, T, Abrahamsson, I, Lang, N, 2003. De novo alveolar bone formation adjacent to endosseous implants. A model in the dog. *Clin Oral Impl Res* 14:251–262.

Block, MS, Kent, JN, 1990. Factors associated with soft and hard tissue compromise of endosseous implants. *J Oral Maxillofac Surg* 48:1153–1160.

Brånemark, P-I, Hansson, B, Adell, R, Breine, U, Lindstrom, J, Hallen, O, Ohman, H, 1977. Osseointegrated implants in the treatment of the edentulous jaw. Experience from a 10-year period. *Scand J Plast Reconstr Surg* 16:1–132.

Brånemark, P-I, 1983. Osseointegration and its experimental background. *J Prosthet Dent* 50:399–410.

Cordioli, G, Zajzoub, Z, Piatelli, A, Scarano, A, 2000. Removal torque and histomorphometric study of four different titanium surfaces. *Int J Oral Maxillofac Implants* 15:668–674.

Davies, J, 2003. Understanding peri-implant endosseous healing. *J Dent Ed* 67:932–949.

De Leonardi, D, Garg, A, Pecra, G, 1997. Osseointegration of rough acid-etched titanium implants: one-year follow-up of placement of 100 minimatic implants. *Int J Oral Maxillofac Implants* 12:65–73.

De Leonardi, D, Garg, A, Pecra G, 1999. Osseointegration of rough acid-etched titanium implants: five-year follow-up of placement of 100 minimatic implants. *Int J Oral Maxillofac Implants* 14:384–391.

Esposito, M, Hirsh, J-M, Lekholm, U, Thompsen, P, 1998. Biological factors contributing to failures of osseointegrated oral implants (1). Success criteria and epidemiology. *Eur J Oral Sci* 106:527–551.

Etter, T, Hakanson, I, Lang, N, 2002. Healing after standardized clinical probing of the periimplant soft tissue seal—a histomorphometric study in dogs. *Clin Oral Impl Res* 13:573–582.

Garg, A, Arun K., 2004. "Bone Physiology for Dental Implantology." In: *Bone Biology, Harvesting, Grafting for Dental Implants*. Carol Stream IL: Quintessence Publishing Co, Inc., p 5–18.

Gotfedsen, K, Berglunh, T, and Lindhe, J, 2002. Bone reactions at implants subjected to experimental peri-implantitis and static load. An experimental study in the dog. IV. *J Clin Periodontol* 29:144–151.

Gröndahl, H-G, 2003. "Radiographic examination." *Clinical Periodontology and Implant Dentistry*. 4th Ed. Oxford: Blackwell Munksqaard, p. 838–851.

Heitz-Mayfield, L, Schmid, B, Weigel, C, 2004. Does excessive occlusal load affect osseointegration? An experimental study of the dog. *Clin Oral Impl Res* 15:259–268.

Hoshaw, S, Brunski, A, 1994. Mechanical loading of Brånemark fixtures affects interfacial bone modeling and remodeling. *Int J Oral Maxillofac Implants* 9:345–360.

Johansson, C, Albrektsson, T, 1987. Integration of screw implants in the rabbit. A 1-year follow-up of removal of titanium implants. *Int J Oral Maxillofac Implants* 2:69–75.

Lazzara, R, Porter, S, Testori, T, 1998. A prospective multicenter evaluation loading of Osseotite implants two months after placement: one-year results. *J Esthet Dent* 10:280–289.

Leonhardt, A, Berglundh, T, Erricsson, I, 1992. Putative periodontal pathogens on titanium implants and teeth in experiential gingivitis and periodontitis in beagle dogs. *Clin Oral Impl Res* 3:112–119.

Martin, Richard M, Carter, Jeffrey B, and Barber, H Dexter, 2000. "Surgical implant failures." In: *Oral and Maxillofacial Surgery: Reconstructive and Implant Surgery*. Raymond J. Fonseca, Michael P. Powers, H. Dexter Barber, eds. Philadelphia: W.B. Saunders Co., 7:275–308.

Marx, R, Ehler, W, Peleg, M, 1996. Mandibular and facial reconstruction: Rehabilitation of the head and neck cancer patient. *Bone* 19(1 suppl):59s–82s.

Marx, R, Sawatari, Y, Fortin, F, Broumand, V, 2005. Bisphosphonate-Induced Exposed Bone (Osteonecroses/Osteopetrosis) of the Jaws: Risk Factors, Recognition, Prevention, and Treatment. *J Oral Maxillofac Surg* 63:1567–1575.

Matarasso, S, Quaremba, G, Coraggia, F, 1996. Maintenance of implants: an in vitro study of titanium implant surface modifications, subsequent to the application of different prophylaxis procedures. *Clin Oral Impl Res* 7:64–72.

Mombelli A, Lang, N, 2000. The diagnosis and treatment of peri-implantitis. *J Periodontol* 17:63–76.

Moon, I, Berglundh, T, Abrahamsson, I, 1999. The barrier between the keratinized mucosa and the dental implant. An experimental study in the dog. *J Clinical Periodontol* 26:658–663.

Park, J, Davies, J, 2001. Red blood cell and platelet interactions with titanium implant surfaces. *Clin Oral Implant Res* 11:530–590.

Schroeder, A, Vander Zyen, E, Stich, K, Sutter, F, 1981. The reaction of bone, connective tissue, and epithelium to endosteal implants with titanium-sprayed surfaces. *J Maxillofac Surg* 9:15–25.

Sclar, Anthony, 2003. "*Soft tissue and Esthetic Considerations.*" In: Implant Therapy. Anthony Sclar, ed. Chicago (IL): Quintessence Publishing Co., Inc., p 4.

Sclar, Anthony, 2003. "Beyond Osseointegration." In: *Soft Tissue and Esthetic Considerations in Implant Therapy*. Carol Stream, IL: Quintessence Publishing Co, Inc., p 1–13.

Shetty, Vivek, Bertolami, Charles, 1992. "The Physiology of Wound Healing." In: *Principles of Oral and Maxillofacial Surgery*. Larry J.

Peterson, A. Thomas Indresano, Robert D. Marciani, Steven M. Roser, eds. Philadelphia (PA): JB Lippincott, p. 3–18.

Silverstein, L, Lefkove, M, Garnich, J, 1994. The use of free gingival soft tissue to improve the implant/soft tissue interface. *J Oral Implantol* 20:36–40.

Silverstein, L, Lefkove, M, 1994. The use of the subepithelial connective tissue graft to enhance both the aesthetics and periodontal contours surrounding dental implants. *J Oral Implantol* 20:135–138.

Smith, D, Zarb, G. 1989. Criteria for success for osseointegrated endosseous implants. *J Prosthet Dent* 62:567–574.

Testori, T, DelFabbro, C, Feldman, S, 2001. A multicenter prospective evaluation of 2-months loaded Osseotite implants placed in the posterior jaws: 3-year follow-up results. *Clin Oral Implants Res* 12:1–7.

Trisi, P, Rao, W, Rebaudi, A, 1999. A histometric comparison of smooth and rough titanium implants in human low-density jawbone. *Int J Oral Maxillofac Implants* 14:689–698.

Wennstrom, J, Bengazi, F, Lekholm, U, 1994. The influence of the masticatory mucosa on the peri-implant soft tissue condition. *Clin Oral Implants Res* 5:1–8.

Zarb, G, Schmill, A, 1990. The longitudinal clinical effectiveness of osseointegrated dental implants: The Toronto study. Part 3: Problems and complications encountered. *J Prosthet Dent* 64:185–194.

Zitzmann, N, Berglundh, T, Marinello, C, 2001. Experimental peri-implant mucositis in man. *J Clinical Periodontol* 28:517–523.

Zoldos, Jozef, and Kent, John, 1995. "Healing of Endosseous Implants." In: *Endosseous Implants for Maxillofacial Reconstruction.* Michael Block and John Kent, eds. Philadelphia: WB Saunders Co., p 40–70.

Index